Practice Management for the Dental Team

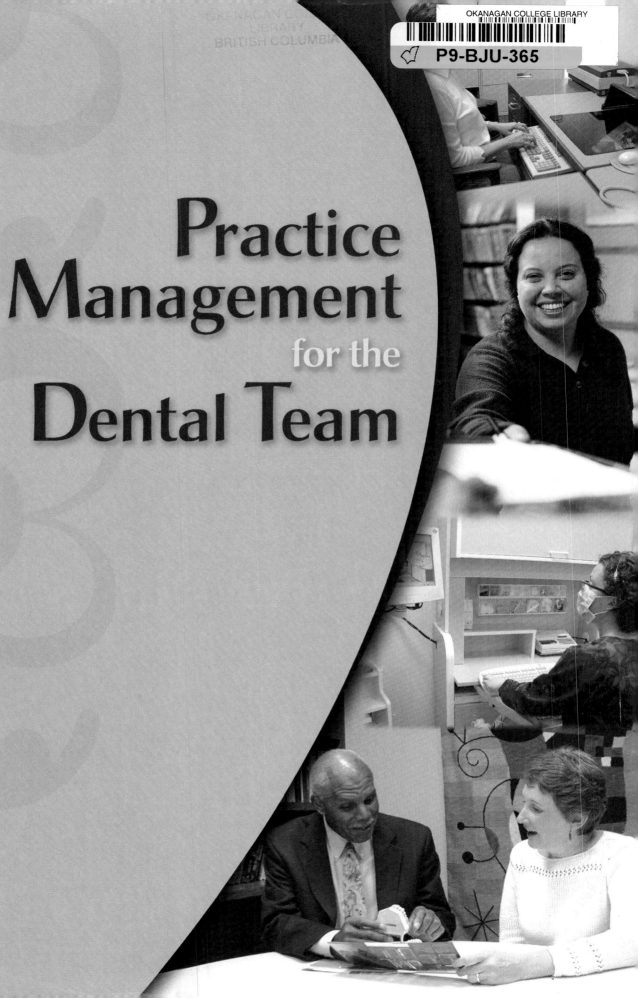

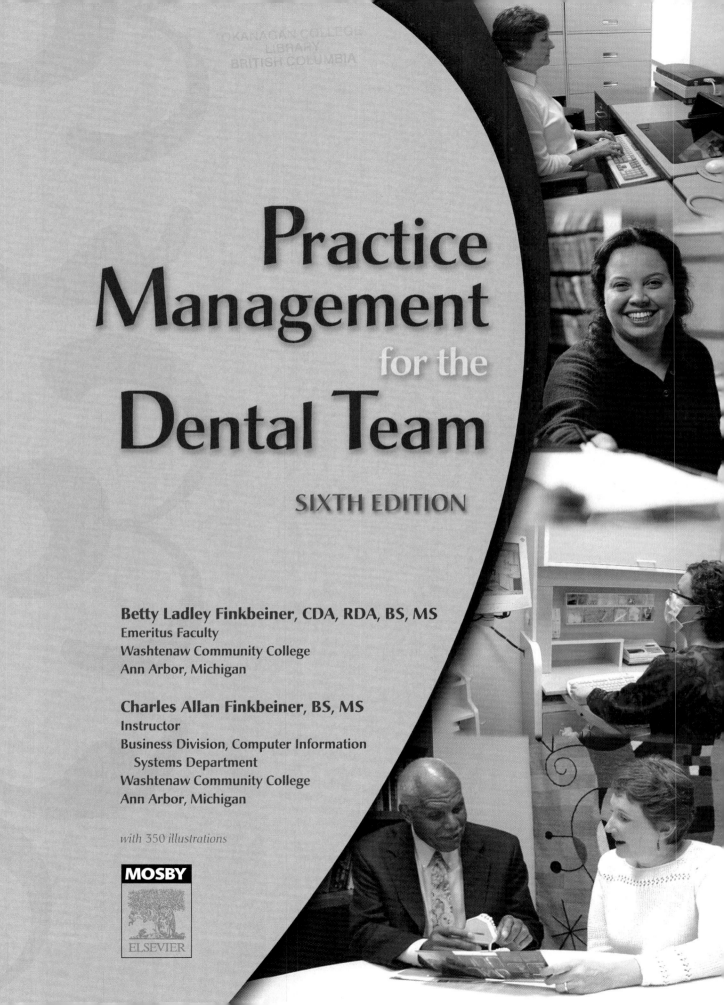

Practice Management
for the
Dental Team

SIXTH EDITION

Betty Ladley Finkbeiner, CDA, RDA, BS, MS
Emeritus Faculty
Washtenaw Community College
Ann Arbor, Michigan

Charles Allan Finkbeiner, BS, MS
Instructor
Business Division, Computer Information
  Systems Department
Washtenaw Community College
Ann Arbor, Michigan

with 350 illustrations

MOSBY

ELSEVIER

MOSBY
ELSEVIER

11830 Westline Industrial Drive
St. Louis, Missouri 63146

PRACTICE MANAGEMENT FOR THE DENTAL TEAM   ISBN-13: 978-0-323-03382-4
Sixth Edition   ISBN-10: 0-323-03382-2

Notice

Knowledge and best practice in this field are constantly changing. As new research and
experience broaden our knowledge, changes in practice, treatment and drug therapy may
become necessary or appropriate. Readers are advised to check the most current information
provided (i) on procedures featured or (ii) by the manufacturer of each product to be
administered, to verify the recommended dose or formula, the method and duration of
administration, and contraindications. It is the responsibility of the practitioner, relying on
their own experience and knowledge of the patient, to make diagnoses, to determine
dosages and the best treatment for each individual patient, and to take all appropriate safety
precautions. To the fullest extent of the law, neither the Publisher nor the Editors/Authors
assume any liability for any injury and/or damage to persons or property arising out or
related to any use of the material contained in this book.

The Publisher

Previous editions copyrighted 1977, 1985, 1991, 1996, 2001

ISBN-13: 978-0-323-03382-4
ISBN-10: 0-323-03382-2

Publishing Director: Linda Duncan
Executive Editor: Penny Rudolph
Managing Editor: Jaime Pendill
Developmental Editor: John Dedeke
Publishing Services Manager: Melissa Lastarria
Project Manager: Ellen Kunkelmann
Designer: Andrea Lutes

Printed in Canada

Last digit is the print number: 9 8 7 6 5 4

This edition is dedicated to

Shirley Wilson

A mentor, colleague, and treasured friend. Her often-solicited advice is given with smiling grace. The measure of our trust in her is that her message is always closed with love from "Aunt Shirley."

Preface

This edition represents more than three decades of education in Dental Practice Management. The first edition evolved from a course team taught by the original two authors. The course continues, as does the concept that dentistry is a twofold profession: it is a health care profession, but it is also a business. Along the way, however, the course has been modified to meet the needs of the modern student and is available online as part of a distance learning program in dental assisting at Washtenaw Community College in Ann Arbor, Michigan.

As in previous editions, we have provided a comprehensive textbook with emphasis on the important role of the business office in the modern dental practice. Although the emphasis in the text relates to the administrative assistant, this text is an excellent reference for the dental student, dental hygienist, or practicing dentist. The title *administrative assistant* replaces business assistant in this edition because the role of the person who manages the business office is so diverse that it warrants a higher level of recognition. This term refers to any person who assumes the primary responsibilities of managing the business office. The administrative assistant's role is changing as technology, managed health care, and federal regulations continue to influence the dental office.

This sixth edition continues to provide the reader with a comprehensive overview of the dental business office. We have modified some of the innovative features that will be of value to the dental, dental assistant, or dental hygiene student, as well as those professionals already in practice. These features include the following:

- Throughout the book, boxes highlight information and specialized terms that relate to specific topics.
- Each chapter begins with a comprehensive list of outcomes to be covered within the chapter.
- Marginal notes denote significant phrases to which the authors wish to draw the reader's attention.
- Key terms are boldfaced upon first mention in the text and are listed and defined in the alphabetical glossary at the end of each chapter.
- Review questions and suggested activities that can be used by students and practitioners to summarize and reinforce important concepts are presented in each chapter. Working Forms are provided on an accompanying Elsevier Evolve Learning Resources website, along with some suggested activities that coincide with chapter materials.

- CD icons at the end of Chapter 11 (Appointment Management Systems) and Chapter 15 (Accounts Receivable) invite the reader to complete the CD-ROM Software Activities by using the interactive electronic software program provided by EagleSoft.
- Chapter 18, "Planning and Managing Your Career Path," prepares readers for a new job by providing helpful tips on interviewing, letter writing, and resume building.

Throughout the book and in the CD-ROM simulations, we have focused on the process rather than specific details. We wish to emphasize that any fees or data cited in this book are only examples and are not to be perceived as a norm for any geographic area. The illustrations include two practicing dentists. Use your imagination; these practicing dentists could be a father/daughter, mother/son, or a husband/wife team practice.

Betty Ladley Finkbeiner
Charles Allan Finkbeiner

How to Use the Patterson EagleSoft Practice Management Software

Each copy of *Practice Management for the Dental Team* is packaged with a complimentary copy of Patterson EagleSoft.

It should be noted that this is a demonstration version of the EagleSoft program that must be installed onto your computer in order to work. This demonstration version allows you to explore and become familiar with the program, as well as work through the Software Exercises found in Chapters 11 and 15. Additional practice exercises are available on the Evolve website.

Before attempting to install this program on a computer in a school's computer lab facility, please discuss with your instructor or administrator to check on your school's installation policy.

System Requirements

Pentium III or higher
64 MB of RAM or better
4x or higher CD-ROM drive
800 x 600, 24-bit (thousands of colors) color display or better
500 MB available hard disk free-space
Printer available to print "Help" topics or documentation as needed
Windows® 98 SE, Windows® 2000, or Windows® XP

Installation

For technical support regarding the **installation** of this program, contact EagleSoft at 800-475-5036 and provide reference code #40726. For assistance with exercises or functions of this program, please talk to your instructor.

Insert the Patterson EagleSoft demonstration disk into your computer's CD-ROM drive. If you have enabled your system's Auto-Start function, the Demonstration window appears automatically and you can skip to Step 5 below. If the start-up wizard does not appear automatically, you must complete Steps 1-4 below.

1. Close all software applications on your computer, including Windows Explorer.
2. Select Run from the Windows Start Menu. The Run window appears.
3. Type "D:\runme.exe" in the open field. (If the CD-ROM drive on your computer is represented by a different letter, substitute the appropriate letter.)

4. Select OK.
5. Select Skip Intro to bypass the opening video.
6. The EagleSoft Demonstration window appears. Select Demo Installation. From the popup menu, select Demo Install Instructions.

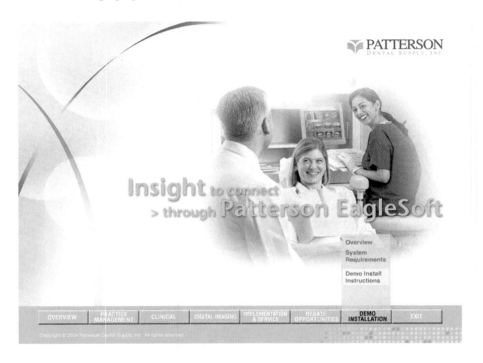

7. After reviewing the Installation Instructions, select Install Demo.

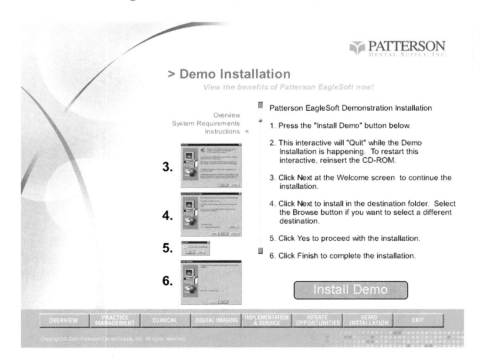

8. The Welcome window appears. Select Next.

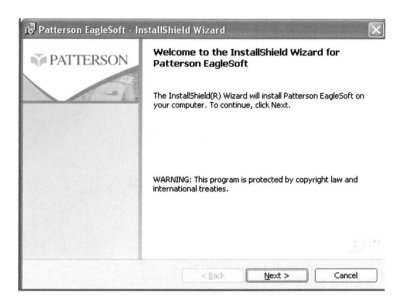

9. Read the License Agreement. If you agree to the terms, click on "I accept the terms in the license agreement." Select Next.

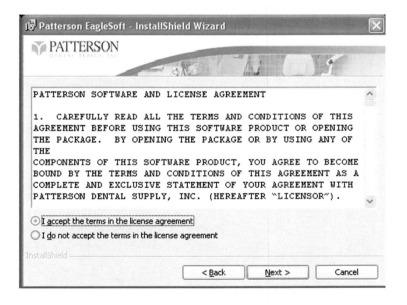

10. When the licensing agreement comes up during the installation process, Windows XP Home Edition users will encounter a warning that the EagleSoft program will install on the system but may not function at appropriate levels.

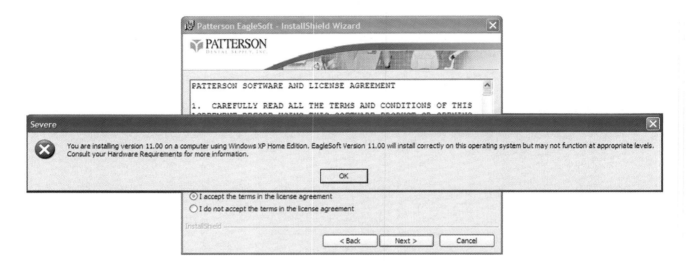

The demonstration CD **is** compatible with Windows XP Home Edition. The EagleSoft program is intended for professional use. This message is a warning that the full version of EagleSoft 11.00 that would be used in a dental practice office may not function ideally with Windows XP Home Edition.

11. Select Install.

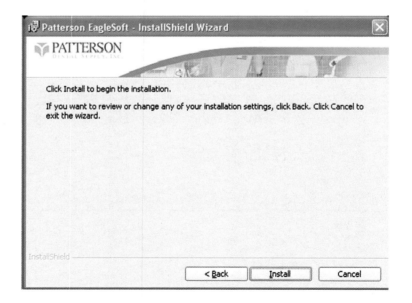

12. The Installation Process window appears. When the installation is completed, select Finish in the Installation Wizard Complete window.

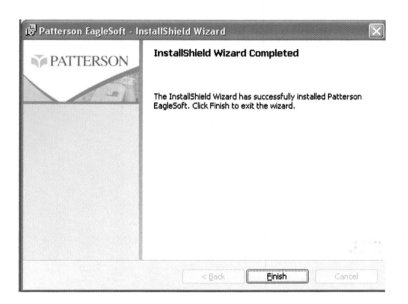

13. Select OK to restart your computer.

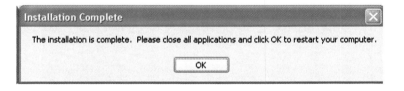

14. You can now remove the disk from the CD drive. It is not necessary to reinsert the disk each time you use the Patterson EagleSoft program.

Installation Troubleshooting

If you are attempting to install the CD-ROM on your computer and receive the following message – **Note: This CD is outdated** – your system may require an alternative form of installation. Please perform the following steps:

1. Run the CD-ROM. Once the error appears, click "OK" and leave the CD-ROM in the drive.
2. Open "My Computer" and then right-click on the CD-ROM drive, which should read "ES Demo 11.36."
3. Double-click to open the DEMO folder.
4. Double-click on the "setup.exe" (setup launcher) file to run the install.

The CD-ROM from this point should install normally.

Using the Patterson EagleSoft Demonstration Program

How to Log In

1. Click on the Patterson EagleSoft desktop icon, or select Start, Programs, EagleSoft, Patterson EagleSoft.
2. A window appears notifying you that this is a demonstration version. Select OK.

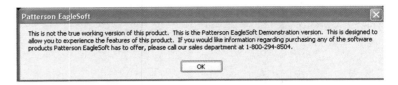

3. The Login window appears. Select James Patton from the Provider drop-down list box. A password is not needed in the Password field. Select Login.

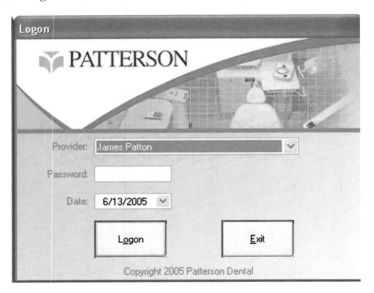

Keyboard Shortcuts

Shortcut	Function
Ctrl key + P	Opens Person List window
Ctrl key + W	Opens Walkout Processing window
Ctrl + Shift +P	Opens Receive Payments window
F1 key	Opens the Online User's Guide
F5 key	Recalls the last patient in the system
F2 key	Opens List windows in various screens

Viewing Modes

The program opens in the Integrated Mode. To view the **Practice Management Mode**, select **Window | Practice Management Mode**. To view the **Clinical Mode**, select **Window | Clinical Mode**.

NOTE: The software exercises in the textbook utilize the EagleSoft demonstration program in the Practice Management Mode or Integrated Mode. For more information about working within this demonstration program in the Clinical Mode, see the Evolve website.

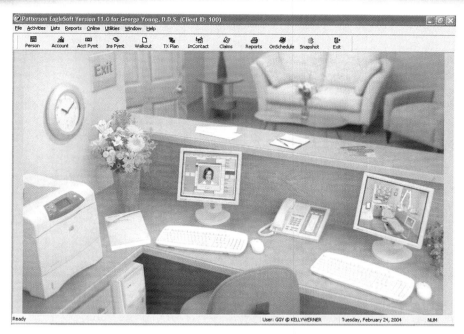

This is the Practice Management Mode.

Viewing and Editing Practice Information

Only information on the Messages, Notes, and Preferences tabs can be edited.

1. From the **Lists** menu, select **Practice Information**. The Practice Information window appears.

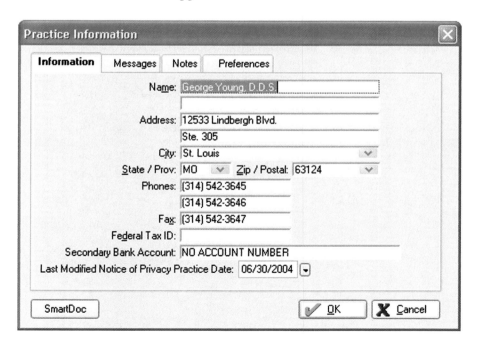

2. Select the **Messages**, **Notes** or **Preferences** tabs to edit any information.
3. Select **OK** to save and exit the Practice Information window.

Viewing and Editing Providers

All information can be edited.
1. From the **Lists** menu, select **Providers/Staff**.
2. Select a **Provider** and select **Edit**.
3. The **Edit Provider/Staff** window appears.

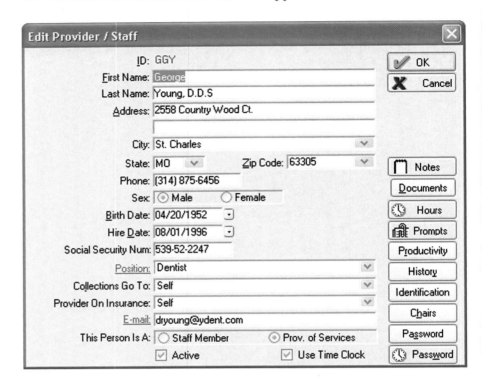

4. If desired, edit any of the information in the fields or drop-down list boxes.
5. The toolbar on the right side of the window offers methods of editing information, such as adding notes, changing hours, editing prompts, viewing productivity and more.
6. Select **OK** to save and exit the **Edit Provider/Staff** window.
7. Select **Close** on the **Provider/Staff** window.

Viewing and Editing Patients

All information can be edited.
1. From the **Lists** menu, select **Person**.
2. Select a person from the Person List. Select **Edit** once a person is selected.
3. If desired, edit any of the information in the fields or drop-down list boxes.

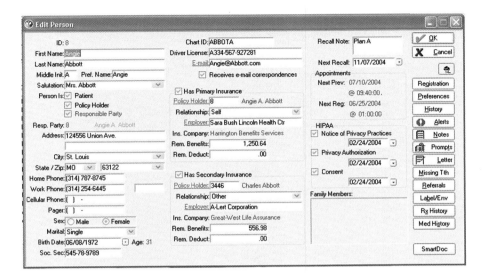

4. The toolbar on the right side of the window offers methods of editing information, such as adding preferences or alerts; viewing patient, medical and prescription history; and entering prompts, referrals and missing teeth.
5. Select **OK** to save and exit the **Edit Person** window.
6. Select **Close** on the **Person List** window.

Attaching an Insurance Company to a Policy Holder

1. From the **Lists** menu, select **Person**.
2. Select a person from the Person List. Select **Edit** once a person is selected.
3. If it is not selected, select the **Policy Holder** check box. The **Policy Holder**, **Relationship**, **Employer, Remaining Benefits** and **Remaining Deductible** fields are now available.
4. Select the checkbox next to **Has Primary Insurance** or **Has Secondary Insurance**. The **Policy Holder Number** appears and **Self** appears in the **Relationship** field.
5. To assign an employer to the patient, select in the **Employer** field and press the **F2** key, or select the underlined word **Employer**. The Employer List window appears.
6. Select the patient's employer (the insurance company appears next to the employer name) and Select **Use**. The employer and insurance information appears with the remaining benefits and deductible.
7. A message will appear asking "Do you want to update the employer information?"; select **Yes** to save and exit.
8. From the Person List window, select **Close**.

Attaching an Insurance Company to a Dependant

1. From the Lists menu, select **Person**.
2. Select a person from the Person List. Select **Edit** once a person is selected.

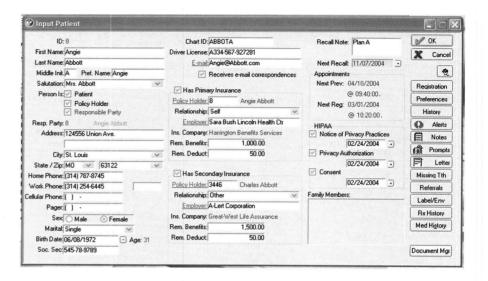

3. If it is not selected, select the **Has Primary Insurance** or **Has Secondary Insurance** check box. The **Policy Holder**, **Relationship**, **Employer, Remaining Benefits** and **Remaining Deductible** fields are now available.
4. Select in the **Policy Holder** field and press the **F2** key, or select the underlined words **Policy Holder**. The Policy Holder List window appears. Select the policy holder for this patient and Select **Use**. Once this is done, a **Policy Holder Number** appears, the type of the relationship appears in the **Relationship** field (use the drop down list to select a relationship) and the policyholder's employer appears. If the employer's insurance information has been entered, the insurance company appears below the **Employer** field.
5. Select **OK** to save and exit.
6. From the Person List window, select **Close**.

Scheduling Daily Appointments

1. From the Practice Management toolbar, select the **OnSchedule** button. The **OnSchedule** window appears.
2. Right-click in the white area. A menu appears with scheduling options.
3. Choose **Schedule Appointment** from the menu. A **Patient List** window appears.
4. Select a patient from the **Patient List** window and Select **Use**.
5. The **New Appointment** window appears for the selected patient. Patient and account information appears in the top portion of the window. If desired, you can change the appointment type, provider, or time units and enter a prefix, amount, or notes.

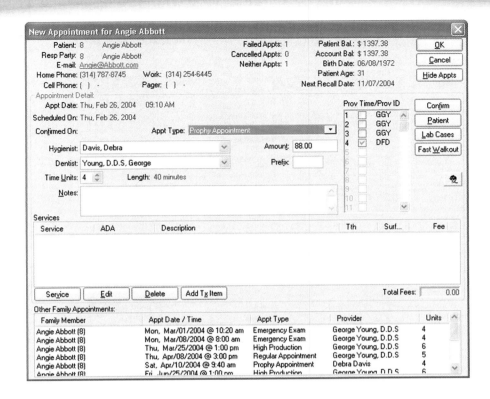

6. Select **Service** to attach a service to this appointment according to the Service or ADA Code, Service Type and Description.
7. Highlight the Service and select the **Use** button.
8. Select **OK** to enter the appointment.

Processing a Walkout Statement

1. From the toolbar, select the **Walkout** button. The Walkout Statement window appears.
2. Select the **Patient** field and press the **F2** key to access the Person List window. You can also select the **Patient** hyperlink.
3. Select a patient and Select **Use**. The patient's information appears in the top portion of the Walkout Statement window. If this patient has a treatment plan, please follow the remaining instructions in this step. If not, proceed to the next step.
   a. A window appears with the following message: "**This patient has planned/scheduled procedures. Do you want to select items to be completed?**" Select **Yes** to select treatment plan items.
   b. From the Treatment Plan Items window, select the items you want to include on the walkout and Select the **Mark** button. To include all items, select the **Mark All** button.
   c. When finished selecting items, select **OK**. The selected items will appear in the Walkout Statement window.
4. The blinking cursor appears in the **Service** field. To add services to the walkout statement, press the **F2** key to access the **Service Codes List** window.
5. Select the **Service Code** radio button to sort the list by the service code.
6. Select a service and select **Use**.
7. Repeat steps 4-6 if you wish to add more services to the walkout statement.

8. Select **Process** once you are ready to begin processing this walkout statement. The Walkout Processing window appears.

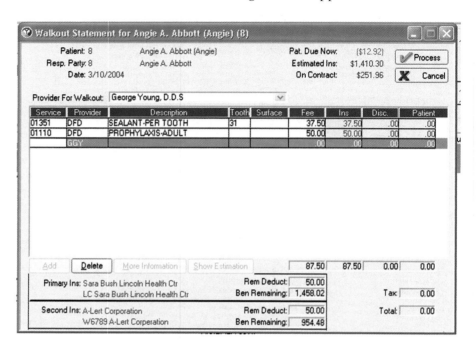

9. From the Walkout Processing window, enter a payment on the walkout or a credit adjustment on the account by entering the payments or credit adjustments in their fields. Select **OK**.
10. A window appears asking if you are ready to process this walkout statement. Select **Yes**.
11. If there is insurance on this walkout, the Insurance Questions window appears. Select the **Print Now** radio button. Select **OK** to print the insurance claim and to finish processing the walkout.

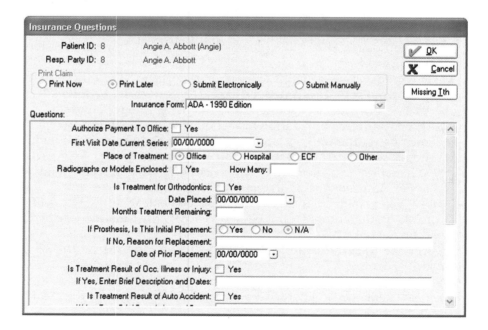

Posting Payments

1. From the Practice Management toolbar, select the **Acct (Account) Payment** button. The Receive Payment window appears.

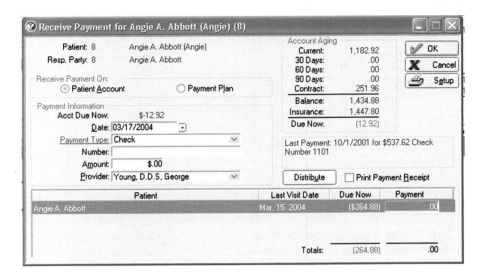

2. The blinking cursor appears in the **Patient** field. Press the **F2** key to access the Person List window. You can also select the underlined word **Patient**.
3. Select a patient and Select **Use**. The patient's information appears in the top portion of the Receive Payment window.
4. The blinking cursor appears in the **Number** field. If applicable, enter a check number, or select a different payment type from the Payment Type drop-down list box.
5. Enter an amount in the **Amount** field. The bottom section of the Receive Payment window displays any other dependants on the account. The account payment is evenly distributed over each balance or you can manually distribute the payment among the account members.
6. Before processing the payment, select the **Print Payment Receipt** check box.
7. Select **OK** to process the payment. A window appears asking if you are ready to apply the payment. Select **Yes**.

EagleSoft Online User's Guide

It is recommended that you become familiar with how to run certain parts of the EagleSoft program before beginning your assignments. You will want to review the **Online User's Guide** for these topics: New Patient Setup; OnSchedule Setup; Scheduling Appointments; Account Ledger; Account Window. A brief summary of how to use EagleSoft's help resource follows.

Online User's Guide – Once you have started EagleSoft, select **Help** above the toolbar, and then select **User's Guide**. To find specific information, select the **Index** tab. You will then be able to enter a keyword to find the appropriate section(s) in Help. Double-click the sub-entry (if present) that best describes the subject you need help with. The requested Help Topic window will appear and may be printed for easy reference.

The most commonly requested topics have been reprinted for your convenience.

Reviewing Account Ledger

The **Account Ledger** section shows all transactions that have been posted to any member in the selected account. The most recent transactions are listed at the top.

- All debit transactions (transactions that increase the patient's balance) and notes are displayed in black (for example, patient services are in black).
- All transactions with outstanding insurance claims appear in blue.
- All credit transactions (transactions that decrease the patient's balance) are displayed in red (for example, patient's payment appears in red).
- Deleted transactions and adjustments are in green. A deletion adjustment refers to the offsetting adjustment that is created by deleting an original transaction. For example:

    Deleting a $100 service, which is a debit amount, creates a $100 Delete Adjustment, which is a credit amount.

    Deleting a $50 payment, which is a credit amount, creates a $50 Delete Adjustment, which is a debit amount to offset the original transaction.

A running balance is kept and displayed. Here is a listing of the various types of **Debit Transactions**: Completed service Debit adjustment Billing charge Finance charge Returned check Here is a listing of the various types of **Credit Transactions**: Account payments Insurance payments Payment plan payments Credit adjustment Write off the account In addition to debit and credit transactions, the account history also displays the following types of account notes: Account note Modified transactions Deleted transactions Submitted insurance notes Payment plans Letters, recalls, and statements.

Accepting an Account Payment or Payment on a Payment Plan

1. From the **Account** window, choose **Acct Payment**. The **Account Payment** window is displayed. You can also access this by right-clicking in the **Patient** window in the **Account** window.
2. If the patient has a payment plan, click the **Payment Plan** radio button.
    *For more information on making Payment Plan payments, see the **Payment Plan** chapter in this unit.*
3. Type in the **Payment Information.** Reminder: Payments are assigned to the oldest patient balance first, unless specified otherwise.
4. Choose **OK** to record the payment and return to the **Account** window.

New Patient Setup

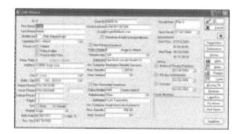

1. From the **Lists** menu, choose **Practice Management Lists** and then **Person**. **-or-**Click **Person** on the toolbar. **-or**

2. In **Practice Management** or **Clinical** modes, select **Person** from the **Lists** menu. The **Person List** window is displayed.

3. To add a new patient, choose **New**. The **New Person** window is displayed.

4. Enter the **ID**. The ID can include numbers or letters up to five characters. If you have chosen auto numbering, the ID is automatically entered for you after you save the information. Once the ID is saved, it cannot be changed without deleting the patient.

5. Enter the name of the patient and type or select the salutation. The salutation is used on letters generated in **EagleSoft**.

6. Enter the patient's preferred name and middle initial.

7. Indicate if this person is a **Responsible Party**, **Policy Holder**, or **Patient** by checking the appropriate boxes. If the person is only a policy holder for the account and not a patient, this person must still be set up within **EagleSoft**; just designate the person as a policy holder only. The same holds true for a person acting as a responsible party. An example might be a parent who is not a patient at your practice, but has a child who is a patient at your practice. In this situation, add the parent to your database and designate the parent as a responsible party for the patient.

8. If the patient is not a responsible party, then type the responsible party's ID (press the **F2** key to choose or create a responsible party). The responsible party's name is displayed.

9. Type or select the patient's other biographical information, such as the social security number and birth date.

10. Enter a Chart ID record for additional sorting and filtering options.

11. Enter the patient's Driver's License number.

12. Type or select the **Recall Note, Next Recall** date, and **Next Prev Appt** (next preventive appointment) date.

    Recall Note is used to identify specific patients. For example, if you type the word **CROWN**, you can later generate a report in Money Finder of all patients with the **CROWN** recall note.

    For more information about The Money Finder, see **The Money Finder** *section in the* **Practice Management** *chapter.*

    Next Prev Appointment date is the manually entered date for the next preventive appointment (if you are not using **OnSchedule**) or the next preventive appointment date with an appointment type marked to update the next preventive appointment (for **OnSchedule** users).

    Next Regular Appointment date is the manually entered date for the next regular appointment (if you are not using **OnSchedule**) or the next regular appointment date with an appointment type marked to update the next regular appointment (for **OnSchedule** users).

13. Mark the box **Has Primary Insurance**, if applicable.

14. Enter the Policy Holder ID (or press **F2** to select or create a policy holder).

15. Specify the **Relationship** to the insured and the **Employer** providing insurance. Press **F2** to select an existing employer or to create a new one.

16. Verify the **Rem. Benefits** (Remaining Benefits) and **Rem. Deduct** (Remaining Deductible), if applicable.

17. If the patient has secondary insurance, choose **Has Secondary Insurance**. You are asked if you would like to assign the person as the secondary policy holder. If someone other than this person is the secondary policy holder, choose **No**; otherwise, choose **Yes**.

18. Type or select the **Recall Note, Next Recall** date, (next preventive appointment). **Next Recall** date is the date in which the patient is due for his/her next prophy appointment.
19. **View the patient's next scheduled appointments.**
20. Select the checkbox, under HIPAA, to save the date of Notice of Privacy Policy, Privacy Authorization, and Consent.
21. View a list of family members with scheduled appointments. Right-click to open **OnSchedule**.
22. Add and view Patient photos in Practice Management. In Edit Person, click the **New Patient Photo** button and browse to the photo location. Select the patient photo file and click **OK**.
23. Choose **OK** to save and return to the **Person List** window.

OnSchedule Setup

Before we begin scheduling appointments, you must first specify some preferences for using **OnSchedule** in your office. To utilize **OnSchedule** to its fullest, please take the time to set up the following:

Scheduler Preferences

To set up your preferences for **OnSchedule**:
1. From the **File** menu, choose **Preferences** and click **OnSchedule**.
2. See the section on **Preferences** for more information on setting up **OnSchedule** preferences.

Provider Hours

To set up provider hours:
1. From the **Practice Management Lists** menu and then **Provider/ Staff**.
2. From the **Providers/Staff List** box, highlight the **Provider** you assign hours to and click **Edit**.
3. From the **Edit Provider/Staff** window, click **Hours**. The **Provider Hours** window is displayed. Adjust the hours as necessary, and click **OK**.
4. The color used in **OnSchedule** to identify this provider is shown in the **Provider Color on Schedule** box.
5. To change the color for the provider, click **Change Color**. The **Colors** window opens. Click on the new color of your choice, then click **OK**. The new color appears in the **Provider Color on Schedule** box.
   Note: We recommend avoiding the use of darker colors for the providers.
6. Modify the **Start**, **Close**, and **Lunch** times for the provider. If the provider does not work on a day the practice is open, uncheck the box next to the name of the day, removing the checkmark next to **Open**.
7. If the provider is unavailable for lunch times, be sure the box next to **Take Lunch** is checked and that the lunch times are accurate for this provider.
8. Complete the steps above for each of the days the provider is/is not available.

Acknowledgments

One of the primary messages with which we preface the beginning of every class we teach is that *dentistry is a team and there is no "I" in the word team.* So it is with the writing of any textbook. It takes an entire team of dedicated people to produce this textbook. This book would not be published if it were not for the dedicated staff at Elsevier, including Penny Rudolph, Executive Editor; Jaime Pendill, Managing Editor; John Dedeke, Associate Developmental Editor; and Ellen Kunkelmann, Project Manager.

It seems that with each edition of this text, some life-changing situation has always presented a challenge. So it has been this time as the authors begin a new phase of their lives in a warmer climate and thoughts turn to more consulting and less classroom experiences. For support during this time, we thank our sister, Pat Neil; nephew and niece Mark and Becke Ladley; and Betty's colleagues in the Dental Assisting Program at Washtenaw Community College—Kathy Weber, Kristina Sprague, and Dean Granville Lee, who have been so very helpful. To Linda Stakley, Betty's administrative assistant for nearly 20 years and the person who has helped to obtain illustrations and provide guidance in word processing for our many projects, we give a very special "thank you." We also thank our friends Charlotte Hanson for her many last-minute consultations and John Blatt for his continued friendship and humor that carry us through life's challenging moments.

And we are most appreciative of the input on the insurance chapter given to us by Becky Nagy, Communications Specialist, Delta Dental Plans of Michigan, Ohio, and Indiana; the ethics chapter, Esther R. Scherb, DMD, JD, Chair, DANB Board of Directors; and the infection control chapter, John Molinari, PhD, Professor of Microbiology at the University of Detroit Mercy.

Lastly, we owe a debt of gratitude to EagleSoft, A Patterson Company, for making it possible to include the interactive CD-ROM that accompanies every copy of this textbook. We extend our sincere appreciation to Pam Hemmen, Technology Marketing Manager; Anne Mansfield, Marketing Specialist; and Kelly Werner, Technical Writer.

Contents

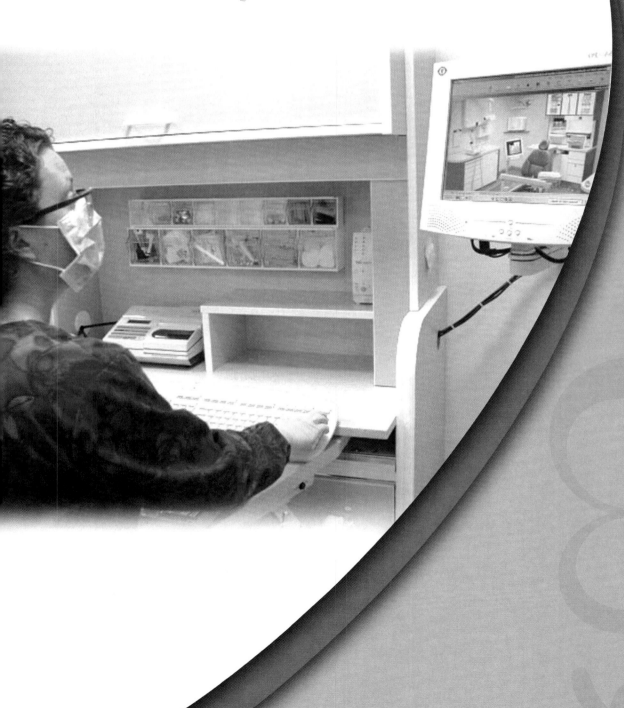

Dentistry as a Business

Chapter

1

The Business of Dentistry

Chapter Outline

Dentistry as a Service Profession
Leadership in the 21st Century
   Authoritative Leadership
   Free-Rein Leadership
   Participatory Leadership
   Today's Leader
Personal Characteristics of an Effective Leader
   Self-Confidence
   Genuineness
   Acceptance of a Culturally Diverse Population
   Enthusiasm
   Assertiveness
   Effective Listening
   Recognition of Others' Needs
   Sense of Humor
   Willingness to Be a Team Player

Learning Outcomes

Mastery of the content in this chapter will enable the reader to:

- Define glossary terms
- Explain the concept of dentistry as a business
- Describe the service concept
- Define communication
- Differentiate between various styles of management
- List characteristics necessary for establishing relationships

The administrative professional's role in the dental office of the 21st century is changing and ever-challenging. The person assigned this role must have the ability to achieve practice objectives, increase productivity, demonstrate skills in computer technology, and effectively use the most important asset of the practice—its human resources. Indeed this is a time of exploding technology, both in the business office and in clinical treatment areas within the practice. Dentistry as a business must face the same issues as other healthcare and business systems and realize that the world is changing. There is diversity in race, ethnicity, gender, and age, and today's dental professional must be able to address these issues.

Dentistry is a healthcare profession that has a twofold role: to provide healthcare service and to make a profit as a small business. As a healthcare service, dentistry provides quality care for the patient, following standards of care established by governmental agencies and the profession itself. As a healthcare profession, dentistry embraces the following objectives:

- Provide relief of pain from dental origin
- Help prevent pain by practicing preventive dentistry
- Help maintain patients' personal appearance
- Help patients masticate their food throughout their lifetimes
- Assist in maintaining good oral health

As a **business**, an enterprise in which one is engaged to achieve a livelihood, the dental practice must meet the following criteria:

- Operate efficiently
- Operate safely
- Be productive
- Utilize technology
- Create a profit

For years, dentists have referred to the business office as the front office. This serves to decrease the importance of this area of the practice. After all, there is no "back office." Dentists refer to other areas of the dental practice according to the work that takes place in them. The clinical areas of the office are referred to as treatment, laboratory, hygiene, or radiographic rooms. The business office should assume its rightful name, since all business activities of the practice take place there, including financial transactions, patient and staff communication, appointment management, recall, inventory, insurance management, and records maintenance.

The traditional education of the dentist has placed great emphasis on developing a highly competent diagnostician and clinician but has often left a noticeable void in the area of practice management. Dentistry in the 21st century faces an ever-changing population, a culturally diverse workforce and patient clientele, heightened consumer rights, increased state and federal regulations, managed care, satellite offices, expanding group practices, and redefinition of dental assistant and dental hygienist utilization and credentialing. Forward-thinking dental practitioners will embrace change as a lifelong, ongoing process for the individual and the practice. The successful dental practice will be lead by individuals who look at all situations as opportunities to create excitement and enthusiasm in meeting new challenges. These individuals will realize that technology alone cannot drive the practice, but that employees are a major asset. Therefore, a greater emphasis must be placed on practice management. The business office manager becomes a vital professional by maintaining records, implementing business systems, managing business operations, and maintaining **communication** (transmitting information from one person to another) between the dentist, the staff, the patient, and the community.

As modern dentists accept the roles of dentist and entrepreneur, they accept the responsibility of delegating expanded intraoral duties to the appropriate clinical assistants, more extraoral duties to the laboratory technician, and additional responsibility to the business manager.

DENTISTRY AS A SERVICE PROFESSION

In the infancy of the 21ˢᵗ century, it is evident that the industrial age that dominated society has given way to a service-oriented age, and dentistry is a major healthcare service. Dental treatment may be the objective for a patient; however, the dental staff must be constantly aware that when patients come to the office to seek treatment or perhaps a restoration (a tangible product), they are also seeking the most important product—**service,** an intangible product in the form of care. Service is a system of accommodating or providing assistance to another person.

Patients will remain with the dental practice only if they are satisfied with the services rendered. Figure 1-1 illustrates the many "ifs" the dental staff will encounter in the retention of a patient in the dental practice. It is important to remember that patients have choices. If patients choose to come to the office from either a recommendation or a random selection, and if they are satisfied with the treatment and care, they may return. If patients are still satisfied at the return visit, they may continue to return. However, if there is dissatisfaction at any stage of the service, patients may opt not to return to the office.

The basis for patient retention is communication, the ability to understand and be understood. A patient seldom leaves a dental practice because of dissatisfaction with the margins of his or her composite restoration. However, the patient may leave because a staff member made it difficult to obtain a completed insurance claim form, was too busy to listen to a concern, made frequent errors on statements, or didn't communicate the treatment plan in advance.

Service is not a result of clinical and cognitive skills but rather attitudinal skills that evolve into a commitment to the welfare of others. Box 1-1 lists a variety of activities that indicate a service-oriented office.

> The basis for patient retention is communication.

LEADERSHIP IN THE 21ˢᵀ CENTURY

Leadership is vital to the success and growth of a practice. Leadership is not about being the boss or being a good manager. According to Hastings and Potter in the leadership management text *Trust Me,* leadership is not *what* we do; it is *who* we are. The authors also state that "Simply put, leadership is influence. Leadership involves influencing others for good, rousing others to action, and inspiring them to become the best they can be, as we work together toward common goals." Think about persons who have influenced

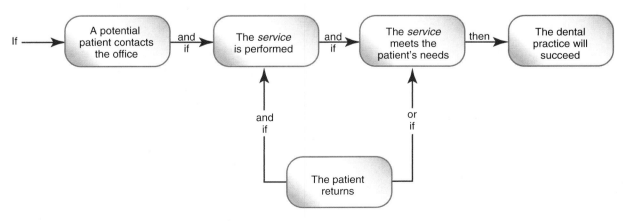

Figure 1-1 The service concept.

Box 1-1
Activities That Promote Service

- Maintaining regularly scheduled office hours
- Providing emergency care during the dentist's absence
- Maintaining the appointment schedule without delays
- Maintaining professional ethics
- Practicing quality care
- Recognizing patient needs
- Taking time to listen to patient concerns
- Respecting the patient's right to choice
- Informing patients of alternative treatment plans
- Allaying fears
- Hiring qualified employees
- Assigning only legally delegable duties to qualified staff
- Seeking staff input in decision making
- Encouraging an environment of caring
- Updating procedural techniques, equipment, and office decor regularly
- Maintaining office equipment
- Maintaining professional skills routinely
- Operating safely
- Maintaining quality assurance
- Attending risk-management seminars
- Participating in community services
- Being genuine and honest

you to work and motivated you to make major decisions. They were leaders; they caused you to take action. A leader in the dental office must be able to motivate the staff to masterful communication, and guide the staff and the dentist in working together to define goals and improve practice strategy.

Traditionally, the dentist may have managed the office in an authoritative, free-rein, or participatory type of leadership. Today the effective leader must have skills in change mastery, technology, and virtual office systems that extend beyond the local domain.

Authoritative Leadership

Authoritative management allows the dentist to make all decisions as the central authority figure. Dental auxiliaries are not involved in most decision making and are directed in what their role is within the system. This atmosphere provides little incentive for staff members, because they are merely figures who carry out specific orders. This is an efficient system that requires less decision-making time than others, but human relations researchers look upon this system with skepticism. This system should be used with caution in a healthcare delivery system such as a dental practice. The dentist in this system generally seeks to hire dental personnel who are passive, lack a desire to make judgments, and look to another person for direction. In an authoritative system, there is little opportunity for communication in the office, since the dentist seldom listens to the staff members' ideas or considers their needs.

Free-Rein Leadership

Free-rein leadership does not place the responsibility of management on any one person. The easygoing dentist does not provide direction for the staff, and everyone just seems to follow along with the current. The dentist is not consistent in policies and procedures and may make erratic changes in schedules. Staff members always seem to do their work without attempting new techniques because they prefer to do their jobs the same old way (why change?). To overshadow a lack of leadership, the dentist may hire assistants who are dependable, dominant, and do not enjoy challenges in their daily routine. Generally, communication in this system is not definitive, because little effort is made to develop understanding among staff members. Often this type of leadership exists because of poor organization and a lack of goals.

Participatory Leadership

Participatory leadership is considered to have the greatest advantages for a dental practice. This form of management recognizes each member of the staff as a person whose skills are necessary in obtaining the ultimate goals for the practice. Participatory management requires that all staff members have a part in making decisions and that the dentist be genuinely interested in the staff. The staff is required to share in the responsibility and decision making. Therefore, such an office will include employees who are eager to accept responsibility, willing to make decisions, and seek challenges in their daily work. This system provides an opportunity for communication: each person seeks to understand the others, and staff members are encouraged to express their ideas.

Leadership can be defined as doing the right thing, whereas management is defined as doing things right. In a dental office the dentist is most commonly referred to as the leader. There can be many leaders in the dental office. In a large multistaffed office, the administrative assistant may be the office manager who is the leader in the business area. A clinical assistant may be the leader in the clinical activities area, and a dental hygienist may assume responsibility for preventive activities and treatment. In such situations the dentist serves as the overall leader, and there is a responsible leader in each office area.

Today's Leader

The leader in the dental office today must embrace trust, a willingness to understand change, humility, commitment, focus, compassion, integrity, peacemaking, and endurance (Box 1-2).

As a business, the dentist/leader of the 21st century will strive to achieve practice goals by:
- Considering long-term results over short-term results.
- Stressing effectiveness over efficiency alone.
- Thinking strategically rather than operationally.
- Being proactive rather than reactive to situations.
- Being driven by plans rather than problems.

The effective dental office cannot think and act independently. Marketing service in a dental practice means considering human, financial, and technical resources in a worldwide market. Patients seen in the dental office come from diverse backgrounds and present complex and diverse treatment options. Likewise, the dental materials and technology used in all facets of the office come from a worldwide market. The dental office of this century must be a virtual office that not only serves the local community but also recognizes its role in the global community.

> ### Box 1-2
> #### Elements That Build Effective Leadership
>
> - **Trust** promotes good relationships and confidence with the staff, as expanded duties are delegated to clinical staff and advanced management techniques are assigned to business staff.
> - **A willingness to understand change** and recognize that disruptions are inevitable, with the willingness to shift gears to pave the way for change.
> - **Humility** is a focus on being open, teachable, and flexible.
> - **Commitment** seeks to develop vision and values in a leader and moves leaders to stand for something greater.
> - **Focus** gives leaders the ability to achieve and direct their time and energy to important goals and objectives.
> - **Compassion** is the desire to understand and care for others, such as staff, family, patients, or community.
> - **Integrity** demands that leaders be responsible for seeking to create quality assurance in their service for patients, as well as in all their relationships.
> - **Peacemaking** leaders bring calmness to the office by listening, learning from others, and seeking good solutions rather than making quick decisions.
> - **Endurance** refers to courage, perseverance, and strength when situations, people, or the environment become chaotic or difficult.

PERSONAL CHARACTERISTICS OF AN EFFECTIVE LEADER

Generally, the first contact a patient has with the office is with a staffperson in the business office, administrative assistant, or office manager. It is difficult to identify a job today that does not include interaction with people. Whether you have a job in education, custodial services, law, science, religion, office technology, or architecture, you will find that productivity is greatly enhanced by an ability to communicate. In fact, it is difficult to find any job today in which communication is not important. It has been found that 80 percent of the people who fail at their jobs do so not because of a lack of technical skills, but because they do not relate well with people.

Your attitude can either give the patient a positive impression or convince the patient to seek dental care elsewhere. Whether communicating with patients, staff, or friends, you must develop basic "people skills" for successful communication. In addition to the elements found in a leader, discussed earlier in this chapter, the office manager must have skills that include self-confidence, genuineness, enthusiasm, assertiveness, honesty, acceptance of others, the ability to be a good listener, and willingness to be a team player.

Self-Confidence

Self-confidence is the ability to believe you can do a job well. To have self-confidence, you must accept yourself. You must have a healthy mental picture of yourself and learn to accentuate your positive attributes. Having self-confidence means identifying your strengths and building on them, and accepting your weaknesses and not dwelling on them.

An administrative assistant with self-confidence assumes responsibility, adapts to change, accepts challenges, and provides input in decision making. For instance, administrative assistants who are self-confident will initiate

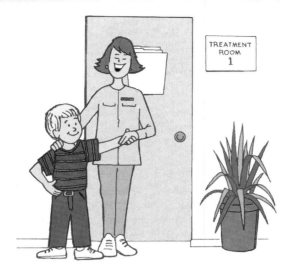

Figure 1-2 An arm resting on a child's shoulder displays caring.

marketing needs, make suggestions for changes, and implement new procedures without hesitancy, confident that they know what is going on. They are willing to take risks and are able to recommend changes in a routine or procedure with confidence that the idea is worthwhile and merits consideration.

Genuineness

Being genuine means being yourself. If you are genuine, you are sincere and straightforward. This is important when dealing with people in a healthcare profession. A genuine, caring person is not afraid to reach out and touch someone. Placing a hand on a shoulder of a frightened patient or holding a frightened child's hand (Figure 1-2) shows you care and displays a genuine concern for another person's feelings. Put yourself in the patient's place, and show the kind of concern you would like to receive.

Patients feel comfortable with a genuinely caring administrative assistant and are likely to open up and share their innermost feelings. When patients express fear or frustration, an assistant with genuine concern says, "I'm sorry to hear you feel this way. Is there anything I can do to help you?" Patients may simply need a person to listen, a friendly smile, or a comforting pat on the shoulder.

Acceptance of a Culturally Diverse Population

Today's administrative assistant must communicate with people who speak English as a second language. You may find it necessary to use another dictionary or reference such as *Spanish Terminology for the Dental Team*, if an interpreter is not available. Such references will aid in communicating with patients to determine basic information for clinical and financial records as well as clinical questions.

You will find that each person's values are established from his or her background and previous experience. To accept others you must be willing to accept them as worthy human beings without a desire to change them to fit into your value system. Accept them for what they are, not for what you think they ought to be. Communication is often difficult when a person acts or appears "different" than what is perceived as the norm. For instance, when a patient with a prosthesis replacing his or her right arm visits the office, the prosthesis may attract your attention, and you may even stare at the device. Your focus is on the disability and not on the patient. In the healthcare profession, it is important to concentrate on seeing the person and not the disability.

Enthusiasm

Being enthusiastic means you are interested in your work, you are expressive, and you leave your problems at home. To be enthusiastic does not mean you are a phony or a constant chatterbox, but that you have a sincere interest in your work and the world around you. Dental assistants who are enthusiastic about their work are likely to read professional journals, seek knowledge about new technology or specific areas of interest, participate in community activities or professional organizations, and become an involved professional. To be enthusiastic you must act enthusiastic.

An enthusiastic dental assistant takes time to learn about the patients and their interests, and when the patients ask questions, seeks to find the answers. An enthusiastic person is happy to get to work, enjoys sharing others' experiences, appreciates good humor, and is not totally exhausted at the end of the day. An enthusiastic person has a positive outlook on life.

> To be enthusiastic, you must act enthusiastic.

Assertiveness

Being assertive does not mean being aggressive. An assertive person is bold and enterprising in a nonhostile manner. An administrative assistant is often called upon to assume new responsibilities and must take the initiative to get the job done. Consider this situation. Staff members in the office where you have been employed for three years have been complaining about salaries, often among themselves at lunchtime. Everyone feels awkward about discussing it with the dentist because they are not sure what to say. An assertive person will take the initiative to research salaries in areas that represent comparable responsibilities, determine the production and value of each staff member, and present the data to the dentist in a nonthreatening manner. To be assertive often requires tact, initiative, and willingness to take a risk.

Effective Listening

Listening is more than hearing. A good listener hears not only the facts but also the feeling behind the stated facts. Good listening is a combination of hearing what a person says and becoming involved with the person who is talking. Sometimes a hearing loss or a preoccupation with your problems, goals, or feelings can make it difficult for you to hear what is really communicated. In a busy dental office, you may ignore what a person is really saying because you are too preoccupied with your work, deadlines, or future activities to listen effectively to a patient's needs. Often you hear only what you want to hear or have time to hear.

Sometimes, too, you forget to listen with your eyes. You need to see what the person is saying; you need to look at the speaker when he or she is talking (Figure 1-3). When you observe a person's body language, you observe facial expressions, gestures, and posture that will give you clues to that person's feelings. Consequently you hear what people are saying by observing the emotions they display.

In reflective listening the listener absorbs what has been said, reflects on it, and restates or paraphrases the feeling or content of the message in a way that demonstrates understanding and acceptance. This type of listening is beneficial to a healthcare professional as both dentist and patient interact to

> Listening is more than hearing.

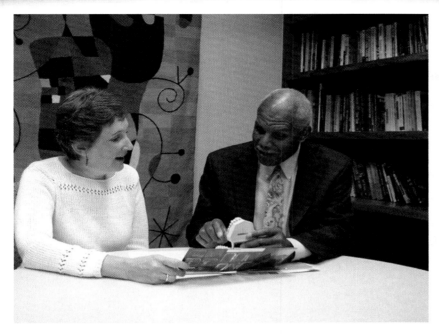

Figure 1-3 A dentist listens with his eyes during a consultation with a patient. (Courtesy Kathy Weber and Cal Williams, Ann Arbor, MI.)

create a better understanding of the situation. A scenario in a dental office might go something like this:

Patient: "I just don't know whether to have a porcelain crown on this front tooth or not. My family has always accepted me like this, but every time I have my picture taken I always worry that this gray tooth will show, so I keep my mouth closed."

Assistant: "You have considered having the crown done, but sometimes feel you shouldn't do it?"

Patient: "Uh, huh."

The assistant has restated the basic statement of the patient. The message was in her own words and wasn't judgmental. When correctly paraphrased, the speaker will generally respond in the affirmative. If not, the paraphrase needs to be restated until the message is received clearly.

Another form of this listening style and paraphrasing is as follows:

Dentist employer: "I don't understand why we haven't received the new impression material that we ordered."

Assistant: "Do I hear you saying that you think maybe I didn't place the order?"

Dentist employer: "No, I was just wondering if maybe the supply house isn't stocking that material."

This conversation could have ended with the original statement of the dentist and with the assistant upset, thinking there was a hidden meaning in the statement. Instead, the assistant queried the dentist to determine what the statement really meant and then realized the true meaning of the statement.

At first, using these techniques may seem cumbersome or artificial. Try them and practice them, and soon you will realize the benefits of reflective listening. Good listening skills require that you understand a person before you speak. Such action will result in improved relations with patients and staff and may result in fewer conflicts.

Recognition of Others' Needs

All people need some form of recognition. Your colleagues within the office have needs for friendship and recognition and a desire to feel they are valued for their contribution to the team's success. This doesn't mean that you and your colleagues have to socialize outside the office. It simply means that you should be willing to work cooperatively with them to accomplish the objectives of the practice. Ignoring another person's needs does not facilitate good interpersonal relations.

Sense of Humor

A dental office can be a stressful setting for staff members who clamor to meet the demands of the daily schedule and the patient who is filled with fears of potential treatment. How you interpret a crisis situation, however, is more important. Look at the situation with a sense of humor, and let yourself lighten up. However, always be careful to laugh at the situation and not at the person. Your patients and colleagues should not be made the brunt of a joke.

Consider adding humor to the office with cartoons on the bulletin board. Remember that humor lessens conflict and eases tension and is perhaps the best dose of medicine that could be prescribed in any dental office.

Willingness to Be a Team Player

> There is no "I" in the word team.

Dentistry is a team-oriented business. There is no "I" in the word team. Building a team is a simple concept when you realize that teams are made up of individuals with diverse skills and talents. Each team member must have clearly defined skills that need to be identified and measured against the skills of other team members. Once a person realizes his or her role on the team and how best to accomplish specific tasks, achieving team goals can be accomplished and eagerly anticipated. Offices that are committed to building a team can achieve results more effectively than offices in which each individual works independently.

Key Terms

Business – An enterprise in which one is engaged to achieve a livelihood.
Communication – The process of transmitting information from one person to another.
Dentistry – A healthcare profession concerned with the care of the teeth and surrounding tissues including prevention, elimination of decay, replacement of missing teeth and structures, esthetics, and correction of malocclusion.
Leadership – The method of influencing others for good, rousing others to action and inspiring them to become

the best they can be, as a group works together toward a common goal.
Management – The act or art of leading a team to accomplish goals and objectives while using skill, care, and tactful behavior.
Service – In dentistry, the process of providing quality care for patients while following standards of care established by governmental agencies and the profession itself.

LEARNING ACTIVITIES

1. Explain the three types of traditional leadership that might be found in a dental office.
2. Consider offices that you have visited, and identify the leadership style of each dentist. What effect does leadership have on the communication in each office?
3. Reflect on past job situations, and determine how various personal characteristics can affect how you develop a positive or negative relationship.
4. Describe situations in a dental office that are more effective when performed as a team.

Bibliography

Abrams R: *Wear clean underwear: business wisdom from mom,* New York, 1999, Villard.
Fulton-Calkins PJ: *General office procedures for colleges,* ed 12, Cincinnati, 2003, South-Western.
Hastings W, Potter R: *Trust me,* Colorado Springs, 2004, WaterBrook.
Mosby: *Spanish terminology for the dental team,* St. Louis, 2004, Mosby.
Thill JV, Bovée CL: *Excellence in business communication,* ed 5, Upper Saddle River, NJ, 2002, Prentice-Hall.

Chapter

2

Dental Team Management

Chapter Outline

Learning Outcomes

Mastery of the content in this chapter will enable the reader to:

- Define glossary terms
- Determine goals and objectives for a dental practice
- Explain staff etiquette
- List duties of an administrative assistant
- Identify the five *R*s of good management
- Identify functions of an administrative assistant
- Identify characteristics of an effective administrative assistant
- Manage interpersonal communications of staff and dentist
- Explain employee empowerment
- Discuss the procedures for conducting a staff meeting
- Explain the importance of hiring a skilled administrative assistant
- Define time management
- Describe how to manage time efficiently
- Explain the purpose of an office procedural manual
- Identify components of an office procedural manual
- Describe recruitment and hiring practices
- Describe the contents of a personnel policy in an office procedural manual
- Explain the use of pre-employment testing
- Describe new employee orientation
- Manage staff conflict

ESTABLISHING PRACTICE GOALS AND OBJECTIVES

Prior to opening a dental practice, the dentist should define a practice philosophy and establish specific objectives for the practice. A lack of goals and objectives results in lack of direction for the dentist and staff and may result in poor relationships with patients. As the practice grows, these goals and objectives will need to be revised. It is vital that the dentist in a participatory healthcare practice seek input from the staff when establishing these objectives.

A common sequence for establishing objectives includes the following steps:

1. **Develop a Practice Philosophy.** The dentist identifies in a broad statement the basic concepts about patient care, business management, auxiliary utilization, health and safety, and continuing education for the practice.
2. **Develop Practice Objectives.** In this stage, each broad goal is broken into a series of specific objectives for the practice. These objectives should be specific positive action statements that will indicate the expected results.
3. **Develop Practice Policies.** These are statements of basic policy that will affect both staff members and patients. These statements may be covered by broad headings, followed by specific policies. It is wise to share these with the patients as shown in the office policy in Chapter 3 and with the staff as shown in the procedural manual later in this chapter.
4. **Develop Procedural Policies.** Each broad statement can be broken down again into specific objectives and further defined into specific tasks for all of the common office procedures. A result of this effort will be most valuable when inserted in the procedural manual.

5. **Develop Business Principles.** These objectives place emphasis on the actual business activities of the office. Here, the dentist outlines in numeric terms the budget process for the practice and procedures for managing business activities.

6. **Develop a Practice Standard.** It is necessary for the dentist to identify a quality standard that will define a self-performance level and performance level expected of the staff. The dentist should provide for the staff an explanation of how this standard is to be maintained.

As a dentist and staff work through the development of objectives for the practice, these objectives become rules by which the office is managed. As the practice expands and new technology is developed, it will be necessary to review and revise these goals and objectives. Most important in participatory management is the involvement of the entire dental team in the development of these objectives.

Develop a Staff Recognition Program. As stated earlier, the staff is the greatest asset a dentist can have in the office. Specific guidelines need to be established for hiring a qualified staff, selecting a wide range of creative benefits, and establishing a competitive salary scale that reflects productivity and cost-of-living increases. Most employees will work hard if they are compensated well and recognized for their efforts. However, a common complaint of dental assistants is lack of recognition. An employee must be given challenging responsibilities, and salaries must be commensurate with the accomplishment of these responsibilities. A frequent thank-you will help to improve rapport, but don't overlook profit sharing, gift certificates, and travel as real incentives in a recognition program.

BUSINESS OFFICE ETIQUETTE

Office etiquette refers to business manners. Rules that applied to social graces 25 years ago or even 10 years ago may no longer work in our society. Many former rules of etiquette were formal and rigid and often do not apply to the more casual lifestyles of today's society. Yet in a professional business office, the fact still remains that your actions and behavior will be observed by clients, patients, visitors, and those who have the potential to promote you.

For a dentist employer, the potential for practice growth and patient acceptance depends on the etiquette of the staff. Good manners can lead to promotions over equally qualified persons with less poise; create a self-confident, successful, professional person; help professionals handle their superiors; and lessen awkwardness among people. They are essential to building good relationships. Specific applications of etiquette are applied to different phases of business activities in many of the ensuing chapters.

THE SHIFTING ROLE OF THE ADMINISTRATIVE ASSISTANT

For many years the administrative assistant's role has been defined with various terms including *secretary, receptionist, business assistant,* and even *front-desk person.* Many of these titles are still used today, but the changing role of this important staffperson shifts the title to a more appropriate one of *administrative assistant.* The duties of the administrative assistant are varied and may be assigned at different levels. As the dental team expands, the dentist is likely to delegate more management duties to the administrative assistant. In a large dental practice, a dentist may employ several staff members in the business office, each with separate responsibilities as an administrative assistant, receptionist, insurance manager, and data clerk. However, in a smaller practice, these duties may be delegated to one person. The administrative assistant title in this text refers to the person whose primary responsibility involves business activities of the dental office. In general, the duties of an administrative assistant include many of the tasks identified in Box 2-1.

Box 2-1
Basic Job Responsibilities of the Administrative Assistant

Maintain Patient and Staff Relations
Schedule appointments
Set up meetings and conferences
Obtain information for and maintain all patient clinical and financial records
Prepare consultation materials
Communicate both verbally and in writing with patients and staff both within and outside the office
Administer computer networks
Set up and administer financial arrangements with patients and other parties
Maintain recall and inventory systems
Implement marketing strategies
Design office manuals and pamphlets
Arrange for and conduct staff meetings and other conferences
Solve day-to-day problems within the role of the administrative professional
Provide support for patients and professional staff
Make travel arrangements
Implement state and federal regulations
Initiate job advertisements, interview, and make recommendations on the employment of office personnel
Set up training and evaluation processes for employees
Organize, assign, and evaluate workloads
Arrange for risk management and OSHA seminars
Supervise appropriate office support staff

Operate Electronic Office Equipment
Use telecommunication technology, including the telephone, voicemail, e-mail, and fax
Manage websites
Help to upgrade and recommend office software
Provide computer and software training

Manage Records
Manage patient records including clinical charts, insurance forms, laboratory requisitions, HIPAA forms, and other clinical data
Maintain employee records
Maintain OSHA records
Maintain MSDSs
Prepare state and federal forms
Maintain an accounts payable system
Utilize a credit bureau and collection agency
Order and receive supplies, and verify invoices

Manage Mail
Manage incoming and outgoing mail
Maintain an e-mail system
Maintain USPS mail

STAFF MANAGEMENT

The term *management* has many definitions, but for the dental office it may be defined as the process of getting things accomplished with and through people, by guiding and motivating their efforts toward common objectives.

Some people may say, "Managers are born, not made." However, individuals can nurture their natural skills into sound management skills through experience, effort, and learning. As you advance into an administrative position you will make mistakes, but remember that you learn from mistakes as well as successes.

The Five *R*s of Management

Successful management can be attributed to five basic *R*s: responsibility, respect, rapport, recognition, and remuneration.

An employee should be delegated all tasks that are legally delegable and for which he or she is properly qualified. Employees cannot work to achieve their maximum productivity if they feel they are not given responsibility for which they are answerable. *Responsibility* denotes duty or obligation. It also denotes follow-through and completion of a project. An employee who is to become a valuable member of the dental health team must be delegated responsibility. If responsibility is withheld, then it is assumed that the administrative assistant or employer does not feel the employee is capable of the task, and concern should be given for retaining this employee.

Respect is consideration or esteem given to another person. Each member of the dental health team must respect the others' education, skills, and values. To not have respect indicates a lack of confidence and again reflects a poor attitude toward another person's capabilities. Each member has a major role on the team and should possess expert skills and credentials that warrant respect.

Rapport is a mutual trust or emotional relationship that exists among the office staff members. Each dentist sets the tone for the rapport in the office. A good rapport in the office is effused to the patients who recognize how well the team members work together during tense times and how they enjoy each other's professional friendship.

Recognition is achievement. A person can be recognized for a task well done or for special achievements. Recognition can come in the form of verbal praise or a sign placed in the office recognizing employment and credentials.

Remuneration is a monetary recognition of achievement. Most employees say that they are willing to work hard if they are compensated for their efforts. Remuneration should be based on education, merit performance, longevity, and cost of living. Dentist employers who affirm that their employees have worked with them for many years, with repeated job satisfaction reviews, are those who delegate responsibility; create good rapport in the office; respect, trust, and recognize their employees; and provide compensation commensurate to other small business and allied health employment.

> Individuals can nurture their natural skills into sound management skills through experience, effort, and learning.

Functions of an Administrative Assistant

The basic functions of an administrative assistant in a dental office are shown in the schematic drawing in Figure 2-1. Some assistants may interpret this diagram to mean that their job is "a vicious circle." In actuality many of these functions overlap, and the basis for each depends on planning. Sound planning before beginning an activity may eliminate the need for crisis management, or handling one crisis after another.

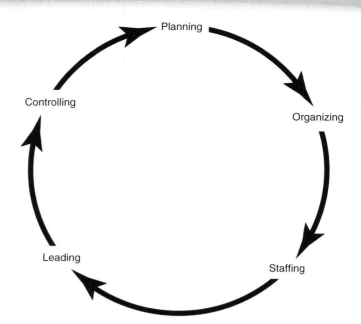

Figure 2-1 Functions of an administrative assistant.

Planning is identifying what is to be done in the future. The goals and objectives discussed earlier are vital to planning. The administrative assistant will be involved in long-range planning as well as daily planning.

Organizing is determining how the work will be divided and accomplished by members of the dental team. After procedures have been identified and tasks enumerated for each procedure, the administrative assistant is required to assign the duties to specific staff members. It is essential that the dentist give this authority to the administrative assistant. Without this authority, the administrative assistant cannot manage effectively.

Staffing includes the recruiting, selecting, orienting, promoting, paying, and rewarding of employees. Cooperation between staff members will be necessary as new employees are integrated into each technical area of the office. Staffing also involves instructing, evaluating, and educating employees and providing opportunities for their future development. Additionally, the business administrative assistant will be responsible for recommendations of an appropriate system of pay and benefit package.

Leading involves directing, guiding, and supervising the staff in the performance of their duties and responsibilities. It consists of exercising leadership; communicating ideas, orders, and instructions; and motivating employees to perform their work effectively and efficiently. This is really the "people" function of management.

Controlling is the function of management that deals with determining whether or not the plans are being achieved and, when necessary, making decisions to modify the plans in order to achieve the specific objective.

Basic Skills of an Administrative Assistant

At this point you may be wondering what basic skills you need to function as an administrative assistant and perform the administrative role effectively. Although many skills are needed, a few of the most important ones are the following:
- Conceptual skills
- Human relations skills

- Administrative skills
- Technical skills

The relative importance of these skills varies according to the type of office in which you are employed; the type of practice, whether it is a specialty or general practice; the job being performed; and the staff being managed.

Conceptual skills involve the ability to acquire, analyze, and interpret information in a logical manner. These skills allow you to put an idea or concept into perspective and to perceive how this idea would affect the whole practice.

Human relations skills aid you in understanding people and allow you to interact with them effectively. These skills are vital in a health profession and involve communication, motivation, and an ability to lead.

Administrative skills are those that help you to use all of the other skills effectively in performing administrative functions. These include the ability to establish and follow policies and procedures, to process paperwork in an organized manner, and to coordinate activities in the office.

Technical skills include understanding and being able to supervise effectively the specific processes, practices, and techniques required of specific jobs in the business office. This is the use of all of the knowledge of dentistry and business that allows you to perform day-to-day operations in the office.

> Human relations skills aid you in understanding people and allow you to interact with them.

The Ethical Administrative Assistant

In addition to the basic skills the administrative assistant should possess, the professional attitude and ethics of this person will have a significant influence on the staff. The following suggestions may identify some attributes of an ethical, caring administrative assistant:

1. **Respect the Dentist and the Practice Concepts.** Being respectful of a dentist employer means not circumventing him or her with issues or concerns. If you have an idea that you believe will improve the practice, discuss it with the employer. If you have problems with a task or a staff-person, share these concerns. You must believe in the dentist and the practice, and support the objectives that have been defined. If you stay in a practice in which unethical conduct occurs, you are essentially supporting this type of practice and thus your ethics become questionable.

2. **Be a Good Listener.** Listen with your eyes; hear what the other person is saying; ask questions; and restate the ideas to be sure you understand the person's message.

3. **Maintain Frequent Communication.** If you want people to follow you, they must know who you are, what you represent, what you can do, and what your vision is. To do this you must tell and show them. Disseminate your ideas in meetings and in day-to-day interactions with the staff. Cultivate relationships outside the office, so you will have a network of contacts from which to draw information **when a task is to be done.** As an administrative assistant, written and verbal communication must be continuous and supportive. Take time to communicate positive responses to the staff. The attitude that you present to others will affect their performance both positively and negatively. You must let the staff know that you possess the skills and knowledge to lead them in their daily workload and that you, too, are capable of performing the tasks that you assign. Frequent communication does not relate to staff interaction only. It must be practiced with patients. They must understand relevant issues that relate to their dental care and must receive frequent communication from and about the office.

4. **Utilize Feedback.** Recognize nonverbal cues; use feedback as a positive source of communication; and transmit feedback between management and staff.

5. **Make Ethical Decisions.** Gather facts and analyze problems; develop alternatives; determine ethical issues involved; brainstorm with staff members; determine what actions should be taken and if they are practical; and evaluate the results of decision making.

6. **Avoid Unnecessary Delays in Decision Making.** Sound decisions should be made as soon as possible; if conflicts go unresolved, greater problems may be created.

7. **Delegate Authority.** Show confidence in the staff members by allowing them to assume responsibility; provide freedom for them to work.

8. **Identify Constraints Within Which Work Must Be Done.** Establish time limits on production needs; allow staff members to develop their own approaches within the framework you have defined.

9. **Exercise Self-Control.** Emotional outbursts don't lead to constructive management; don't "talk down" to staff members.

10. **Make Time Available to Staff.** Don't be too busy to listen to a staff-person. This doesn't mean you have to drop everything to listen, but make time available for staff input.

11. **Respect Diversity.** The ethical administrative assistant will understand that the world is diverse and that it will continue to become even more diverse in the future. This means that the administrative assistant must respect diversity of all people whether it is in ethnicity, race, gender, or age.

12. **Build and Develop Strong Followers.** One of the hallmarks of a successful administrative assistant is to surround oneself with action-oriented, dedicated followers. By showing confidence in the followers' abilities, providing challenging assignments, and being genuinely concerned, the administrative assistant will garner respect, loyalty, and commitment while inspiring high-quality performance. In essence, the administrative assistant makes it easier to delegate and free himself or herself to devote more energy to issues that require his or her time. The key in this characteristic is for the administrative assistant to be genuine and honest in delegation and simply not delegate duties that have no challenge or are not recognized.

13. **Make Yourself Visible.** As an administrative assistant, you cannot hide behind a desk and be a leader. There is nothing arrogant or inappropriate about letting others know what you and other members of the staff have accomplished. Share a complimentary memo with the staff or patients when significant achievements have been made. Participate and encourage staff members to participate in activities that place you and the office in the spotlight. Be cautious not to take on too much. However, what you take on should be done with quality and panache.

14. **Learn from Your Mistakes.** Everyone makes mistakes, so don't agonize over them. Find ways to avoid making the same mistake again. Avoid assigning the blame to others. Some individuals will consistently blame others for their mistakes. This characteristic does not make a good administrative assistant. Leadership is about accepting the mistake, moving forward, and not wallowing in the past.

15. **Expand Your Leadership Role.** As an administrative assistant or office manager, you must extend your leadership role beyond the dental office. Make an effort to become involved in other professional or business groups that will provide valuable information for your office and offer you the opportunity to place your office in the spotlight.

STAFF COMMUNICATION

Communication is an essential element in management and becomes a vital link in establishing a meaningful relationship between you, the dentist, other members of the staff, and the patient.

The basic definition of communication is to understand and to be understood by another person. Bob Adams states in his book *Streetwise Managing People: Lead Your Staff to Peak Performance,* that "Quality Communication = Positive Interaction." When an office staff employs positive, constructive communication, it is sending a consistent message. The relative success of a dental practice is measured by the ability of the staff members to communicate with each other and with the patient. The form that communication takes in an office may be dictated by the type of leadership in the office, as described in Chapter 1.

Communicating with staff members is in many ways like communicating with patients. You are transmitting information to another person and therefore understanding that person. However, the difference in communication with staff members is that the status of the persons involved has changed and the channels of communication may be more complex. To achieve quality communication, consider following the simple steps suggested in Box 2-2.

Channels of Communication

As a dental practice increases in size, the channels of communication become more complicated. Formal and informal communication exists. A formal communication channel is dictated by the type of management that exists in the practice. Formal communication may be downward, upward, or horizontal.

Downward communication is exemplified when a dentist issues an order, or mandate, that is disseminated to the staff member at the next level. The basic channel is shown in Figure 2-2. A more complex system, as shown in Figure 2-3, illustrates an office as it increases in staff size, including several dentists and auxiliaries. Downward communication includes instructions, explanations, and communication that will aid the employee in performing work.

Upward channels of communication are vital in a formal setting. Employees should be free to express attitudes and feelings. This type of communication reverses the flow of information in Figures 2-2 and 2-3 and is generally of a reporting nature. It may include suggestions, complaints, or grievances. A lack of upward communication may result in dissatisfied employees.

Box 2-2
Suggestions for Creating Positive Staff Interactions

- Help others to be right, not wrong.
- Whenever possible, have fun.
- Be enthusiastic.
- Seek ways for new ideas to work, not reasons whey they won't.
- Be bold and courageous; take chances.
- Help others achieve success.
- Maintain a positive mental attitude.
- Maintain confidentiality.
- Verify information given to you before you repeat what you hear; avoid gossip.
- Speak positively about others whenever the opportunity arises.
- Say "thank you" for kind gestures or a job well done.
- Express a happy attitude in your nonverbal communication.
- If you don't have anything positive to say, don't say anything.

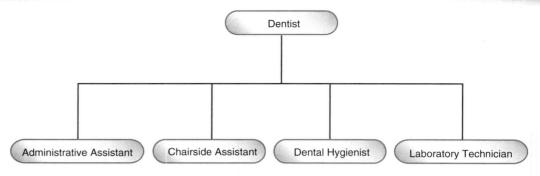

Figure 2-2 Downward communication as exemplified in a traditional dental practice.

Horizontal communication is essential for a larger organization. This type of communication involves transmittal of information from one department to another. This type of communication exists within large offices, clinics, hospitals, and dental schools.

Informal channels of communication can also be referred to as the "grapevine." This form of communication is often feared by administrative assistants but, if handled effectively, can provide the assistant with insight into staff emotions. Frequently, the grapevine carries rumors, personal interpretations,

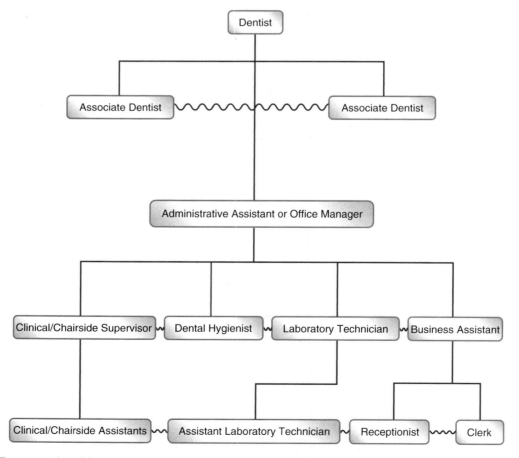

Figure 2-3 Downward and horizontal communication shown in an organizational chart of a group practice. Note that the levels of the dentists may vary according to the organization of the practice.

or distorted information. Fear often causes an active grapevine. It becomes the responsibility of the administrative assistant to listen to the grapevine and eliminate rumors by explaining the true facts. Thus the administrative assistant develops skill in handling tension created by the grapevine.

Employee Empowerment

As in most businesses, dentistry is confronted with the issue of how to obtain a high degree of employee productivity and yet maintain cost-effectiveness. One sure way to meet this objective is to maximize the utilization of the skills of each employee. Most dentists will include in the office objectives a statement "to support and encourage each staff member to reach his or her potential." When this objective is supported in every action and deed within the office, the practice is highly successful.

What exactly is employee empowerment? According to *Webster's New World Dictionary,* Third College Edition, *empower* means to give power or authority to; to authorize; to give ability to; to enable; to permit. For a dental practice, this means giving employees:

- The power and authority to accomplish office objectives and all legally delegable duties independently.
- The ability to accomplish objectives and all legally delegable duties independently.
- Permission to accomplish objectives and all legally delegable duties independently.

The dentist who gives employees the power, ability, and permission to accomplish office objectives and perform legal tasks independently will have the edge over the competition. To be successful, the dentist must be able and willing to recognize the value that each employee brings to the office. In Bob Adams's book *Streetwise Managing People: Lead Your Staff to Peak Performance,* the author declares that "empowered employees attempt to work above and beyond their anticipated capabilities." He recommends that to empower employees, an environment must be created where the staff does the following:

- Behaves as an owner of the job and company.
- Behaves in a responsible manner.
- Sees the consequences of the work they do.
- Knows how they are doing and how they are valued in the practice.
- Is included in determining solutions to problems.
- Has direct input into the way in which the work they do is done.
- Spends a good deal of time smiling.
- Asks others if they need help.

Many concepts that Adams introduces seem to show common sense. When applied to a dental practice, these concepts seem to fit like a glove. Box 2-3 lists concepts that can easily be adapted to any dental practice to empower each member of the staff to become a meaningful member of the dental team.

> To be successful, the dentist must be able and willing to recognize the value that each employee brings to the office.

Conducting a Staff Meeting

Regularly scheduled staff meetings should become a routine part of the dental practice. They are an effective means of keeping communication channels open. The staff meeting provides an opportunity to define and review the goals for the practice. Although criticism may be part of a staff meeting, such a meeting should not be designed as a gripe session. The time and length of the staff meeting will vary, according to the needs of the staff. Some offices schedule an hour per week, others close the office for a half or a full day for a retreat session, and still others find luncheon or breakfast meetings effective.

Box 2-3
Concepts to Empower Employees

- Create a communication process that is complete, consistent, and clearly understood by all members of the staff.
- Ensure that all employees understand what is expected of them in their respective job positions.
- Provide each employee with the appropriate training, information, and materials to successfully accomplish their job duties.
- Clearly define and establish evaluation instruments for the responsibilities for each job.
- Create controls that are guidelines that allow flexibility.
- Encourage and practice behaviors that promote encouragement, support, and clear feedback to employees.
- Encourage and promote a sense of responsibility in each employee.
- Encourage and promote continuing education and credentialing.
- Create opportunities for staff members to work together in teams.
- Make it easy for people praise each other. Make the office one that recognizes and acknowledges praiseworthy actions.
- Listen to employees at all times. Make the office systems listen to the employees.
- Trust the employees.

> The staff meeting provides an opportunity to define and review the goals for the practice.

An agenda may be used in planning a staff meeting. The agenda, combined with the list of rules below, will serve to expedite the business objectives of the staff meeting.

Notify each staff member of the time and place of the staff meeting. Request a return reply for attendance. Determine the priority of agenda items. Obtain suggestions for these items from the staff members. Provide a copy of the agenda to each staff member, and adhere to the agenda items. Review accomplishments. Determine goals and needs for change. Establish a method for accomplishing these goals. Review outcome of the meeting and provide keyboarded minutes to the staff. Maintain a strict meeting schedule. Don't allow one person to monopolize the meeting. Don't turn the meeting into a gripe session.

Staff Etiquette

Chapter 1 describes the importance of business etiquette. Etiquette or the application of good manners can be applied to daily interactions with each member of the staff. Etiquette must be practiced with each of your colleagues on a daily basis, and it cannot simply be turned on and off when patients are around. The statement "Good manners begin at home," can be adapted to the dental office by remembering that good manners begin with the staff. The failure to promote good manners with each other can be detrimental. Employers subconsciously take the pulse of relationships among their employees, and such readings often reveal poor relationships among the staff.

> Good manners begin with the staff.

Furthermore, as discussed later in this chapter, poor relationships relate directly to productivity. Box 2-4 lists several suggestions for implementing good staff etiquette.

Managing Conflict

Some administrative assistants become defensive and irritated when confronted with a complaint. Some individuals feel that a complaint is a reflection

> ## Box 2-4
> ### Suggestions for Improving Staff Etiquette
>
> - Determine the office code of behavior.
> - Extend a friendly greeting to coworkers each day.
> - Make introductions when individuals are not acquainted.
> - Extend friendly greetings to people who enter the office; stand when you greet the person. Introduce yourself.
> - Extend a cordial "thank you" or "goodbye" when someone leaves the office for the day.
> - Maintain good relations with your peers.
> - Learn how to handle your rivals with tact.
> - Be a team player.
> - Avoid becoming a do-gooder who seeks constant recognition.
> - When conflict exists, learn to mend fences.
> - Dress and act professionally when representing the office at conferences or seminars.

on them personally. However, conflicts are normal between an administrative assistant and an employee or between a patient and a member of the staff. Concern should be raised if numerous complaints arise, because this may indicate a serious problem.

Regardless of the nature of the complaint, the administrative assistant should review the details of the complaint and seek to resolve the problem quickly. Steps in resolving the problem might include the following:

- Make time available as soon as possible to discuss the problem. A delay may result in additional conflict or may be interpreted to mean that you are not interested in listening to the problem.
- Listen patiently to all the issues, keeping an open mind. You can gain the staff member's confidence by encouraging the person to talk and indicating that you want to provide fair treatment.
- Determine the real issue. Frequently, a complaint is made about a problem, when in reality a deeper concern is the real issue. For example, a person may be complaining about unfair work assignments, when actually the source of the problem is a personality clash between two staff members.
- Exercise self-control. Avoid arguments or expressions of personality conflicts between the complaining parties. Emotional outbursts generally do not lead to constructive resolution of the problem. Should this result, it is wise to terminate the meeting until a future meeting can be scheduled, and the problem can be discussed in a calm manner.
- Avoid a delay in decision making. A dental office is a relatively small business organization, and allowing a conflict to go unresolved can cause undue stress on the entire staff. If it is necessary to delay a decision, let the persons involved know the status of the problem.
- Maintain a record. Documentation of meetings or discussions is helpful should future conflict arise over the same problem. It is impossible for you to recall all of the issues about an incident. Therefore information should be retained in the employee file or appropriate area for future reference.

It is not easy to resolve conflict. Most of us wish to avoid it. However, we must realize conflict will arise whenever we have two or more people working together. As an administrative assistant, you should try to be fair and objective. If you follow these suggestions, you will have at least attempted to resolve the complaint in a professional manner and will possibly avoid minor conflicts that can escalate into major crises.

Barriers to Staff Communication

Barriers that exist in patient communication are prejudice, poor listening, preoccupation, impatience, and even impaired hearing. These barriers all exist within the staff. Additional barriers, such as status or position, resistance to change and new ideas, or attitudes about work, compound communication difficulties with coworkers. Because these barriers exist, administrative assistants should never assume that the message being sent will be received as it was intended. They should be aware of potential misinterpretations and work to overcome barriers to improve channels of communication with the staff.

Periodically, the staff should evaluate its exchange of information and determine if all channels of communication are open to everyone. During a staff meeting, an agenda item might be the completion of a questionnaire that would indicate each staff member's feelings about office communication.

ADVANTAGES OF HIRING A SKILLED ADMINISTRATIVE ASSISTANT

A dentist today can ill afford the risk of hiring inexperienced personnel to manage the business office. In addition to having a broad knowledge of dentistry, the administrative assistant should be curious, highly organized, and able to accept responsibility and make decisions, as well as have an understanding of computers and other automated business equipment, possess skills in management, and communicate with people.

Few statistics are available, but it seems that in the past dentists have hired persons with a little knowledge of dentistry and minimal experience, or they have promoted chairside/clinical assistants to administrative assistants. Because administrative assistants need a broad background in dentistry, it would appear that the last arrangement would have a distinct advantage if the assistant were willing to accept the transition. It is more desirable to hire a person with education in both business and dental assisting. For the administrative assistant with the appropriate education and background, a special credential as a Certified Dental Practice Management Assistant (CDPMA) is available through the Dental Assisting National Board (DANB). Successful completion of this national credentialing examination will verify one's credibility in the dental business office and can be valuable in applying for a position in a dental office. Inquiries about the criteria for taking this examination can be directed to the Dental Assisting National Board, 676 N. St. Clair, Suite 1880, Chicago, IL 60611, or visit their website at www.danb.org. The advantages of hiring an educated administrative assistant are listed in Box 2-5.

TIME MANAGEMENT

A vital aspect of the job as an administrative assistant is time management. There is more to working efficiently than just knowing how to perform a specific task. Administrative assistants also need to know when to perform each task, how to choose which job to do first, and how long each project will take. Understanding the relationship of time to production is also important. All of these together make up time management.

Much research has been done over the years on time and motion studies in the dental treatment room. These studies have resulted in the dental

> ### Box 2-5
> #### Advantages of Hiring an Educated Administrative Assistant
>
> **An educated administrative assistant has the following attributes:**
> Understands basic dental terminology
> Understands interpersonal communication
> Understands clinical data
> Is able to transpose clinical data to financial data
> Is able to explain treatment procedures to a patient
> Can promote or sell dental care
> Understands the consequences of dental neglect
> Practices infection-control procedures
> Implements OSHA regulations
> Understands appointment sequencing for various dental procedures
> Is able to manage emergency procedures
> Is less likely to make common errors

profession implementing the concepts of four-handed dentistry and the utilization of a chairside/clinical assistant to increase productivity and reduce stress. Less emphasis has been placed on production in the dental business office. However, much can be learned from the research general business has done on time management. Remember, although dentistry is a healthcare system, it is still a small business and has profit as its objective. Thus time management becomes a vital component to the dental practice.

Time management in the dental business office involves planning and scheduling your work and avoiding wasted time. The behaviors that waste time in the business office are failing to plan and budget time, giving in to interruptions, failing to follow through and complete a task, slowness in reading and making decisions, performing unnecessary work, and failure to delegate. Other time wasters are lack of privacy and desk clutter. Solutions to many common time wasters are suggested in Box 2-6.

To determine the effectiveness of your own time management, you must assess the way you are currently working. Determine ways to use your time more effectively, or confirm that you are already using your time efficiently. Evaluation of time management is an ongoing process and can be done routinely by recording the way you currently spend your time; analyzing how you spend your time; determining what activities can be adjusted to make you a more effective worker; scheduling your activities daily, weekly, monthly, and long-range; and adhering to the schedule. Efficient time management requires that you organize individual tasks, maintain daily schedules, analyze daily tasks, schedule major projects, establish deadlines, and organize workflow.

Maintaining Daily Schedules

To efficiently maintain a daily schedule, it is necessary to utilize a calendar of activities and tasks and a "to-do" list, determine priorities, show flexibility, use free time, and review the schedule with the dentist.

The use of a calendar and personal appointment book as well as the office appointment book is necessary in maintaining a daily schedule. A desk or electronic calendar provides a method for keeping track of your daily schedule and is used for short- and long-range scheduling. Make entries neatly if done manually, be consistent in making entries, and avoid making confidential entries if you use an electronic calendar that is accessible to others.

Box 2-6
Solutions to Eliminate Time Wasters

Time Waster	Solution
Lack of goals	Prepare a to-do list and use it.
Telephone interruptions	Use an answering machine or voicemail during specified work times.
Procrastination	Do it first!
Feeling tired, stressed, or irritable	Schedule a thorough physical examination; develop a wellness plan; enroll in a stress-management course.
Lack of future plans	Develop short- and long-range plans.
Disorganized work area	Purchase organizers; put away work when finished; don't begin a new project until one is complete.
Accepting too many jobs	Learn to say no!
Waiting for information/ return calls	Use an answering machine or voicemail.
Incomplete work	Plan time to finish projects with no interruptions.
Socializing with coworkers	Avoid the situations; restrict others from too much socializing.
Unnecessary work	Analyze the task; eliminate it if not necessary.

A to-do list should provide a summary of all pending tasks, not just those to be done on a specific day. This list need not include routine daily tasks, such as opening and closing the office or opening mail. Delete each task upon completion, and transfer tasks not completed to a list for the following day.

Determine priorities by ranking each task on the list by its priority or its level of urgency and importance. Items on the list can be ranked by giving a 1 to tasks that must be completed immediately, 2 to tasks that must be completed that day, and 3 to tasks that must be done whenever you have time.

Be flexible in your plans for the day, because emergencies arise and new priority tasks will be identified. For instance, the dentist may need you to produce an important document immediately that was not on your list. At this point, it may be necessary to seek help from other staff members to complete other pressing tasks. With total team effort, a reprioritizing of previously identified tasks can be quickly accomplished to meet unplanned needs.

In addition to the routine to-do list, another list could be kept that details various tasks that should be completed when time permits. Such a list provides tasks to do when there is a slow time or when there are no patients scheduled.

DESIGNING A PROCEDURAL MANUAL

The procedural manual is a valuable instrument in maintaining maximum efficiency in the dental office while providing a means of communication. It includes the dentist's philosophy of the practice and defines the job responsibilities for each team member. The manual also states in specific detail the technique to be implemented for each procedure in both the business and clinical areas of the office. Although the manual should be written under the direction of the dentist, each member of the team should contribute equally in the development of the manual to provide a total team effort.

The following list of guidelines provides subjects to be included in an office procedural manual. You can purchase basic office manual formats and add inserts for the dentist's philosophy and specific duties relating to the practice.

GUIDELINES FOR A PROCEDURAL MANUAL

I. Statement of purpose or objective of the manual
II. Statement of philosophy for the practice
III. Table of contents
IV. Office communications
    A. Vocabulary
    B. Telecommunications
    C. Reception techniques
    D. Written communication
    E. Patient education
V. Staff policies
    A. Conduct
    B. Grooming and appearance
    C. Dress codes: clinical and business office attire
    D. Staff meetings
VI. Employment policies
    A. Probationary period
    B. Promotion
    C. Hours of work
    D. Overtime
    E. Holidays
    F. Vacations
    G. Absences and leaves
    H. Salaries
    I. Insurance
    J. Additional benefits
    K. Termination of employment
    L. Personal telephone calls and personal mail
VII. Office records
    A. Infection control in records handling
    B. Patient records
    C. OSHA records
    D. Material Safety Data Sheets (MSDSs)
    E. Employee records
    F. Transfer of records
    G. Accounts receivable
    H. Accounts payable
    I. Filing
VIII. Infection-control policy
    A. OSHA guidelines
    B. Health risk categories
    C. Nomenclature
    D. Disinfection and sterilization guidelines
    E. Waste management
    F. Medical history procedures
    G. Universal precautions
    H. Preventive vaccinations
IX. Clinical procedures
    A. Emergencies
    B. Tray setups

Writing a Personnel Policy

As part of the office procedural manual, a well-defined personnel policy must be established. A fair and equitable personnel policy may help to eliminate conflicts that could arise among team members. The material in Box 2-7 illustrates a suggested personnel policy. This policy may be altered to satisfy the needs of an individual office.

Box 2-7
Personnel Policies for the Office of Joseph W. Lake, DDS, and Ashley M. Lake, DDS

Probationary Period
Your first 3 months will be considered a probationary period, during which Drs. Joseph and Ashley Lake will see how you progress with the new work. During this period your employment may be terminated without notice. The dentist will create a Merit Rating Report at the termination of the probationary period and periodically thereafter. This report will be used as the basis for salary increases and promotions.

Promotion
Your demonstrated ability to perform your job well, your attendance and punctuality record, and your relationships with employees will all have a bearing on your opportunities for promotion and advancement in salary. Any outside courses of study that result in skills in addition to those noted on your application will be added to your record to ensure complete information when reviewing your record for advancement. All employees will be reviewed every 6 months.

Hours of Work
The office is open from 8:00 AM to 5:00 PM Monday and Wednesday, and 8:00 AM to 9:00 PM on Tuesday and Thursday. On Fridays the office is closed. Lunch hour is from 12:00 PM to 1:00 PM. The basic week totals 35 working hours that will be assigned by each dentist.

Overtime
Overtime salary is paid for units of ½ hour. Fractions of less than ½ hour of overtime are not reported. If your salary is less than $2150 per month, compensation for work authorized by the dentist in excess of 35 hours is at the rate of time and one half beyond 35 hours in any week, or for work on Saturdays, Sundays, and holidays.

Holidays
You will have the following legal holidays with pay: New Year's Day, Memorial Day, Independence Day, Labor Day, Thanksgiving Day, and Christmas Day. When the office is closed for a religious holiday or other holiday, an announcement will be made in advance.

Vacations
Requests for vacation time in excess of 1 day must be made 30 days in advance. You will be entitled to 2 weeks of vacation after completing

Box 2-7
Personnel Policies for the Office of Joseph W. Lake, DDS, and Ashley M. Lake, DDS—cont'd

12 months of continuous employment, and 4 weeks of vacation after 10 years of employment. A legal holiday that falls within the vacation period adds 1 day to your vacation. When a vacation falls within a vacation period, salary will be paid in advance to the latest regular salary payment date falling within the vacation period.

Absences and Leaves
Regular attendance and punctuality are necessary for smooth functioning of the dental office, and your record in this respect will be considered in determining your advancement and salary adjustment. However, there are certain absences that are unavoidable and for which provision will be made. In each case, the dentists should be notified in advance when possible, or before 7:30 AM on the day of your absence. If you fail to make proper notification, the unadvised absence will be counted as absence without salary.

Sick leave for your own confining illness
When absence is for your own illness, salary is paid for up to 1 day for each month of employment, cumulative to 30 days. If you need sick leave in addition to the above, such a request should be made to Dr. Lake for additional time without pay.

Court duty
If you are required to serve as a juror or witness, your absence is considered as a leave with salary.

Death in the immediate family
If there is a death in your immediate family, up to 3 days of leave may be granted with salary.

Leave of absence for other reasons
If you request a leave of absence for other reasons or for a longer period than is provided with salary, various factors will be taken into consideration, including your previous work and attendance records, the length of leave you are requesting, the work needs of the office, and any other pertinent factors.

Salaries
Payment of your salary is by check on a weekly basis, covering salary through Wednesday of the current week. Salary checks are distributed each Friday. Salary increases are considered every 6 months. The quality of your work, the amount of responsibility you assume, your attendance and punctuality records, your attitude toward the staff and patients, and your length of service are factors that enter into the consideration. Deductions from salary regularly include withholding tax and Social Security. Deductions for group insurance, hospital care, and other benefits are made only upon written request.

Insurance
To help provide security in times of sickness and hospitalization, health insurance is available as follows: membership in a group health insurance plan is available to all those employed up to 1 year on a payroll deduction basis.

Box 2-7
Personnel Policies for the Office of Joseph W. Lake, DDS, and Ashley M. Lake, DDS—cont'd

Staff members may select this insurance at their own expense for the first 12 months of employment. Deductions for hospital care are made the first payday of each month. At the end of 12 months, Dr. Lake will pay this coverage upon a successful merit rating evaluation. Coverage of your spouse and dependent children under 19 years of age may be included in your hospital care contract.

Social Security is provided through payments by you and Dr. Lake to the U.S. government. Your share of the cost is deducted from each salary payment.

Additional benefits
In addition to regular salary increases, the members of the staff are eligible for several additional benefits.

Uniform stipend
Dr. Lake will provide a uniform stipend as follows:

Chairside or clinical assistants/hygienists will wear surgical scrubs with outer laboratory coats provided by the office, for which all laundry will be provided. At the end of 6 months of successful employment, Dr. Lake will issue an additional stipend to the Central Uniform Shop for the cost of shoes.

Administrative assistants will receive a dress stipend not to exceed $1200 at the end of 6 months. At the end of 12 months, an additional dress/uniform stipend will be issued not to exceed $2000. Thereafter, a stipend will be issued annually not to exceed $2750.

Professional organizations
At the end of 12 months of successful employment, the dues of your professional organization will be paid by Dr. Lake. The statement and proof of membership must be submitted to Dr. Lake for payment.

Education and travel
You are encouraged to increase your skills at all times. To ensure your exposure to current changes in dentistry, Dr. Lake will provide the following benefits: After 6 months of employment, payment not in excess of $450 for any educational seminar; after 12 months of employment, 3 days absence with pay and $1200 applicable to coursework or educational travel; after 5 years of employment, 5 days absence with pay and $2500 applicable to coursework or educational travel.

Profit sharing
After completion of 2 full years of successful employment, Dr. Lake will provide the following profit-sharing bonus to each staff member: 2% of total business in excess of $125,000, plus 2% of total receipts in excess of $125,000.

Infection-control policy
An effective infection-control program has been implemented in the office for the protection of staff members, patients, and family members. It is recommended that you adhere to the *Infection Control Policy Handbook* and that you are aware of all updates of this manual as they occur. The cost of Hepatitis B vaccine and TB vaccine will be covered by the office.

Box 2-7
Personnel Policies for the Office of Joseph W. Lake, DDS, and Ashley M. Lake, DDS—cont'd

It is highly recommended that you receive other protective vaccines for childhood diseases not previously contracted. You will be compensated for such immunization. All staff in this office is classified as to the health risk involved according to one of the following categories identified by the Occupational Health and Safety Administration (OSHA) guidelines.

In the past there have been three categorizations of tasks to differentiate exposure contact with blood, body fluids, and tissues. In reality there are only two. Either a person has *no* contact with blood, or they have some or continuous exposure. Thus, in reality, the definitions look more like the following:

Category I

Tasks that involve exposure to blood, body fluids, or tissues. Most, although not necessarily all, tasks performed by the dentist, dental hygienist, dental assistant, and laboratory technician would fall in this category. This category also includes clerical or nonprofessional workers who may perform unplanned clinical tasks.

Category II

Tasks that involve no exposure to blood, body fluids, or tissues. An administrative assistant, business office receptionist, bookkeeper, or insurance clerk who does not handle dental instruments or materials would be a Category II worker.

Termination of employment

Resignation

You are asked to give 2 weeks written notice of resignation. If you have been employed for 6 months or more and you resign during the vacation period having given 2 weeks notice, you will be compensated for your vacation according to the vacation schedule.

Release

If you are released from your position for reasons other than misconduct, in which case no notice is given, you will have notice or salary in lieu of notice as follows: If you have been employed for at least 6 but less than 12 months, 1 week; If you have been employed for 13 months or more, 2 weeks.

Personal telephone calls and personal mail/e-mail

Telephone traffic is heavy at the Joseph W. Lake, DDS, and Ashley M. Lake, DDS, practice. Personal telephone calls affect the workload in 2 ways: they prohibit incoming calls from patients, and they take time from your job. Limit the number of personal calls, and receive incoming calls only in an emergency. Personal cell phones should be turned off or set on "silent" mode during office hours. Similarly, the volume of mail is heavy at the office; therefore, do not use the office address for personal mail/e-mail.

HIRING PRACTICES

Writing a Job Description

A current, accurate job description should exist for each position in the dental office. These job descriptions will aid employees in telling prospective employees what will be expected of them on the job and will aid in training new staff members.

To write a job description you need to do a job analysis. A job analysis involves observing the employee and gathering information about the job. List the tasks that make up the job, and determine the skills, personality characteristics, and educational background needed for the employee to perform this job satisfactorily. The staff then reviews the job description. It is revised as necessary and placed in the procedural manual. An outline for a job description is shown in Figure 2-4.

Writing a Job Advertisement

The content of an advertisement for new staff members should be the result of a well-thought-out job description. List the skills you expect the person to have, require a resume, and identify attractive features of the job such as benefits, salary, and working conditions. If you expect to attract highly qualified candidates, your advertisement cannot be a mundane, brief statement seeking inexperienced people. Periodically look at the classified ads in the local paper for ideas in other allied health professions. Compare the two advertisements in Figures 2-5 and 2-6. Which advertisement presents a greater challenge for a prospective employee? The ad seeking an inexperienced person will probably get more response, but this isn't a contest to get the largest response. The procedure of advertising should seek to screen potential candidates. A request for an educated person cuts down on potential training costs for the dentist and can ensure a minimal level of education.

Interviewing Prospective Employees

Part of the management role for the administrative assistant may be interviewing applicants for a position on the staff. This is an important responsibility and requires a great deal of skill. The suggestions in Box 2-8 may aid you when conducting an interview.

Legal Considerations in Hiring

There are several legal factors to be considered in hiring an employee. These include application forms, citizenship status, and testing.

An employer must ensure that application forms avoid any questions regarding race or ethnic background. Furthermore, each applicant who completes an application form must be provided with the same type of form. Be certain that the application form used in the office does not violate any state requirements. For example, a state may deem it unlawful to use a lie-detector test. Thus, such a question on an application asking the applicant to take a lie detector test could be in violation of state law.

It is in violation of federal law to hire an unauthorized (illegal) alien. An employer must require proof of an applicant's legal status, and the Immigration and Naturalization Service (INS) Form I-9 (Employment Eligibility Verification form) must be filled out before employment. Documents accepted for verification include an original U.S. passport, a certificate of U.S. citizenship or naturalization, an alien registration card with photograph, a state-issued driver license, a Social Security card, or a birth certificate.

Job Title _____
You will report to _____

GENERAL OBJECTIVES:

The administrative assistant will manage the day-to-day activities of the business office. This person will be responsible for maintaining office documents, patient, employee, and governmental records; scheduling patients; interviewing and managing staff; managing accounts receivable and payable; managing inventory and recall systems; operating electronic office equipment; and maintaining various types of telecommunications systems.

SPECIFIC OBJECTIVES:

Maintain office documents
- Select and complete patient clinical records
- Manage insurance claim forms
- Establish and maintain a recall system
- Maintain employee records
- Complete and maintain governmental forms

Maintain an accounts receivable system
- Maintain accounts receivable activity
- Prepare bank deposits
- Prepare statements
- Follow up delinquent accounts

Perform accounts payable activities
- Verify invoices with monthly statements
- Write checks
- Reconcile the bank statement
- Prepare materials for the accountant

Supervise staff personnel
- Prepare job descriptions
- Interview and screen potential employees
- Determine staff needs and schedules
- Orient new staff
- Evaluate staff

Perform support duties
- Establish equipment maintenance program
- Plan for update and risk management seminars
- Implement state and federal regulations
- Help support staff as needed

JOB CRITERIA:

Education
- Certified/Registered Dental Assistant, Certified Dental Office Manager, or a minimum of 5 years experience in business management
- Knowledge of electronic office automation
- Formal business courses
- Knowledge or experience in management

Personal requirements
- Must be able to work with any employee and be able to resolve conflicts between employees
- Must be able to discuss all dental/financial needs with patients and be objective and pleasant to them
- Must be able to cooperate with other dental office staff personnel
- Must be able to work with the doctor and convey needs to the staff in a participatory manner

SALARY:

$35,500 - $57,700 plus benefits
Salary based on the salary chart in the office procedure manual
Date prepared: 01/25/--

Figure 2-4 Job description.

Registered Dental Assistant who is ambitious and skilled in ergonomic four-handed dentistry. Duties require clinical, laboratory, and business office management skills in a general practice. Must have expanded functions credential. Attractive salary and benefits. Write to: Joseph W. Lake, D.D.S., 611 Main St. S.E., Grand Rapids, MI 49502

Figure 2-5 Newspaper advertisement.

Pre-Employment Testing

A variety of employment testing may include standardized tests, polygraph tests, and drug and alcohol tests. Although a small dental office will seldom use all these tests, it is possible that an institution or larger corporation with dental facilities may take advantage of all the tests.

Businesses such as a dental practice may legally use professionally developed standardized tests to verify knowledge, aptitude, and skills during a selection process. Tests used to screen applicants can become discriminatory when they serve to disqualify members of a minority culture who are unfamiliar with the language or concepts but are fully qualified for the job. Dentistry can avail itself of standardized tests developed by the Dental Assistants National Board and various state regulatory agencies. To create a new test when many such tests already exist can place a practitioner at potential legal risks.

Many private sector employers are considering drug and alcohol testing as a pre-employment requirement. The main type of test is a urinalysis, which is likely to be part of a pre-employment physical examination.

An employer refusing to hire someone with AIDS violates federal and state disability discrimination laws. Protection under Title VII of the 1964 Civil Rights Act has been extended to disabled persons, including those infected with the AIDS virus or who have tested positive for the HIV virus. An employer probably would not be justified in refusing to hire an individual with AIDS, unless the employer could establish that the prospective employee would endanger the health and safety of others. This issue is controversial for the dental care profession and must be met with a thorough understanding of both legal and ethical ramifications.

Conducting an Interview

Prior to conducting an interview, gather all of the information about each candidate, develop an outline of questions, and determine the physical setting for the interview. Often a neutral location such as a lounge or conference room will make the candidate feel more at ease.

Dental Office Administrative Assistant: Interested in an exciting position you find in a large, diverse, professional office? A group dental practice is expanding its clinical facilities. Position demands strong supervisory skills, ability to work effectively under pressure, use good judgment, and be able to accept responsibility. Forward your resume to: Box #2589, Grand Rapids News, Grand Rapids, MI 49502

Figure 2-6 Blind ad.

> **Box 2-8**
> **Suggestions for Job Interview Preparation**
>
> Perform a task analysis of the proposed job.
> Determine the competencies needed to fulfill the job requirements.
> Prepare a well-defined job description.
> Have the applicant complete a job application.
> Determine how to measure an applicant's ability. Tests may be utilized to measure certain abilities, such as keyboarding speed and accuracy.
> Explain the requirements of the job completely.
> Determine key questions to ask in the interview.
> Review reactions toward the applicant. Were you comfortable? Was the applicant an active participant in the conversation? Was the individual shy or domineering?
> Make accurate observations about the applicant's answers, grammar, and nonverbal cues during the interview. Use a check-off form to ensure that each candidate is evaluated on the same basis.
> Record evaluations as soon as the interview is completed to assure that you don't forget the responses.
> Investigate references the applicant has provided. This confirms the accuracy of the applicant's statements.

As the interview begins, establish rapport with the candidate by introducing yourself and creating a sense of pleasantness between you and the candidate. Explain the purpose of the interview, and generate a relaxed atmosphere. During the interview, motivate the candidate to participate.

The main part of the interview consists of asking questions, listening to responses, answering questions, and providing a transition from one discussion topic to another. Gain confidence in questioning the applicant to reflect each facet of the individual's background. Ask such questions as, "Tell me about your previous job experiences," "What is your attitude toward your previous working experience?" or "What do you feel your strengths and weaknesses are for the position available in this office?"

Common types of questions asked during an interview include direct, indirect, and hypothetical. The direct question will generally elicit an expected response. An indirect question does not imply a yes or no response. The following examples illustrate the differences in these types of questions.

Direct: "Would you be opposed to traveling to a satellite office?"

Indirect: "How would you feel about traveling to a satellite office?"

A hypothetical question describes an actual situation and elicits a response from the candidate.

Hypothetical: "If one of our patients told you he refused to pay an account because he didn't like the way he was treated, how would you respond?"

This type of question is valuable because it is as close as the interviewer will get to observing the candidate's behavior.

During the interview you have two major functions: to gather information about the candidate's qualifications for the job in a nondiscriminatory manner and to convey information to the candidate about the office and specific job responsibilities (Box 2-1). By keeping questions and discussion relevant to the job, you will achieve the first task. The first task requires that you be aware of certain legal considerations related to interviewing. Rules of thumb for asking interview questions are shown in Box 2-9. Guidelines by the U.S. Department of Labor and the U.S. Equal Employment Opportunity

---

Box 2-9
Three Rules of Thumb for Interviewing

When asking interview questions, consider these rules of thumb:
1. Ask only for information that you intend to use to make hiring decisions.
2. Know how you will use the information to make a decision.
3. Recognize that it is difficult to defend the practice of seeking information that you do not use.

Commission (EEOC) prohibit discriminatory hiring based on race, creed, color, sex, national origin, handicap, or age. Questions related to any of these as well as marital status, children, ownership of a house or car, credit rating, or type of military discharge can also be considered discriminatory. Questions that should and should not be asked during an interview include many of those shown in Box 2-10, and topics that should be avoided are listed in Box 2-11. The second task of the interview can be met if you include all of the following areas:
- Specific job responsibilities
- Orientation procedures
- Opportunities for advancement
- Management procedures

Box 2-10
Questions to Ask and Not to Ask During an Interview

Do Ask

What was your absentee record at your prior place of employment?
Do you know of any reason (for example, transportation) why you would be unable to get to work on time and on a regular basis?
Are you available to work overtime?
We are looking for employees with a commitment to this position. Are there any reasons why you might not stay with us?
What are your career objectives?
Do you foresee any reasons why you could not be assigned to a branch or satellite office?
Where do you see yourself in five years?

Don't Ask

1. Where were you born?
2. Where and when did you graduate from high school?
3. Do you have any handicaps?
4. What religious holidays do you practice?
5. Are you married?
6. Do you plan to have children? How many?
7. Do you own a home?
8. Do you own a car?
9. Do you have any debts?
10. Can you provide three credit references?
11. Is your spouse likely to be transferred?
12. Is your spouse from this area?
13. How old are you?
14. How do you feel about working with members of a different race?
15. What language(s) do your parents speak?

> **Box 2-11**
> **Topics to Avoid During the Interview Process**
>
> Arrest records
> Marital status
> Maiden name
> Spouse's name
> Spouse's education
> Spouse's income
> Form of birth control
> Child care arrangements
> Lawsuits or legal complaints
> Ownership of car or residence
> Loans
> Insurance claims
> National origin
> Mother's maiden name
> Place of birth
> Disabilities
> Weight
> Age
> Date of high school graduation
> Religion
> Social organizations

- Professional responsibilities
- Work hours, salary, and fringe benefits

Concluding an Interview

The conclusion of the interview is a good opportunity for the applicant to tour the office. This is a good time, if convenient, for the rest of the staff to meet the candidate. Inform the applicant of the plans for arriving at a decision and a date by which the decision will be made. Factors to avoid in making a decision are listed in Box 2-12.

Once all of the candidates have been interviewed and the decision made about each, the person to be hired should be contacted promptly. A letter of confirmation should be sent to the new employee stating the conditions of

> **Box 2-12**
> **Factors to Avoid in Making Staff Selections**
>
> In making a selection or recommendation for hiring a staffperson, avoid making assumptions such as the following:
> 1. The dentist or staff members might prefer employees of certain ethnic or racial origins.
> 2. Those who come in contact with your employees might not want to deal with women or minorities.
> 3. Coworkers might object.
> 4. The job might involve unusual working conditions that would disqualify the applicant.

employment, that is, wages, hours, promotions, beginning date, and other conditions agreed upon during previous discussions. The letter should identify probationary periods, which allow either party to terminate employment within an established period of time, without fear of penalty. It is wise to have the employee sign the letter. A copy is then retained by the employee and a copy is placed in the employee file. A letter should also be sent to candidates not being hired, and their applications may remain on file if desired.

New Employee Training

A well-organized dental team will provide a smooth transition for the new employee into the practice. Time for the new employee to become well established in the office will vary according to the individual office. Among the many activities involved in new employee training, you should be able to do the following:

- Describe how the practice is run and what standards are required of the staff.
- Explain the organizational chart and job descriptions.
- Complete employee documents, including federal and state tax forms.
- Review procedural techniques.
- Allow time for observation, but let the skills and responsibilities of the new employee be utilized as soon as possible.
- Identify areas of strengths and weaknesses. Positive reinforcement is necessary to create confidence. However, poor performance should be altered to avoid reinforcement of less-than-quality work. It is easier to correct poor performance early in training rather than later, when it seriously affects the office production.
- Provide additional training beyond the educational experiences already achieved. This may be accomplished within the office or may require a more formal setting in a nearby school.
- Evaluate the performance of the new employee regularly. This allows changes to be made in performance and provides the staffperson with knowledge of his or her status.
- Review progress with adequate promotion via benefits or a pay increase.
- Terminate an employee if substandard performance continues. If all efforts to improve the employee's performance have failed, it is wise to terminate the employee promptly rather than to continue with substandard performance.

Key Terms

Administrative assistant – A person whose role is often defined as secretary, receptionist, business assistant, or "front desk person," and whose responsibilities include the day-to-day management of the dental practice.

Communication – The ability to understand and be understood.

Manager – A term often used to refer to an administrative assistant.

Time management – The ability to prioritize tasks, determine how long each project will take, and work effectively in managing time to production.

LEARNING ACTIVITIES

1. Write job descriptions for a chairside/clinical assistant, administrative assistant, and dental hygienist. What tasks should be identified for each of these jobs in a job analysis? Review classified advertisements in a local paper.
2. Compare the content of ads in various health occupations. What characteristics appeal to you in these ads? Why?
3. Create an interview outline that lists the sequence of events of an interview. Develop a series of questions that will determine a candidate's skills for a job.
4. Describe how you would handle the following conflict situations:
   a. Dr. Lake reprimands you for having forgotten to make a telephone call he requested you to make. What would you do?
   b. A chairside/clinical assistant criticizes another assistant for wearing facial piercings, which is a violation of the office procedural manual for clinical assistants. What would be your response?
   c. Office hours for the staff are 8:15 A.M. to 5:00 P.M. An assistant is chronically late, arriving 15 to 20 minutes after the assigned time each day. This person always leaves by 5:00 P.M. and seldom is late leaving for lunch. Friction is occurring among the staff. The dentist doesn't seem to be concerned. Is this really a problem? What are the issues involved? Can there be a resolution? What action should be taken, and who should take action?

Bibliography

Adams B, et al: *Streetwise managing people: lead your staff to peak performance,* Holbrook, MA, 1998, Adams Media Corporation.

Fulton-Calkins PJ: *General office procedures for colleges,* ed 12, Cincinnati, 2003, South-Western.

Hastings W, Potter R: *Trust me,* Colorado Springs, 2004, WaterBrook Press.

Thill JV, Bovée CL: *Excellence in business communication,* ed 5, Upper Saddle River, NJ, 2002, Prentice Hall.

Chapter

3

Patient Management

Chapter Outline

Learning Outcomes

Mastery of the content in this chapter will enable the reader to:

- Define glossary terms
- Understand patient needs
- Explain the special needs of patients
- Identify barriers to communication
- Recognize nonverbal cues
- Manage interpersonal communication in the reception area
- Design an office policy statement
- Explain marketing techniques in dentistry
- Describe external and internal marketing
- Understand patient rights

People are an essential part of the dental practice. The most important person in a dental practice is the patient. You must never overlook the fact that each patient has a different background and different needs. Therefore, while communicating with patients, it is important that you recognize each as an individual with specific needs and that you determine how to be sensitive to those needs. Remember that dentistry is a helping profession. Not only must every effort be made to alleviate patients' discomfort, but patients must be taught to help themselves.

> The most important person in a dental practice is the patient.

UNDERSTANDING PATIENT NEEDS

Each person who comes in contact with patients should have an understanding of the basic drives involved in motivating patients. Unless the dentist and staff have a basic understanding of these drives, they will become discouraged after numerous attempts fail to motivate patients to appreciate good dental health and quality dentistry.

With concern for humanism in this healthcare profession, it seems appropriate that you should be aware of the contributions of two humanistic psychologists, Abraham Maslow and Carl Rogers.

Maslow's Hierarchy of Needs

Dr. Abraham Maslow has described a "Hierarchy of Needs" (Figure 3-1) that aids in understanding how a person's needs motivate his or her behavior. Maslow identified five basic levels of needs ranging from basic biological needs to complex social or psychological drives.

1. **Physiological or biological.** These are bodily needs, and they are the first to be satisfied. You must satisfy these physical needs, or you won't live long enough to satisfy any social or psychological needs. If you are healthy, eat regularly, and are housed adequately, you can advance to the next level of the hierarchy with a sense of well-being.
2. **Safety or security needs.** Once the basic biological needs are met, you are ready for the second level of the hierarchy. This level allows you to explore your environment. Just as small children begin to explore their environment once their food and comfort needs have been met, you as an adult begin to explore. This is the level at which you feel safe and free from danger, threats, or other deprivation. If you have a job that is nonthreatening and live in a safe environment, you will feel secure and will be able to advance to the next level.

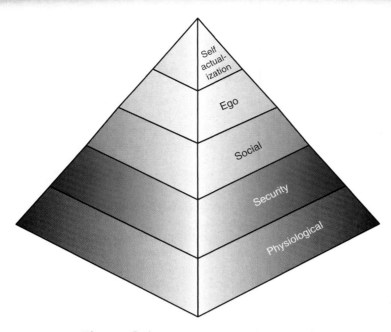

Figure 3-1 Maslow's Hierarchy of Needs.

3. **Social or love needs.** Once you are secure in your environment, you can advance to the level of social interaction. The poet John Donne wrote, "No man is an island, complete to itself." Donne realized that to be human means to interact with others. At this level on the hierarchy, Maslow realized that you need to interact with others with whom you share similar beliefs and who provide you with reinforcement to continue your social relationships. This love or social interaction gives you confidence to advance to the next level on the hierarchy.

4. **Esteem needs.** From interaction with others at the previous level, you will generate goals for yourself. Your peers often consider these needs as ego needs that relate to your self-esteem, reputation, and recognition. Here you look forward to achieving your goals, and from accomplishment you will receive self-esteem. Typically the self-satisfaction you receive from accomplishing these goals provides an impetus to establish new goals and begin the cycle again.

5. **Self-actualization.** Self-actualized people are motivated by the need to grow. To achieve this need, you must have achieved self-esteem and have confidence in yourself. Later in life, Maslow expanded his thoughts on the self-actualized person and explained that to achieve this level people must be relatively free of illness, sufficiently satisfied in their basic needs, positively using their capacities, and motivated by some existing or sought-after personal values. A person at this level often wants to help others achieve their goals by teaching them lessons he or she learned in the earlier stages. Some people never reach this level because they have not aspired to its recognition.

Relating this hierarchy to dentistry means getting to know your patients and the individuals with whom you are associated. Before a dentist can motivate a patient to accept a certain type of dental treatment, it must be understood where the patient is on the hierarchy of needs.

To help realize the application of these needs to dentistry, consider this situation. One of your patients is a bank president who is respected for his civic activities and has a warm, loving family and a fine home. The patient develops severe pain in the maxillary anterior area. The pain is sudden, sharp, and excruciating. It is difficult for him to eat, and there is a great deal of swelling in his upper lip. This person has dropped from perhaps a self-esteem level to the physiological, and the dentist must satisfy this physiological need immediately before attempting to suggest any further treatment.

Setting up payment plans for a patient often exposes a conflict of needs. A patient must ensure that basic needs of food, housing, and clothing are met, yet there may be a desire to meet social needs by improving appearance with some form of dental treatment. A conflict arises in the decision-making process when the patient is confronted with conflict on how to satisfy all of these needs with a specified income. The dentist and staff must make an effort to determine the patient's needs, realize the patient's potential conflict, and consider presenting an alternative treatment plan so the patient has some options.

This theory need not only apply to relationships with patients. It also can be applied to interactions between staff members. The dentist, assistant, and hygienist all have the same needs, and each is concerned, like the patient, about security today and in the future. Often conflict arises when a person becomes fixed at one level. There may appear to be no change in motivation, and the person remains unchanged in his or her perspective. This is evidenced often when a person has an interest in making money or increasing a social status without regard for other people's levels of motivation.

Perhaps one of the best lessons you can learn from Maslow's theory is that an individual has a choice in determining his or her behavior. Although basic physiological and environmental needs have a strong influence, an individual makes choices voluntarily.

Rogers' Client-Centered Therapy

Dr. Carl Rogers, another humanistic psychologist, believed that "it is the client who knows what hurts, what directions to go, what problems are crucial, what experiences have been deeply buried." Rogers also suggests that you must accept the patient or other person as a genuine person with his or her own set of values and goals, and that these people must be treated with "unconditional positive regard."

Client-centered therapy assumes that patients know how they feel, what they want, and what their priorities are. Applied to dentistry, this philosophy encourages you to listen to the patient. Further, this concept suggests that you must respect patients as human beings, not just numbers, case studies, or research projects. These people have needs, and their desires should not be repressed. The combined concepts of Maslow and Rogers provide the groundwork for a humanistic, caring attitude, which should be a requisite for all healthcare providers.

BARRIERS TO PATIENT COMMUNICATION

Often we are unable to communicate with patients because barriers have been established. One of the first barriers you may create is prejudging a patient. A dentist may hesitate to present an extensive treatment to a patient because of the way the patient dresses or the type of car he or she drives. As a result, the patient is never told about alternative forms of treatment because his or her economic status has been prejudged. Often a person with a disability is prejudged. When a patient who has an artificial limb, is in a wheelchair, or has a visible birthmark on the face enters the dental office, frequently the first noticeable feature is the disability. If this patient is with a spouse or another person, the patient may go unnoticed while questions are directed to the accompanying person. As a dental healthcare worker, it is important to treat people with disabilities as you would treat any other patient and direct all of your communication to them.

Another barrier occurs when you hear but do not *listen*. A dental professional should never be too busy to listen with understanding to a patient. Don't just listen to the words. Listen to the *meaning* of the words and the feeling behind the meaning. Before presenting your point of view, you must be able to restate what has been said to the patient's satisfaction. This may sound easy, but have you ever tried it? Often people are too eager to present their own point of view and fail to understand the real meaning of what the patient is attempting to say. What is the patient who says, "I think I'll wait to have that treatment done" really saying? If you say, "Oh, that's okay, Mrs. Gates, I understand," you won't find out what the patient is really saying. You may cut off communication. The patient may really be saying, "I'm scared," "I can't afford it," or "I don't like the way you treat me." The best way to arrive at the real meaning is to continue the dialogue until you discern the patient's true feelings. For example:

Assistant:

"Mrs. Romano, do you feel that you want to wait with the treatment?"

Patient:

"Yes."

Assistant:

"Do you want to wait because you are too busy now?" (*The patient may say yes and terminate the conversation at this point, or the conversation may continue.*)

Patient:

"No, it's just that I don't know if I should spend that much money right now."

Assistant:

"Do you feel that the bonding is a greater investment than you planned?"

Patient:

"Well, it's not that I can't afford it. I guess what it boils down to is that I've never had that type of treatment, and I'm not certain what it's going to involve."

Assistant:

"In other words, you don't understand the procedure?"

Patient:

"Yes, I guess that's it. I'm really a bit skeptical about what's going to happen." *(The hidden meaning becomes evident.)*

Notice in this dialogue that the assistant never offered a solution to the problem, such as an alternative payment plan or a later appointment date. Rather, the assistant continued the dialogue with the patient and rephrased what the patient said to arrive at the real meaning.

A third barrier is preoccupation. During daily routines, many demands are placed on your time, and suddenly you begin to think about other activities while trying to communicate with a patient. Everyone has been in that position at one time or another. A patient is trying to explain why an appointment time is not convenient, and suddenly you realize you haven't heard a word that was said because you were concentrating on another problem. This often happens in an office that is understaffed. Each staff member has so much work to accomplish that listening to a patient sometimes just becomes an additional burden. Unfortunately, patients are quick to recognize such preoccupation and may suddenly stop talking or eventually may even stop coming into the dental office. This type of situation re-emphasizes the service model illustrated in Chapter 1. As mentioned earlier, the patient is the most important person in the office and should be given your complete attention.

Unawareness of importance, impatience, and even hearing loss is a barrier to communication. You may not realize how important the problem is to a patient and simply ignore it as a whim. Likewise, you may inadvertently find yourself becoming impatient with a chatty young child or an older person who is slow. Furthermore, it is possible that you may not be hearing everything a person says because of a hearing loss of which you are not aware.

It is not beneficial just to know about these barriers. You must be willing to do something to evaluate yourself. Before each contact with a patient, decide to ignore extraneous activities and be willing to listen and understand a patient's problem before you offer a solution.

Recognizing Nonverbal Cues

Many books have been written in recent years defining and guiding the reader to recognize nonverbal communication cues. Nonverbal cues refer to the gestures and body movements a person makes in a given situation.

Every member of the dental staff should have some awareness of this area. Just as a "picture is worth a thousand words," so a gesture can give meaning to a person's inner feelings. Nonverbal communication provides feedback on the patient's reactions.

The alert assistant is able to pick up these cues and interpret them while communicating with a patient. Care should be taken not to be misled by one gesture. A series of gestures will generally give a more realistic indication of a person's attitude. A dental office presents many opportunities to use and to receive nonverbal cues.

NERVOUSNESS. A patient who enters the reception room and sits down, locking the ankles together and clenching the hands, may be expressing fear by holding back emotions (Figure 3-2). This may occur in the dental chair when

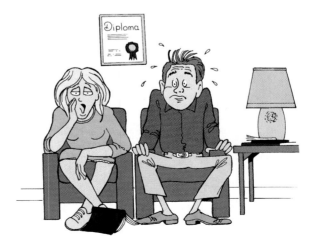

Figure 3-2 The difference between a bored patient and a "scared-to-death" patient.

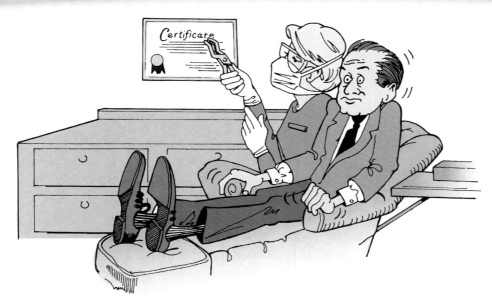

Figure 3-3 A patient displaying nervousness in the dental chair.

a person clenches the armrests and locks the ankles together (Figure 3-3). When the patient relaxes, he or she will automatically unlock the ankles.

DEFENSIVENESS. A patient or staff member may use a gesture of crossed arms and clenched fists as signals to indicate disagreement or defensiveness. This gesture may even indicate the person has withdrawn from the conversation (Figure 3-4). This may occur when a patient is being ignored by the dentist and assistant as they communicate with each other (Figure 3-5).

TOUCHING. An assistant has many opportunities to use this gesture, which indicates caring or loving (Figure 3-6). A hand on a small child's shoulder may show concern, or an arm around the shoulder of a senior citizen may give reassurance (Figure 3-7).

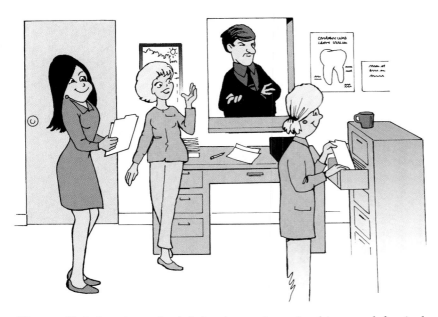

Figure 3-4 A patient who is being ignored crossing his arms defensively.

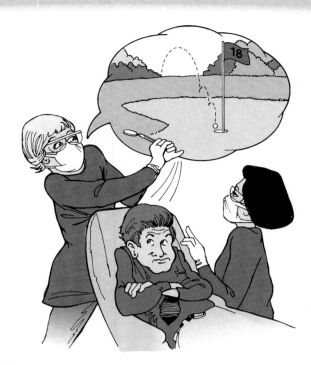

Figure 3-5 A dentist and an assistant ignoring a patient.

OPENNESS. During a consultation with a patient, a dentist should express openness rather than assume an authoritative posture behind a desk. Having the patient seated beside the desk removes this barrier and allows the dentist an opportunity for more open gestures, as in Figure 3-8.

EMBARRASSMENT. A patient's hand covering the mouth may indicate a wish to avoid the embarrassment of exposing an unsightly oral condition. A similar signal may be tightening of the upper lip to conceal the teeth (Figure 3-9).

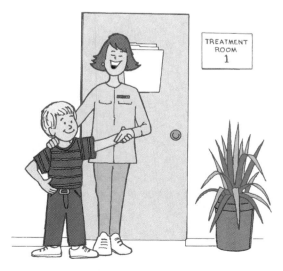

Figure 3-6 An assistant displaying caring by touching a child.

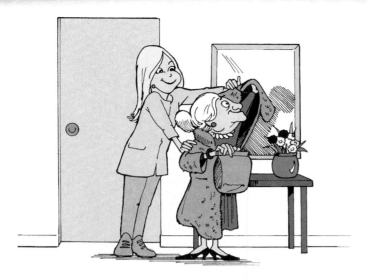

Figure 3-7 Assisting an older adult patient with her coat indicates caring.

Many more nonverbal cues exist. It is vital that you become aware of the meaning of these valuable tools in communication. No one tool or technique will assure successful communications. Communication is based upon a leader who has well-defined goals and a staff working as a team. These efforts, combined with a sincere interest in satisfying a patient's needs, will provide a successful communication system in the dental office.

IMPROVING VERBAL IMAGES

A health professional has an obligation to allay fears and comfort patients. The most obvious way of accomplishing these tasks is to create a good image in the patient's mind. In a dental office you need to eliminate the use of words or phrases that conjure a negative thought. For instance, when you say,

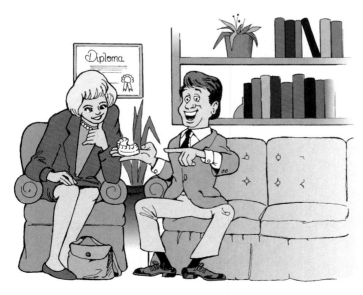

Figure 3-8 A dentist in consultation with a patient.

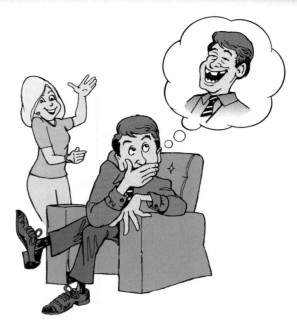

Figure 3-9 A patient covering his mouth to indicate embarrassment.

"This won't hurt," you have told the patient there is a possibility that it will "hurt." If you had said, "We will make you as comfortable as possible," or "You may feel this," you would have let the patient know you were there to help him or her be comfortable. In Chapter 10, terms and phrases frequently used in a dental office are discussed in greater detail. Try replacing discomforting terms or phrases with words that create a more positive environment. Also use language the patient will understand when discussing treatment.

THE PATIENT

As mentioned earlier, the most important person in the dental office is the patient. Although it is obvious that dentistry is a business, it should never be forgotten that it is first a healthcare profession. A great deal is expected of a patient: following directions, keeping appointments, and paying the fee promptly. In return, we must take time to recognize the patient as a person and realize that the patient has some special needs and inherent rights.

Patient Rights

The phrase "patient rights" is much used today. The result has been action on the part of most healthcare professions to design "A Patient's Bill of Rights." It is unfortunate that in some healthcare agencies, the care has become so impersonal that it is necessary for a professional association or agency to formally document the things that are naturally considered patient rights. Some healthcare workers see this action as confirmation of a patient's inherent rights, not the result of a lack of consideration.

As our society becomes increasingly concerned with individual rights, members of the dental healthcare team cannot afford to neglect patient rights. You must be considerate of the patient as a human being rather than as just a subject of a dental procedure. Take time to recognize the patient as a person and consider the list of rights in Box 3-1 as rights of the patient and not as threats to the profession of dentistry.

> A health professional has an obligation to allay fears and comfort patients.

Box 3-1
Patient Rights

Patients in a dental practice are entitled to:
1. Be treated with adequate, appropriate, compassionate care at all times and under all circumstances.
2. Be treated without discrimination based on race, religion, color, national origin, sex, age, handicap, marital status, sexual preference, or source of payment.
3. Be informed of all aspects of treatment.
4. Be informed of appointment and fee schedules.
5. Review their financial and clinical records.
6. Obtain a thorough evaluation of their needs.
7. Be treated as a partner in care and decision making related to treatment planning.
8. Receive current information and be assured of quality treatment.
9. Be able to refuse treatment to the extent provided by law and to be informed of the medical/dental consequences of that refusal.
10. Expect confidentiality of all records pertinent to their dental care.
11. Be informed if the dentist participates in different third-party payment plans.
12. Request and expect appropriate referrals for consultation.
13. Be taught how to maintain good oral health for a lifetime.
14. Receive treatment that will prevent future dental or oral disease.
15. Expect continuity of treatment.
16. Be charged a fair and equitable fee.
17. Have appointment schedules and times maintained.
18. Be treated by a staff of professionals who maintain good health and hygiene.
19. Be respected for requesting a second opinion.
20. Be respected as a human being who has feelings and needs.

Managing the Patient's Special Needs

Many patients with special needs enter a dental practice. Your attention was drawn to some of these earlier, during the discussion of barriers to communication. A patient who is physically or psychologically challenged, an older adult, a child, a single parent, or a homeless person may visit the office for various types of treatment.

The Americans With Disabilities Act of 1990, commonly known as the ADA, sets specific guidelines for businesses. Several issues regarding structural design of a building are discussed in Chapter 6. Other factors in this law require the dentist not to discriminate against a person who requires dental care. For most disabled persons, if they can get into a treatment room, they can receive treatment. Perhaps the biggest problem a dentist faces in treating a challenged patient is when the patient can't mentally or physically cooperate. For example, a dentist faces several compromises when a patient has cerebral palsy and the mouth is uncontrollably moving, or is a quadriplegic whose high neck injuries would make moving from a wheelchair to a dental chair dangerous. Even though there are times when some dental treatment can be done in a wheelchair, the law allows a dentist to make referrals for the patient's safety.

It may be necessary for you to make a special effort in communication with some patients. For instance, if the disabilities include vision or hearing impairments or the patient uses a wheelchair or walker, you may find it necessary to take special care when communicating. For patients who have hearing difficulty, you may need to stand in front of them when talking to ensure that they are able to read your lips. For patients with poor vision, you may need to read questions or have a guardian review materials that require a response, such as a health questionnaire. For people using wheelchairs, walkers, or crutches, it may be necessary to take extra time when asking them to move about, or you may even need to go to them directly with forms that need to be signed.

Recognizing Abuse

In our society, abuse is evident in many forms, most commonly child and adult abuse. Each year more than 2.7 million children are abused or neglected by caregivers, relatives, or strangers. More than 1000 children die annually as a result of this abuse. Child abuse may be classified as physical, sexual, emotional, or overall neglect. Adults, those who are elderly and dependent on others for care, as well as people from a volatile relationship, may also be victims of abuse.

Dentists are faced with abuse in two ways. The forensic dentist may be presented with a postmortem case of a victim who has bite marks or tooth marks. In addition, a dentist may treat victims of abuse in the office.

Abused children or adults may show overall signs of neglect, abnormal fears or neuroses, or evidence of extraoral or intraoral anomalies such as bite marks, scars, lacerations, fractured teeth, burns, and bruises of varying colors on exposed areas of the body.

The dentist has an obligation to examine the patient thoroughly, ask reasonable questions about existing conditions, and document the injuries on the dental record. Reports of suspected abuse should be made to the state or county social services office. In most states, failure to report suspected abuse is a misdemeanor.

RECEPTION ROOM TECHNIQUES

Since the duties of the administrative assistant include many facets of communication, continual awareness of communication barriers is necessary.

The impression that the administrative assistant makes upon patients is usually lasting and, of course, should be favorable. Remember that you represent the dentist and the practice; a patient who feels comfortable with you will probably feel comfortable with the dentist.

The Role of the Receptionist

As a receptionist, you will be the first person to greet patients as they enter the office. You should appear neat and professional. In many business offices today, the administrative assistant wears professional businesslike clothing rather than a uniform. You should be certain that your clothing or uniform is clean, your shoes are well-polished, and your hair neatly styled. The positive image you create as a receptionist indicates a clean and well-organized office (Box 3-2). The image portrayed in this role must remain with the patient, so this is no place to try out new clothing styles, experiment with garish jewelry, or wear facial and oral piercings.

As the patient enters the office, you should be seated, acknowledge the patient immediately with a pleasant smile and cheerful "hello," and call him or her by name. Everyone likes the feeling of being known and recognized.

> **Box 3-2**
> **Tips for Professional Etiquette in the Dental Office**
>
> - Use correct grammar; pronounce words correctly; expand your vocabulary.
> - Explain technical terms in understandable language without being demeaning.
> - Make patients feel important; discuss issues of interest to them.
> - Perform proper introductions of the patient and staff members.
> - Introduce yourself to a new patient; shake hands heartily to extend a warm welcome.
> - If a patient is engaged in a conversation with another person, avoid standing within hearing range. If you wish to talk to one of them, leave the area and return later.
> - Don't eat or drink in front of patients.
> - Say "thank-you" when a patient is helpful, has cooperated during treatment, or has complimented you.
> - Send thank-you notes for referrals or other thoughtful acts.
> - Respect the patient's privacy.
> - If the telephone rings while you are talking to a patient, excuse yourself to answer it. If a lengthy conversation is expected, ask the caller if you can return the call; then complete the business with the patient.

Even though you may be busy with a telephone call, at least look up and smile. This will inform the patients that you are aware of their presence.

Reception Room Appeal

A bright, cheerful, and pleasantly decorated office will usually make a favorable impression on the patient. If the room appears to have a warm and friendly atmosphere, the patient will relax. (Design of the reception room for the patient's comfort is discussed in Chapter 6.) Offering a cup of coffee or tea or other beverage may put the patient at ease.

Reading material in the reception room should be current and geared toward a wide variety of interests. A good selection might include gourmet cooking, sports, travel, community and world news, and health magazines. Recipe cards can be placed in an attractive holder (Figure 3-10) to aid patients in copying information from magazines and assorted health-related cookbooks (Figure 3-11). This will prevent them from tearing pages from books and magazines. Avoid dirty carpet, frayed furniture, and unsightly plants. Also, children's books, as well as quiet games and toys, should be available. An area designated as a children's play area is helpful. If background music is played in the office, be sure to select music that has a soothing effect rather than loud rock or heavy concert music.

Waiting Patients

One of the responsibilities of the receptionist is to keep patients informed of delays or indicate what the waiting time will be. Unexpected delays or emergencies should be explained honestly. Be careful not to make excuses or to say that the dentist is running late (Figure 3-12). Be honest about the length of time the patient will have to wait to be seen.

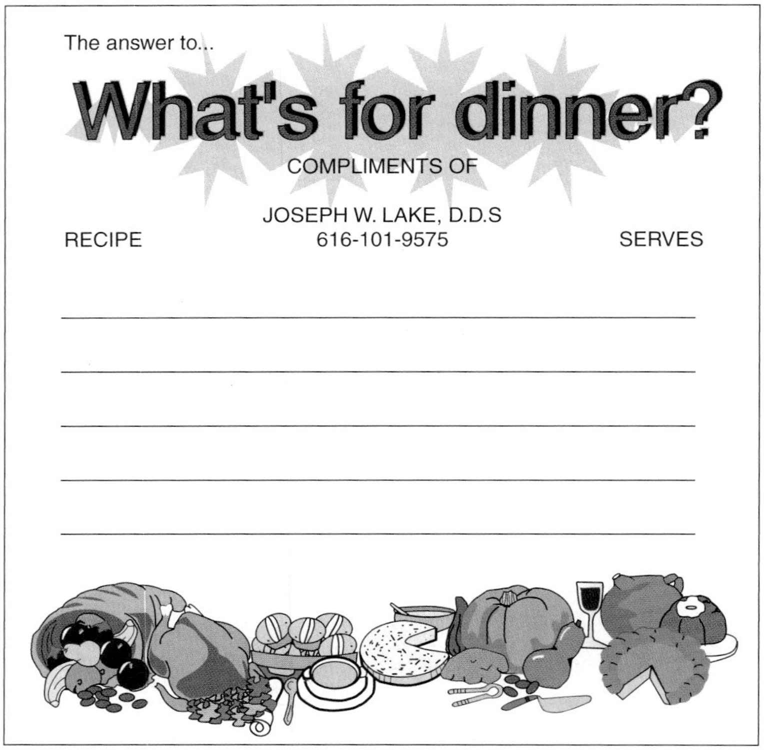

The answer to...
What's for dinner?
COMPLIMENTS OF
JOSEPH W. LAKE, D.D.S
616-101-9575
RECIPE
SERVES

Figure 3-10 A recipe card for copying information from magazines.

American Heart Association
Low-Fat, Low-Cholesterol cookbook
Over 1 million copies sold
third edition

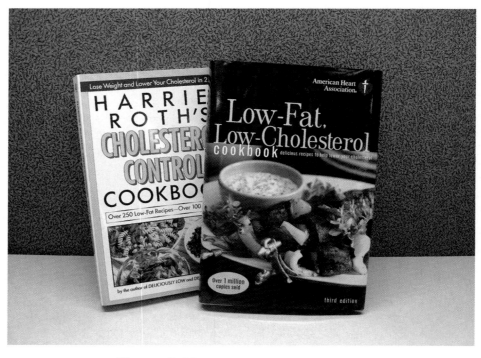

Figure 3-11 Cookbooks related to health.

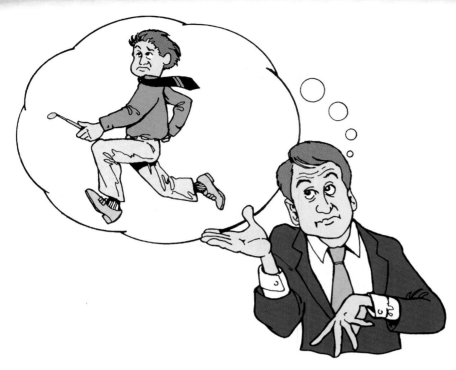

Figure 3-12 "The dentist is running late."

OFFICE POLICY

The office policy pamphlet is the key to establishing an understanding between the patient and the office staff. The office policy should be a written statement of the dentist's philosophy and policies, defining the responsibilities of both the patient and the dental office staff. It is given to a new patient at the first visit and serves not only as an informational device but also as a good public relations tool.

Often a new practitioner will neglect to establish an office policy only to be confronted with misunderstandings with patients at a later date. The office policy should be implemented when the office is first opened and revised as the practice grows and changes. However, such a policy can be integrated into an established practice with minimal effort.

Contents of an Office Policy

Each practice will have its own specific needs, but every policy should include the following elements:

1. *Philosophy.* This is a statement of the dentist's attitude toward the practice of dentistry and, more specifically, the moral and ethical obligation to the patient. It is in this section that the dentist can make a statement about how the practice is unique and what gives it something special that will attract and retain patients.
2. *Office hours.* Although these may occasionally vary, specific hours should be listed for the patient's benefit. It is advisable to inform patients of times available for emergency appointments. This will avoid a congested schedule and unnecessary calls at inconvenient times.
3. *Appointment control.* A statement should be included designating the person who controls appointment making. It should also be noted that

patients are seen by appointment only to discourage "drop ins." A broken appointment policy should be included in the office policy and should be adhered to consistently.

4. *Payment policy.* The dentist should outline acceptable specific payment plans. These plans should be described in detail, and the person responsible for implementing them should be identified. Finally, a statement should be made regarding parental responsibility for the treatment of minors.

5. *Hygiene.* The value of hygiene, self-care, and preventive dentistry through the periodic recall system should be emphasized. The system utilized in the office should be explained thoroughly to each patient.

6. *Attitude toward children.* The roles of the dentist, staff, and parent in the treatment of children must be explained. The preparation of a child before treatment and management of the parent and child during treatment should be well defined to avoid future conflicts.

7. *Auxiliary utilization.* The dentist has the responsibility to define the relationship of each staff member to patients, thus explaining the value of team dentistry for quality care and maximum efficiency. The dentist should identify the credentials and responsibilities of each staff member.

8. *Infection-control policies.* Such policies can be explained to assure patients that the latest barrier techniques and most current preventive concepts are being used for their protection.

9. *Quality assurance.* This is an explanation of efforts taken to ensure that procedures and techniques used in the office are routinely evaluated to maintain good quality.

10. *Staff continuing education.* This explains the efforts the dentist makes to continuously update himself or herself and the staff in life support, infection control, and other technological advances.

11. *Office data.* The dentist's name, address, phone number, fax, and e-mail address should appear on the cover or be easy to find within the policy for the patient's convenience.

Designing an Office Policy Statement

The administrative assistant can be invaluable to the dentist in designing the office policy statement. Once the basic policy has been established, the assistant makes the final draft and aids in designing several styles for final selection. The final style will be the dentist's choice but should be attractive, well-organized, brief, and sized to be easily handled by patients (Figure 3-13).

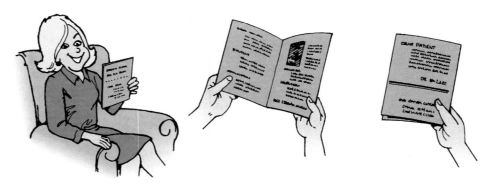

Figure 3-13 A patient reading the office policy.

Welcome to our office...

Joseph W. Lake, DDS
Ashley M. Lake, DDS

611 Main Street, SE
Grand Rapids, MI 49502
Phone: 616-101-9575
Fax: 616-101-9999
e-mail: office@dapc.com

INITIAL EXAMINATION...

Each patient that we have the privilege to serve is entitled to and will receive a thorough examination. This examination includes necessary x-rays, diagnostic models, and an oral examination as required to make an accurate analysis of your mouth. An estimate of the fee involved will be given.

OFFICE HOURS...

Office hours are from 9 to 12 and 1 to 5 on Monday and Wednesday and 9 to 12 and 1 to 7 on Tuesday and Thursday. There are no office hours on Friday or Saturday though on those days, a recorder will answer your call, take messages, and refer you to emergency numbers.

APPOINTMENTS...

The administrative assistant has complete charge of appointments in the office. We will reserve a time that is convenient for you. We will make every effort to keep our schedule on time.

When a change of appointment is necessary, 24 hours advance notice is required.

EMERGENCY TIME...

Time is specifically reserved for emergency care at 10:15 A.M. and 4:45 P.M. We will treat your immediate problem and re-schedule you for further necessary treatment.

MINORS...

Parental approval of the dental treatment is necessary. Parents are requested to wait in the reception room except for consultation.

Small children are more receptive to dental care in the morning. We will request cooperation in having them excused from school.

Figure 3-14 An office policy.

Many offices prefer to use a professional printer to achieve a professional-looking pamphlet. In Figure 3-14, the policy has been printed on both sides of heavy 8½-by-11-inch bond paper folded in half. A simpler, less expensive statement printed on office letterhead is shown in Figure 3-15. Remember, that the office policy has two primary purposes: it is a practice builder, and it informs the patient about office procedures and the dentist's philosophy. When it achieves both purposes, the office policy becomes a valuable public-relations device.

MARKETING

When advertising was first legalized in 1977 by action of the Supreme Court, many dentists perceived this action to be demeaning to the profession. Today, dentists across the country have come to realize that in a competitive, consumer-oriented society, they must become involved in marketing to increase their practice loads. No matter how you attempt to change it, marketing is advertising, and all dentists practice some form of advertising.

PAYMENT POLICIES...

When extensive treatment is necessary, an estimate of the fee will be presented before services are rendered. The administrative assistant will explain our payment policies and make financial arrangements that are mutually satisfactory.

The fee for treatment requiring a single office visit is payable at the conclusion of the appointment. Other treatment is billed monthly and payable upon receipt of the statement.

Please feel free to make inquiries about our fees, or your dental treatment. You will find the staff most capable, sympathetic, and courteous in providing this information.

Our fees are related directly to the cost of office operation and to strict attention to office efficiency.

INFECTION CONTROL POLICY...

In this office we use a variety of barrier techniques for your individual protection. These techniques include gloves, masks, protective eye shields and coverings, protective clothing, and when necessary specialized intra-oral devices. Our staff regularly attends meetings on safety standards and we implement all of the latest OSHA standards and recommendations of the American Dental Association.

DENTAL STAFF...

The administrative and clinical assistants in this office are Certified or Registered Dental Assistants and they are highly skilled in the areas of office management and clinical assisting. The administrative assistant is in charge of all payment arrangements, insurance forms, billing, and appointment scheduling. The clinical assistants are the doctor's operative assistants and with the utilization of these skilled assistants is able to increase efficiency in treatment, thus enabling you to receive complete and thorough dentistry.

While all assistants may assume responsibility for patient education, the Registered Dental Hygienist is in charge of dietary analysis and the oral prophylaxis. After the defective areas are charted, the doctor will do a complete oral examination. The extensive education and experience of our hygienist establishes this professional as an authority in the field of oral hygiene.

PERIODIC EXAMINATION...

We share the desire of all of our patients to minimize the need for extensive dental treatment. This can only be done by regular examinations which detect dental disease before it becomes extensive.

At the conclusion of your treatment, you will be placed on our Preventive Recall Program, which requests you to return at a specified time for a re-examination. Your current dental treatment will be inspected, your home care program reviewed, and your teeth cleaned and polished.

The goal of this program is to:
• Maintain your attractive appearance
• Provide good dental comfort and health
• Prevent unnecessary loss of teeth

To keep abreast of new techniques, our staff enrolls in four to eight days of continuing education each year. During the time that the doctor and the staff attend meetings, a recorder will direct you to a colleague who will take emergency calls for this office.

Our office is always receptive to suggestions that might be useful to improve our services to you.

Figure 3-14, cont'd

Marketing Skills

Marketing should be a natural habit that is practiced at all times. Team members must work together to educate patients about the practice and procedures, provide quality treatment in a comfortable, safe environment, offer outstanding customer service, and make patients want to tell their family and friends about their great dentist and staff. To market a dental practice effectively, the staff needs a specific set of skills that will aid them in promoting the practice.

THE OFFICE TRADEMARK. The dentist needs to verbalize an identity. What makes the practice different? Large corporations such as 3M, Sony, Starbucks, Microsoft, and Amazon.com all have an identity. For instance, a dentist might sum up the office identity by using words such as *thorough, caring,* or *leading edge.* The word *thorough* denotes that each patient will be given quality time. *Caring* suggests old-fashioned commitment to the patient, regardless of business pressure. The phrase *leading edge* indicates that the dentist and staff are progressive and keep abreast of new materials and techniques. These messages must be driven home at every opportunity.

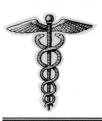

Dental Associates, PC

Joseph W. Lake, DDS – Ashley M. Lake, DDS

Dear Patient:

On behalf of the staff and myself, I welcome you to our office. You are important to us. We pride ourselves in making dentistry a pleasant experience for our patients. You can always expect to be treated as a guest when visiting us.

It is our desire to provide the most thorough and efficient treatment as possible. Complete oral health care comprises not only the elimination of existing dental disease but also the prevention of future disease. Except in emergency cases, new adult patients receive a thorough dental examination consisting of the following:

1. Record of medical/dental history
2. Visual mouth examination
3. Complete x-ray examination
4. Prophylaxis (preventive cleaning)
5. Any other diagnostic aids necessary to render a thorough diagnosis
6. Oral hygiene instructions

The requirements for children vary according to age and dental needs.

After the examination is completed, an appointment will be made to discuss the conditions present and the most thorough treatment plans for you. Also at this visit, appointments will be scheduled, estimated fees given, payment plans presented, and all financial arrangements completed. The practice depends upon reimbursement from patients for the costs incurred in their care and financial responsibility on the part of the patient must be determined before treatment. If you require a consultant at this time, we require that he or she accompany you for this important appointment. The responsible adult must be present at a consultation involving children.

We sincerely believe that one of the most important services that we have to offer is a plan for preventive dentistry. All patients are notified at periodic intervals for preventive examinations and the oral prophylaxis.

Except for emergency cases, you may expect us to be on time. Likewise, we will expect the same courtesy. Should it be necessary for you to reschedule an appointment, we require 24 hours notice, except in case of an emergency. This allows us to use your reserved time for another patient.

It is our hope that your dental visits will be prompt and pleasant so that in the future you will want to help increase our fine family of patients through your recommendations.

To continue improving our service, we invite your comments and suggestions at all times.

Sincerely,

Joseph W. Lake, DDS

611 Main Street, SE – Grand Rapids, MI 49502   Phone: 616.101.9575 Fax: 616.101.9999
E-mail: office@dapc.com or Visit us at: www.Lakedental.com

Figure 3-15 Policy statement printed on office letterhead.

For instance, when a patient contacts the office for the first appointment, the administrative assistant can take the opportunity to promote the thoroughness of the practice. Instead of first asking what time of day is most convenient, you can start the conversation with "Mrs. Timmon, let me be the first to welcome you to Dr. Lake's practice. She is a very caring and thorough dentist who takes time to be current with all of the leading technology and materials. I promise you that all members of our team will go out of our way to provide you with dental care and to make your visits pleasant."

> The single most important characteristic in a staff member is an enthusiastic attitude.

ENTHUSIASTIC ATTITUDE. The single most important characteristic in a staff member is an enthusiastic attitude. The employee with an enthusiastic attitude shows up for work every day on time, is willing to help others, maintains a cheery disposition all day, and ensures that patients come first. This enthusiastic attitude means the "no whining" rule is always in place, because whining is contagious. The enthusiastic attitude means the patient's problems come first and personal problems are kept to yourself or shared with a friend in private.

SEIZING OPPORTUNITIES. There are many ways to get the word out about a practice. For instance, when a new patient makes an appointment, you could say, "Mrs. Timmons, we are looking forward to seeing you at 3 PM on Wednesday. By the way, would you like to make an appointment for any other members of the family at this time?"

PRACTICE AMBASSADORS. Each member of the staff is expected to be an ambassador to the practice. Each staff member should be provided with his or her own business cards, and they should promote the practice to family and friends. It may even be possible to suggest that the office be used after hours for community group meetings if office space is adequate. When a new staff member joins a practice, the dentist should prepare an announcement that can be sent to the new team member's circle of family, friends, or other professional associates.

Internal Marketing

Marketing can be divided into two forms, internal and external. Internal marketing is what one does within the office to retain patients. Internal marketing is that "first impression." It is how the patient perceives that the dental staff is caring and enjoy their work; it is the patient's feeling that the dentist is willing to listen to his or her individual dental problem. Internal marketing is how you retain patients once you have attracted them to the practice.

As mentioned in Chapter 2, one of the most important assets a dentist has in an office is the dental staff. When the staff members are committed to the practice, highly motivated, and enthusiastic, they become the impetus to a successful internal marketing program. Look at Figure 3-16, and note that most of the ideas for internal marketing for patient retention are staff-oriented. Staff members should be given specialized duties in which they perform well as part of an internal marketing program. For instance, a staff-person who writes well could manage written communication, whereas another who has a good understanding of insurance could explain insurance benefits to patients.

Patients who know that the dentist and staff care about them and don't consider them as merely case numbers or blank checks will return to the practice and, more important, will refer friends and colleagues.

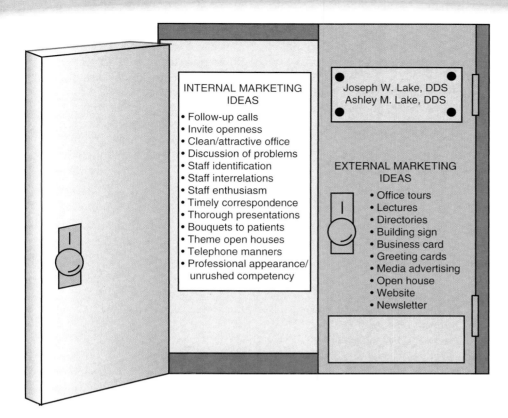

Figure 3-16 Internal and external marketing ideas.

External Marketing

External marketing is met with greater skepticism by the profession. The key to successful external marketing is to determine prospective patients and the best method to attract them. The dentist must identify his or her objectives, define the strengths of the practice, determine the budget, and review all the sources for external advertising. Some forms of such marketing can be as simple as offering lectures to local organizations or as complex as media advertising. A review of Figure 3-16 illustrates other potential sources of external marketing. When using any source of advertising, the dentist must realize that the results will not be immediate and that a consistent and repetitive message must be directed to prospective patients in order to obtain results.

The most important factor to remember in any form of marketing is that you must be able to produce what you claim. No matter where or how much the dentist advertises, if quality dental care is not delivered in a caring, sensitive manner, the patient will not return. A good motto for a dentist to remember is "You may attract them, but you won't keep them."

Key Terms

Client-centered therapy – A form of therapy that when applied to dentistry encourages listening to patients to learn about their feelings, desires, and priorities.

Hierarchy of needs – Five basic levels of needs described by Abraham Maslow, which are used to aid in understanding how a person's needs motivate behavior. They are physiological, safety or security, social or love, esteem, and self-actualization.

Marketing - Marketing is a form of advertising, and in dentistry it is what one does within the office to retain patients.

Nonverbal cues - Gestures and body movements a person makes in a given situation to denote a feeling.

Office policy - A form of written communication that identifies the dentist's philosophy and policies and defines the responsibilities of the patient and dental staff.

Patients' rights - Inherent rights of a patient to be informed of services being performed, the cost, and the consequences of such treatment.

LEARNING ACTIVITIES

1. Identify and give examples of barriers in communication.
2. Describe the duties of a receptionist in communicating with patients and putting them at ease.
3. Explain Maslow's Hierarchy of Needs and Carl Rogers' client-centered therapy as they relate to dentistry.
4. What is marketing?
5. Explain two basic types of marketing procedures that could be used in a dental practice.
6. What ideas could be implemented in a practice to increase marketing for existing patients? What could be done to attract new patients?
7. List five rights of the patient that should be considered during a treatment procedure.
8. If a clinical facility is available, observe nonverbal behavior. Silently stand out of sight of a patient, dentist/dental student, and a dental auxiliary. Observe as many forms of nonverbal communication as possible. Did the participants pick up these clues? If so, what was the reaction?
9. During your daily activities, become aware of nonverbal cues given to you. What types of facial expressions, hand movements, and torso movements do you notice? Do they affect your behavior?
10. List the preconceptions that a patient might have about a dental office and the staff.
11. List attitudes that a dental assistant, a dental hygienist, and a dentist might have about a patient. Are there similarities or differences in the perceptions of each of these people?

Bibliography

Bernstein DA, Nash PW: *Essentials of psychology*, ed 2, Boston, 2002, Houghton Mifflin.
Frazier GL: *Connecting with customers*, ed 2, Upper Saddle River, NJ, 2004, Prentice Hall.
Locker KO, Kyo Kaczmarek S: *Business communication: building critical skills*, ed 2, New York, 2003, Irwin/McGraw-Hill.
Mosley DC et al: *Supervisory management*, ed 4, Cincinnati, 1998, South-Western.
Rathfus SA: *Psychology in the new millennium*, ed 7, Orlando, 1999, Harcourt Brace.
Schwab D: What your staff needs to know about marketing your practice, *Dental Economics*, January 1999, pp. 51–53.

Chapter 4

Legal and Ethical Issues in the Dental Business Office

Chapter Outline

Learning Outcomes

Mastery of the content in this chapter will enable the reader to:
- Define glossary terms
- Explain the impact of ethics and law on the dental business office

- Differentiate between the various types of law that affect the practice of dentistry
- Explain various types of consent
- Describe situations in the dental business office that would lead to potential litigation
- Describe the code of ethics of professional dental organizations
- Identify 12 steps in making ethical decisions

Each day dental professionals are faced with issues involving the legal requirements and standards of care, voluntary and involuntary, in the delivery of dental treatment. The **Dental Practice Act** of each state defines the requirements necessary to practice dentistry and the scope of dental practice for that particular state. Standards for dental care may arise from both **common law** (judicial decisions) and statutory law (enacted by a legislative body), such as the state Dental Practice Act. The dental professional is governed also by voluntary standards, such as the principles of ethics, developed and implemented by the dental profession itself. Both legal and voluntary requirements and standards are implemented for the protection of society and, ultimately, the patient. This process of regulation is illustrated in Figure 4-1.

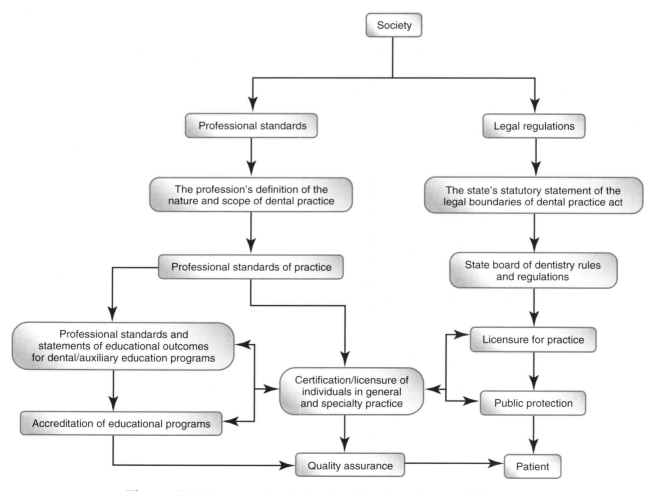

Figure 4-1 Diagram of professional and legal regulations of dentistry.

An administrative assistant practicing in a dental office today needs to have an understanding of the effect of law on the dental practice and an awareness of its importance on his or her performance of daily duties. Further, each member of a professional organization should be familiar with the code of ethics for its professional group.

Membership in a professional organization is voluntary, and thus the standards of these organizations are considered voluntary. However, these standards are used as guidelines in peer review. Professional organizations continually reassess the functions of their standards and the qualifications of their members. The standards of professional health organizations reflect the assessment of the need for dental care and the public's expectations for dentistry and its auxiliaries. Examples of voluntary standards are illustrated in the profession's code of ethics, professional standards for accreditation of educational programs, standards for credentialing, and standards of various service organizations. Legal standards for dental care are determined through common law and result in standards such as the Informed Consent Doctrine, which is discussed later in this chapter. Legislative action through the Dental Practice Act establishes the legal requirements and scope of the practice within the state. This action establishes education, credentialing, and licensure requirements for the dentist and any dental auxiliaries recognized in the state Dental Practice Act.

Copies of the principles of ethics for any of the dental professional organizations may be obtained from their national offices or official websites. To obtain a copy of the state Dental Practice Act, contact the Board of Dentistry in your state. You may also purchase a *State Fact Booklet* from the Dental Assisting National Board (DANB) website, available at www.DANB.org.

DEFINITION OF LAW

Law consists of enforceable rules governing relationships among individuals and between individuals and their society. A broad definition of the law implies that there must be established rules, such as constitutions, statutes, administrative agency rules, and judicial decisions. Rules of law must be enforceable and establish limits of conduct for governments and individuals in society.

In many states, the Board of Dentistry is an administrative agency at the state level. The executive officers of an administrative agency perform specific functions, including enforcing laws within their agency. The state boards have the power to make rules and regulations that conform to enacted laws, such as the Dental Practice Act. Rules and regulations adopted by the board are components of the body of law, referred to as administrative laws. State statutes must conform to the state's constitution and the federal constitution. The Dental Practice Act is an example of state statutory law.

Classifications of Law

Law can be divided into two classifications: civil and criminal. **Civil law** relates to duties between persons or between citizens and their government. **Criminal law** deals with wrongs committed against the public as a whole.

In a civil case, one party tries to correct an interference with his or her interest by another party. The other party may have failed to comply with a duty or otherwise breached an acceptable standard of conduct. The other party may be required to pay for the damages caused by failure to comply with that duty. In criminal law, the interests of society are at stake and the government may seek to impose a penalty, such as a fine or imprisonment, on the guilty person.

CRIMES AND TORTS

A **crime** is a wrongdoing against the public at large, and is prosecuted by a public official. In most cases when a crime is committed, there is intent to do wrong. However, a person or entity that breaks certain laws may be guilty of a crime whether there was intent or not. Criminal liability typically involves both the performance of a prohibited act and a specified state of mind or intent on the part of the actor. In some cases, the omission of an act can be a crime if the person or entity has a legal duty to perform the act, such as failure to file a federal income tax return.

A crime can be classified as a misdemeanor or a felony. A **misdemeanor** is less serious than a felony and is punishable by a fine or imprisonment up to one year. A **felony** is a more serious crime and generally is punishable by imprisonment for longer period of time.

A **tort** is a civil wrongdoing. It is an interference with a recognized interest or a breach of a legal duty owed by a defendant to a plaintiff. The plaintiff in most instances must show that the defendant's action or omission was a cause of loss or harm to the plaintiff. A tort is generally resolved through a civil trial with a monetary settlement for damages. Included in torts are the areas of negligence, assault and battery, infliction of mental distress, defamation, and fraud.

Torts may be intentional or unintentional acts of wrongdoing. If intentional, this means that the person committing the tort intended to commit the wrongful act. Intentional torts for which a dental assistant could be held liable include assault and battery, defamation of character, invasion of privacy, immoral conduct, and fraud.

Unintentional torts do not require a particular mental state. Failure to exercise a **standard of care,** such as performing a treatment that a reasonably prudent professional would perform in similar circumstances, is an example of an unintentional tort. Thus, even if a dental professional neither wishes to bring about the consequences of the act nor believes that they will occur, negligence may be alleged whereby someone suffers injury because another failed to live up to a particular standard of care. Questions relating to the failure to exercise a standard of care need to be answered. The following four elements make up the unintentional tort of negligence:

1. Was there a duty to follow a standard of care?
2. Was this duty breached?
3. Did the plaintiff suffer injury?
4. Was the injury a direct result of that breach of duty?

Strict liability is an unintentional tort. It relates to a person being liable for actions regardless of the care exercised and for damages or injuries caused by the act.

Negligence is the performance of an act that a reasonably careful person under similar circumstances would not do, or the failure to perform an act that a reasonably careful person would do under similar circumstances. Professionals usually consider malpractice a form of negligence, but it can mean, in a broader sense, any wrongdoing by a professional. **Malpractice** can refer to any professional misconduct, evil practice, or illegal or immoral conduct, not just negligence. Malpractice can be either unintentional or intentional. Box 4-1 contains a list of negligent acts that might occur in a dental office.

Litigation

Litigation is the process of a lawsuit. A **lawsuit** is a legal action in a court. The person or party that institutes the suit in court is the **plaintiff.** The person being accused of the wrongdoing is the **defendant.**

> Failure to exercise a **standard of care**, performing treatment that a reasonably prudent professional would perform in similar circumstances, is an example of an unintentional tort.

> Professionals usually consider malpractice as a form of negligence, but it can mean, in a broader sense, any wrongdoing by a professional.

Box 4-1
Common Negligent Acts in a Dental Office

Abandonment
Burns
Mistaken identity
Foreign objects left in patients after surgical procedures
Use of defective equipment
Failure to observe patient reactions and take appropriate action
Medication errors
Drug administration errors
Failure to exercise good judgment
Failure to communicate
Loss of or damage to patient's personal property
Disease transmission

During malpractice litigation, the patient may be the plaintiff. The dentist or person who is being sued is the defendant. It is likely that other individuals in the dental office, such as a dentist associate, dental assistant, or hygienist might be named as a defendant, fact witness, or an expert witness in the legal proceedings. A **fact witness,** when placed under oath, must provide only firsthand knowledge, not hearsay. In such testimony, the fact witness describes what he or she saw or did during a specific act. For instance, if the fact witness is being questioned about the administration of a local anesthetic for a patient, the witness may be asked if he or she was told what type of anesthetic to prepare, if he or she prepared the anesthetic and passed it to the dentist, how much anesthetic was administered to the patient, and what the patient's reaction was following the anesthetic administration. If the fact witness only received the directions and prepared the anesthetic for the setup but did not participate in its administration, only the initial questions can be answered. To describe any further action not observed would be inappropriate and may be considered speculation or hearsay.

An **expert witness** is called to testify and explain to the judge and jury what happened based on the patient's record and to offer an opinion as to whether or not the dental care, as administered, met acceptable standards. Standards may vary by state. Often a dentist may be called as an expert witness to testify in malpractice litigation because of his or her educational background and strong clinical expertise. A strong knowledge of dental law and dental standards, as well as an understanding of malpractice liability, is beneficial in such cases.

DENTAL PRACTICE ACT

The legal requirements necessary to practice dentistry as well as the scope of what can be practiced are developed through legislative action within the state and are identified in the state Dental Practice Act. This act defines the minimum educational standards, requirements for credentialing, and the criteria for license revocation or suspension for a dentist, hygienist, and in several states the dental assistant. Other legal requirements are enacted by the government in the form of rules and regulations and, like the Dental Practice Act, also regulate the practice of dentistry. An example of a government agency that makes requirements that affect the practice of dentistry is the state Department of Labor.

A state Dental Practice Act is not frequently changed. However, as changes take place in technology and standards of dental care are modified, it may be necessary to apply new rules and regulations to the state Dental Practice Act. An administrative assistant should regularly obtain a copy of any changes in the Dental Practice Act or new rules and regulations and retain it on file.

Many state Dental Practice Acts define conditions under which a dental assistant or hygienist may perform specific duties. Each state provides a list of definitions within the law, and the descriptive language may vary significantly from state to state. Examples of such terminology include patient of record, assignment, and supervision. **Patient of record** refers to a patient who has been examined and diagnosed by a licensed dentist and whose treatment has been planned by that dentist. **Assignment** commonly refers to the dentist assigning a specific procedure to a dental assistant or hygienist that is to be performed on a designated patient of record. For certain procedures, the dentist does not need to be physically present in the office or in the treatment room at the time the procedure is being performed. **Supervision** refers to the conditions under which a patient of record may be treated by an assistant or hygienist and the protocol to be followed after the treatment is rendered. One type of supervision is referred to as *direct supervision* and generally means that the dentist has designated a patient of record upon whom services are to be performed and has described the procedure to be performed. The dentist examines the patient before prescribing the procedures to be performed and again upon completion of the procedure. Under the definition of direct supervision, the dentist generally must be physically present in the office at the time the procedures are being performed. It is important to remember that the legal standards within a dental law are for the protection of the general public, and interpretations of requirements for the protection of the general public may differ in each state.

PROFESSIONAL STANDARDS

Over the last half-century, the dental assisting profession has taken several steps to ensure the competence of its practitioners in such areas as the credentialing process. *Credentialing* is a generic term that refers to the ways in which professionals can measure and maintain their competence.

The processes used in credentialing include accreditation, certification, and licensure. Accreditation generally is the process by which an entity or educational program is evaluated and recognized by an outside agency for having attained a predetermined set of standards. These standards are identified by the professional and educational organization, including peer groups. In dentistry, the Commission on Dental Accreditation of the American Dental Association is responsible for accrediting educational programs in dentistry, dental assisting, dental hygiene, and dental laboratory technology. When a program is accredited by the American Dental Association (ADA), the program makes public its accreditation status. Such accreditation validates that a specific educational program has met a set of standards to address the needs of the profession and the public. In many instances, a criterion for obtaining a credential such as certification or licensure is contingent on successful completion of an ADA-accredited educational program.

National certification in dental assisting is a voluntary procedure and may be achieved through the DANB. This organization provides credentialing for the clinical dental assistant, the orthodontic assistant, and the administrative assistant as described in Chapter 2. The process of credentialing requires prerequisites involving education and clinical experiences and measures whether the person has met certain criteria established by the non-governmental organization for the dental assisting profession.

Licensure is the credential granted to a candidate by the state after the candidate has met the state's designated requirements to practice in the profession. Generally this license is granted after the person has met certain educational requirements and has completed some form of state testing. Licensure is intended to protect the consumer and is designed for the clinical dental assistant who has direct patient care responsibilities.

CODE OF ETHICS

Ethics is a branch of philosophy and is a systematic, intellectual approach to the standards of behavior. The purpose of a professional code of ethics is to help members of the profession achieve high levels of behavior through moral consciousness, decision making, and practice by members of the profession. Ethics in daily professional practice challenges a practitioner to differentiate between right and wrong. Morals are considered voluntary personal commitments to a set of values. Values are the standards used for decision making that endure over a significant period of time. The expected behaviors of the dental professional are based on a set of standards derived from aspired acceptable behaviors. Every health professional must realize that there is right and wrong and that there is no right way to do a wrong thing.

ADA Principles of Ethics

Each organized group within the profession of dentistry, including the ADA, ADAA (American Dental Assistants Association), and ADHA (American Dental Hygienists' Association), has a code of ethics for its members. This code of ethics is based on moral principles that reflect concern for care of the patient.

> There is no right way to do a wrong thing.

Dentistry as a profession enjoys a certain right of independence, in decision making and self-governance, as a result of the training and education of its members. However this right carries with it an obligation to maintain quality standards and be responsible to one's patients and peers. This right does not allow a member of the profession to disregard professional standards or laws governing the practice of dentistry. The profession's primary goal is to provide quality care to patients in a competent and timely manner. To maintain high standards of care, the dental professional can continue to improve the quality of care through education, training, research, and maintenance of a stringent code of ethics and professional conduct. Figure 4-2 is the official publication of the ADA, which includes the ADA Principles of Ethics and Code of Professional Conduct. This document identifies five basic categories of ethics and professional conduct for a dentist. An overview of these principles is included in Box 4-2.

ADAA Principles of Ethics

Like the ADA, the ADAA has addressed the issue of ethics by preparing the following statement as the principles of ethics for its members:

> Each individual involved in the practice of dentistry assumes the obligation of maintaining and enriching the profession. Each member may choose to meet this obligation according to the dictates of personal conscience based on the needs of the human beings the profession of dentistry is committed to serve. The spirit of the Golden Rule is the basic guiding principle of this concept. The member must strive at all times to maintain confidentiality and exhibit

American Dental Association

PRINCIPLES OF

Ethics

AND

CODE OF

Professional

Conduct

With official advisory opinions revised to January 2005.

Figure 4-2 Official publication of the ADA. (Courtesy American Dental Association, Chicago, IL.)

respect for the dentist/employer. The member shall refrain from performing any professional service that is prohibited by state law and has the obligation to prove competence prior to providing services to any patient. The member shall constantly strive to upgrade and expand technical skills for the benefit of the employer and the consumer public. The member should additionally seek to sustain and improve the local organization, state association, and the ADAA by active participation and personal commitment.

ETHICAL AND LEGAL CONSIDERATIONS FOR THE ADMINISTRATIVE ASSISTANT

Each day the dental professional is confronted with ethical and legal decisions. The basis for each of these decisions may change as laws and societal influences affect the delivery of dental care. As mentioned previously, each member of the dental profession must constantly be vigilant of the changes taking place in laws affecting dentistry. Even though the administrative

Box 4-2
Overview of ADA Principles of Ethics and Code of Professional Conduct

SECTION 1 — Principle: Patient Autonomy ("self-governance")

The dentist has a duty to respect the patient's rights to self-determination and confidentiality.

This principle expresses the concept that professionals have a duty to treat the patient according to the patient's desires, within the bounds of accepted treatment, and to protect the patient's confidentiality. Under this principle, the dentist's primary obligations include involving patients in treatment decisions in a meaningful way, with due consideration being given to the patient's needs, desires, and abilities, and safeguarding the patient's privacy.

SECTION 2 — Principle: Nonmaleficence ("do no harm")

The dentist has a duty to refrain from harming the patient.

This principle expresses the concept that professionals have a duty to protect the patient from harm. Under this principle, the dentist's primary obligations include keeping knowledge and skills current, knowing one's own limitations and when to refer to a specialist or other professional, and knowing when and under what circumstances delegation of patient care to auxiliaries is appropriate.

SECTION 3 — Principle: Beneficence ("do good")

The dentist has a duty to promote the patient's welfare.

This principle expresses the concept that professionals have a duty to act for the benefit of others. Under this principle, the dentist's primary obligation is service to the patient and the public-at-large. The most important aspect of this obligation is the competent and timely delivery of dental care within the bounds of clinical circumstances presented by the patient, with due consideration being given to the needs, desires, and values of the patient. The same ethical considerations apply whether the dentist engages in fee-for-service, managed care, or other practice arrangement. Dentists may choose to enter into contracts governing the provision of care to a group of patients; however, contract obligations do not excuse dentists from their ethical duty to put the patient's welfare first.

SECTION 4 — Principle: Justice ("fairness")

The dentist has a duty to treat people fairly.

This principle expresses the concept that professionals have a duty to be fair in their dealings with patients, colleagues, and society. Under this principle, the dentist's primary obligations include dealing with people justly and delivering dental care without prejudice. In its broadest sense, this principle expresses the concept that the dental profession should actively seek allies throughout society on specific activities that will help improve access to care for all.

SECTION 5 — Principle: Veracity ("truthfulness")

The dentist has a duty to communicate truthfully.

This principle expresses the concept that professionals have a duty to be honest and trustworthy in their dealings with people. Under this principle, the dentist's primary obligations include respecting the position of trust inherent in the dentist-patient relationship, communicating truthfully and without deception, and maintaining intellectual integrity. Codes of professional conduct can be found for each section in the Principles of Ethics and Code of Professional Conduct handbook (an ADA publication), or on the ADA website, available at www.ada.or/prof/law/code/index.asp.

Box 4-3
Common Business Activities That Lead to Potential Litigation

Making false accusations about another person in verbal or written communication
Providing another party or agency with confidential information without patient consent
Entering inaccurate data on patient records
Duplicating copyrighted material without permission
Using unauthorized software
Gaining illegal access to computer data
Maliciously or deliberately damaging data in a computer
Falsely entering data on insurance claims
Failing to follow federal or state disease-transmission or waste-management regulations
Failing to maintain accurate local, state, or federal governmental records

assistant has contact with the clinical areas of the office, emphasis in this text is placed on only those areas that directly relate to activities of the dental administrative assistant. Box 4-3 lists those activities that the administrative assistant may encounter that could lead to potential litigation. The following discussion provides the administrative assistant with a practical understanding of various issues. These situations also should provoke your critical-thinking processes to consider other situations that might be common to a dental practice.

Assignment of Duties

As described in the section on the state Dental Practice Act, it is the responsibility of the licensed dentist to assign specific procedures to dental auxiliaries. If a duty that is illegal within the state is assigned to the dental assistant, the dentist is liable for this illegal action. Further, if a dental assistant performs a procedure that is not legally delegable to be performed by the assistant, the assistant is liable for such action.

Several factors should be considered in the issue of assignment. First, before an employee is hired, copies of the appropriate credentials should be reviewed to assure the person does indeed have the specified credentials. Second, the administrative assistant or office manager must be responsible for retaining on file current copies of all employee credentials. Third, the employer-employee relationship often creates conflict in such assignments. An assistant may feel that if a dentist assigns a task, it must be performed because the dentist is an authority figure, or the assistant may feel that his or her job will be jeopardized if the assignment is not carried out. To perform a task that is not legally delegable or for which an assistant is not qualified or has no credentials simply because it was assigned by the dentist can place the assistant in a position of potential negligence.

> If a duty that is not legal within the state is assigned to the dental assistant, the dentist is liable for this illegal action.

CONSENT

Consent is the voluntary acceptance or agreement to what is planned or done by another person. To examine or treat a patient without consent constitutes an unauthorized touching and makes the person committing the act guilty of battery as discussed above. Two forms of consent exist in the delivery of dental care: *informed* and *implied*.

Informed Consent

Informed consent is a concept that has evolved for decades as courts and legislatures have demanded more disclosure on the part of the provider of care to a patient. The idea behind the concept of informed consent is that every adult of sound mind has the right to determine what can and cannot be done with his or her body. For that person to make a proper judgment, he or she must be given information by the healthcare provider. The patient must be given enough information about the proposed treatment, in understandable language, in order to make an intelligent decision as to whether to proceed with the treatment. Moreover, the patient must have ample opportunity to ask questions and have them answered.

In general, courts and legislatures have defined specific elements that describe informed consent. These elements state that consent must be given freely; treatment and diagnosis must be described in understandable language; risks, benefits, and estimate of success of treatment must be described; prognosis if no treatment is elected and alternative treatment plans must be explained; and the patient must be given the right to ask questions and have them answered.

It is important to remember that if these conditions are not met, then the courts may conclude that the patient did not consent to the procedure and therefore the dentist may be liable for actions such as battery or negligence (depending on the individual state).

For consent to be legally valid, it must be informed and given freely, and the patient must be an adult of sound mind. Patients under the influence of alcohol, drugs, or severe stress may not have sufficient mental capacity to grant permission for treatment. When a dentist treats a minor, only the parent or guardian of the minor may grant consent. This excludes grandparents, baby-sitters, and siblings. However, parents may authorize another party to grant consent for treatment during the parents' absence. Such authorization must be signed prior to treatment consent. A variety of consent forms are available and need to be used during all invasive procedures.

Specialty practices such as endodontics and oral surgery have forms designed specifically for their specialties. Figure 4-3 shows an example of a common form for a general practice. These forms must be signed, dated, and retained in the patient record.

> Consent is the voluntary acceptance or agreement to what is planned or done by another person.

Implied Consent

Other agreements that flow automatically from the relationship between the patient and the dental professional fall under the category of implied consent. These agreements trigger responsibilities that work in two ways; those that the dentist owes to the patient and those that the patient owes to the dentist. Accepting a patient for treatment implies that the dentist agrees to accept certain responsibilities for that patient's dental care. Likewise, if a patient agrees to accept treatment by the dentist, it is considered that the patient assumes certain responsibilities. Boxes 4-4 and 4-5 list implied responsibilities for each of these parties.

MANAGED CARE

Managed care refers to a cost-containment system of healthcare insurance that may direct utilization of health benefits by restricting the type, level,

CONSENT TO TREATMENT ▬▬▬▬▬

CHRIS A. BROWN, D.D.S.
19 E. Center St. — Madison, WI 53701
608.123.4567

Date _____

I was informed by the abovenamed doctor(s) of the risks, possible alternative methods of treatment, and possible consequences involved in the treatment by means of:

_____
_____
_____

for the relief of _____

_____

Understanding this, I hereby authorize the above named doctor(s) or whomever s/he (they) may designate, to administer such treatment to

me (or _____)
Name of Patient if Minor

Signed _____
Patient or Person Authorized to Consent for Patient

Witness _____

Date _____

Form 4554 • 3/86 SYCOM Madison, WI Printed in U.S.A.

Figure 4-3 Informed consent form. (Courtesy SYCOM, Madison, WI.)

and frequency of treatment; limiting access to care to certain entities or practitioners; and basing the level of reimbursement for services on a capitation or other risk basis. Limitations imposed by managed care companies generally are directed at payment for services, but the policies may also limit the actual services received by a patient. In this way, managed care systems raise several legal and ethical issues for the dentist and healthcare professional. Patients may ask dentists to render only the treatment that is covered by the insurance plan, rather than the necessary treatment. Insurance companies are profit-driven and may not sufficiently consider the healthcare professional's responsibilities. Capitated plans can cause an ethical dilemma for a dentist when, for example, a dentist is paid for patient care whether or not it is provided, because it is obvious that it is not in the dentist's short-term economic interest to provide that care. Further, if certain care is not reimbursed, a patient may forgo needed treatment due to financial concerns. For the patient's interest to be protected, the dentist must be relied upon to adhere to both legal and ethical principles.

RISK MANAGEMENT PROGRAMS

A dental professional teaches preventive concepts to patients with a firm conviction that such practice will prevent future disease. This concept can be applied to prevention of malpractice claims. Most dental societies, organizations, and institutions are taking an active role in providing seminars and programs in risk management. The dental administrative assistant commonly assumes the responsibility for scheduling risk-management seminars and maintaining records of such attendance.

Box 4-4
Implied Duties Owed by the Dentist to the Patient

Use reasonable care in the provision of services as measured against acceptable standards set by other practitioners with similar training in a similar community.

Be properly licensed and registered, and meet all other legal requirements to engage in the practice of dentistry.

Obtain an accurate health (medical and dental) history of the patient before a diagnosis is made and treatment is begun.

Employ competent personnel and provide for their proper supervision.

Maintain a level of knowledge in keeping with current advances in the profession.

Use methods that are acceptable to at least a respectable minority of similar practitioners in the community.

Refrain from performing experimental procedures.

Obtain informed consent from the patient before instituting an examination or treatment.

Refrain from abandoning the patient, and ensure that care is available in emergency situations.

Charge a reasonable fee (by community standards) for services.

Refrain from exceeding the scope of practice authorized by your license or permitting those acting under your direction to engage in unlawful acts.

Keep the patient informed of his or her progress.

Refrain from undertaking any procedure for which you are not qualified.

Complete care in a timely manner.

Keep accurate records of the treatment rendered to the patient.

Maintain confidentiality of information.

Inform the patient of any untoward occurrences in the course of treatment.

Make appropriate referrals, and request necessary consultations.

Comply with all laws regulating the practice of dentistry.

Practice in a manner consistent with the codes of ethics of the profession.

Use universal precautions in the treatment of all patients.

Box 4-5
Implied Duties Owed by the Patient to the Dentist

Cooperate in your care by following home care or other reasonable instructions, taking prescribed medications, and showing up for recalls.

Keep appointments, and notify the office of cancellations or appointment delays.

Provide honest answers to questions asked on the history form and by the dentist and office personnel.

Notify the office staff or dentist of any change in health status.

Pay a reasonable fee for the service if no fee is agreed upon in writing or orally.

Remit the fee for services within a reasonable time.

Risk-management programs primarily show where dentists have been found liable in the past and try to teach dentists how to avoid exposing themselves to such liability. Often these programs accomplish this goal by reviewing real cases where dentists have been successfully sued. This method has a great impact on the dentists and auxiliaries. Risk-management programs aid the dental professional in identifying, analyzing, and dealing with risks in the dental office.

Risk-management programs generally include information on operating safety, product safety, quality assurance, and waste disposal. Operating safety programs emphasize methods of operating in an environment that ensures the safety of the patient, staff, and visitors. Programs about product safety update the dental team on the use of current materials and equipment and methods of evaluation and maintenance of these products. Quality assurance programs provide information on evaluating all systems used in the care of a patient. Waste-disposal programs provide the most current information on disposing of medical and dental wastes. Risk-management education combined with competent practice can be great insurance to the dental professional for avoiding potential litigation.

ABANDONMENT

Abandonment is defined as the severance of a professional relationship with a patient who is still in need of dental care and proper transfers or referrals. Though this legal concept primarily affects the dentist, the administrative assistant should be aware of its existence and aid the dentist in ensuring that no patient is abandoned in mid-treatment.

An example of abandonment might arise when a dentist who has been in practice for many years is suddenly diagnosed with a terminal illness. Many patients are in mid-treatment stages, and it appears that the dentist will be unable to resume work immediately. The future is uncertain for the dental practice. In this situation, arrangements must be made by the dentist and his or her family or staff to provide treatment for the patients. It may be necessary to hire a dentist for interim professional coverage of the patients or provide the names of dentists who are willing to accept the patients into their practices. The practice may ultimately need to be sold to another dentist. The administrative assistant plays a major role in this situation, since patients should be informed of the transition. Further information on patient care must be provided or transferred to the new treating dentists in an efficient manner. When informing patients of such changes, the administrative assistant must tell patients where their dental records are located. Patients should be given a reasonable period of time, typically 30 to 60 days, to contact the office to have their records transferred elsewhere if they do not wish to be seen by the new dentist. The administrative assistant should also ensure that the transfer of information meets federal and state law requirements on patient records, including meeting privacy requirements. Be certain to refer to the latest privacy guidelines by the Health Insurance Portability and Accountability Act of 1996 (HIPAA) for legal protocol.

Another abandonment situation could occur when a patient in the practice has been very irritating. For example, a patient may have failed to keep multiple appointments or give advance notification for broken appointments. The dentist may become very distressed with the patient and state that the patient is no longer desired in the practice.

To refuse to treat this patient is abandonment. Therefore the administrative assistant needs to inform the patient in writing why the dentist is no longer able to treat him. A letter should be sent, stating that if the patient needs a referral in his geographical area, he may contact the local dental society (include the name, address, and phone number of the dental society). The letter should also include a statement indicating that the dentist is willing to provide emergency care, including treatment for pain and infection, for 30 days from the date of the letter. The letter should be sent by certified mail with a return receipt requested. A copy of the letter and the returned receipt should be retained in the patient record. It would be prudent for the dentist to have a written policy on this issue. The policy should be posted or otherwise communicated to all patients so that there are no surprises, and liability is mitigated, when a patient receives such a letter.

FRAUD

Fraud is a deception that is deliberately practiced in order to secure unfair or unlawful gain. One of the most common practices of fraud is in the obtaining of fees through third-party payments by misrepresentation.

An example of a fraudulent action occurs when a patient has insurance coverage from July 1 of the past year until June 30 of the current year, after which time the patient would no longer receive this benefit. The patient had a maximum benefit coverage of $1200 for the year and to date had only used $450 of the benefit. Toward the end of June, it was determined that the patient needed a fixed bridge. The patient was informed of the fee for the bridge. The patient was further informed that after June 30 the services would not be covered and that she would be responsible for payment. The patient argued that it was the responsibility of the dentist to alter the date on the claim form, since she still had a $700 available benefit and in the future would bring her business to the dentist.

It is fraud to change the date on the claim form to indicate that the bridge was inserted before June 30 when indeed the bridge would not be inserted until mid-July. Though efforts might be made to complete the case prior to the deadline, a common solution is to explain to the patient that she is asking you to commit fraud. At this point, the patient will usually refrain and apologize.

Another example of a fraudulent act occurs when a patient's dental fee is covered by two insurance carriers requiring the coordination of benefits. The claim forms are processed. A check is received from the primary carrier for the correct amount of money. However, when a check is received from the secondary carrier, the amount is in excess of the fee and it appears the carrier has paid as a primary carrier. Consequently there is extra money received. The assistant enters the fee as it should have been on the patient's financial record but enters the entire check into the deposit, leaving an excess of funds in the account.

To avoid this situation, the administrative assistant should have informed the insurance carrier immediately after the check in excess of the correct payment was received. It is possible to enter the check into a deposit, but then a check for the amount of overpayment must be written and returned to the insurance carrier with the appropriate information concerning the overpayment.

RECORDS MANAGEMENT

Nothing can be more valuable in defending against potential litigation than adequate records. These are a vital responsibility of the administrative assistant. Though discussed in other areas of this text, the importance of including complete and thorough information in a patient's record cannot be overemphasized. You should record not only the exact date, type of treatment, materials used, complications, and special notations about the treatment but also any untoward incidence regarding patient comments or reactions. Initials of the treating operator(s) and recorder must be included. Remember that the better the documentation is, the less the legal risk will be.

You should also document any irregularities or unusual incidents occurring between patients, employees, and employers. All employee reports need to be retained in employee records. Such documentation might include narratives of episodes of accidental needle punctures. These incidents require a report that includes the name of the employee, the name of the patient being treated, and the date and time of the injury. Other incidents that may warrant documentation might include unusual behavior on the part of a patient or a verbal confrontation between staff members. Thorough, accurate, and objective documentation is your best defense in litigation.

DEFAMATION OF CHARACTER

Defamation of character is the communication of false information to a third party about a person that results in injury to that person's reputation. Such communication can be verbal (slander) or written (libel). The false statement could be about a person's product, business, profession, or title to property. A dental professional should make statements about a patient or other professional only as it relates to the rendering of dental care and only to other dental care providers involved in that care.

NEGLIGENCE

Negligence is an act of omission (neglecting to do something that a reasonably prudent person would do) or commission (doing something that a reasonably prudent person would not do). To prove negligence, it is necessary to prove that there has been a breach of duty owed, including deviation from the standard of care. In a dental negligence case, it is often necessary to provide expert testimony. To prove negligence, the plaintiff must show that there is an obligation to provide care according to a specified standard; that there was failure to meet that standard; that the failure to meet the standard led to injury; and that there was in fact an actual injury to the patient.

Though most often this action involves direct patient care, indirect patient care can also be a basis for finding negligence. Therefore by the way of example, the administrative assistant who may be assigned to such tasks as sterilization or other supportive clinical tasks should be aware that negligence can occur as a result of activities that do not involve direct contact with the patient.

The Health Care Quality Improvement Act of 1986 authorized creation by the federal government of a **National Practitioner Data Bank** as a central repository to collect and release information on professional competence and conduct. The repository includes information on paid malpractice claims and adverse reports of healthcare licensees. In most states, when a dentist is found negligent, the adverse act is reported to the NPDB. The administrative assistant may review this act and research the NPDB at the website www.npdb-hipdb.com//index.html.

INVASION OF PRIVACY

Invasion of privacy is a tort that refers to a number of wrongs involving the use of otherwise private information. As relevant here, tort may involve the publishing or otherwise making known or using information relating to the private life or affairs of a person without that person's approval or permission; prying into private affairs; or appropriating the plaintiff's identity for commercial use.

When an insurance company employee contacts an administrative assistant to clarify information about a patient on a claim form, the potential for invasion of privacy is present. The insurance clerk asks for verification of data from the patient's chart, specifically the date of birth of the child patient and the father's name and social security number. The administrative assistant offers to fax this to the insurance company. To save time, the assistant simply transfers a copy of the entire patient record, including information about a communicable disease. This action has now placed the patient record in a setting not requested nor otherwise authorized by the patient. Thus the patient's privacy has been invaded.

The administrative assistant should have requested that the incomplete form be returned to the dental office or that a written request for information clarification be made by the insurance company. Only the information requested should have been given, and it should have been reviewed to be certain the information was part of the claim form that the patient had signed.

Another potential invasion of privacy situation could occur when an administrative assistant is having difficulty collecting an account in a dental office. The patient had failed to make payment on the account of $3000 for the past 12 months. During a private conversation about the account, the patient informed the administrative assistant that her business was about to enter bankruptcy, and that her spouse had just been diagnosed with schizophrenia and was recovering from a serious alcohol dependency. During a discussion with a friend who worked in a local business, the assistant shared the story about the patient, who was a well-known member of the community.

Disparaging remarks and personal information about the patient were passed on to the listener. The story came back to the patient, and the source of information was traced to the assistant.

To avoid this situation, you must remember that any information a patient gives to the dental staff remains confidential within the office. No information about a patient should be shared outside the office. When a patient requests a transfer of records of dental treatment, a signed authorization to transfer should be completed by the patient. The administrative assistant, once again, must adhere to the regulations of the HIPAA.

GOOD SAMARITAN LAW

In the last 2 to 3 decades, every state in the United States has passed some form of legislation that grants immunity for acts performed by a person who renders care in an emergency situation. This concept, called the *Good Samaritan* law, was considered necessary to create an incentive for health care providers to provide medical assistance to the injured in cases of automobile accidents or other disasters without the fear of possible litigation. This law is intended for individuals who do not seek compensation but rather are solely interested in providing care to the injured in a caring, safe manner, with no intent to do bodily harm. This law does not provide protection for a negligent healthcare provider who is being compensated for services.

AMERICANS WITH DISABILITES ACT

In 1990, the federal government enacted legislation to ensure that persons with some degree of disability are not discriminated against. The **Americans with Disabilities Act** (AwDA), not to be confused with the ADA (American Dental Association), affects the dental office in the area of prohibitions against employment discrimination and by requiring facilities be accessible to physically and mentally compromised patients. This law identifies five categories of persons who are protected from discrimination. The categories protect individuals who have a physical or mental impairment that substantially limits one or more major life activities, those who have a record of such impairment, and those who are regarded as having such impairment. The categories include:

1. Persons whose physical or mental impairment substantially limits one or more major life activities, such as seeing, hearing, speaking, walking, breathing, performing manual tasks, learning, caring for oneself, or working. Included in this category are persons who have disabling conditions such as AIDS, HIV infections, heart disease, diabetes, cancer, learning disabilities, and mental retardation.
2. Persons who have a record of impairment, such as a history of heart disease or mental illness.
3. Persons who, while fully functional and not actually disabled, are regarded as having such an impairment due to severe disfigurement.
4. Persons who are discriminated against because they have a known association or relationship with a disabled individual.
5. Persons who currently participate in or who have completed a drug or alcohol rehabilitation program.

Box 4-6 shows a list of Titles that describe the provisions of the AwDA. This federal mandate is aimed at the elimination of discrimination against individuals with disabilities and clearly defines enforceable standards. Attention should be given to Title III and Title V as they relate to the dental office. It is wise for the office manager to obtain a copy of this act for the office and routinely update the office policies as required. The address for the Office of Americans with Disabilities is listed on page 192 and is also available at www.usdoj.gov/crt/ada/adahom1.htm.

Box 4-6
Provisions of the Americans with Disabilities Act

Title I	Prohibits discriminating employment policies
Title II	Prohibits discrimination against disabled persons in the use of public transportation.
Title III	Requires that public accommodations operated by private entities do not discriminate against persons with disabilities
Title IV	Prohibits discrimination against disabled individuals in the area of communication, especially hearing-impaired and speech-impaired individuals.
Title V	Contains miscellaneous provisions regarding the continued viability of other state or federal laws that provide disabled persons with equal or greater rights than the Act. Specifically, this section prohibits state or local governments from discriminating against individuals with disabilities.

COMPUTER SECURITY

The administrative assistant may be exposed to potential activities that would cause illegal or unethical activity while using a computer. **Computer security** refers to safeguards that are implemented to prevent and detect unauthorized access or deliberate damage to a computer system and data. A computer crime is the use of a computer to commit an illegal act.

In a dental office, the most common activity that would violate computer integrity is software theft, or piracy. Some people make an illegal copy of a disk or tape instead of paying for an authorized copy. Software theft is a violation of copyright law and is a crime. For large users, such as dental schools or other healthcare institutions, most software companies provide a site license and multiple copy discounts.

Though most dental offices use personal computers rather than a mainframe, the potential for gaining unauthorized access to data can still exist. If you inadvertently gain access on the computer to unauthorized or confidential data, you should exit the file including this data and report to the appropriate supervisor that you accidentally entered a confidential file. However, to make changes in a confidential file without authorized permission constitutes an unethical and possibly illegal act. Refer to the HIPAA standards in Chapter 7 to ensure information integrity.

TWELVE STEPS TO MAKING ETHICAL DECISIONS

The administrative assistant has much to consider when carrying out routine duties in the dental business office. During all activities, you must keep in mind questions about the tasks being performed. Routinely ask yourself the questions in Box 4-7.

Box 4-7
Twelve Steps to Making Ethical Decisions

1. Is the task I am performing legally delegable to me?
2. Do I have the necessary credentials to perform this task?
3. Am I physically and emotionally competent to perform this task?
4. Am I performing this procedure in a safe working environment that meets OSHA standards?
5. Has the patient been informed about his or her treatment?
6. Am I respecting the patient's right to privacy and confidentiality?
7. Do I maintain complete and accurate records, and have I documented special problems arising with patients, employees, or an employer?
8. Do I maintain professional liability insurance?
9. Do I participate in risk-management programs?
10. Am I willing to maintain appropriate standards at the risk of losing a job when confronted with a lack of ethics or legal responsibility on the part of an employer or fellow employee?
11. Do I maintain current knowledge of changes in reporting methods and occupational safety required by the Dental Practice Act?
12. Do I actively participate in my professional organization and contribute to community dental health?

Key Terms

Abandonment - The severance of a professional relationship with a patient who is still in need of dental care and attention without giving adequate notice to the patient.

Americans with Disabilities Act - A federal law that affects the dental office by prohibiting employee discrimination and by requiring facilities to be accessible to physically and mentally compromised patients.

Assignment - Refers to the dentist assigning to a dental assistant or hygienist a specific procedure that is to be performed on a designated patient of record.

Beneficence - The principle of ethics that refers to "doing good." The dentist has a duty to promote the patient's welfare.

Civil law - Law that relates to duties between persons or between citizens and their government.

Common law - Law that relates to judicial decisions.

Computer security - Refers to illegal or unethical use of computer software either by theft or piracy.

Consent - Voluntary acceptance or agreement to what is planned or done by another person.

Crime - A wrongdoing against the public at large that is prosecuted by a public official.

Criminal law - Law that refers to wrongs committed against the public as a whole.

Defamation of character - Communication of false information to a third party about a person that results in injury to that person's reputation.

Defendant - The person or party that is being sued in a lawsuit.

Dental Practice Act - The law in each state that defines the scope of dental practice and the requirements that are necessary to practice dentistry.

Ethics - Branch of philosophy that identifies a systematic, intellectual approach to the standards of behavior.

Expert witness - A witness who is called to testify and explain what happened based on the patient's record and to offer an opinion as to whether the dental care, as administered, met acceptable standards.

Fact witness - A witness who describes what he or she saw or did during a specific act.

Felony - A serious crime that is punishable by imprisonment generally for more than one year.

Fraud - A deliberately practiced deception that is committed in order to secure unfair or unlawful gain.

Informed consent – Consent for treatment that is given by a patient of sound mind after being informed in understandable language about such treatment by the healthcare provider.

Invasion of privacy - Publishing, making known, or using information relating to the private life or affairs of a person without that person's approval or permission.

Justice - The concept of fairness and integrity.

Lawsuit - A legal action in court.

Litigation - The process of a lawsuit.

Malpractice – Intentional or unintentional professional misconduct, evil practice, or illegal or immoral conduct.

Managed care - A cost-containment system that directs utilization of health benefits by restricting the type, level, and frequency of treatment; limiting access to care; and controlling the level of reimbursement for services.

Misdemeanor - A crime of a less serious nature than a felony.

National Practitioner Data Bank - An agency that was implemented as a central repository for information about paid malpractice claims and adverse reports of healthcare licensees.

Nonmaleficence - Refers to the "do no harm" clause in the principle of ethics. The dentist has a duty to refrain from harming the patient.

Negligence - An act of omission (neglecting to do something that a reasonably prudent person would do) or commission (doing something that a reasonably prudent person would not do).

Patient of record - A patient who has been examined and diagnosed by a licensed dentist and whose treatment has been planned by that dentist.

Plaintiff - The person or party that institutes a lawsuit.

Standard of care - Treatment that a reasonably prudent professional would perform in similar circumstances.

Supervision - Refers to the conditions under which a patient of record may be treated by an assistant or hygienist and the protocol to be followed after the treatment is rendered.

Tort - A civil wrongdoing that is a breach of legal duty owed to the plaintiff by the defendant and that must be the primary cause of harm to the plaintiff.

LEARNING ACTIVITIES

1. Explain the application of the two forms of consent that apply to the delivery of dental care.
2. What four questions should be asked to determine an unintentional tort of negligence in dental care?
3. Identify ten steps that should be followed when making ethical decisions.
4. Identify ten implied duties that a dentist owes a patient.
5. List five business office activities that could lead to potential litigation.
6. Explain the element of informed consent.
7. Explain the function of a state Dental Practice Act and its impact on a consumer.
8. Describe the role of the dental assistant in the state in which you practice.
9. Would the dental assistant be liable for any legal liability in the state in which you practice?
10. Search the Americans with Disabilities Act website to determine how this act would affect the renovation of a dental office building built in 1995.

Bibliography

ADA principles of ethics and code of professional conduct, Chicago, 2005, American Dental Association.

Davison JA: *Legal and ethical considerations for dental hygienists and assistants*, St. Louis, 2000, Mosby.

State fact booklet, Chicago, 2004, Dental Assisting National Board.

Recommended Websites

http://www.danb.org
http://www.npdb-hipdb.com//index.html
http://www.usdoj.gov/crt/ada/adahom1.htm
http://www.ada.org/prof/prac/law/code/index.asp

Chapter

5

New Technology in the Business Office

Chapter Outline

Learning Objectives

Mastery of the content in this chapter will enable the reader to:

- Define glossary terms
- Differentiate between a manual office and an office using new technology
- List types of electronic office equipment used in new technology
- Describe the elements of information systems
- Explain the four operations of a computer
- Explain how technology can be used to increase profitability
- Describe the application of technology to a dental practice
- Explain the purpose of a feasibility study
- Explain the difference between general and specific task software
- Discuss dental software, word processing, electronic spreadsheet, database, graphics, and Internet software
- List guidelines to follow when selecting software
- Explain why implementing a change to a computer system is important to all staff members

---

Box 5-1
Applications of New Technology in the Business Office

Electronic charting
Computerized scheduling
Online office procedures manuals
Add progress notes to online records
Automated insurance claims
Buying supplies from online supply warehouses
Telemarketing with webpages
E-mail staff and patients
Enroll in online college courses
Provide a means for continuing education
Allow for "virtual group practices" where solo practitioners share one
   set of records
Consult with experts from all over the world

Just ten years ago in the traditional dental business office, the typewriter served as the central piece of equipment. Today, however, **new technology** has replaced manual systems with online, interconnected commerce. New technology in the office is the application of **computers** and associated electronic equipment to prepare and distribute information. Indeed the computer has made an impact on the profession of dentistry and is used routinely in the clinical and business applications of the office.

Few businesses today can avoid the explosion in the need for more information. The prudent selection of technology equipment is a major component of dental office productivity and efficiency. Presently, there are millions of electronic workstations in all types of offices in the United States, and the numbers are growing. In fact, office automation using the **Internet** has been called the "primary way to do business in a high-tech world." Some form of computer usage is now installed in more than 75% of dental offices in North America. Today, little understanding of manual office systems and equipment is necessary for effective application of the latest technology to the modern business office.

The **electronic office** is a workplace where sophisticated computers and other electronic equipment carry out many of the office's routine tasks and provide more options for gathering, processing, displaying, and storing information. Some applications of technology in the electronic office are outlined in Box 5-1.

The technological revolution that led to the information age has had a profound effect on the business office. The use of electronic office technology in the dental business office allows the staff to be more organized and efficient. It can help to automate routine office tasks, improve cash flow, and increase accuracy. Today, a patient in a general practice can have a radiograph digitally processed and transferred to the oral surgeon before the patient even leaves the general dentist's office. This concept can be likened to the application of four-handed dentistry in the clinical setting, because both result in improved patient care, increased productivity, and reduction of stress on the dental staff.

INFORMATION SYSTEMS

An **information system** is a collection of elements that provide accurate, timely, and useful information. To understand the procedure of an

Box 5-2
New Technology Terms

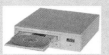

CD/DVD Drives: Most computers come with a 32X to 48X speed CD-ROM drive that can read CDs. If you plan to write music, audio files, and documents on a CD or DVD, then you should consider upgrading to a CD-RW. An even better alternative is to upgrade to a DVD+R/+RW combination drive. It allows you to read DVDs and CDs and to write data on (burn) a DVD or CD. A DVD has a capacity of at least 4.7 GB versus the 650 MB capacity of a CD.

Card Reader/Writer: A card reader/writer is useful for transferring data directly to and from a removable flash memory card, such as the ones used in your camera or music player. Make sure the card reader/writer can read from and write to the flash memory cards that you use.

Digital Camera: Consider an inexpensive point-and-shoot digital camera. They are small enough to carry around, usually operate automatically in terms of lighting and focus, and contain storage cards for storing photographs. A 1.3 to 2.2-megapixal camera with an 8 MB or 16 MB storage card is fine for creating images for use on the Web or to send via e-mail.

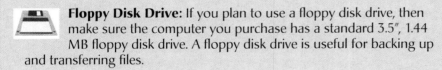**Digital Video Capture Device:** A digital video capture device allows you to connect your computer to a camcorder or VCR and record, edit, manage, and then write video back to a VCR tape, a CD, or a DVD. The digital video capture device can be an external device or an adapter card. To create quality video (true 30 frames per second, full sized TV), the digital video capture device should have a USB 2.0 or FireWire port. You will find that a standard USB port is too slow to maintain video quality. You will also need sufficient storage: an hour of data on a VCR tape takes up about 5 GB of disk storage.

Floppy Disk Drive: If you plan to use a floppy disk drive, then make sure the computer you purchase has a standard 3.5", 1.44 MB floppy disk drive. A floppy disk drive is useful for backing up and transferring files.

Hard Disk: It is recommended that you buy a computer with 40 to 60 GB if your primary interests are browsing the Web and using e-mail and Office suite-type applications; 60 to 80 GB if you also want to edit digital photographs; 80 to 100 GB if you plan to edit digital video or manipulate large audio files even occasionally; and 100 to 160 GB if you will edit digital video, movies, or photography often, store audio files and music, or consider yourself to be a power user.

Joystick/Wheel: If you use your computer to play games, then you will want to purchase a joystick or wheel. These devices, especially the more expensive ones, provide for realistic game play with force feedback, programmable buttons, and specialized levers and wheels.

Box 5-2
New Technology Terms—cont'd

 Keyboard: The keyboard is one of the more important devices used to communicate with the computer. For this reason, make sure the keyboard you purchase has 101 to 105 keys, is comfortable, easy to use, and has a USB connection. A wireless keyboard should be considered, especially if you have a small desk area.

 Microphone: If you plan to record audio or use speech recognition to enter text and commands, then purchase a close-talk headset with gain adjustment support.

 Modem: Most computers come with a modem so that you can use your telephone line to dial out and access the Internet. Some modems also have fax capabilities. Your modem should be rated at 56 Kbps.

 Monitor: The monitor is where you will view documents, read e-mail messages, and view pictures. A minimum of a 17″ screen is recommended, but if you are planning to use your computer for graphic design or game playing, then you may want to purchase a 19″ or 21″ monitor. The LCD flat panel monitor should be considered, especially if space is an issue.

 Mouse: As you work with your computer, you use the mouse constantly. For this reason, spend a few extra dollars, if necessary, and purchase a mouse with an optical sensor and USB connection. The optical sensor replaces the need for a mouse ball, which means you do not need a mouse pad. For a PC, make sure your mouse has a wheel, which acts as a third button in addition to the top two buttons on the left and right. An ergonomic design is also important because your hand is on the mouse most of the time when you are using your computer. A wireless mouse should be considered to eliminate the cord and allow you to work at short distances from your computer.

 Network Card: If you plan to connect to a network or use broadband (cable or DSL) to connect to the Internet, then you will need to purchase a network card. Broadband connections require a 10/100 PCI Ethernet network card.

 Printer: Your two basic printer choices are ink-jet and laser. Color ink-jet printers cost on average between $50 and $300. Laser printers cost from $300 to $2,000. In general, the cheaper the printer, the lower the resolution and speed, and the more often you are required to change the ink cartridge or toner. Laser printers print faster and with a higher quality than an ink-jet, and their toner on average costs less. If you want color, then go with a high-end ink-jet printer to ensure quality of print. Duty cycle (the number of pages you expect to print each month) also should be a determining factor. If your duty cycle is on the low end – hundreds of

Box 5-2
New Technology Terms—cont'd

pages per month – then stay with a high-end ink-jet printer, rather than purchasing a laser printer. If you plant to print photograph s taken with a digital camera, then you should purchase a photo printer. A photo printer is a dye-sublimation printer or an ink-jet printer with higher resolution and features that allow you to print quality photographs.

 Processor: For a PC< a 2.0 GHz Intel or AMD processor is more than enough processor power for application home and small office/home office users. Game home, large business, and power users should upgrade to faster processors.

 RAM: RAM plays a vital role in the speed of your computer. Make sure the computer you purchase has at least 256 MB of RAM. If you have extra money to invest in your computer, then consider increasing the RAM to 512 MB or more. The extra money for RAM will be well spent.

 Scanner: The most popular scanner purchased with a computer today is the flatbed scanner. When evaluating a flatbed scanner, check the color depth and resolution. Do not buy anything less than a color depth of 48 bits and a resolution of 1200 x 2400 dpi. The higher the color depth, the more accurate the color. A higher resolution picks up the more subtle gradations of color.

 Sound Card: Most sound cards today support the Sound Blaster and General MIDI standards and should be capable of recording and playing digital audio. If you plan to turn your computer into an entertainment system or are a game home use, then you will want to spend the extra money and upgrade from the standard sound card.

 Speakers: Once you have a good sound card, quality speakers and a separate subwoofer that amplifies the bass frequencies of the speakers can turn your computer into a premium stereo system.

 Video Graphics Card: Most standard video cards satisfy the monitor display needs of application home and small office users. If you are a game home user or a graphic designer, you will want to upgrade to a higher quality video card. The higher refresh rate will further enhance the display of games, graphics, and movies.

 PC Video Camera: A PC video camera is a small camera used to capture and display live video (in some cases with sound), primarily on a Web page. You also can capture, edit, and share video and still photos. The camera sits on your monitor or desk. Recommended minimum specifications include 640 x 480 resolution, a video with a rate of 30 frames per second, and a USB 2.0 or FireWire connection.

Box 5-2
New Technology Terms—cont'd

 USB Flash (Jump) Drive: If you work on different computers and need access to the same data and information, then this portable miniature mobile storage device that can fit on your key chain is ideal. USB flash drive capacity varies from 128 MB to 4 GB.

 Wireless LAN Access Point: A Wireless LAN Access Point allows you to network several computers, so they can share files and access the Internet through a single cable modem or DSL connection. Each device that you connect requires a wireless card. A wireless LAN Access Point can offer range of operation up to several hundred feet, so be sure the device has a high-powered antenna.

 Zip Drive: Consider purchasing a Zip disk drive to back up important files. The Zip drive, which has a capacity of up to 750 MB, is sufficient for most users. An alternative to purchasing a backup drive is to purchase a CD-RW or DVD+R/+RW and burn backups of key files on a CD or DVD.

(From Shelly GB, Cashman TJ, Vermaat ME: *Discovering computers: fundamentals edition,* Boston, 2004, Course Technology.)

information system, the administrative assistant must understand basic terminology related to this concept. A glossary of terms and definitions will help the novice understand the terminology of the modern electronic office and will be useful in selecting contemporary office equipment. Box 5-2 contains a detailed list of basic information system terms.

Figure 5-1 depicts the five elements that make up the information system:
- Hardware (the equipment)
- Software (programs)
- Data
- Personnel
- Procedures

Hardware

Hardware is the information system's physical equipment. The central piece of hardware in the information system is the computer. A computer is a device that electronically accepts **data,** processes the data arithmetically and logically, produces output from the processing, and stores the result for future use. Computers are generally classified in three categories: (1) mainframe, (2) minicomputers, and (3) microcomputers.

The mainframe computer is a large system that handles numerous users, stores large amounts of data, and processes data at very high speeds. This type of system may be found, for example, in an insurance company in which the mainframe computer is used to process many claim forms, with large amounts of data that must be processed quickly.

A midrange system (or minicomputer) is compact and has a slower processing speed and more limited storage capacity than the mainframe system,

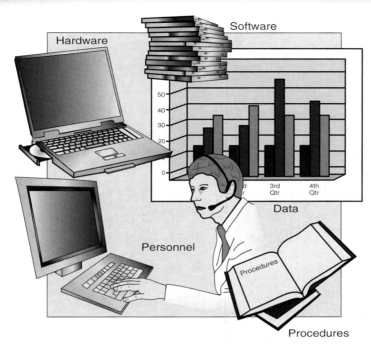

Figure 5-1 Five elements of an information system.

but it is more powerful than the microcomputer. This type of system is often found in large dental practices in which computer resources are shared. A centralized processing area may be implemented with this system, and processing can be done for several dentists in one practice or different dentists throughout an office building.

The microcomputer (also called a *personal computer*) is the smallest computer of the systems mentioned and is self-contained with regard to the circuitry and components for arithmetic, logic, and control operations (Figure 5-2). These machines are generally priced under $2000, and the cost continues to decrease. This kind of system is becoming increasingly popular in many small dental practices and can be connected together to form a Local Area Network **(LAN)**.

In addition to the computer system just described, other technologies prevalent in the business office today include telephone systems with the capacity for voicemail or paging, voice equipment, fax (facsimile) machines, copy machines, calculators, electronic typewriters, dental imagers, and scanners.

- Voicemail allows both incoming and outgoing telephone messages to be recorded and processed. A telephone connected to the **word processing** center can serve as the input system for dictation. This allows a person to record dictation from telephones either within or outside the office.
- Pagers carried by members of the office staff allow them to be signaled when needed.
- Voice equipment records voice sounds as input for a voice-activated system or for later transcription using magnetic belts, magnetic tapes, and plastic or magnetic disks. The latter type of equipment can be used for referral letters or for recording information to be transferred to the clinical records, or to record research reports, minutes of a staff meeting, or the summary of a conference.
- Fax machines send and receive documents or other graphic images over the telephone systems.

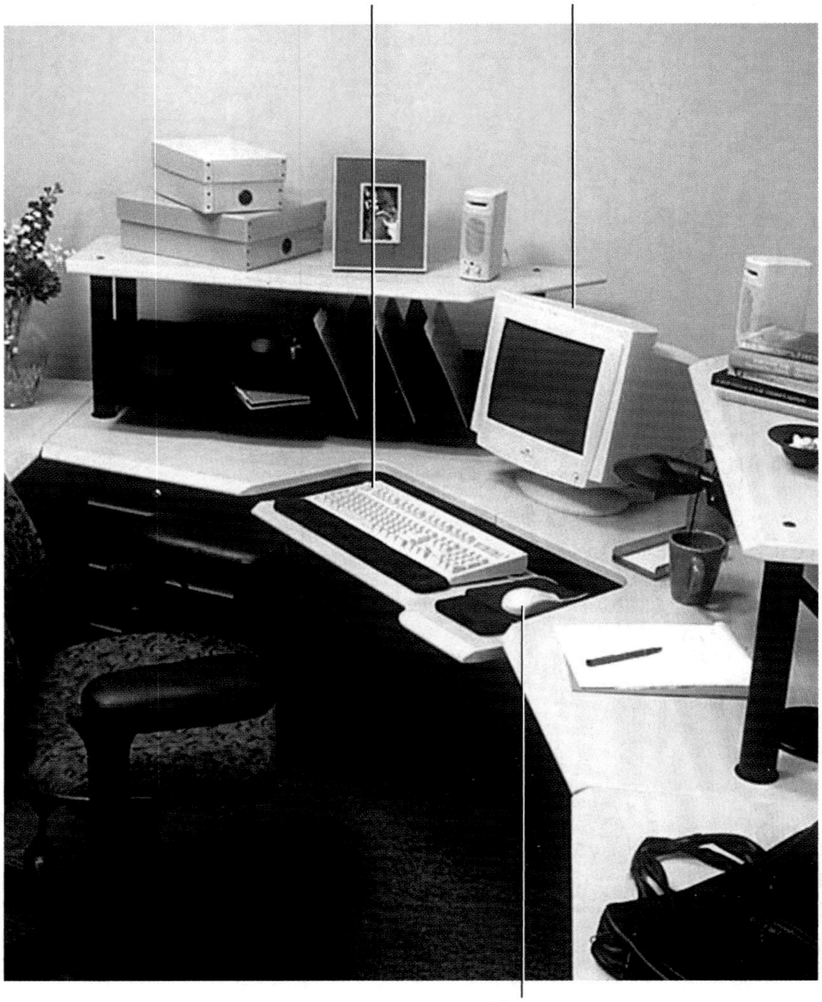

Keyboard   Monitor

Mouse

Figure 5-2 Components of a microcomputer. (Courtesy Steelcase, Inc., Grand Rapids, MI.)

- Copy machines reproduce letters, pages from magazines and books, charts and drawings, financial reports, clinical records, and statements from the patients' ledger cards. See Box 5-3 for features of copiers.
- Calculators found in computer **software** or those purchased separately are a great help to assistants with many routine duties that require mathematical skill. Except for the computer calculators, many are inexpensive enough to be sold at department and discount stores and also at office machine dealers. The price of a calculator is not determined entirely by the number of its functions, although this is an important factor. The types of components and materials used to produce the machine also affect the price (Box 5-4).
- Electronic typewriters, single components containing keyboard, internal **processor,** storage unit (may be a mini-diskette), and printer, are designed for general office automation work at one workstation. Box 5-5 describes various features of electronic typewriters.
- Dental imagers input graphic data into the computer memory by using intraoral cameras. Data are stored, and a hard copy of the intraoral condition

Box 5-3

Features to Consider When Selecting or Using Copiers

See also Figure 5-3.
1. Style of copiers—tabletop size or stand-alone floor models
2. Volume of work to be done—low-volume, mid-volume, high-volume
3. Quality of copy desired—clear and sharp
4. Selection of paper size for reports, ledger cards, and letters
5. Ability to reproduce from a colored original or colored ink
6. Speed and output—number of copies per minute
7. Capability to make copies on regular office forms and paper
8. Availability of outside copying business to handle a large volume of documents (such as a new office policy) or other specialized copying services

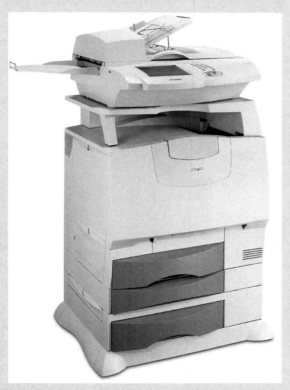

Figure 5-3 Multi-task machine. Performs four functions in one—a true multi-task machine: color printer, scanner, plain-paper FAX, copier.

can be printed. Cosmetic imagers are capable of displaying proposed changes that will result from specific treatment.

- Scanners input text or graphical data directly into computer storage without keying. Any of these devices may be directly connected to the computer system and provide a centralized source for information. Chapter 10 includes detailed descriptions of telecommunications systems and techniques.

Software

The computer system is directed by a series of instructions called a *computer program*, or *software*, that directs the sequence of operations the system is

Box 5-4
Features to Consider When Selecting a Calculator

See also Figure 5-4.
1. Type of display
2. Printing capabilities
3. Quality of keyboard
4. Type of batteries. On portable models, are they easily obtained? Are they throwaway or rechargeable?
5. The durability of components and materials. Factors other than cost will influence the selection of a calculator.
6. Ease of operation. The calculator should allow for the basic computations of addition, subtraction, multiplication, and division. Some machines can solve difficult trigonometry problems that only an accomplished mathematician could answer accurately.
7. Decimal functions. A fixed decimal restricts the number of decimals; a floating decimal puts no restriction on the position of the decimal point.
8. Repeat and constant operations. This feature allows the operator to add or subtract a series of identical numbers by depressing the *add* or *subtract* function key repeatedly.
9. Memory register. Figures can be added to or subtracted from and are available until the register is cleared.

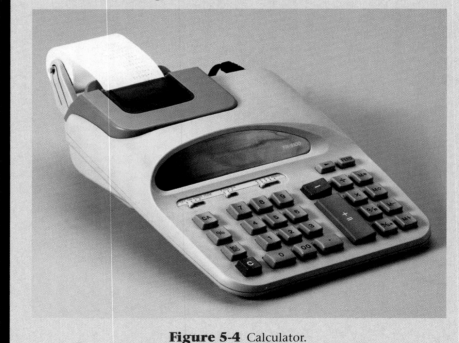

Figure 5-4 Calculator.

Box 5-5
Questions to Consider When Preparing to Automate

1. Is there a manual system in place that gives all the data needed to evaluate the practice monthly?
2. Do the dentist and staff understand the significance of the data?
3. Is the staff organized?
4. Does the work get done in a timely manner?
5. Do the patients receive current and accurate information?
6. Is the staff stable and team oriented?

to perform. Software in the dental office might include general-purpose software, such as word processors, spreadsheets, or **database** systems; or it may include software specifically designed for dental practice management. Software may be provided with the computer system or be purchased as individual or bundled packages. The parts of the desktop window that need to be identified are shown in Figure 5-5.

Data

Data refers to the facts or figures that the information system needs to produce accurate and timely information. Data are the raw material of the information system and are manipulated or processed by the computer to produce the finished product—information. For instance, the administrative assistant enters data such as fees, treatment rendered, and payments on a financial record. The finished product can result in a statement or an insurance claim form. If the data are incorrect, the resulting information will be incorrect: "garbage in, garbage out."

Personnel

In some larger computer installations, properly trained data processing personnel are required to operate and maintain the information system. However, in most dental practices, the administrative assistant is responsible for the accuracy of both the input and output of the information system as well as the setup and maintenance. When a system is installed in an office, most system vendors will provide a training session for the staff. As updated versions are released, seminars on system operations are offered.

Procedures

Procedures are the written documentation or policies that help maintain the information system efficiently. Specialized manuals can be assembled, or these procedures may be included in the office procedures manual described in Chapter 2.

Figure 5-5 Parts of a typical desktop window.

If any of the elements –
hardware, software, data,
personnel, or procedures
– are missing or flawed,
the entire information
system may be affected.

If any of the elements—hardware, software, data, personnel, or procedures—are missing or flawed, the entire information system may be affected.

OPERATIONS OF AN INFORMATION SYSTEM

Regardless of the computer that is selected for business office use, computers are capable of performing four general operations known as the *information processing cycle*. These four operations are (1) input, (2) process, (3) output, and (4) storage. By using these four processes, the computer will process the data into information.

Parts of a Computer

INPUT DEVICE. The most common means of entering information and instructions into the computer is the keyboard (Figures 5-6 and 5-7). Special keys on the enhanced 101-key keyboard may include a numeric keypad, cursor control keys, and function keys. In addition to the keyboard, a host of other data collection devices include the mouse or trackball, touch screens, graphic input devices, scanners, and voice input. These devices may input data directly without any keystrokes.

PROCESSOR. The processor is the controlling unit of the system that contains the electronic circuitry to manipulate data. This unit is known as the *central processing unit (CPU)* (see Figure 5-6), and it directs and controls all of the computer's activities. As the data are accepted from the input device, the data are processed according to the program. The program is a series of instructions directing the computer to perform a sequence of tasks. The number of programs and data that can be stored in the processing unit depends on the main memory of the system. The memory capacity of computers varies, but the computer has a fixed memory capacity. One byte of computer memory could be considered equivalent to one character of storage. The memory capacity is expressed in terms of kilobytes, megabytes, or gigabytes, which roughly represent 1 thousand, 1 million, or 1 billion bytes of storage, respectively. The typical office system might have 8 megs (megabytes) of main memory and a 4-gig (gigabytes) hard drive for storing patient records.

OUTPUT DEVICE. The printer and the monitor are the two most commonly used output devices (see Figure 5-6). If a paper copy (hard copy) is needed, the computer will be directed to print a copy. When no permanent record is needed, the output is displayed on the monitor (soft copy).

There are two classifications of printers: impact and nonimpact. The **impact printer** creates images on the paper as the mechanism strikes the paper, ribbon, and characters together. The two most common impact printers are the dot matrix and letter-quality printers. Most dot matrix printers print bidirectionally and can print text and **graphics.** The quality of the dot matrix printer depends on the number of pins used to form the character. For example, near-letter-quality (NLQ) printers with a 24-pin print head produce a better quality than a 9-pin print head. Another impact printer is the daisy-wheel printer, which has a printing element resembling the flower of a daisy. This printer has letter-quality printing; many different type styles can be selected, but the printer cannot print graphics.

The **nonimpact printer** creates images on the paper without characters striking the sheet of paper. Nonimpact printers are almost noiseless, because the characters are shaped with the use of light or a spray of ink. The two most

Nonimpact printers are
almost noiseless, because
the characters are shaped
with the use of a light or a
spray of ink.

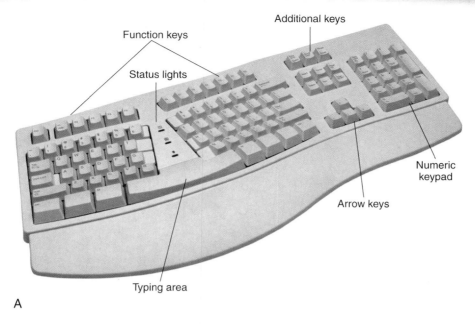

A

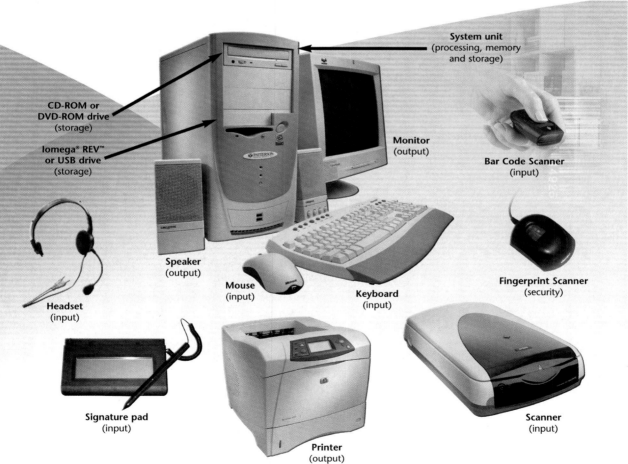

Figure 5-6 A, Computer keyboard. **B,** Computer system. (**B,** Courtesy Patterson-EagleSoft, Effingham, IL.)

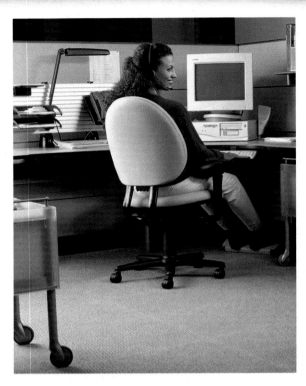

Figure 5-7 Workstation—keyboard and monitor. (Courtesy Steelcase, Inc., Grand Rapids, MI.)

common nonimpact printers are ink jet and laser printers. To create the characters, the ink jet printer uses nozzles to spray ink onto the paper. The laser printer, often called an *intelligent printer,* combines both printing and photocopying features to make it the most economical choice. These printers shape characters through the use of light (laser beams). The intelligent printer is able to collate, stack, and place images on both sides of the paper. The cost of these printers have decreased and so they now produce multiple copies more economically. Some printers in both categories are now able to print color images, which greatly enhances the visual effect of the output.

As the information is entered, it is displayed on the video display screen, also known as a *monitor* or **CRT** (*cathode-ray tube*). Terminals are classified as **dumb terminals** or **intelligent terminals.** Dumb terminals depend upon the system to which they are connected for memory and processing circuitry. Intelligent terminals have their own processing capabilities (see Figure 5-7).

STORAGE MEDIA. Auxiliary storage will be used to store data and programs that are not being processed on the computer (see Figure 5-6). Types of storage include floppy disk, hard disk, disk, Zip disk, tape cartridge, compact disk, and jump drive (Figure 5-8). Other devices for storage are also used, but they usually require a large computer system. The floppy disk or diskette used with most personal computers is the 3½-inch high-density (HD) size. This disk consists of a thin, flexible plastic circle enclosed in a protective jacket. The hard disk is a rigid metal disk coated with magnetic material that makes it suitable for recording and storing data. Zip disks are similar to floppy disks but can hold over 100 times more data. Disks and tape cartridges are used primarily for backup purposes. The optical compact disk system uses a laser to burn microscopic holes on the surface of a hard plastic disk. The most popular optical disk formats used for data storage are the recordable compact

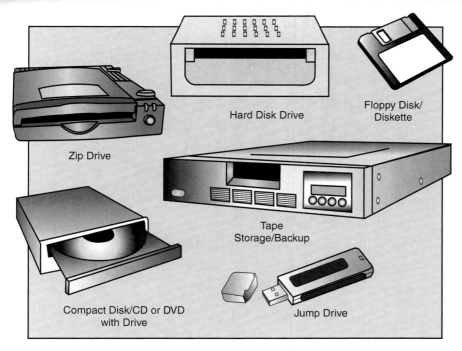

Figure 5-8 Different types of storage media.

disk (CD-R) and rewritable compact disk (CD-RW), which can hold even more data than a Zip disk. Another small optical disk format used for storage is the CD-ROM, which stands for compact disk read-only memory. Most software is distributed on the CD-ROM format. Another type of storage becoming more popular are jump drives, which are portable storage devices that plug directly into computers, hold large amounts of data and do not require any type of disk.

PROFITABILITY OF THE INFORMATION SYSTEM

All of the high-tech equipment available today will not make the private dental office, clinic, or dental laboratory more efficient if proper procedures are not followed before investing in the information system. Before the office acquires new equipment of any kind, the needs of the office should be identified. The major categories of equipment you may need to consider include computers dedicated to such tasks as word processing, records management, and accounting; copying machines; calculators; dictation/transcription equipment; and electronic typewriters. Other specific types of equipment used to handle mail and telephone systems are discussed within the content of specific chapters of this book.

A **feasibility study** is one of the most reliable ways to determine what type of computer a dental practice needs and if new technologies are needed. This study can be conducted within the office by a vendor (usually an equipment manufacturer), an organization, or a qualified individual (such as the administrative assistant). A feasibility study must involve everyone who will use the system and other support staff. Some factors to consider when doing the feasibility study include (1) type and size of the practice, (2) cost, (3) ability of the staff, and (4) training requirements. Investing in a computer is unwise if it simply becomes a billing machine. An office is prepared for automation if the questions in Box 5-6 can be answered in the affirmative.

> All of the high-tech equipment available today will not make the private dental office, clinic, or dental laboratory more efficient if proper procedures are not followed before investing in the information system.

Box 5-6
Common Features of Word Processors

Insert
Insert character(s)
Insert word(s)
Insert line(s)
Insert document(s)

Delete
Delete character(s)
Delete word(s)
Delete sentence(s)
Delete paragraph(s)
Delete page(s)
Delete entire document

Keyboard and Screen
Control Printing
Cursor movement
Page up and down
Word wrap
Upper- and lower-case display
Function keys
Control keys
Status line
Line
Column

Format
Top and bottom margins
Left and right margins
Tab stops
Single and double spacing

Move
Move sentence(s)
Move paragraph(s)
Move blocks

Search and Replace
Search to specific text
Search and replace word
Search and replace character strings

Printing
Print columns
Subscripts
Superscripts
Underline
Boldface
Headers
Footers
Page numbering
Document title

Once the need for a system has been established, it will be time to begin selecting equipment and software, setting up the procedures for using the equipment, training personnel, and entering the initial data.

SOFTWARE SELECTION

The first part of the chapter can be used as a guideline in selecting the hardware components of the information system for the office needs, with the help of equipment manufacturers. The next task is the selection of software. Software is the computer program(s) written to meet specific user needs.

Selecting software that will perform the jobs specific to your office is important. Software is available that performs a general task such as word processing, spreadsheets, database, graphics, electronic, and desktop publishing. Software can also perform specific tasks for dental offices, including account reports, patient reports, patient history, transactions, prescription history, insurance claim processing, appointment scheduling, treatment planning, summary reports, billing and aging receivables, referral tracking, income analysis, recall, and inventory management. Figures 5-9 through 5-22 include illustrations of some of the various screens that can be accessed in a commonly used software system.

The **patient information screen** (Figure 5-9) includes comprehensive patient information. The accounts screen includes accounts payable information (Figure 5-10). A variety of payment and remittance information is found on this screen including the minimum monthly payment, date of the

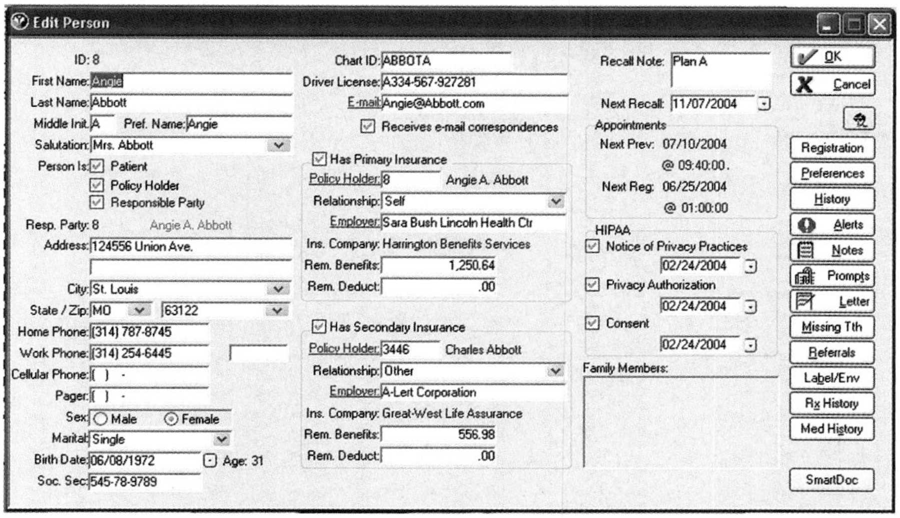

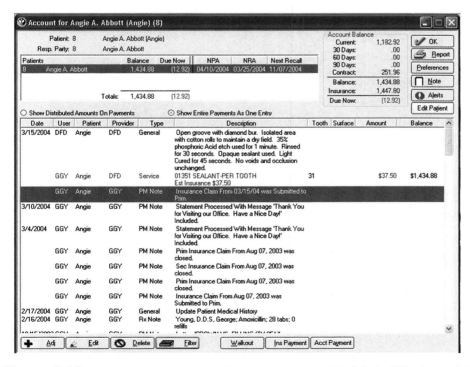

Figure 5-9 Patient information screen. (Courtesy Patterson-EagleSoft, Effingham, IL.)

last statement, current account balance, and outstanding insurance or budget plan balances.

The **Patient Master report** (Figure 5-11) can be filtered or sorted using different criteria, such as patient zip codes, birthdays, phone numbers, insurance coverage, and more.

Prescription window (Figure 5-12): This window has a pull down section that enumerates the patient medication history.

Transaction entry screen: Various modes of this screen can be obtained. Figure 5-13 is a transaction window with the ADA window showing the ADA codes for the completed treatment.

Figure 5-10 Patient accounts screen. (Courtesy Patterson-EagleSoft, Effingham, IL.)

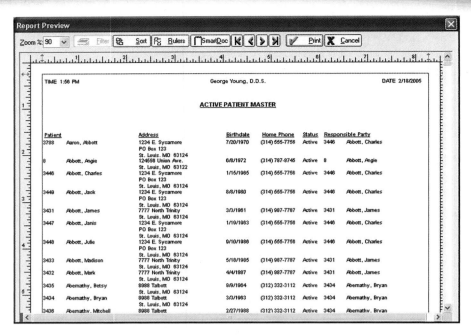

Figure 5-11 The Patient Master report can be filtered or sorted using a variety of criteria: patient zip code, birthday, phone number, insurance status, and more. (Courtesy Patterson-EagleSoft, Effingham, IL.)

View claim for transaction window (Figure 5-14): By clicking the "claim stat" in this software, the assistant can view the status of an insurance claim. By clicking on claims, the "process insurance claim form" window will open, and you then mark the claims and click on process; the form is automatically sent to the insurance company.

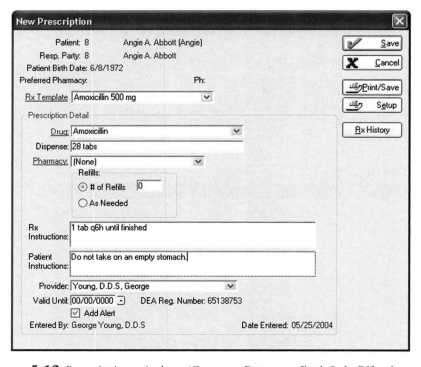

Figure 5-12 Prescription window. (Courtesy Patterson-EagleSoft, Effingham, IL.)

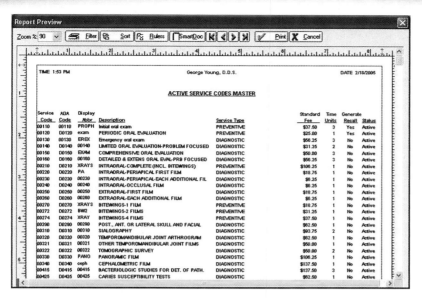

Figure 5-13 Service codes list with ADA codes. (Courtesy Patterson-EagleSoft, Effingham, IL.)

Treatment plan screen (Figure 5-15): This screen enables you to produce a treatment plan for the patient and to track all of the planned treatment to completion.

Appointment screens: The daily appointment screen with an expanded view to indicate various treatment rooms (Figure 5-16).

Schedule versus goal screen: From OnSchedule, you can view a provider's scheduled appointments versus the goal for each day (Figure 5-17).

Family recall: This can pull up everyone in a family and identify the exam due date (Figure 5-18).

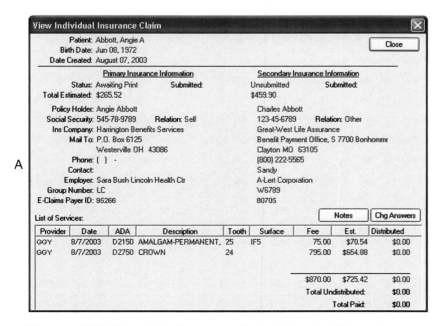

Figure 5-14 View claim for transaction window. **A,** Claims view.

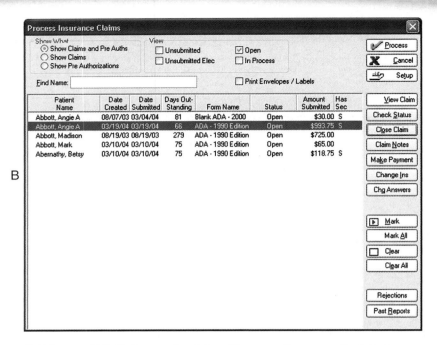

Figure 5-14, cont'd B, Process in claim. (Courtesy Patterson-EagleSoft, Effingham, IL.)

Tickler file: This is provided in the appointment section of the program to collect and store information on patients who have missed, canceled, or broken appointments (Figure 5-19).

Clinical charting: This may be linked to the software system. Charting can be done in the treatment room using a graphic format. Charting can be done in a basic format or may include complex charts for periodontics and other specialty areas. This chart can even be e-mailed to another dentist for evaluation (Figure 5-20).

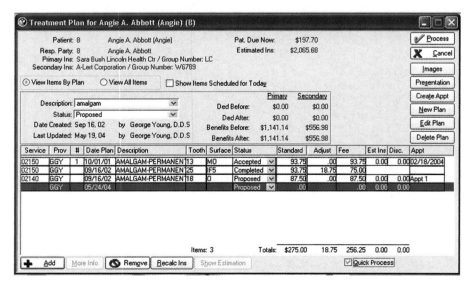

Figure 5-15 Treatment plan screen. (Courtesy Patterson-EagleSoft, Effingham, IL.)

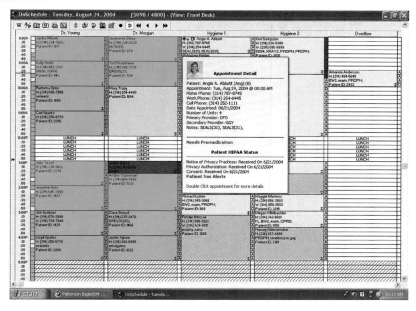

Figure 5-16 Daily appointment screen. (Courtesy Patterson-EagleSoft, Effingham, IL.)

Daily treatment room schedule: This includes the amount of time and type of treatment to be rendered.

Day sheet report: summarizes practice activity for a period of time (Figure 5-21).

Annual graphic reports: These are generated to illustrate categorical treatment production (Figure 5-22).

Appropriate selection of a software package is extremely important. For the software to be effective, the computer functions must be applicable to the specific dental practice. Stored data and information must be usable and easily accessible. The required applications should be presented to the vendor rather than asking the vendor what the dental practice should do. To be more specific, take a routine accounts receivable task and have the vendor

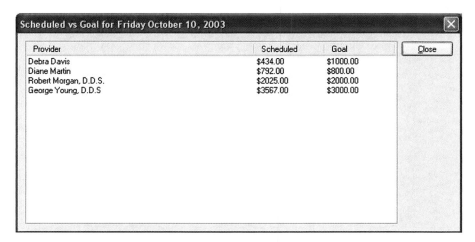

Figure 5-17 Schedule versus goal screen. (Courtesy Patterson-EagleSoft, Effingham, IL.)

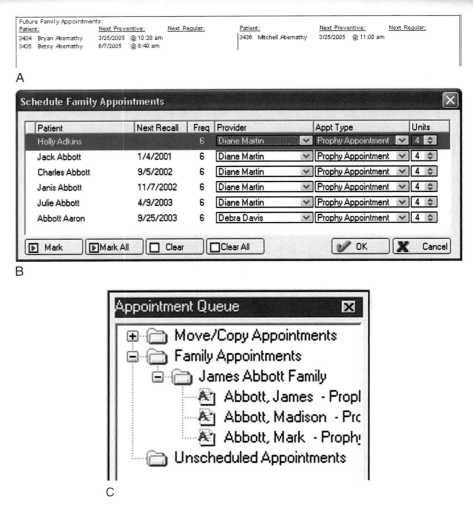

C

Figure 5-18, Family recall. **A,** Future dates of family member appointments. **B,** Next recall dates of each person in family group. **C,** Appointment query screen for a family. (Courtesy Patterson-EagleSoft, Effingham, IL.)

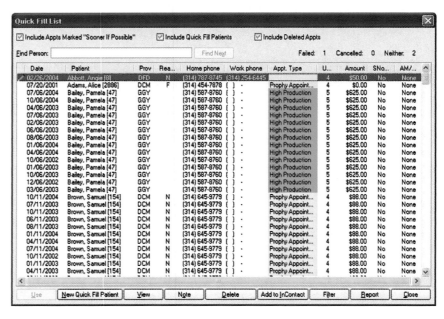

Figure 5-19 Tickler file. (Courtesy Patterson-EagleSoft, Effingham, IL.)

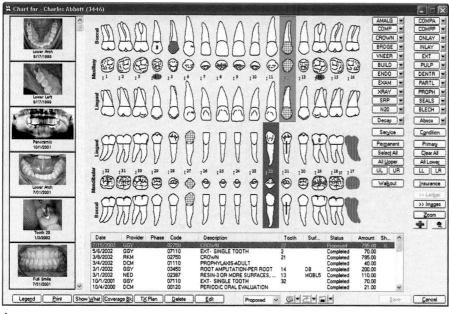

A

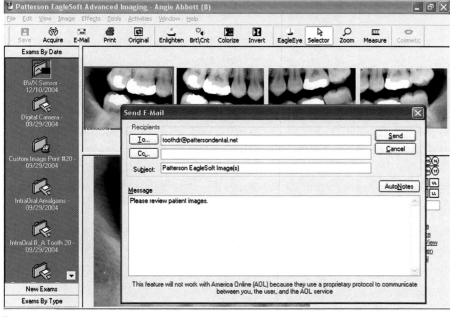

B

Figure 5-20 A, Presentation manager. **B,** Chart e-mail screen. (Courtesy Patterson-EagleSoft, Effingham, IL.)

explain how it would be processed with that company's equipment and software. Inquire how different procedures (e.g., billing, payments, appointment notification) can be combined. Another option is starting with basic software packages, such as insurance estimating and billing, and then adding appointment tracking, treatment planning, marketing, and payroll.

Select those functions of the software that will satisfy the most pressing needs first. For example, if an assistant is plagued with a backlog of insurance

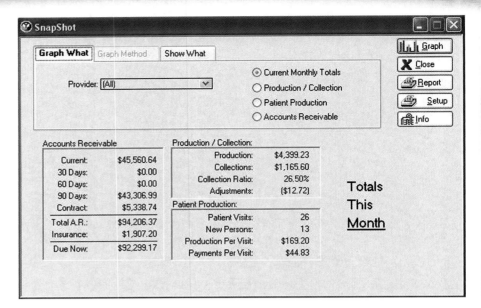

Figure 5-21 Summary of activities. (Courtesy Patterson-EagleSoft, Effingham, IL.)

claim forms, resulting in a serious cash flow problem, the software packages directly related to relieving this situation should be explored first.

The preceding text illustrates a sampling of dental software, all of which help to improve cash flow and increase productivity. The list goes on, however; the word processing function is also invaluable to the dental practice and can be integrated with the information system to improve communications with the patients. The computer, when used to produce welcome letters, treatment letters, and special greetings, can be a very effective marketing tool.

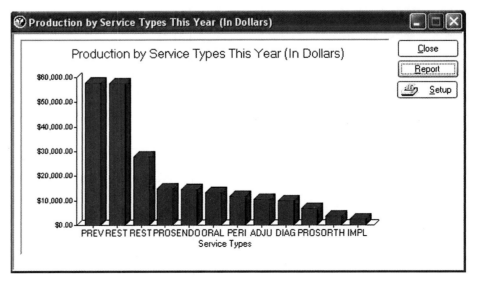

Figure 5-22 Provider production forecast by service. (Courtesy Patterson-EagleSoft, Effingham, IL.)

When using word processing software on the computer, the document is prepared electronically and the text is entered on the computer keyboard in the same manner as on a typewriter. As the text is entered, it is displayed on the screen (monitor) and stored in the computer's memory. This is an electronic format, and it is easy to edit a document by making changes in the text. Text can be corrected by using a backspace or delete key. Words, sentences, paragraphs, or pages may be added or deleted from a document. Text can be moved from one section to another. The document is formatted according to your specifications. For example, margins, type style, double or single spacing, underlining, boldface or italics, and page length are determined by the user. When the document is finalized and all corrections made, a command is made to have the document printed. You can have more than one copy printed, and each copy is an original. These documents are stored in the computer's memory, and can be used again in their original text or edited and brought up to date.

Many word processing packages include other features such as spell check, grammar check, and a thesaurus. Some spell-check software will enable you to add words common to your specific dental practice.

Word processing software can be a very productive tool for the dental practice and should be selected wisely. Box 5-6 lists common features of word processing software packages.

Software that has been written specifically for the dental office may include the capabilities of **electronic spreadsheet** calculations, database, and graphics. If these functions are not included but are needed, then additional commercial software packages may be another option.

An electronic spreadsheet software package allows the user to organize numeric data in a worksheet or table format. The user enters the data into the formula that has been typed in specific rows and columns, known as *cells*. As the data are entered into the proper cells, the electronic calculations are performed automatically. Daily postings and updates can be made very easily. An electronic spreadsheet's ability to recalculate data makes this an invaluable tool for business office management.

Database software allows the user to create electronic files that can be retrieved, manipulated, and updated as necessary. A database is a collection of data that is stored in multiple files. Database software features include (1) operations to create the database, copy, delete, and sort the data; (2) data editing and updating capabilities; (3) mathematical functions; and (4) the ability to retrieve data and produce a report. Such a software package is a valuable tool in an inventory control or recall system.

A graphics software package allows the user to create graphs from numeric data; this is sometimes part of the spreadsheet software package. The most common forms of graphics are pie charts, line diagrams charts, and bar charts (Figure 5-23). Graphs are good management tools for reviewing information and helping to communicate information more effectively. When using graphics in a presentation, select the type of graph that is most appropriate for your purpose. Don't try to present too much information, use few words, be consistent, and keep the graphics simple.

INTEGRATED APPLICATIONS

Electronic spreadsheet software and word processing are usually used independently of each other, but what if you wanted some of the information from the spreadsheet in a word processing document? Integrated software combines these applications into a single set of programs that allow the user to share data between applications.

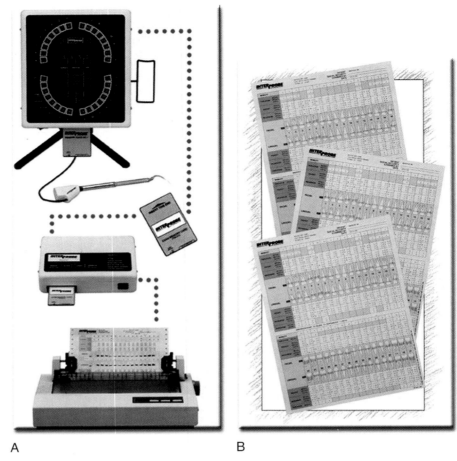

A   B

Figure 5-23 A, The Interprobe Periodontal Exam and Charting System provides highly accurate and repeatable periodontal measurements with superior charting capabilities. The system requires only a single operator and records, stores, and prints the examination automatically. **B,** Samples of the periodontal charts automatically produced by the Interprobe system. Objective measurements of pocket depth and gingival recession from the CEJ are ensured by the probe's constant 15-gram pressure. (Courtesy The Dental Probe, Inc., Glen Allen, VA.)

Clinical Records Applications

Although it may appear that the bulk of record management is generated only in the business office, one cannot overlook the computer as a communication tool between the treatment room and the business office. A variety of charting systems allows a clinical assistant to enter data directly on a keyboard at chairside, which then provides a printout in the business office. An example of this system is shown in the periodontal examination and charting system in Figure 5-23. Systems are available for patient histories, general and specialty charting, and treatment completed. Such a system also eliminates record contamination, because barrier covers may be placed over the keyboard and the chances of disease transmission through record management are decreased.

GUIDELINES FOR MAKING THE RIGHT SOFTWARE SELECTION. As stated previously, choosing the right software for the specific need of the dental practice can be difficult. The information in Box 5-7 should help.

Box 5-7
Guidelines for Choosing the Right Software

1. Determine the needs of the dental practice—type of practice, size of practice, ability of staff, cost, and training required for the doctor and support staff.
2. Select a vendor who is reputable and provides fast and efficient support when you have questions. Ask about other dental practices that use the system. How many systems have they installed within your geographic area? Are the insurance forms that are processed through the system accepted by participating insurance companies?
3. Know what you want the computer to do—process insurance claims, improve billing, improve practice management, improve office efficiency and auditing, track delinquent accounts, compute monthly finance charges, and aid in communications as a marketing device.
4. What type of backup does the system have in case of computer failure?
5. If security of information is a concern, how is it managed?
6. Know what type of training is available from the vendor. Systems are available that have tutorial software. This software uses a text and recorded instructions for the learner.
7. The computer and software selection process requires a great deal of thought and time, so make the selection carefully. Everyone will have to live with the decision that is made.

IMPLEMENTING THE CHANGE TO COMPUTERIZATION

To implement the applications on a computer and make the transition to the computerized system, a total team effort is necessary. The computer operation will affect all staff members, and they need to know how their individual jobs are affected.

Resistance to the use of computers can be expected if employees are not made aware of and involved in the change. Begin communicating with other staff members early in the planning stages. You will gain their cooperation and support if they are made aware of the computer system's advantages. The staff needs to know that the workload can be distributed to more than one individual, that it lessens tedious and repetitive work, that it produces higher-quality work, increases production, and helps cut office costs.

Establishing Procedures

Establishing procedures is necessary to make sure that work flows smoothly through the entire process—from origination to completion. A procedures manual for computer tasks is beneficial for all staff members. This manual provides detailed information about how various tasks are completed and by whom, as well as the purpose of each task.

Software manuals that are provided with the software should be carefully evaluated. If the documentation and instructions are difficult to follow and understand, the individual will not use the system properly and efficiently.

SUMMARY OF NEW TECHNOLOGY IN THE BUSINESS OFFICE

A computer's primary advantage is the accuracy and quality of its finished results, but without proper management and usage, the computer becomes a costly investment with poor returns. A well-planned information system will help make the office more efficient, and the combination of an experienced staff and high-technology equipment will result in higher productivity, better patient relations, and a happier staff.

LEARNING ACTIVITIES

1. Describe the importance of an information system to dentistry.
2. List and explain the operations a computer can perform.
3. Explain the difference between an impact and a nonimpact printer.
4. Describe how a feasibility study aids in determining the need for automation.
5. Describe computer software.
6. Explain the difference between general-task and specific-task software.
7. Describe how word processing, electronic spreadsheet, database, and graphics software can be used effectively in the dental office.
8. List six guidelines used in making the right software selection.
9. Explain why computer procedures are important when setting up a new computer system within the dental practice.
10. Select an activity such as recall management, accounts receivable, or letter writing and determine an approximate time saving that can be achieved from using the computer versus producing the end result in a traditional manual manner.

Key Terms

See Box 5-2.

Bibliography

Fulton PJ: *General office procedures for colleges*, ed 12, Cincinnati, 2003, South-Western Publishing Co.

Lavine L: Proper positioning of monitors, *Dental Economics*, November 2004.

Neilburger EJ: Computers: 10 rules for selecting a computer system, *Dental Economics*, 8:96, 1998.

Shelly GB et al: *Discovering computers 2006; a gateway to information*, Boston, 2005, Course Technology.

Shelly GB et al: *Discovering computers: fundamentals*, ed 2, Boston, 2005, Course Technology.

Office Design and Equipment Placement

Chapter Outline

Physical Environment
Office Design and the Americans with Disabilities Act
Seasonal Affective Disorder
Design of the Reception Room
Design of the Business Office
Principles of Time and Motion
Body Positioning
Health and Safety Issues
Selecting Office Supplies

Learning Outcomes

Mastery of the content in this chapter will enable the reader to:
- Define glossary terms
- Define ergonomics as it applies to the dental business office
- Describe classifications of motion
- Describe the implementation of time and motion in a dental business office
- Describe Seasonal Affective Disorder
- Explain the effect of the Americans with Disabilities Act on office design
- Identify criteria for reception room design
- Identify criteria for business office design
- Describe factors involved in office design that relate to the Americans with Disabilities Act
- Describe the arrangement of common business equipment

At some point in your career it is likely you will be asked to help design, remodel, or improve the efficiency of the dental business office. These responsibilities demand an understanding of the principles of motion economy and of the placement of office equipment to create an environment in which you can work smarter and not harder.

In the past, more emphasis was placed on the design of the dental treatment rooms than on the design of the business office. However, planning of the business office workspace is equally important. This area should be ergonomically designed so that the business staff can perform its tasks with the greatest efficiency. **Ergonomics** is the science that studies the relationship between people and their work environments. Interrelated physical and psychological factors are involved in the creation of a stress-free work environment. By understanding the abilities that people have and their work patterns, it is possible to design work environments that conform to the abilities and work needs of the employee. The appropriate use of ergonomics can make the job more productive and efficient and can reduce work-related discomfort and injuries.

> **Ergonomics** is the study of the effects of the work environment on health and well-being.

PHYSICAL ENVIRONMENT

Physiological factors include color, lighting, acoustics, heating and air conditioning, space, and furniture and equipment. Color plays a major role in how a patient perceives a practice and in the staff's health, productivity, and morale. An attractive, cheerful, and efficient office inspires confidence in the staff and comfort in the patient. A drab, dirty, or untidy office can create an attitude of doubt or mistrust. Light colors are more appealing than dark colors. Some decorators work with dark colors for walls but use lighter accent colors to downplay the dark base color. Grays are often used with tones of mauves. Certain tones of gray can be tiring, and they tend to put workers to sleep. Light hues of warm colors can create cheerful surroundings. Cool colors, such as light greens and blues, can produce a tranquil atmosphere.

> An attractive, cheerful, and efficient office inspires confidence in the staff and comfort in the patient.

Dental offices no longer need to present a stark, sterile image. Designers today are adding warmth and beauty to the office, while providing comfort and efficiency. A comfortable patient is a happier patient. Moreover, staff productivity is likely to be greater in a pleasant working environment. Many office plans are available; the one chosen should reflect the dentist's personality and satisfy the needs of the staff and patients.

Office Design and the Americans with Disabilities Act

For years patients have had difficulty gaining access to dental treatment rooms because of poorly designed offices. The Americans with Disabilities Act of 1990 has affected the design of dental offices in patient treatment. Special attention should be directed to this act to ensure that the office design complies with state and federal guidelines. The Justice Department issues accessibility specifications for offices, but some states have even stricter standards. Accessibility features must be incorporated into renovations of a building, and those features must be accessible from elsewhere in the building. For example, making a lobby bathroom accessible to a wheelchair patient is not adequate if the patient cannot get to the lobby. Box 6-1 presents a list of recommendations for designing a barrier-free office.

The government estimates that the cost of incorporating accessibility features into new construction is less than 1% of construction costs. Because remodeling existing buildings usually is more costly, the requirements for them are less stringent. Currently the law requires only "reasonable modifications" that are "readily achievable," both terms that may lead to litigation. Further information on any part of the Americans with Disabilities Act is available from the sources listed in Box 6-2. You may also visit the website at http://www.ada.gov or http://www.access-board.gov.

Box 6-1
Design Features of a Barrier-Free Office

The following modifications for creating a barrier-free environment comply with the Americans with Disabilities Act:
- Designate handicapped parking areas.
- Install sidewalk and curb access to accommodate wheelchairs or other devices.
- Install access ramps to building and office areas.
- Widen doors and doorways to accommodate wheelchairs and other devices.
- Install raised letters and Braille on elevator controls.
- Provide visual and sound alarms.
- Install grab bars.
- Install raised toilet seats and wider stalls.
- Make paper towel dispensers accessible.
- Install paper cup dispensers at existing water fountains.
- Eliminate plush, low-density carpeting.

Seasonal Affective Disorder

In geographic locations where there are extremes of sunshine and darkness, often patients or staff may be affected by Seasonal Affective Disorder (SAD). Sunlight serves to keep our body's internal "circadian" clock in sync, so a person is alert and awake in the day and ready to sleep at night. A person's health, mood, and behavior can be affected when the quality and quantity of sunlight is lessened. A direct consequence of SAD can be winter depression or sleep disorders.

There are many companies that provide lighting systems to overcome SAD. If staff members are affected by SAD, it may be worth the investment to increase the health of the staff. Most of the lights are designed for the brightness needed for light therapy. With a brightness level of 10,000 lux at 24 inches, these lights have been proven to be a fast and effective light therapy at a comfortable distance. Most lights are easy to use and safe (no harmful UV rays).

Box 6-2
Sources of Information on the Americans with Disabilities Act

Office of the Americans with Disabilities Act
U.S. Department of Justice
P.O. Box 66118
Washington, D.C. 20035-6738
1-800-514-0301 (voice)
1-800-514-0383 (TDD)
Internet website (ADA home page): http://www.ada.gov

Architectural and Transportation Barriers Compliance Board
1111 18th Street NW, Suite 501
Washington, D.C. 20036
1-800-872-2253 (voice)
1-800-993-2822 (TDD)
Electronic bulletin board: 202-272-5448
Internet website: http://www.access-board.gov

Design of the Reception Room

The **reception room** (the term waiting room has a negative connotation) is the gateway to the dental office and provides the patient's first impression of the dentist. A warm atmosphere can be created in the reception room, furnishing a comfortable, "living room" environment. The office should reflect the theme originating in the reception room (Figure 6-1, *A* and *B*).

Patients should be able to check in with the administrative assistant at the desk as soon as they arrive. For privacy, patients should have access to a restroom off the reception room, and appropriate signs should direct them to this area.

Seating in the reception room varies from office to office, depending on individual practice styles. A general rule is to provide two seats for each dental chair in a general practice. High-volume practices, such as orthodontics or pediatrics, will require three or four seats per dental chair, whereas an oral surgery or endodontic practice needs only one or two seats per chair.

Seating space is an important consideration. People generally do not like to have others sitting too close to them. When completing forms or other business activities, a person needs some privacy. Comfort should be the major concern when selecting furniture for this area. It needs to be sturdy but not too formal or too casual. Low, cushiony couches and armless chairs are sometimes difficult for even an agile person to get out of and even more difficult for an older adult or arthritic patient. Figure 6-2 illustrates comfortable armchairs with a sturdy base.

Special amenities are a thoughtful gesture, such as a desk-height table with an electrical outlet that makes it convenient for businesspeople or students to bring laptop computers to use while waiting. A self-serve coffee or juice bar is a considerate gesture toward busy patients. These amenities send a message that the dentist respects the patient's time and wants to make the office a friendly place to visit (Box 6-3).

> The reception room is the gateway to the dental office and provides the patient's first impression of the dentist.

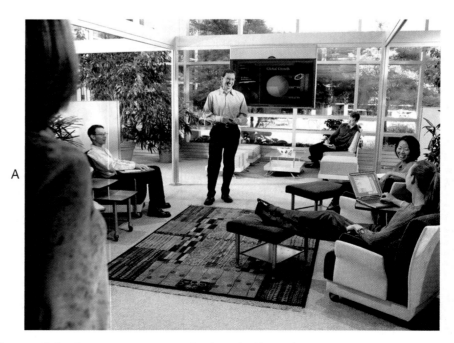

Figure 6-1 The reception room of a dental office reflects a theme. **A,** Full-length windows bring the outdoors into this reception room. (Courtesy Steelcase, Inc., Grand Rapids, MI.)

Continued

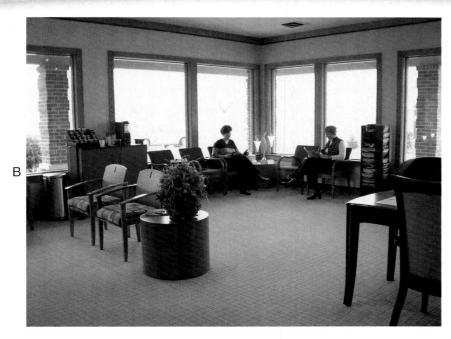

Figure 6-1, cont'd B, Open areas allow a patient personal space as well as work areas (Courtesy Dr. Neil Smith, Bridgman Family Dental Care, Bridgman, MI.)

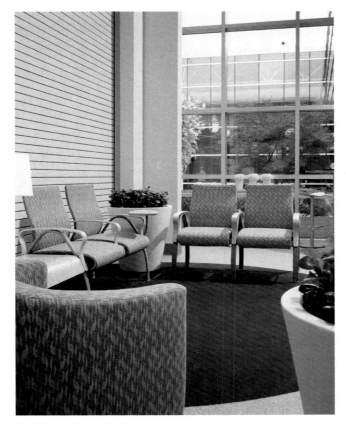

Figure 6-2 A reception room with comfortable chairs provides adequate seating space. (Courtesy Steelcase, Inc., Grand Rapids, MI.)

Box 6-3
Keys to Creating a Comfortable Reception Room

1. A soft warning bell or chimes should announce the patient's arrival in the reception area.
2. The patient's arrival should be acknowledged immediately. A clear glass window affords privacy, yet allows the administrative assistant to see all the activity in the reception room. When a window is used, it commonly is 44 inches from the floor and at least 36 by 36 inches. A barrier-free environment can be created with the open concept. A desk area for physically challenged patients is positioned 27 to 29 inches from the floor (Figure 6-3).
3. Coat racks should be convenient for both children and adults. A nearby bench benefits older adults, small children, and anyone putting on boots.
4. Magazine racks can be placed on a wall or table. They also should be convenient for both children and adults (Figure 6-4).
5. If necessary, a small children's corner can be included. In many specialty offices, such as orthodontics or pediatric dentistry, an office theme can be created.
6. The style and number of seats and tables depend on the patients' requirements. A combination of sofas and chairs also provides a comfortable seating arrangement. Chairs should be of a height and depth that afford easy seating and exiting.
7. An automatic air freshener eliminates "dental" odors, and cordial "no smoking" signs can be posted at the entrance and in the reception room.
8. An adjoining restroom eliminates trips to the inner office.
9. Wood paneling, fabric, textured wallpaper, antiques, live plants, artwork, and mirrors add warmth to the reception room and reflect the dentist's personality.
10. Signs directing patients to various rooms should be large and easy for all patients to read.
11. Lighting intensity and color should be adequate for easy reading of printed materials in any part of the room.

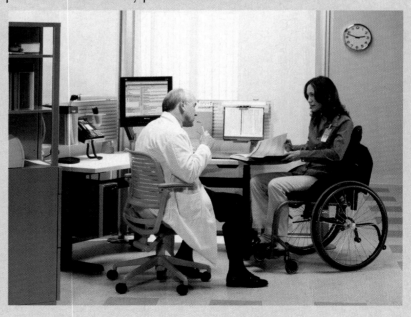

Figure 6-3 Countertops are situated for the convenience of physically challenged patients. (Courtesy Steelcase, Inc., Grand Rapids, MI.)

Box 6-3—cont'd

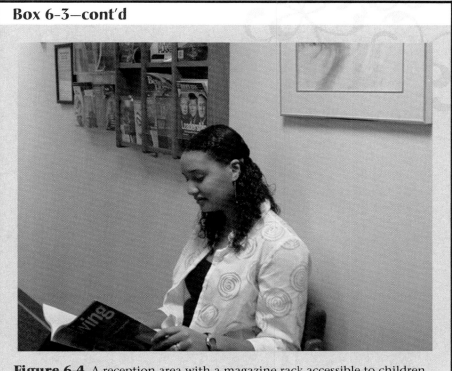

Figure 6-4 A reception area with a magazine rack accessible to children and adults. (Courtesy Ona Erdt, Ann Arbor, MI.)

Design of the Business Office

The business office work space should provide a healthful, enjoyable environment that minimizes disruption and distraction. The business office should be centrally located between the reception room and the dental treatment rooms. This central location is convenient for the patient and allows the administrative assistant to be aware of the activities in the office. Figure 6-5 illustrates three different floor plans that use a central location for the business office. The first two are examples of small dental offices; the third is a basic floor plan for a team concept that uses advanced functions dental staff. The factors involved in designing a business office work environment are motion economy, space planning, health issues, safety, and security. The following suggestions should be considered:

1. The administrative assistant should be seated facing the reception room.
2. Two desk heights ensure comfort and efficiency. The keyboard level should be approximately 27 inches, and the writing level about 29 inches (Figure 6-6). Twenty inches is an adequate depth for most working areas. A depth over 30 inches is excessive; it makes reaching inconvenient and reduces the amount of floor space in the office.
3. A counter approximately 44 inches high provides a writing area for patients and privacy for the assistant and for documents on the desk (Figure 6-7).
4. The business office clock should be out of view of patients in the reception room.
5. Central controls for an intercom system should be integrated with the telephone or mounted on the wall as a separate unit within easy reach

of the assistant (Figure 6-8). Auxiliary units should be connected with the private office, laboratory, and treatment rooms.

6. Master controls for the music system, heating, cooling, and lighting also should be located in the business office. Labeling these controls prevents accidental shutoff of any of the utilities.
7. Lateral or open files (Figure 6-9), at a depth of 18 inches, require less space than vertical files. These files are supplied in 30-, 36-, and 42-inch widths with two to five drawers.
8. Cupboard space is necessary for storage of paper and supplies.
9. Small compartmentalized areas above the desk provide easy access to items such as appointment cards and telephone message pads.
10. Telephones should be installed at each workstation and should be made hands free whenever possible.
11. Desk drawers should have full suspension for maximum use.

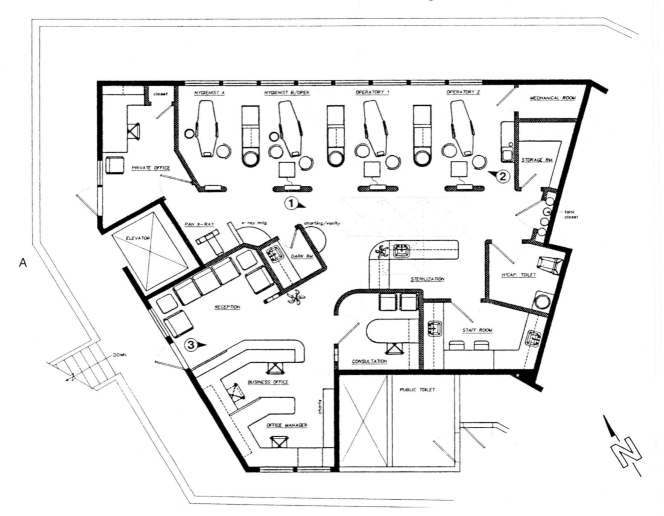

Figure 6-5 A, An irregularly shaped dental suite that uses the concept of openness. The isolating effect of doors between clinical and business areas is eliminated, yet modular dividers separate these areas and provide privacy for the patient. (Courtesy Design for Health, Mitchell Goldstein, Santa Cruz, CA.)

Continued

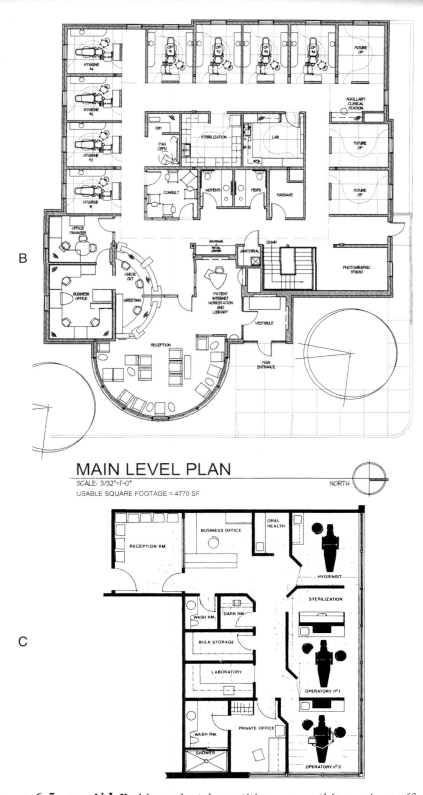

MAIN LEVEL PLAN

SCALE: 3/32"=1'-0"

USABLE SQUARE FOOTAGE = 4770 SF

NORTH

Figure 6-5, cont'd B, Many dental practitioners use this spacious office for patient and staff comfort. The office suite includes an open concept and multireception areas; it also provides patient privacy. (Courtesy *Dental Economics,* PennWell, Tulsa, OK.) **C,** A small office designed for efficiency and patient comfort includes all basic rooms and also provides openness. (Courtesy Health Science Products, Birmingham, AL www.hspinc.com 1-800-237-5794.)

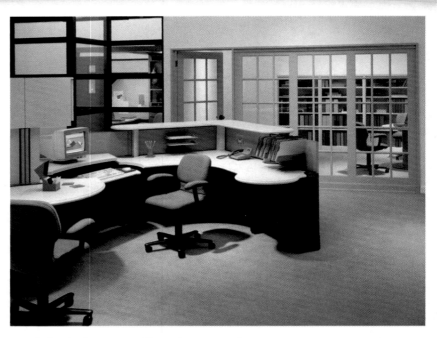

Figure 6-6 The business office adjacent to the reception room provides adequate desk space, sufficient lighting, a filing area, comfortable seating, and direct access to computer and telecommunication systems. (Courtesy Steelcase, Inc., Grand Rapids, MI.)

12. Inserts and dividers in drawers aid in organization of materials.
13. A small area adjacent to the business office set up for private calls and conversations with patients is convenient and can be used for completion of insurance forms.

Many of these criteria have been incorporated into the design of the business office shown in Figures 6-6 and 6-7.

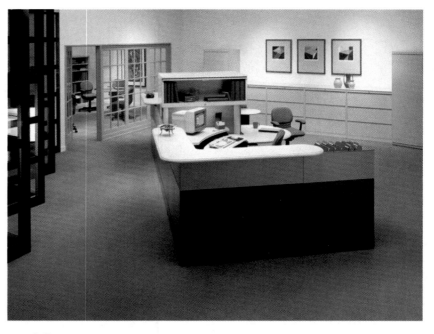

Figure 6-7 Counter space in the business office allows the patient a comfortable position for business transactions. (Courtesy Steelcase, Inc., Grand Rapids, MI.)

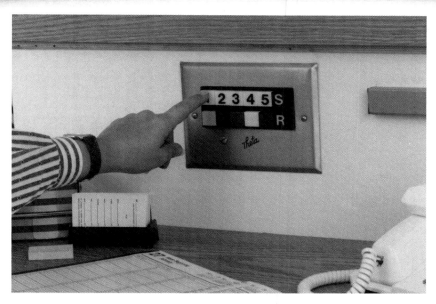

Figure 6-8 Wall-mounted non-verbal intercom system. (Courtesy Theta Corp., Niagara Falls, NY.)

PRINCIPLES OF TIME AND MOTION

When determining the placement of office equipment and supplies, the principles of time and motion should be considered. **Time and motion** refers to the amount of time and degree of motion required to perform a given task. This principle is as important in the business office as in the dental treatment rooms. Many studies and much research have gone into minimizing the amount of time and motion it takes to perform basic chairside tasks. However, these principles have not always been applied to the dental

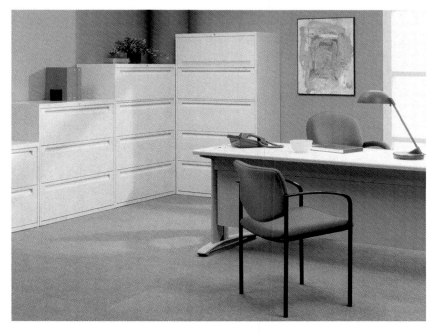

Figure 6-9 Lateral files. (Courtesy Steelcase, Inc., Grand Rapids, MI.)

> **Box 6-4**
> **Classifications of Motion**
>
> Class I: Fingers-only movement
> Class II: Fingers and wrist movement
> Class III: Fingers, wrist, and elbow movement
> Class IV: Fingers, wrist, elbow, and shoulder movement
> Class V: Arm extension and twisting of the torso

business office. Because the dentist seldom spends time in the business office, the staff's suggestions should be considered when designing the area. Before positioning equipment and supplies, staff members should determine the most common tasks and routinely used materials and should attempt to classify the motions used during those tasks.

In the early 1950s, researchers at the University of Alabama classified motions according to the amount of energy required to perform various chairside tasks. These classifications (Box 6-4) can also be applied to the business office. The administrative assistant should try to use only Class I, II and III motions, which require the least amount of energy and reduce stress.

To improve motion economy, it is often necessary to eliminate unnecessary steps or tasks, rearrange equipment and materials, organize procedures, simplify tasks, and evaluate the outcomes. The principles of motion economy (Box 6-5) can aid in accomplishing each of these goals, thereby reducing stress and increasing productivity in the practice.

BODY POSITIONING

The administrative assistant must consider proper seating arrangements during routine daily activities. When possible, all activities should be performed in a seated position to avoid undue stress on the neck, back, and legs. A chair with a broad base, four or five casters, and a well-padded seat and back support is helpful (Figure 6-10). Improper posture while standing or

> **Box 6-5**
> **Applying the Principles of Motion Economy in the Business Office**
>
> 1. Position materials as close to the point of use as possible.
> 2. Use motions that require the least amount of movement.
> 3. Minimize the number of materials to be used for a given procedure.
> 4. Use smooth, continuous motions, not zigzag motions.
> 5. Organize materials in a logical sequence of use.
> 6. Position materials and equipment in advance whenever possible.
> 7. Use ergonomically designed stools or chairs to provide good posture and body support.
> 8. Use body motions that require the least amount of time.
> 9. Minimize the number of eye movements.
> 10. Provide lighting that eliminates shadows in work areas.
> 11. Avoid abrupt contrasts in room lighting to minimize eyestrain.
> 12. Position computer monitors to allow for line of sight to screen within 10 to 40 degrees horizontal.
> 13. Provide work areas that are elbow level or 1 to 2 inches lower.

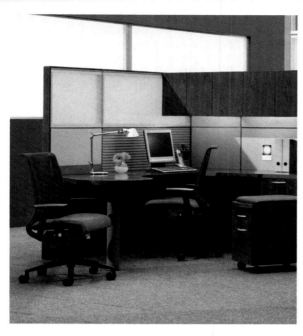

Figure 6-10 Ergonomically designed office chair: The Think™ Chair. (Courtesy Steelcase, Inc., Grand Rapids, MI.)

sitting can lead to fatigue, which in turn affects productivity. The suggestions presented in Box 6-6 can help ensure the greatest comfort and efficiency. Figure 6-11 illustrates proper seated posture while using a computer with a tabletop monitor.

An alternative position for the computer monitor is to recess it beneath the desk as shown in Figure 6-11, *B*. The schematic drawing in Figure 6-11, *C* illustrates the positioning of a person in an ergonomic chair using the recessed monitor.

Tilt and glare are both factors in monitor placement. When the recessed monitor position is used, it is necessary to follow the manufacturer's recommended position in order to avoid any neck problems. Two side benefits of recessed monitor placement are the elimination of the patient observing the monitor screen and additional space made available on the desktop.

Box 6-6
Ergonomically Correct Body Positioning

1. When a person is seated, the thighs should be parallel to the floor, the lower legs vertical, and the feet firmly on the floor.
2. When a person is using a keyboard, the arms should be positioned so that the forearms and wrists are as horizontal as possible.
3. The eye to computer screen distance should be 16 to 24 inches.
4. The keyboard should tilt 0 to 25 degrees.
5. The back and neck should be erect, and the upper arms perpendicular to the floor.
6. The buttocks should be well supported on the chair seat, which should be 16 to 19 inches from the floor.

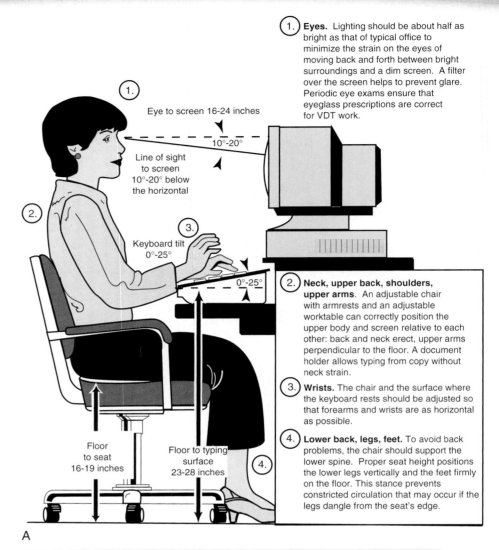

1. **Eyes.** Lighting should be about half as bright as that of typical office to minimize the strain on the eyes of moving back and forth between bright surroundings and a dim screen. A filter over the screen helps to prevent glare. Periodic eye exams ensure that eyeglass prescriptions are correct for VDT work.

Eye to screen 16-24 inches

10°-20°

Line of sight to screen 10°-20° below the horizontal

Keyboard tilt 0°-25°

0°-25°

2. **Neck, upper back, shoulders, upper arms.** An adjustable chair with armrests and an adjustable worktable can correctly position the upper body and screen relative to each other: back and neck erect, upper arms perpendicular to the floor. A document holder allows typing from copy without neck strain.

3. **Wrists.** The chair and the surface where the keyboard rests should be adjusted so that forearms and wrists are as horizontal as possible.

4. **Lower back, legs, feet.** To avoid back problems, the chair should support the lower spine. Proper seat height positions the lower legs vertically and the feet firmly on the floor. This stance prevents constricted circulation that may occur if the legs dangle from the seat's edge.

Floor to seat 16-19 inches

Floor to typing surface 23-28 inches

A

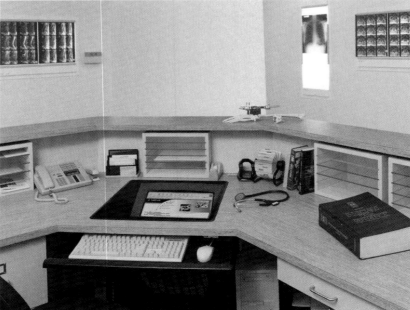

B

Figure 6-11 **A,** Posture and positioning in relation to equipment promotes high-level productivity. **B,** Recessed monitor provides ergonomic positioning and increased work surface on the desk. (Courtesy Nova Solutions, Inc., Effingham, IL.)

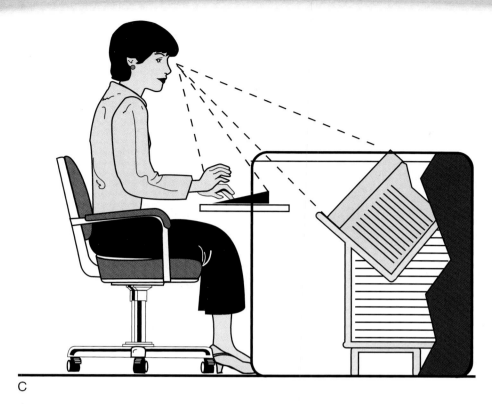

C

Figure 6-11, cont'd C, A schematic illustrates the ergonomic position of an operator using a Nova Station.

Persons who have used this system often wonder why they have always used the desktop monitor. For further information on this system, refer to the website for Nova Desks later in this chapter. Refer to Box 6-6 for recommendations for desk height and foot clearance using any of these systems. Much of the success of an office may be attributed to its efficiency and productivity without loss or waste. Again, the goal in ergonomic body positioning should be to work smarter and not harder.

Health and Safety Issues

A variety of factors can affect the health and safety of business office personnel. For example, spending hours each day looking at a computer screen can result in eyestrain and fatigue. Repetitive keyboarding can lead to wrist discomfort and possibly carpal tunnel syndrome, although use of an ergonomically designed keyboard (Figure 6-12) can help reduce this stress. The following tips can help reduce fatigue and eyestrain when working at a computer:
- Make sure the screen is neither too dark nor too bright.
- If you are using the computer continuously, take a 10- to 15-minute break every two or three hours.
- Use good posture.
- Stand up every half hour.
- Periodically look away from the screen for a few minutes.
- Use an ergonomically designed mouse, such as a track ball.
- Use an ergonomically designed chair.
- Consider a recessed monitor system.
  Safety hazards can exist in the dental business office. In 1970 the Occupational Safety and Health Act was passed to ensure that workers in

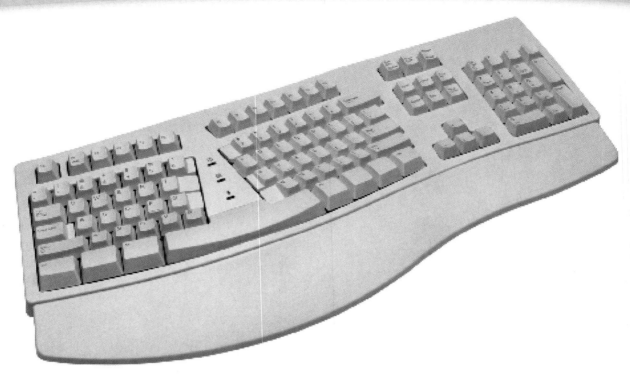

Figure 6-12 An ergonomic keyboard.

the United States have a safe working environment. Much has been discussed in terms of the relation of this act to the dental treatment room, but often the impact on the business area is overlooked. The Occupational Safety and Health Administration (OSHA) requires employers to provide a hazard-free work environment, that is, one without recognized dangers that can cause death, injury, or illness. Box 6-7 presents a list of hazards that might be found in business offices. Of course, in dental and medical offices, this list is compounded by the possibility of disease transmission (see Chapter 17). The lists in Boxes 6-7 and 6-8 can be used periodically to check for possible hazards.

Box 6-7
Potential Hazards

- Frayed or loose telephone cords or electrical wires
- Wires loosely secured to the floor
- Improperly grounded wall or floor switches
- Use of improper electric current to electronic equipment
- Spilled beverages or food on the floor
- Paper cutters, knives, or spindle files
- Loose floor covering on the stairs or floor
- Wearing of jewelry that can be caught in electronic equipment such as copiers
- Open files or drawers

Box 6-8
Hazard Checklist

The following points should be evaluated routinely to ensure that safety measures have been observed:
- Floor coverings are durable and in good repair.
- Floor surfaces in clinical areas are hard and uncarpeted.
- Antislip protection is available on smooth floor surfaces.
- Electrical equipment and cords are in safe operating condition.
- Employees have been trained in proper operation of equipment.
- Only one drawer of a file cabinet is opened at a time.
- Office furniture has no sharp edges but does have stable arms and legs.
- The locations of eyewash areas are posted in laboratory and clinical areas.
- First aid kits are well stocked and readily accessible.
- "No smoking" signs are posted in visible locations.
- All guidelines on infection control from the Occupational Safety and Health Administration (OSHA) are followed and are posted in visible locations.
- Hazard information is posted and available for all employees.

SELECTING OFFICE SUPPLIES

When first setting up a business office, determining what supplies will be needed may be an overwhelming task. Many dental suppliers assist in stocking the clinical area, but they seldom consider the "nuts and bolts" of the business office. Box 6-9 presents a basic list of the various forms and office supplies needed in a dental business office. Most office supply companies can assist you, and a variety of stationery suppliers can provide samples of stationery and forms. A walk through your favorite office supply discount store can be fascinating, but buy only the supplies most needed, not one of everything available.

Box 6-9
Basic Office Supplies

General Supplies
    Ballpoint pens
    Calendar and calendar holder
    Clear tape and tape dispenser
    Erasers
    Felt-tip markers
    Hole puncher; three-hole puncher
    Letter opener
    Masking tape
    Paper clips (small and large)
    Pen holder
    Pencil sharpener
    Pencil tray
    Pens and pencils
    Rubber bands
    Rubber stamps and pad

Continued

Box 6-9
Basic Office Supplies—Cont'd

Scissors
Stapler, staples, staple remover
Utility tray (for paper clips, pens, pencils, and other small items)
Wastebasket

Paper Supplies
Adhesive notes
Assorted envelopes (e.g., coin and large mailing envelopes)
Business cards
Copy paper (assorted sizes)
Drug reference
Fax paper
File folders
File folder labels
File guides
Index cards
Index tabs
Letterhead (second sheets)
Letterhead and envelopes
Medical and dental dictionaries
Message reply forms
Note pads
Plain white paper
Preprinted office forms
Report covers
Ring binders
Ruled letter- and legal-size writing pads
Standard dictionary
Storage cartons
Telephone message pads

Appointment Management Supplies
Appointment book (optional if not computerized)
Appointment cards
Appointment schedule forms (optional if not computerized)
Replacement sheets for appointment book (optional if not computerized)
Work or school excuse forms

Clinical Forms
Clinical charts
Colored filing labels
Consent forms
File guides
Health alert labels
Health questionnaire forms
Laboratory requisition forms
Patient file envelopes and folders
Prescription pads
Referral forms
Registration forms
Update forms
OSHA reporting forms
Safety management forms

Continued

Box 6-9
Basic Office Supplies—Cont'd

Financial Record Forms
   Application for Employer Identification Number (SS-4)
   Bank deposit slips
   Bookkeeping forms (optional if not computerized)
   Checkbook and replacement checks
   Citizenship Eligibility Form (I-9)
   Employee's Withholding Allowance Certificate Form (W-4)
   Employer's quarterly tax return form (941)
   Employer's annual federal unemployment tax return form (940)
   Insurance claim forms
   Ledger cards and forms (optional if not computerized)
   Payroll forms
   Statements
   Transmittal of income and tax statements form (W-3)
   Wage and tax statement form (W-2)
Microcomputer Supplies
   Disks
   Cleaning materials
   Disk cases
   Disk labels
   Disk mailers
   Mouse pad
   Printer ribbon
   Toner cartridges

When available, ergonomically designed supplies and materials should be purchased.

Key Terms

Classifications of motion system
Refers to the amount of energy it takes
to perform various tasks.

Ergonomics The science that studies
the relationship between people and
their work environment.

Reception room This room is the
gateway to the dental office and provides
the patient's first impression of the dentist.

Time and motion Refers to the
amount of time and the extent of
motion it takes to perform a given task.

LEARNING ACTIVITIES

1. List eight suggestions for the design of a reception room.
2. Discuss 10 factors to consider when designing a business office.
3. Describe the impact of the Americans with Disabilities Act on a dental practice.
4. Describe the concept of time and motion as it applies to a dental business office.
5. Using equipment suggested from the previous chapter and suggestions for office
   design from this chapter, develop an office design that might be used for a typical
   dental practice in your geographic area. Consider the latest electronic equipment,
   and include suggestions for color and texture of flooring, walls, and lighting.

Bibliography

BIFMA Ergonomics guideline, Nova, Effingham, IL, http://www.novadesk.com.
Fulton PJ: *General office procedures for colleges,* ed 12, Cincinnati, 2003, South-Western.
Levin R, Blaes J: Dental practice of the year, *Dental Economics,* June 1999.

Recommended Websites

http://www.access-board.gov
http://www.ada.gov
http://sad.com
http://www.novadesk.com

Communication Management

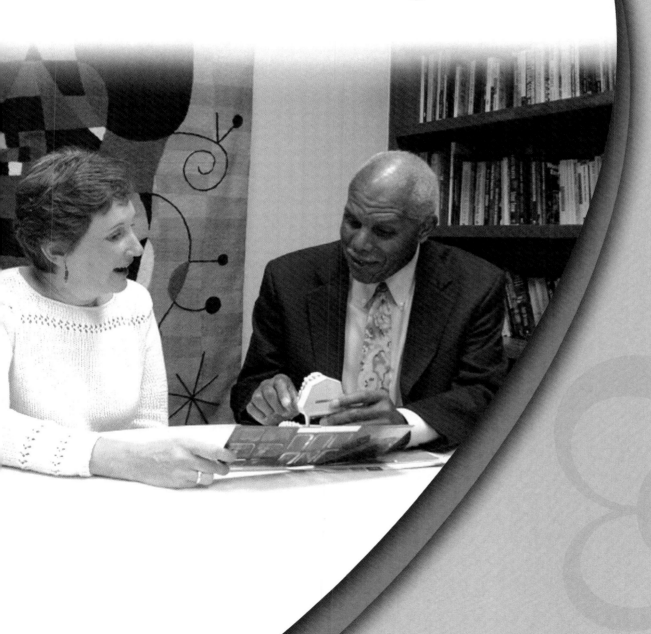

Chapter Outline

Learning Outcomes

Mastery of the content in this chapter will enable the reader to:

- Define key terms
- Define HIPAA
- Describe how to implement HIPAA regulations in the dental office record management system
- Identify the types of records maintained in a dental office
- Categorize the various types of records
- Distinguish between active and inactive records
- List the components of a clinical record
- Describe the function of the components of a clinical record
- Explain the rules for data entry on patient records
- Explain the use of symbols and abbreviations in clinical records
- List the components of patient financial records
- Identify various types of records required by the Occupational Safety and Health Administration (OSHA) that must be maintained in a dental office
- Identify the various types of employee records
- Explain the importance of maintaining accurate records
- Describe methods of records retention and transfer

Every dental professional dreams of a paperless office. However, when reality strikes, one generally concludes that it is not possible to achieve this longed-for dream. The dental office is inundated with a plethora of records and forms, all needed as part of the total dental business practice. Maintaining complete and accurate documents is an important part of successful management of a dental practice. The administrative assistant is required to maintain clinical, financial, employee, state, and federal records. Failure to perform any of these tasks can be a costly experience for the dental practitioner. Therefore, the administrative assistant who can pay routine special attention to detail in maintaining all types of records becomes an immeasurable asset to the dental practice.

HEALTH INSURANCE PORTABILITY AND ACCOUNTABILITY ACT

The Health Insurance Portability and Accountability Act (HIPAA) of 1996, which became effective in April 2003, has impacted the dental profession.

Administrative Simplification provisions of the **Health Insurance Portability and Accountability Act of 1996 (HIPAA)** have affected the dental profession. These provisions require national standards for electronic healthcare transactions. Dentists who transmit health information in an electronic transaction are required to use a standard format. Plans and providers who do not use electronic standards can use the Employee Retirement Security Act (ERISA) healthcare clearinghouse to comply with the requirement. Providers' paper transactions are not subject to this requirement. Primarily, the most affected area in the dental office is the area of transmission of dental claim forms, which are reviewed in Chapter 14. However, as one begins to study the management of patient records, the impact of privacy is one of primary concern.

HIPAA laws may seem daunting at first. However, when you realize that the purpose is to protect and enhance patient rights, it becomes a positive action since everyone is a patient at one time or another. Protecting health information is the right thing to do, and it promotes safe practice for everyone on the dental team, especially the patient. It is also good risk management, helping each dental professional to prevent potential litigation. Security regulations, which the Department of Health and Human Services released under HIPAA, were conceived to protect electronic patient health information. Protected patient health information is anything that ties a patient's name or Social Security number to that person's health, healthcare, or payment for healthcare, such as radiographs, charts, or invoices. Each dental professional should become familiar with state as well as federal laws as these laws are often more stringent than federal laws.

The American Dental Association (ADA) and most state dental associations have done an excellent job of preparing its members for the implementation of HIPAA. The ADA and many dental office stationers provide a HIPAA Security Tool Kit for Medical Practices™, as shown in Figure 7-1. This kit contains most of the forms needed for privacy practices, including the following:

The Notice of Privacy Practices form (Figure 7-2) presents information that the dental professional is required to give patients regarding the office's privacy practices. This form may need to be changed to reflect the dental practice's particular privacy polices or stricter state laws. The name of the practice should be on the notice, and it must be given to each patient at the date of the first service. In addition, the notice should be posted in a clear and prominent location in the office that is visible to any patient seeking service.

Acknowledgement of Receipt of Notice of Privacy Practices (Figure 7-3) is the form the patient signs to acknowledge that he or she has received a copy

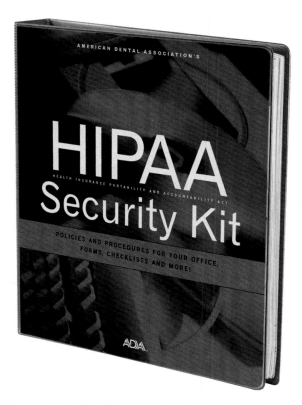

Figure 7-1 HIPAA Security Kit. (Courtesy American Dental Association, Chicago, IL.)

DENTAL ASSOCIATES, PC
Joseph W. Lake, DDS – Ashley M. Lake, DDS
611 Main Street, SE
Grand Rapids, MI 49502
(616) 101-9575

Privacy Officer: Mary Smith, Office Manager   **Effective Date:** November 15, 2002

Notice of Privacy Practices
This Notice describes how medical information about you may be used and disclosed and how you can get access to this information. Please review it carefully.

We care about our patients' privacy and strive to protect the confidentiality of your medical information at this practice. New federal legislation requires that we issue this official notice of our privacy practices. You have the right to the confidentiality of your medical information, and this practice is required by law to maintain the privacy of that protected health information. This practice is required to abide by the terms of the Notice of Privacy Practices currently in effect, and to provide notice of its legal duties and privacy practices with respect to protected health information. If you have any questions about this Notice, please contact the Privacy Officer at this practice.

Who Will Follow This Notice
Any health care professional authorized to enter information into your medical record, all employees, staff and other personnel at this practice who may need access to your information must abide by this Notice. All subsidiaries, business associates (e.g. a billing service), sites and locations of this practice may share medical information with each other for treatment, payment purposes or health care operations described in this Notice. Except where treatment is involved, only the minimum necessary information needed to accomplish the task will be shared.

How We May Use and Disclose Medical Information About You
The following categories describe different ways that we may use and disclose medical information without your specific consent or authorization. Examples are provided for each category of uses or disclosures. Not every possible use or disclosure in a category is listed.

For Treatment. We may use medical information about you to provide you with medical treatment or services. Example: In treating you for a specific condition, we may need to know if you have allergies that could influence which medications we prescribe for the treatment process.

For Payment. We may use and disclose medical information about you so that the treatment and services you receive from us may be billed and payment may be collected from you, an insurance company or a third party. Example: We may need to send your protected health information, such as your name, address, office visit date, and codes identifying your diagnosis and treatment to your insurance company for payment.

For Health Care Operations. We may use and disclose medical information about you for health care operations to assure that you receive quality care. Example: We may use medical information to review our treatment and services and evaluate the performance of our staff in caring for you.

Other Uses or Disclosures That Can Be Made Without Consent or Authorization
* As required during an investigation by law enforcement agencies
* To avert a serious threat to public health or safety
* As required by military command authorities for their medical records
* To workers' compensation or similar programs for processing of claims
* In response to a legal proceeding
* To a coroner or medical examiner for identification of a body
* If an inmate, to the correctional institution or law enforcement official
* As required by the US Food and Drug Administration (FDA)
* Other healthcare providers' treatment activities
* Other covered entities' and providers' payment activities
* Other covered entities' healthcare operations activities (to the extent permitted under HIPAA)
* Uses and disclosures required by law
* Uses and disclosures in domestic violence or neglect situations
* Health oversight activities
* Other public health activities

We may contact you to provide appointment reminders or information about treatment alternatives or other health-related benefits and services that may be of interest to you.

(over)

Figure 7-2 Notice of Privacy Practices form. (Courtesy American Dental Association, Chicago, IL.)

DENTAL ASSOCIATES, PC
Joseph W. Lake, DDS – Ashley M. Lake, DDS
611 Main Street, SE
Grand Rapids, MI 49502
(616) 101-9575

Notice of Privacy Practices
Patient Acknowledgement

Patient Name: _____ Date of Birth: _____

I have received and understand this practice's Notice of Privacy Practices written in plain language. The notice provides in detail the uses and disclosures of my protected health information that may be made by this practice, my individual rights and the practice's legal duties with respect to my protected health information. This includes, but is not limited to:

- A statement that this practice is required by law to maintain the privacy of protected health information.
- A statement that this practice is required to abide by the terms of the notice currently in effect.
- Types of uses and disclosures that this practice is permitted to make for each of the following purposes: treatment, payment, and health care operations.
- A description of each of the other purposes for which this practice is permitted or required to use or disclose protected health information without my written consent or authorization.
- A description of uses and disclosures that are prohibited or materially limited by law.
- A description of other uses and disclosures that will be made only with my written authorization and that I may revoke such authorization.
- My individual rights with respect to protected health information and a brief description of how I may exercise these rights in relation to:
  - The right to complain to this practice and to the Secretary of HHS if I believe my privacy rights have been violated, and that no retaliatory actions will be used against me in the event of such a complaint.
  - The right to request restrictions on certain uses and disclosures of my protected health information, and that this practice is not required to agree to a requested restriction.
  - The right to receive confidential communications of protected health information.
  - The right to inspect and copy protected health information.
  - The right to amend protected health information.
  - The right to receive an accounting of disclosures of protected health information.
  - The right to obtain a paper copy of the Notice of Privacy Practices from this practice upon request.

This practice reserves the right to change the terms of its Notice of Privacy Practices and to make new provisions effective for all protected health information that it maintains. If changes occur, this practice will proved me a revised Notice of Privacy Practices upon request.

Signature: _____ Date: _____

Relationship to patient (if signed by a personal representative of patient): _____

Figure 7-3 Acknowledgement of Receipt of Notice of Privacy Practices. (Courtesy SYCOM, Madison, WI.)

of the Notice of Privacy Practices. If the patient refuses to sign the form, the administrative assistant can indicate that an attempt was made to have the patient sign in the *in-office* section on the form. The patient may also opt to sign a separate refusal form that may then be placed in the record.

Business Associate Contract Terms is a contract form that satisfies the obligation under the HIPAA and its implementing regulations issued by the U.S. Department of Health and Human Services. This form ensures the integrity and confidentiality of protected health information that a business associate may create or receive for or from the dental practice. Other forms such as the Health Information Access-Response/Delay, Complaint, and Staff Review of Policies and Procedures, are available in the ADA manual or from the state dental society.

In order to ensure that records are maintained for patients, a preprinted chart divider provides a permanent record of important HIPAA information for patient files (Figure 7-4).

RECORDS MANAGEMENT

A dental office operates on information; it is created, processed, stored, printed, and distributed in many forms to various sites. Therefore, the dental administrative assistant must establish a logical, functional system for storing and retrieving information. This process is known as **records management** or **information management**. Records have a life cycle, which begins with inception and ends with disposition (Figure 7-5). The life cycle proceeds as follows:

> Records have a life cycle that begins with inception and ends with disposition.

1. Creation. This is the origination of the data. In the case of a patient record, creation begins with the completion of a patient registration form and health questionnaire. At the time of creation, a decision is made as to what information must be retained and the format of the record. If the patient is to continue treatment with the office, a permanent record usually is started on paper or the data are entered into the computer. If the person is a transient patient, the form for recording the data may be different from the standard form, and the record may not be stored with the active clinical charts.

2. Distribution. In this stage, the information may be distributed manually or electronically. It includes sending the patient's clinical record to the dentist for diagnosis once the record has been completed.

3. Use. The dentist evaluates the data and makes a diagnosis or refers the data to an appropriate location for maintenance.

4. Maintenance. This stage of the cycle involves determining if the data or information should be retained. If it is to be retained, the administrative assistant must decide the best way to store it for easy retrieval and how long it should be stored. If the patient is to be seen again and become a patient of record, the clinical record is filed alphabetically either electronically or in a file folder and envelope in a protected file. Some components of the record, such as notes the dentist may have made during evaluation, probably could be destroyed and only the pertinent data kept.

5. Disposition. At this stage, it must be determined if the record should be destroyed because it no longer has value to the office or if it should be stored permanently as an important document. The clinical record is vital and must be retained for a period consistent with the state statute of limitations. Electronic data can be transferred to disks for storage. Paper records, which have no backup, must be kept in a safe, dry area.

DENTAL ASSOCIATES, PC

Joseph W. Lake, DDS – Ashley M. Lake, DDS
611 Main Street, SE
Grand Rapids, MI 49502
(616) 101-9575

Patient Disclosure Authorization Form

Patient Name: _____   Date of Birth: _____

I authorize disclosure of my protected health information only in the specific manner, for the named reason, and to the specific individual(s) described below.

Specific description of information to be used or disclosed:

_____

_____

_____
(use additional sheet if necessary)

Reason for requested use or disclosure:

_____

_____

_____
(use additional sheet if necessary)

Name of the person or entity at this practice authorized to disclose my information:

_____

Name of the person or entity to whom this practice will give my information:

_____

This authorization will expire on the following:

☐ Date: _____

☐ Event (relating to patient or the purpose of the disclosure): _____

This authorization provides that:
- I may revoke this authorization at any time, provided that the revocation is in writing to the Privacy Officer at this practice, except if this practice has taken action relying on this consent or if the authorization was obtained as a condition of obtaining insurance coverage.
- Information used or disclosed pursuant to this authorization may be subject to redisclosure by the recipient and no longer be protected by HIPAA privacy rules.
- This practice will not condition treatment, payment, enrollment in a health plan, or eligibility for benefits on my providing authorization for the requested use or disclosure.
- I have the right to access my protected health information to be used or disclosed.
- I will receive a copy of this completed and signed authorization form.

Signature: _____   Date: _____

Relationship to patient (if signed by a personal representative of patient): _____

Figure 7-4 Preprinted HIPAA Record of Disclosures forms for patient charts. (Courtesy SYCOM, Madison, WI.)

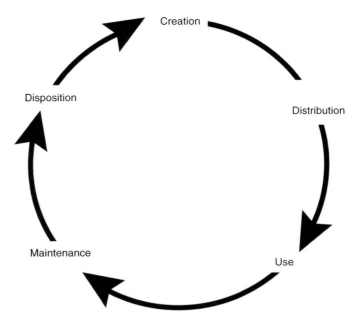

Figure 7-5 Life cycle of a record.

CATEGORIES OF RECORDS

As the administrative assistant, you must decide which records to keep, how to organize and store them, how long they legally must be retained, and when to dispose of them. In general, records can be categorized as *vital, important, useful,* or *unimportant,* and as *active* or *inactive.*

Vital Records

Vital records are essential documents that cannot be replaced. These include patient clinical and financial records and the office's corporate charter and deed, mortgage, or bill of sale. These records should be kept in a fireproof theft-proof vault or safe, and copies often are kept in a protected, off-site location.

> Vital records are essential documents that cannot be replaced.

Important Records

Important records are extremely valuable to the operation of the office, but they are not vital. They include accounts payable and receivable, invoices, canceled checks, inventory and payroll records, and other federal regulatory records. Such records may be needed for a tax audit or if a question arises about a financial transaction. Important records generally should be retained for five to seven years. Most offices keep them for about seven years or in accordance with federal or state regulations.

Useful Records

Useful records include employment applications, expired insurance policies, petty cash vouchers, bank reconciliations, and general correspondence. This category is difficult to define, because one office may consider a document useful, whereas another might find it indispensable. These records usually are retained for one to three years. Before discarding a document, it is always wise to check with the dentist or other staff members to see if it is still needed.

Unimportant Records

Unimportant records are the documents that lie around, have little importance, and take up space. They include such items as notes to you, reminders of meetings, outdated announcements, and pamphlets. Common sense dictates when these materials may be discarded.

TYPES OF PATIENT RECORDS

Patient records generally fall into two categories, clinical and financial. A recall system is another type of record that is retained separate from the clinical chart but which could be considered a type of clinical record. Clinical records are reviewed in this chapter; financial records are discussed in Chapter 15.

Clinical Record

The **clinical record** is a collection of all the information about the patient's dental treatment. Although each patient's clinical record is used during dental treatment, updating and maintaining this record is the administrative assistant's responsibility. Success in maintaining clinical records requires cooperation and efficiency from each member of the dental healthcare team.

Accurate clinical records are vital for several reasons:

1. In treatment of the patient, clinical records serve as a road map. They contain the patient's history and outline future treatment.
2. In a malpractice suit, the dental record is legally admissible as evidence. It can be used for or against the dentist.
3. In third-party payment plans, the dental consultants representing the carrier may review the clinical chart and other parts of the clinical record to determine if services have been rendered adequately.
4. The record acts as verification of treatment rendered for Internal Revenue Service purposes.
5. Components of the clinical records are vital in forensic odontology, the field of dentistry concerned with identification of individuals based on dental evidence.

A patient's clinical record commonly has the following components:
- Patient file envelope or folder
- Registration form
- Health questionnaire and update forms
- HIPAA acknowledgment form
- Clinical chart
- Consultation and referral reports
- Dental diagnosis, treatment plan, and estimate sheet
- Medication history and prescription forms
- Laboratory requisitions
- Consent forms
- Letters
- Postal receipts
- Treatment record/progress notes
- Radiographs
- Copies of laboratory tests

Bulkier materials, such as diagnostic models, generally are stored in an area other than the business office. A cross-reference on the patient record makes these materials easier to locate. Although the dentist chooses the components of the clinical record, staff members' opinions are important when selecting the forms because the staff members must maintain them. With more dental practices moving toward computerized systems, patient

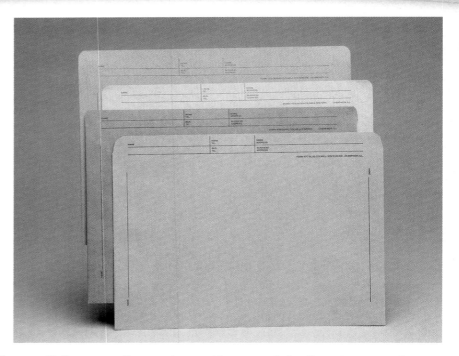

Figure 7-6 Patient file envelopes. (Courtesy Colwell, a Division of Patterson Companies, Inc., Champaign, IL.)

records and files are changing. More of the data will be stored in the computer, and the need for paper copies of these documents will decline.

PATIENT FILE ENVELOPE OR FOLDER. In most dental practices, use of an 8½-by-11-inch file envelope or folder guards against misplacement of records. In practices in which patients are seen by the dentist only or do not return on a regular basis, such as in an oral surgeon's office, a smaller envelope (5 by 8 inches) may be desirable, or the envelope may be eliminated. File envelopes may be plain or color-coded. They are supplied in a preprinted format with spaces for patient information including the patient's name, address, and telephone number (Figure 7-6). This type of envelope is widely used and satisfies the needs of many practices.

Another very common type of storage for patient records is an end-tab file folder with one or two two-hole fasteners (Figure 7-7, *A* and *B*). This type of folder requires the use of vertical-style records. The folders generally have a reinforced tab for easy label placement. They also are precut for quick insertion of a two-hole file fastener. Options include folders with pockets and diagonal cuts and expandable folders. Other auxiliary aids for these records include the hole punch, perm-clip fasteners, and polyvinyl pockets to hold small materials such as radiographs and CDs (Fig. 7-7, *C* to *E*).

Whether folders or envelopes are used, some form of color-coding is necessary to make sorting, storing, and retrieval easier. Color-coding can be done as an alphabetical system or, in a group practice, can be categorized by dentist. In addition to the traditional label (Figure 7-8), either an alpha or numeric label system can be used to sort the records. Year aging labels can be used to identify inactive patient records that may need to be purged from the active storage system (Figure 7-9). In Figure 7-9, *B*, the letters *MA* are the first two letters of the patient's last name, and *E* is the first letter of the patient's first name. The two-digit number indicates the year of the patient's last visit to the office.

PATIENT REGISTRATION FORM AND HEALTH HISTORY FORM. Although they are often combined, these two forms contain two different types of data. They should be retained because they provide more detailed information about the patient.

The patient **registration form** contains general information such as addresses and telephone numbers, as well as employment and insurance information. Figure 7-10 presents two common types of registration forms. This form enables the staff members to become better acquainted with the patient and can provide information for third-party payments and credit checks. Incomplete information on this form can complicate account collection later. Experienced business managers know that an account properly opened is half collected.

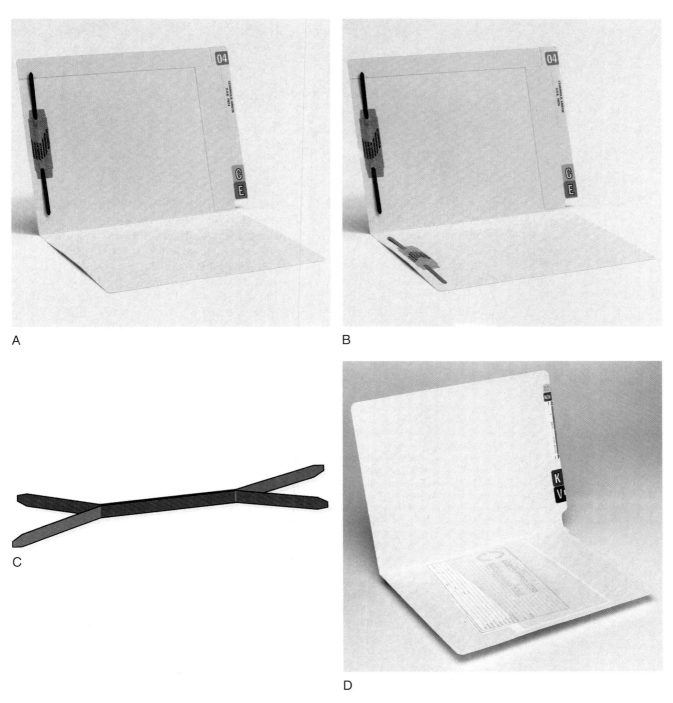

Figure 7-7 A, File folder with one two-hole fastener. **B,** File folder with two two-hole fasteners. **C,** Twin-prong fasteners for fastening pages to either side of a file folder. **D,** Polyvinyl pocket. (**A** through **D** courtesy Colwell, a Division of Patterson Companies, Inc., Champaign, IL.)

Figure 7-8 Traditional name label on file folder.

Each patient should fill out a **health history form** (Figure 7-11) and date and sign it. If the dentist prefers to ask these questions in person, the patient should verify the answers recorded and sign the form. Figure 7-12 shows a combination health history and adult registration form. Figure 7-13 shows the pediatric version of this form. With children, the health history form should be completed by a parent or guardian, not by the child or a baby-sitter. Make sure no nicknames are used and that all data are accurate, because this information is used later to complete insurance forms.

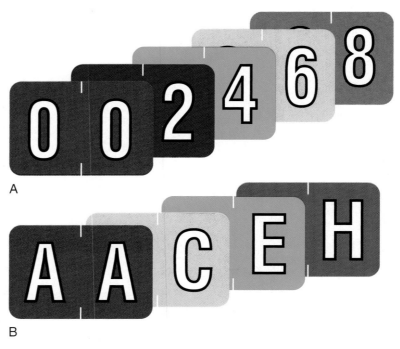

Figure 7-9 A, Numeric and year aging labels on a clinical chart. **B,** Alpha and year aging labels on a clinical chart. (Courtesy SYCOM, Madison, WI.)

WELCOME TO OUR OFFICE

JOSEPH W. LAKE, D.D.S.
611 Main Street, S.E.
Grand Rapids, MI 49502
616. 101. 9575

TODAY'S DATE

_____

Thank you for choosing our office.
In order to serve you properly we will need the following information. (Please print.) All information will be strictly confidential.

Patient's name	Birth date	Marital status
		Single ☐ Married ☐ Widowed ☐ Divorced ☐

Residence address	City	State	Zip	Home phone

If child, parent's name or guardian's name

Name of employer	Address	Business phone

Social security number	Driver's license	Occupation

Do you have medical insurance? ☐ Yes ☐ No	If no, how do you intend to pay? ☐ Check ☐ Cash ☐ Credit card	Ins. co. name & address

Subscriber name	Policy no.	Certificate no.	Is it through your employer? ☐ Yes ☐ No

Name of spouse	Birth date	Social security number

Is there secondary ins., spouse 2nd carrier, etc.? ☐ Yes ☐ No	Name & address of spouse employer	Business phone

Secondary ins. name & address	Policy no.	Certificate no.

Medicaid no.	Medicare no.

Workmen's compensation	Name of company

Address of company	Company phone	Treatment authorized by

Person financially responsible for this account	Address	Relationship to patient

Nearest friend or relative not residing with you	Relationship to patient	Phone

Whom may we thank for referring you?	Address

What is your chief complaint?

I authorize this office to release any information necessary to expedite insurance claims. I understand that I am responsible for all charges, regardless of insurance coverage.

Patient, Parent, or Guardian Signature _____   Date _____

Item 4590 • 12/93 SYCOM® 1-800-356-8141

A

Figure 7-10 A, Common patient registration form. (Courtesy SYCOM, Madison, WI.).

PATIENT REGISTRATION

Patient's name _____ Birth date _____

Name of spouse _____ Birth date _____

If a child, parent's name _____

Single ☐
Widowed ☐
Married ☐
Divorced ☐
Separated ☐

Street address _____ Phone _____

City _____ State _____ Zip _____

Patient employed by _____ Phone _____

Business address _____

Present position _____ How long held _____

Spouse employed by _____ Phone _____

Business address _____

Present position _____ How long held _____

Purpose of this appointment _____

In case of emergency, who should be notified _____ Phone _____

Person responsible for this account _____

Social Security number _____

Drivers License number _____

Spouse's Social Security number _____

Spouse's Driver's License number _____

If using Charge Card, name _____ Card no._____ Exp. date _____

If Medicaid, your number _____ County of _____

If you have insurance, name of insured _____

Name of insurance company _____ Policy no. _____

Is policy connected with a Union   Yes _____ No _____   If yes, name of Union _____

Local no. _____ Group no. _____

If spouse has insurance, name of insured _____

Name of insurance company _____ Policy no. _____

Is policy connected with a Union   Yes _____ No _____   If yes, name of Union _____

Local no. _____ Group no. _____

Whom may we thank for referring you _____

Your Signature _____ **Date** _____

Comments: _____

_____

_____

_____

_____

_____

Item 4047V · 05/94 **SYCOM®** 1-800-356-8141

B

Figure 7-10, cont'd B, Alternative form.

HEALTH HISTORY

Correct answers to the following questions will allow your dentist to treat you on a more individual basis, providing the care appropriate for your particular needs.

Name_____ Birth date _____ Age_____

Why are you now seeking dental treatment?_____

Please answer each question. Check yes or no. If in doubt, leave blank.

	YES	NO
1. Are you in good health now?	☐	☐
2. Are you now under the care of a physician?	☐	☐
If so, what is the condition being treated? _____		
3. Have you ever been hospitalized or had a serious illness?	☐	☐
If yes, explain _____		
4. Have you ever had excessive bleeding following an extraction, or do cuts take longer to heal now than previously?	☐	☐
5. (Women) Are you pregnant? If so, give due date _____	☐	☐
6. Do you use tobacco in any form? If yes, how much _____	☐	☐
7. Do you use alcoholic beverages (more than 2 drinks per day)?	☐	☐

8. Do you have or have you ever had any of the following?

GENERAL	YES	NO	HEART/BLOOD VESSELS	YES	NO
Tire easily, weakness	☐	☐	Rheumatic fever	☐	☐
Marked weight change	☐	☐	Heart murmur	☐	☐
Night sweats	☐	☐	Chest pain/discomfort	☐	☐
Persistent fever	☐	☐	Heart attack/trouble	☐	☐
SKIN			Shortness of breath	☐	☐
Eruptions (rash) hives	☐	☐	Swelling of ankles	☐	☐
Change in skin color	☐	☐	High blood pressure	☐	☐
EYES			Congenital heart disease	☐	☐
Visual change	☐	☐	Mitral valve prolapse	☐	☐
Glaucoma	☐	☐	Artificial heart valve	☐	☐
EARS			Pacemaker	☐	☐
Loss of hearing	☐	☐	Heart surgery	☐	☐
Ringing in ears	☐	☐	Other	☐	☐
NOSE			**BONE/MUSCLES**		
Frequent nosebleeds	☐	☐	Arthritis/rheumatism	☐	☐
Sinus problems	☐	☐	Artificial joints/limbs	☐	☐
THROAT			**DIGESTIVE SYSTEM**		
Soreness/hoarseness	☐	☐	Hepatitis	☐	☐
NERVOUS SYSTEM			Jaundice	☐	☐
Stroke	☐	☐	Ulcers	☐	☐
Headaches	☐	☐	Change in appetite	☐	☐
Convulsions/epilepsy	☐	☐	Black, bloody or pale stools	☐	☐
Numbness/tingling	☐	☐	**URINARY**		
Dizziness/fainting	☐	☐	Kidney disease	☐	☐
Psychiatric treatment	☐	☐	Increase in frequency		
RESPIRATORY			of urination (night)	☐	☐
Tuberculosis	☐	☐	Burning on urination	☐	☐
Emphysema	☐	☐	Urethral discharge	☐	☐
Asthma/hay fever	☐	☐	Bloody urine	☐	☐
Persistent cough	☐	☐	Venereal disease	☐	☐
Sputum production (phlegm)	☐	☐	**BLOOD**		
Cough up bloody sputum	☐	☐	Bruise easily	☐	☐
Difficulty breathing while lying down	☐	☐	Anemia	☐	☐
ENDOCRINE			Blood transfusion	☐	☐
Diabetes	☐	☐	**OTHER**		
Family history of diabetes	☐	☐	Radiation therapy	☐	☐
Thyroid condition/goiter	☐	☐	Chemotherapy	☐	☐
Other	☐	☐	Tumors or growths	☐	☐
			Cancer	☐	☐
			HIV+	☐	☐
			AIDS	☐	☐

Item 4046V • 05/94 SYCOM® 1-800-356-8141   *(Please complete reverse side)*

Figure 7-11 Adult patient health history form. (Courtesy SYCOM, Madison, WI.)

9. Are you ALLERGIC or have you ever experienced any reaction to the following?

	YES	NO		YES	NO
Local anesthetics (e.g., novocaine)	☐	☐	Aspirin or codeine	☐	☐
Barbiturates/sedatives/sleeping pills	☐	☐	Sulfa drugs	☐	☐
Penicillin/other antibiotics	☐	☐	Other allergies _____		

10. Are you taking any of the following?

	YES	NO		YES	NO
Antibiotics/sulfa drugs	☐	☐	Tranquilizers	☐	☐
Blood thinners	☐	☐	Insulin/other diabetes drugs	☐	☐
Blood pressure medication	☐	☐	Recreational drugs	☐	☐
Thyroid medicine	☐	☐	Digitalis/other heart medications	☐	☐
Cortisone/steroids	☐	☐	Nitroglycerin	☐	☐
Antihistamines/allergy drugs/			Aspirin	☐	☐
cold remedies	☐	☐	Other medication _____		

If yes to any of the above, list *name* of medication and *dosage* below:

1._____

2._____

3._____

4._____

11. Is there any disease, condition, or problem not listed above that you think we should know about, or is there any activity your doctor says you cannot do? If so, explain _____

_____

12. Physician's name _____ Phone _____

13. Have you ever had any serious trouble associated with previous dental treatment? _____

_____

14. Does dental treatment make you nervous? No _____ Slightly _____ Moderately _____ Extremely _____

15. Date of last dental visit _____

16. Have you ever been treated for periodontal disease (gum disease, pyorrhea, trench mouth)? _____

    If so, when? _____

17. Do you have or have you ever had any of the following?

MOUTH

	YES	NO
Bleeding, sore gums	☐	☐
Unpleasant taste/bad breath	☐	☐
Burning tongue/lips	☐	☐
Frequent blisters, lips/mouth	☐	☐
Swelling/lumps in mouth	☐	☐
Ortho treatments (braces)	☐	☐
Biting cheeks/lips	☐	☐
Clicking/popping jaw	☐	☐
Difficulty opening or closing jaw	☐	☐

TEETH

	YES	NO
Loose teeth	☐	☐
Sensitive to hot	☐	☐
Sensitive to cold	☐	☐
Sensitive to sweets	☐	☐
Sensitive to biting	☐	☐
Food impaction	☐	☐
Clenching/grinding	☐	☐
Shifting of teeth	☐	☐
Change in bite	☐	☐

ORAL HYGIENE

Do you use the following?

	YES	NO
Brush	☐	☐
Dental floss	☐	☐
Fluoride rinse	☐	☐
Other _____		

How often do you brush _____

Brush is: Soft ☐   Medium ☐   Hard ☐

To the best of my knowledge, all of the preceding answers are true and correct.
If I ever have any change in my health or change in my medication, I will inform the dentist at the next appointment.

Signature of Patient
Parent, or Guardian _____ Date _____

Figure 7-11, cont'd

REGISTRATION AND HEALTH HISTORY

Name	Single	Married	Divorced	Separated	Widowed
Mary Sue Harden			X		

Social Security number	Birthdate	Home phone	Business phone
000-00-0113	*4-17-71*	*419-285-9276*	*216-285-9271*

Residence address	City	State	Zip
415 Sycamore Street	*Pine Bluff*	*Michigan*	*48134*

Employed by	City	State	Zip
Pine Bluff Schools	*Pine Bluff*	*Michigan*	*48134*

Present position	How long held	Your driver license no.	State
Director, Adult Education	*6 years*	*H 721924621*	*Michigan*

Spouse's name
NA

Spouse's Social Security number	Spouse birthdate	Business phone
NA	*NA*	*NA*

Spouse employed by	City	State	Zip

Present position	How long held	Spouse driver license no.	State

Referred by	Address
Jeremy Thompson	*481 Cutler, Grand Rapids, MI*

Who will pay for this account?	Credit card name	No.	Expiration date
Cash / Insurance			

Name of your dental insurance company
Delta Dental of Michigan

Union local	Group no.	Policy no.
742		

Name of your spouse's dental insurance company

Union local	Group no.	Policy no.

It is important that I know about your dental and medical history. Many things have a direct bearing on your dental health. I will review the questionnaire and discuss it with you in detail. Information you give me is strictly confidential and will not be released to anyone without your written permission.

YOUR DENTAL HISTORY

Are you having any discomfort at this time _____

How long since you have been to a dentist *1½ years*

What was done then *Cleaning, x-rays*

Did you have X-Rays *Yes* **How** often did you visit a dentist before then _____ *Every six months*

Have you lost any teeth *No* Why _____

Any complications with extractions _____

Have they ever been replaced by: (1) A Fixed Bridge _____

(2) Removable Partial _____ (3) Denture _____

How many of (1) (2) (3) _____

Are your teeth sensitive to heat _____ to cold ✓ to sweets _____ to sour _____

Have you had your teeth straightened *No* When _____

How often do you brush your teeth *2 X day* When *Morning and night*

How *Press and roll* _____

How long do you use a toothbrush before replacing it *4 X a year*

Do you use dental floss *Yes* How often *3 X a week*

Between-the-teeth stimulator *No* Water jet *No*

Do you have bleeding gums *Sometimes* When *No specific time*

Do you eat between meals *Sometimes*

Do you brush teeth after snacks *Not always*

Does food wedge between your teeth *Yes* Where *Upper right*

Do you grind or clench your teeth *No* When _____

Have you ever had gum treatments *No* When _____

Do you feel you have bad breath at times *Sometimes*

Unpleasant taste in mouth *No*

Any pain in or around your ears *No*   **Do** you hear popping, clicking

or snapping noises when you chew *No*   **Do** you have any nasal

obstruction *No*   **Are** you aware of any swelling

or lump in your mouth *No*

(Other side, please.)

Item 1014V • 04/94 SYCOM® 1-800-356-8141

Figure 7-12 Combination history and registration form. (Courtesy Colwell, a Division of Patterson Companies, Inc., Champaign, IL.)

Do you now have or have you had any of the following habits: Thumbsucking __No__   Fingersucking __No__

Cheek or tongue chewing __No__   Chewing on Pencils __No__   Pens __No__   Lips __No__   Fingernails __Yes__

Do you have any fear of having dentistry done __No__

If yes, why _____

How do you feel about your teeth __They're good to me if I'm good to them__

How do you feel about dentures __Don't want them__

Do you want to avoid the dental discomfort you may have experienced in the past __Haven't had any__

Do you want to avoid dentures __Yes__

Do you want to have pleasant breath __Yes__

Do you want to know how you can keep the natural teeth you still have __Yes__

If you have children, do you want to learn how they may keep their natural teeth for a lifetime without discomfort _____

MEDICAL HISTORY

Physician's name __Marsha Huckins, MD__   Date of last physical exam __1 year ago__

Birthdate __4-17-71__   Age __24__

Do you have or have you had any of the following. Please indicate with check mark (✔).

_____ Any heart problems	_____ Allergies to anesthetics	_____ Hepatitis	__X__ Sinus Problems
_____ High blood pressure	__X__ Allergies to medicines or	_____ Herpes	_____ Stroke
_____ Low blood pressure	drugs	_____ Malignancies	_____ Typhoid Fever
_____ Circulatory problems	__X__ Allergies to __Codeine__	__X__ Measles	_____ Tonsillitis
__X__ Nervous problems	_____ Anemia	__X__ Mumps	_____ Tuberculosis
_____ Radiation treatments	_____ Arthritis	_____ Psychiatric care	_____ Ulcer
_____ Excessive bleeding	_____ Asthma	_____ Rheumatic Fever	_____ Venereal Disease
_____ AIDS	__X__ Diabetes	_____ Scarlet Fever	_____ Other

Are you pregnant _____   Blood Pressure: S _____ /D _____ / _____

Please describe any current medical treatment, impending operations, or any other medical or dental information that may possibly affect your dental treatment.

_____

_____

_____

_____

_____

_____

_____

_____

_____

_____

Date _____   Your signature _____

Figure 7-12, cont'd

thank you for selecting us.

Patient ID # _____

Today's Date _____

We strive to make each of your child's visits pleasant and comfortable. Please fill out this form completely in ink.

Your Child

Child's Name _____   Sex _____ Age _____

Nickname _____ Social Security # _____   Birthdate _____

School _____   Grade _____

Child's Home Address _____

City, State, Zip _____   Phone _____

Responsible Party

Name _____   Relationship _____

Address _____

City, State, Zip _____   Phone _____

Social Security # _____   DL # _____

Who is Responsible for Making Appointments? _____

Parent or Guardian Information   ☐ Mother   ☐ Stepmother   ☐ Guardian

Name _____

Home Phone _____   Work Phone _____

Employer _____   Occupation _____

Social Security # _____   DL # _____

Marital Status   ☐ Single   ☐ Married   ☐ Divorced   ☐ Separated   ☐ Widowed

Parent or Guardian Information   ☐ Father   ☐ Stepfather   ☐ Guardian

Name _____

Home Phone _____   Work Phone _____

Employer _____   Occupation _____

Social Security # _____   DL # _____

Marital Status   ☐ Single   ☐ Married   ☐ Divorced   ☐ Separated   ☐ Widowed

Primary Insurance

Insured's Name _____   Relationship _____

Birthdate _____ Social Security # _____

Employer _____ Date Employed _____ Occupation _____

Insurance Co. _____ Group # _____ Employee # _____

Ins. Co. Address _____ City _____ State _____ Zip _____

Deductible _____ Copay _____ Amount already used _____ Max. annual benefit _____

Additional Insurance

Insured's Name _____   Relationship _____

Birthdate _____ Social Security # _____

Employer _____ Date Employed _____ Occupation _____

Insurance Co. _____ Group # _____ Employee # _____

Ins. Co. Address _____ City _____ State _____ Zip _____

Deductible _____ Copay _____ Amount already used _____ Max. annual benefit _____

Over Please

Figure 7-13 Registration and health history form for children. (Courtesy SYCOM, Madison, WI.)

The patient's history should be reviewed when the person returns for treatment if several months have elapsed since the last visit. A **health history update form** should be completed periodically to keep both the health history (Figure 7-14, *A*) and the personal information (Figure 7-14, *B*) current. The patient should sign and date this form.

HEALTH HISTORY UPDATE ████████████████

Patient: _____   Date: _____

1. Have there been any changes in your health since your last visit?

    _____

    _____

2. Have you recently required other health services? _____

    If yes, nature of care _____

3. Physician's name: _____

4. Have you been hospitalized since your last visit? _____

    If yes, nature of problem _____

5. Any new illnesses?_____

    _____

6. Are you taking any medication(s) now? _____

    To treat: _____

    Name & dosage: _____

7. Do you have any new allergies or reactions to any medications or drugs?

    _____

8. Women only: Are you pregnant?_____ If yes, due date:_____

9. Any other new diseases, conditions, or problems you think we should know

    about? _____

    _____

Patient Signature: _____

Doctor Signature: _____

Form 4051 • 12/93 **SYCOM®** 1-800-356-8141

A

Figure 7-14 A, Health history update form. (Courtesy SYCOM, Madison, WI.)

PERSONAL INFORMATION UPDATE

Name_____ Date _____

1. Has your name changed since your last visit here? _____ yes   _____ no
   If yes, what was the old name? _____
   What name do you use for insurance if different than above? _____
   _____

2. If you have a new or different address since your initial visit here, please
   indicate below:

   _____
   _____
   _____

   Please indicate if any apartment # or P.O. Box # _____

3. Has your marital status changed? _____ yes   _____no

4. Has your telephone number changed? _____ yes   _____no
   Please indicate your correct telephone number _____

5. Has your employment changed? _____yes   _____no
   Please indicate your new employer name and address:

   _____
   _____
   _____

   New employer telephone #: _____

6. Have you changed insurance companies? _____yes   _____no
   If yes, please indicate your new insurance carrier and address.

   Primary _____   Secondary _____
   _____   _____
   _____   _____
   Group Nos. _____   Group Nos._____
   Subscriber Nos. _____   Subscriber Nos. _____

7. Who is responsible for this bill? _____

8. Signature _____

Thank you for your assistance.

Item 4595 • 08/94 • **SYCOM®** 1-800-356-8141

B

Figure 7-14, cont'd B, Personal information update form.

Many types of patient registration and health history forms are available. For example, the form in Figure 7-15 can be used for children. Figure 7-16 shows a short-form style, which combines an abbreviated patient information form and health history form, which may be used for a transient patient. Regardless of the form used, it is important to remember that a current, accurate health history serves as a preventive measure in patient treatment and as a defense in malpractice suits. When collecting the data on these forms, consider the following points:

- Give the patient the form on a clipboard to which a ballpoint pen (not a pencil) has been attached.
- Do not ask the questions in the business office. Some answers may be embarrassing if overheard by other patients in the reception room. Patients often give more information if they do not have to respond orally.
- When making appointments for new patients, ask them to arrive 15 minutes early to allow time for completion of these forms.
- Make sure a parent or legal guardian completes the form for a child.
- Keep the information absolutely confidential. The patient record is not for public review and should not become a feature of lunchtime gossip.
- Review the form to ensure that it has been completed and signed. Patients may avoid questions they do not understand or do not want to answer. If the patient says, "I don't think this question has anything to do with my teeth," explain how it relates to dental care. If the question cannot be justified, it should not be on the form.

Remember, a person's privacy is protected by law. Several questions on forms shown as examples may be considered discriminatory or in violation of a patient's rights. Consequently, the administrative assistant must be aware of the state laws that protect a person's rights and change the form to accommodate these rights. As legal changes occur, most suppliers try to produce forms that are in accord with the laws protecting patient rights.

Clinical Chart

A wide selection of dental charts is available for use in the dental office. Obviously, the needs of specialty practices are different from those of a general practice, and several choices are available for each type of practice. The dentist may purchase a standard form or may design one specifically suited for the needs of the practice. Most supply companies offer a special service for dentists who want to design their own charts.

Most charts are 8½ by 11 inches, made of heavy paper stock, and printed on both sides. Many of these charts are die-punched to fit into a file folder. One side of the record contains a dental chart, a review of the patient's health history, and general patient information. The reverse side provides space for entering the treatment plan and recording services rendered. Some charts have space for entering the fee, but this should not become the patient's financial ledger card, and it need not include a record of payments and balances.

A review of Figures 7-17 to 7-19 will help familiarize you with some of the different types of dental charts. Figures 7-17 and 7-18 show general practice charts that provide similar basic information. Figure 7-19 is a periodontal specialty chart. Figure 7-20 is a separate form that is added to the chart as a progress sheet for treatment entries.

Figure 7-21 is a pediatric clinical chart that emphasizes clinical conditions unique to pediatric patients. A smaller form may be used as an oral surgery chart (Figure 7-22). Re-examination charts (Figure 7-23) may be used at the time of the periodic examination; these forms may be supplied individually or in pads of 50 or more. Many companies also provide self-adhesive anatomical labels to make charting and communication easier (Figure 7-24, *A* to *C*).

CHILD REGISTRATION

Child's name _____ Date _____

Birth date _____ Age _____

Nickname _____ Hobbies _____

Parent's name _____

Residence-street _____

City _____ State _____ Zip _____

School _____

Telephone: Residence _____ School _____

Father employed by _____

Present position _____ How long held _____

Mother employed by _____

Present position _____ How long held _____

Referred by _____

Who will pay this account _____

Purpose of call _____

Name of father's dental insurance co. _____

Policy number _____

Name of mother's dental insurance co. _____

Policy number _____

Parents' Social Security numbers: Father _____

                                          Mother _____

Parent's birth dates: Father _____

                                          Mother _____

Item 539 • 12/93 **SYCOM**● 1-800-356-8141

Figure 7-15 Alternative registration and health history form for children. (Courtesy SYCOM, Madison, WI.)

Information For Emergency Treatment

Date of last medical examination _____

Does child have or has child ever had: Yes   No

    Anemia .... _____ _____

    Diabetes... _____ _____

    Hepatitis .... _____ _____

    Allergies .... _____ _____

        To penicillin .... _____ _____

        To local anesthetic .... _____ _____

    Abnormal heart condition.. _____ _____

    Abnormal bleeding from a cut.................................... _____ _____

    Rheumatic fever... _____ _____

    Heart murmur.. _____ _____

    Is your child under the care of a physician now....................... _____ _____

    Is any medication being taken now... _____ _____

    If so, what _____

        _____

    Other physical conditions_____

        _____

        _____

    Name of physician _____

    Telephone number_____

    Information given by (signature) _____

Date	Service Rendered	Charge	Credit	Balance

Figure 7-15, cont'd

Birthdate _____ Age _____

Date of last medical examination _____

Do you have or have you ever had: Yes   No

REGISTRATION/HEALTH HISTORY ▰▰▰▰▰▰▰▰▰▰▰

Patient's name _____

If a child, parent's name _____

Single ____ Married ____ Widowed ____ Divorced ____ Separated ____

Address _____

City _____ State _____ Zip _____

Business address _____

Telephone: Residence _____ Business _____

Patient employed by _____

Present position _____

In case of emergency, who should be notified _____

Phone _____

Referred by _____

Who will pay this account _____

Purpose of call _____

Spouse's name _____

Spouse's birthdate _____

Spouse employed by _____

Do you have insurance that may cover any part of our services   ☐ Yes   ☐ No

If so, name of primary company _____

Is policy connected with your union   ☐ Yes   ☐ No

If yes, name of union _____

Policy no. _____ Group no. _____

Local no. _____

Social Security no. of person covered _____

Any secondary insurance _____

Name of company _____

Social Security no. of person covered _____

Your signature _____ Date _____

Item 119 • 12/89 SYCOM® Madison, WI Printed In U.S.A.

Charge	Credit	Balance

Figure 7-16 Short-form registration and health history form. (Courtesy SYCOM, Madison, WI.)

EXAMINATION RECORD

Name	Birthdate	Exam date	Medical alerts	Account #

| X-rays |
| Date |
| Diagnostic models |
| Date |
| Photograph |
| Clinical exam |
| Vitality test |
| Blood pressure |

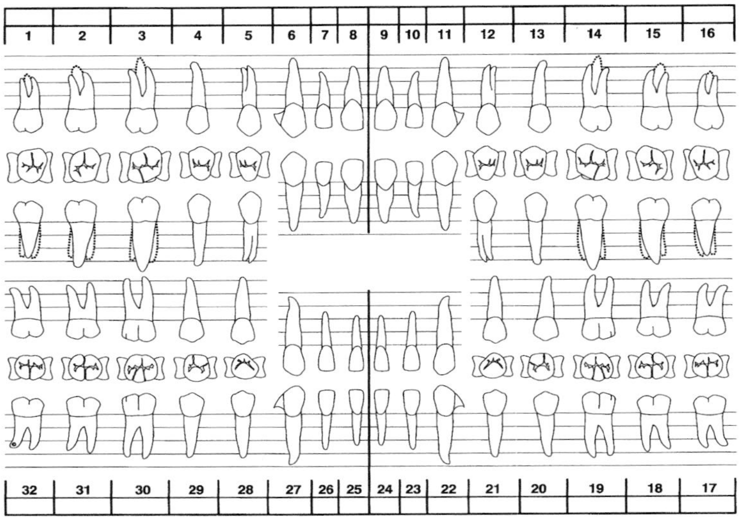

Health Alerts

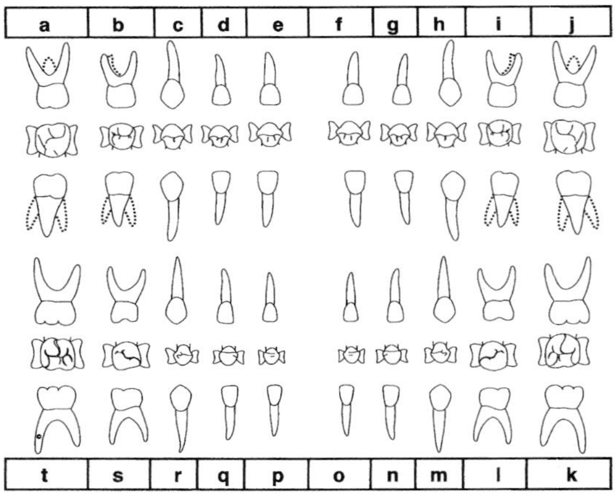

Tooth	Services necessary	
1		
2		
3		
4		
5		
6		
7		
8		
9		
10		
11		
12		
13		
14		
15		
16		
17		
18		
19		
20		
21		
22		
23		
24		
25		
26		
27		
28		
29		
30		
31		
32		

CLINICAL DATA

General condition of teeth _____

Plaque _____ Stains _____ Abrasions _____

Condition of present restorations _____

Overhangs _____ Contact points _____

Condition of the floor of mouth _____

Palate: Hard _____ Soft _____ Cheeks _____ Lips _____

Frenum _____ Tongue _____ Ridges _____

Calculus: Slight _____ Moderate _____ Excessive _____ Oral cancer exam _____

TMJ _____ Neck _____ Occlusion _____

Item 1057V © 3/93 **SYCOM** ® 1-800-356-8141

Figure 7-17 Adult clinical chart (general practice). (Courtesy SYCOM, Madison, WI.)

Name		Address to send statements to		Zip	Daytime phone		
Date	Tooth No.	Service rendered	Insurance ☐	Charges	Payments	Balance

Figure 7-17, cont'd

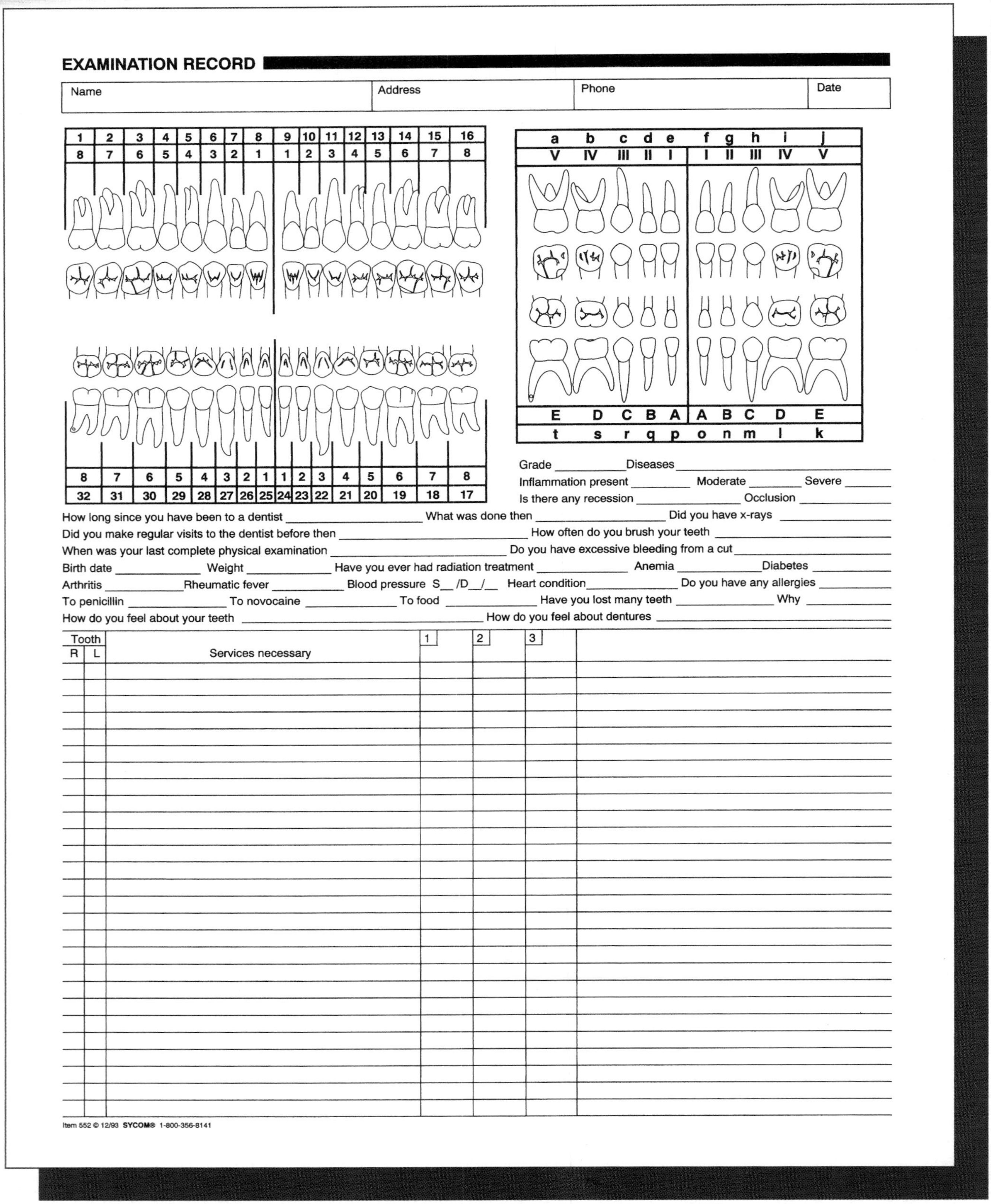

EXAMINATION RECORD

Name	Address	Phone	Date

1	2	3	4	5	6	7	8	9	10	11	12	13	14	15	16
8	7	6	5	4	3	2	1	1	2	3	4	5	6	7	8

a	b	c	d	e	f	g	h	i	j
V	IV	III	II	I	I	II	III	IV	V

E	D	C	B	A	A	B	C	D	E
t	s	r	q	p	o	n	m	l	k

8	7	6	5	4	3	2	1	1	2	3	4	5	6	7	8
32	31	30	29	28	27	26	25	24	23	22	21	20	19	18	17

Grade _____ Diseases _____
Inflammation present _____ Moderate _____ Severe _____
Is there any recession _____ Occlusion _____

How long since you have been to a dentist _____ What was done then _____ Did you have x-rays _____
Did you make regular visits to the dentist before then _____ How often do you brush your teeth _____
When was your last complete physical examination _____ Do you have excessive bleeding from a cut _____
Birth date _____ Weight _____ Have you ever had radiation treatment _____ Anemia _____ Diabetes _____
Arthritis _____ Rheumatic fever _____ Blood pressure S__ /D__/__ Heart condition_____ Do you have any allergies _____
To penicillin _____ To novocaine _____ To food _____ Have you lost many teeth _____ Why _____
How do you feel about your teeth _____ How do you feel about dentures _____

Tooth		Services necessary	1	2	3	
R	L					

Item 552 © 12/93 **SYCOM®** 1-800-356-8141

Figure 7-18 Alternative adult clinical chart (general practice). (Courtesy SYCOM, Madison, WI.)

Name					Address		Phone	
Mo.	Day	Yr.	R	L	Service rendered	Fee	Credit	Balance

Figure 7-18, cont'd

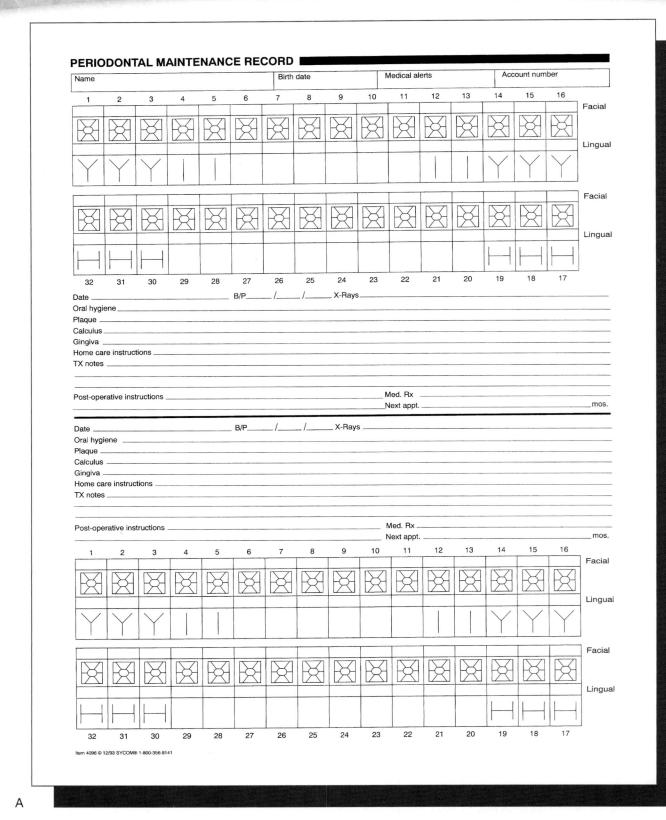

Figure 7-19 A, Periodontal specialty clinical chart, front. (Courtesy SYCOM, Madison, WI.)

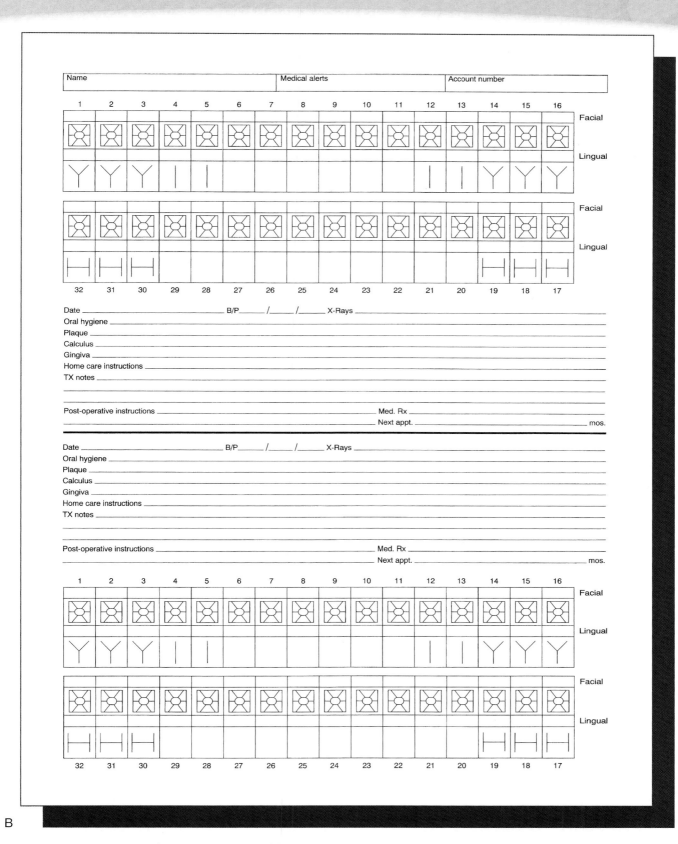

Figure 7-19, cont'd B, Periodontal specialty clinical chart, back.

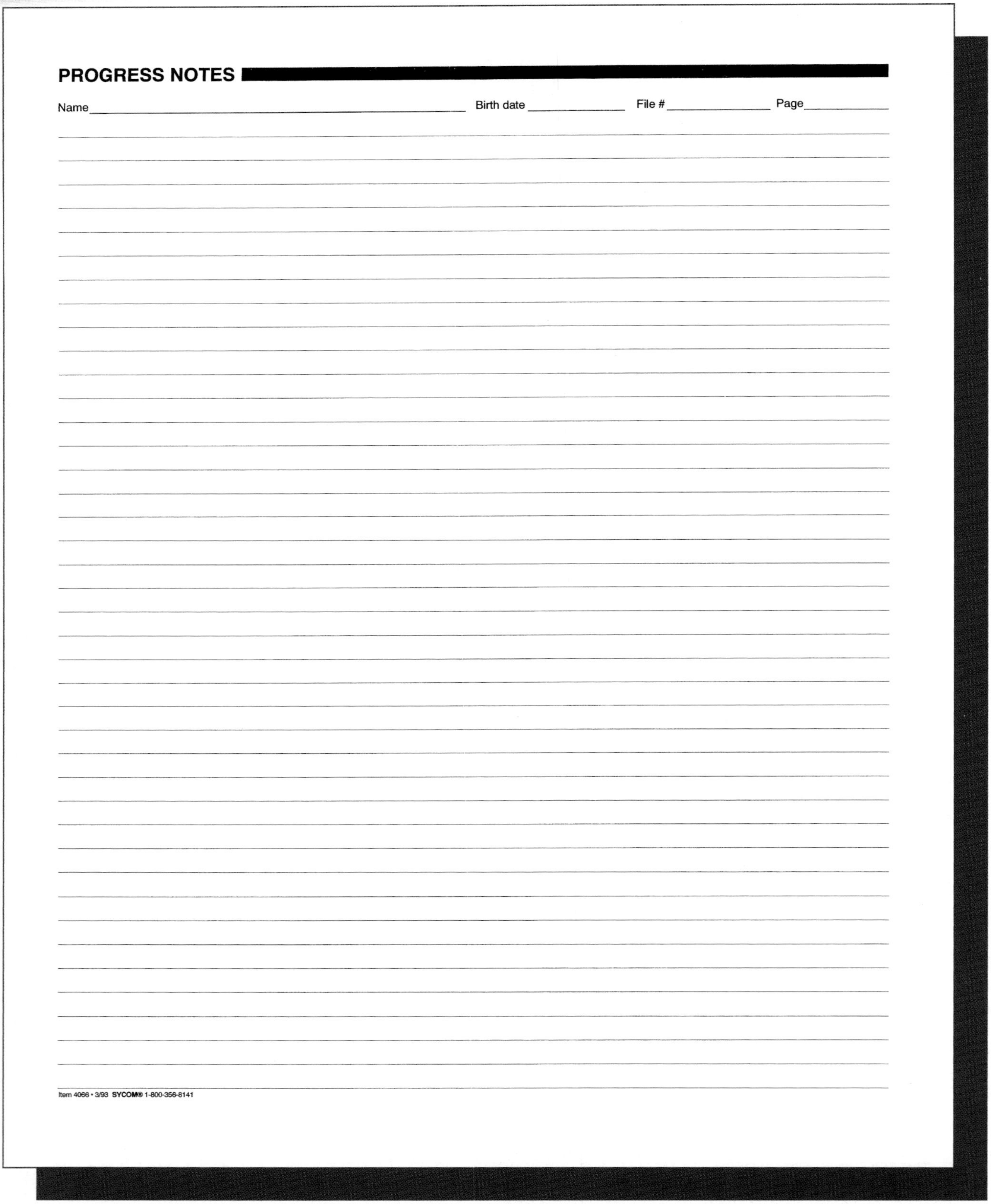

PROGRESS NOTES

Name_____   Birth date _____   File # _____   Page_____

Item 4066 • 3/93 **SYCOM®** 1-800-356-8141

Figure 7-20 Progress sheet added to a clinical chart to record treatment data. (Courtesy SYCOM, Madison, WI.)

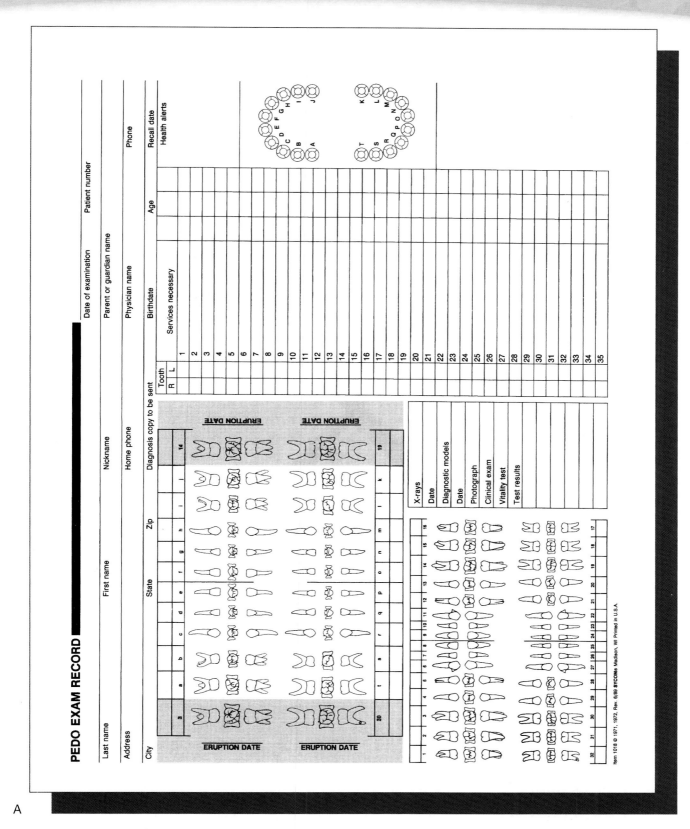

Figure 7-21 A, Pediatric chart, front. (Courtesy SYCOM, Madison, WI.).

Name _____

DENTAL HISTORY — SUMMARY

Attitude _____

Home care _____

MEDICAL HISTORY — SUMMARY

General health _____

Existing illness _____

Medicine/drugs _____

Allergies _____

CLINICAL DATA

General condition of teeth _____

Plaque _____ Stains _____ Abrasions _____ Traumatic injury _____

Occlusion _____ Overbite _____ Crossbite _____

Open-bite _____ Over-jet _____ Mid-line _____

Anterior crowding _____ Facial profile _____

Condition of present dentistry _____

Overhangs _____ Contact points _____ Space management _____

Condition of periodontum _____ Color _____

Recession _____ Palate _____ Floor of mouth _____

Lips _____ Tongue _____ Frenum _____

Tonsil area _____ Papillae _____ Presence of exudate _____

Areas of food retention _____ Saliva _____ Calculus _____

X-ray findings _____

Supernumerary _____ Abscesses _____ Eruption pattern _____

Other anomalies _____

GROWTH AND DEVELOPMENT PATTERN

Patient age _____ Birthdate _____

	Primary	Adult
Date		
3 yrs*		
9 yrs*		
12 yrs*		
Over		

* + or − 6 months

1. Congenitally missing _____ 3. Crowns complete _____

2. Exfoliation _____ 4. Roots complete _____

ORAL HYGIENE

	Above avg.	Avg.	Below avg.
Muscular coordination			
Brushing (sulcular)			
Flossing			
Plaque			
Fluoride - (need)			

Phase microscope findings _____

Disclosing results _____

Food impaction _____

DIETARY ANALYSIS

	High	Normal	Low
Carbohydrates			
Fats			
Proteins			
Milk products			
Meat group			
Vegetable-fruit			
Bread-cereal			
Snacking			
Vitamins			
Minerals			

Summary _____

B

Figure 7-21, cont'd B, Pediatric chart, back.

Figure 7-21, cont'd C, Alternative pediatric chart.

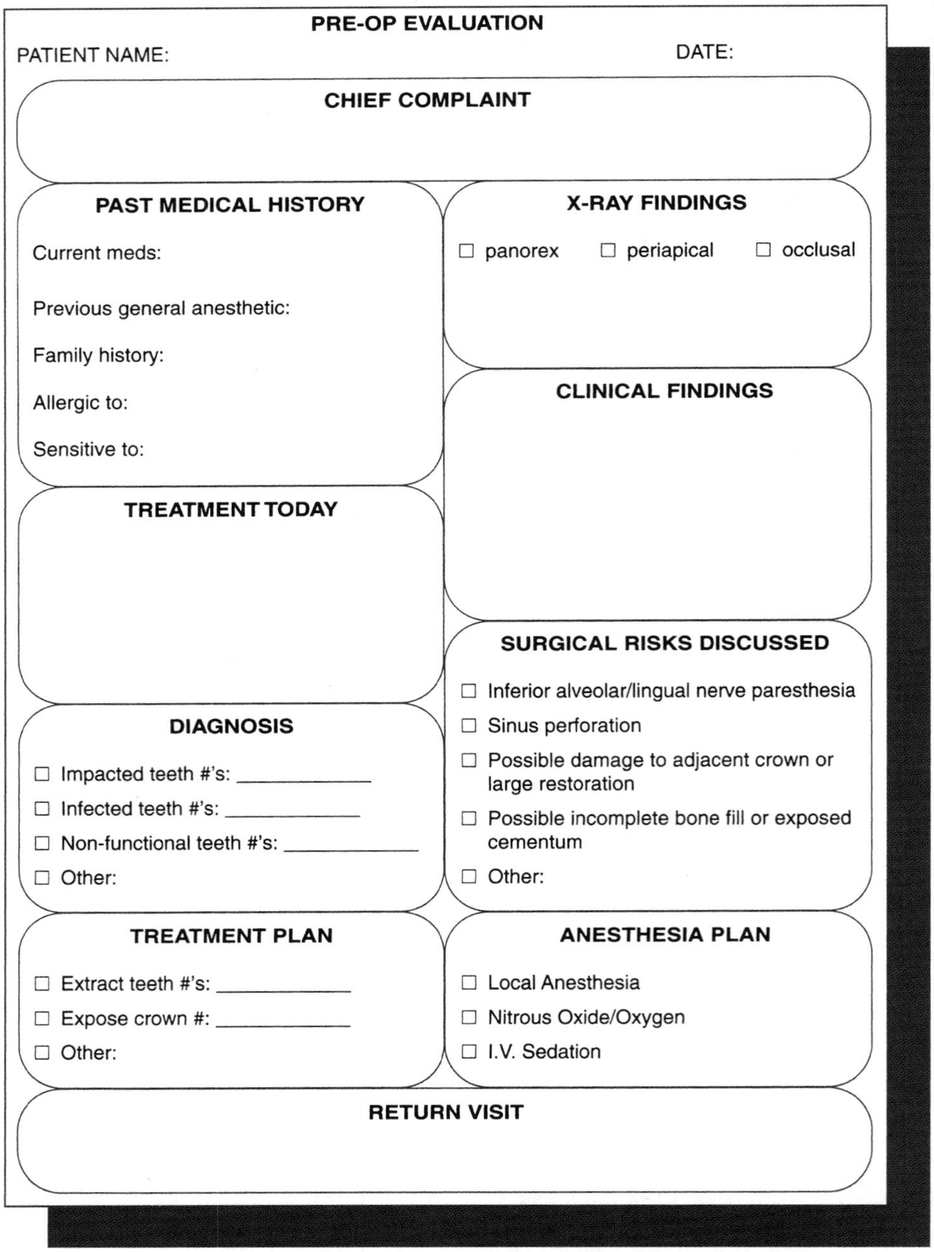

PRE-OP EVALUATION

PATIENT NAME: DATE:

CHIEF COMPLAINT

PAST MEDICAL HISTORY

Current meds:

Previous general anesthetic:

Family history:

Allergic to:

Sensitive to:

X-RAY FINDINGS

☐ panorex ☐ periapical ☐ occlusal

CLINICAL FINDINGS

TREATMENT TODAY

SURGICAL RISKS DISCUSSED

☐ Inferior alveolar/lingual nerve paresthesia
☐ Sinus perforation
☐ Possible damage to adjacent crown or large restoration
☐ Possible incomplete bone fill or exposed cementum
☐ Other:

DIAGNOSIS

☐ Impacted teeth #'s: ____________
☐ Infected teeth #'s: ____________
☐ Non-functional teeth #'s: ____________
☐ Other:

TREATMENT PLAN

☐ Extract teeth #'s: ____________
☐ Expose crown #: ____________
☐ Other:

ANESTHESIA PLAN

☐ Local Anesthesia
☐ Nitrous Oxide/Oxygen
☐ I.V. Sedation

RETURN VISIT

Figure 7-22 Chart that might be used in an oral surgery office. (Courtesy SYCOM, Madison, WI.)

Dental Diagnosis and Estimate Form. This form includes the dentist's diagnosis and the treatment plan recommended for the patient (Figure 7-25). In many cases the patient can select options in the treatment plan. After the consultation has been completed and treatment has been accepted by the patient, the form is signed by the person responsible for the account. Often a clause is included explaining that the fee quoted is an estimate and that unforeseen circumstances may affect the final fee for the service.

Consultation and Referral Report. In some cases, the dentist refers a patient to another dentist for examination, evaluation, and diagnosis. The form shown in Figure 7-26 includes information about the patient, the reason for the referral, and an anticipated treatment plan. This form is sent to

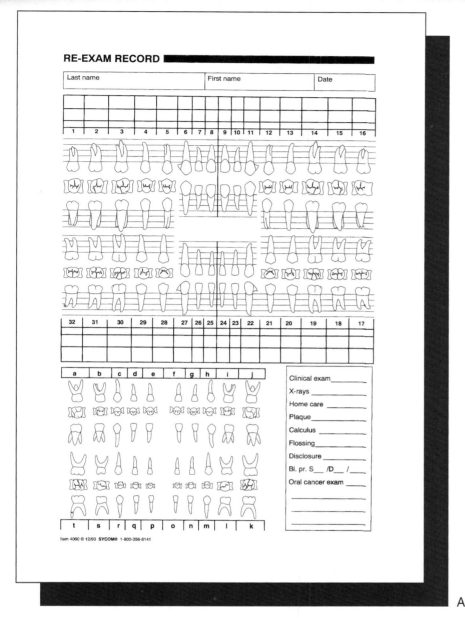

Figure 7-23 A, Re-examination chart. (Courtesy SYCOM, Madison, WI.)

the referring dentist with a copy to the patient. The consultant enters an evaluation and recommendation on the form and returns it to the dentist.

MEDICATIONS HISTORY FORM. As in medical practice, medications are prescribed for a dental patient on a prescription form (Figure 7-27, *A*). Having a history of a patient's medications helps prevent the prescription of drugs that could lead to unsafe interactions. The form in Figure 7-27, *B* is used to record a patient's medication history.

LABORATORY REQUISITIONS FORM. Many states require that a prescription or **laboratory requisition form** (Figure 7-28) accompany each case a dentist sends to a dental laboratory. This blueprint improves communication between the dentist and the laboratory technician and helps eliminate illegal dental practices, thereby protecting the patient.

RE-EXAM RECORD ■

Last name   First name   Date

Address

City   State   Zip   Mould

1	2	3	4	5	6	7	8	9	10	11	12	13	14	15	16
8	7	6	5	4	3	2	1	1	2	3	4	5	6	7	8

Teeth	Upper	Lower
Centrals		
Laterals		
Cuspids		
Posteriors		

Shade

Teeth	Upper	Lower
Centrals		
Laterals		
Cuspids		
Posteriors		

Calculus deposits   Slight _____ Moderate _____ Excessive _____

8	7	6	5	4	3	2	1	1	2	3	4	5	6	7	8
32	31	30	29	28	27	26	25	24	23	22	21	20	19	18	17

Blood pressure S___/D___/__

X-Rays _____

Date _____

Study model _____

Photograph _____

Transillumination
area _____

a	b	c	d	e	f	g	h	i	j
V	IV	III	II	I	I	II	III	IV	V

E	D	C	B	A	A	B	C	D	E
t	s	r	q	p	o	n	m	l	k

Summary

Item 4057 © 1960, 6/89 **SYCOM**® Madison, WI Printed in U.S.A.

B

Figure 7-23, cont'd B, Alternative re-examination record.

CONSENT FORM. A **consent form** (Figure 7-29, *A* to *D*) is commonly used in dentistry as a preventive measure against malpractice suits. The form, which is signed by the patient or by the parent or guardian of a pediatric patient, grants permission for administration of an anesthetic and other specified procedures. It is impossible to have a consent form for every phase of treatment, and it is unrealistic to believe that a general consent form covering every possible procedure would be upheld in court. Therefore a written summary of the treatment plan, as agreed upon by the patient and dentist, dated and signed by both parties, is a more acceptable format for such consent. Chapter 4 reviews the use of various types of consent forms in the dental office.

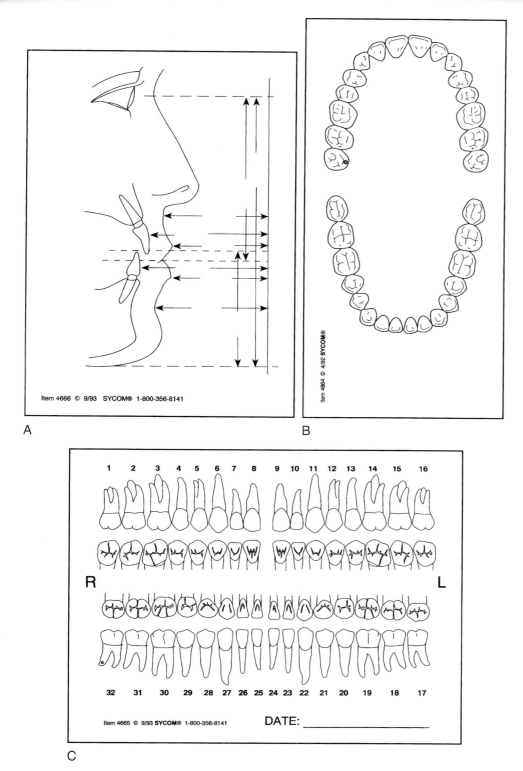

Figure 7-24 A to **C,** Self-adhesive anatomical labels can be used to make special notations on a clinical chart. (Courtesy SYCOM, Madison, WI.)

DENTAL DIAGNOSIS AND ESTIMATE

Name: _____

Date Proposed: _____

JOSEPH W. LAKE, D.D.S.
611 Main Street, S.E.
Grand Rapids, MI 49502
616.101.9575

Tooth #	Conditions	Service Code	Recommendations	Option #1	Option #2

Total Estimate★

★ Estimate, cost may vary due to unforseen circumstances.
These fees are valid for _____ days without reevaluation of
conditions.

Remarks:

Acceptance of treatment:

Option Accepted: _____

Responsible party _____

Date _____

Figure 7-25 Dental diagnosis and estimate form. (Courtesy SYCOM, Madison, WI.)

CONSULTATION/REFERRAL REPORT ▆▆▆▆▆▆▆▆▆▆▆▆▆▆▆▆▆▆▆▆

JOSEPH W. LAKE, D.D.S.
611 Main Street, S.E.
Grand Rapids, MI 49502
616.101.9575

Date:

Referral to:

Patient:

Age

Sex

Family physician:

Patient history:

Planned treatment:

Reason for referral:

Appointment scheduled for: _____ AM
PM

_____
Signature of Attending Doctor

Consultant's reply: _____

_____
Date

_____
Signature of Consulting Doctor

White - To recipient of referral - return to referral source   *Yellow* - To recipient of referral for retained copy   *Pink* - Retain as file copy until white is returned

Form 4052 • 8/88 **SYCOM**® Madison, WI Printed in U.S.A.

Figure 7-26 Consultation and referral report form. (Courtesy SYCOM, Madison, WI.)

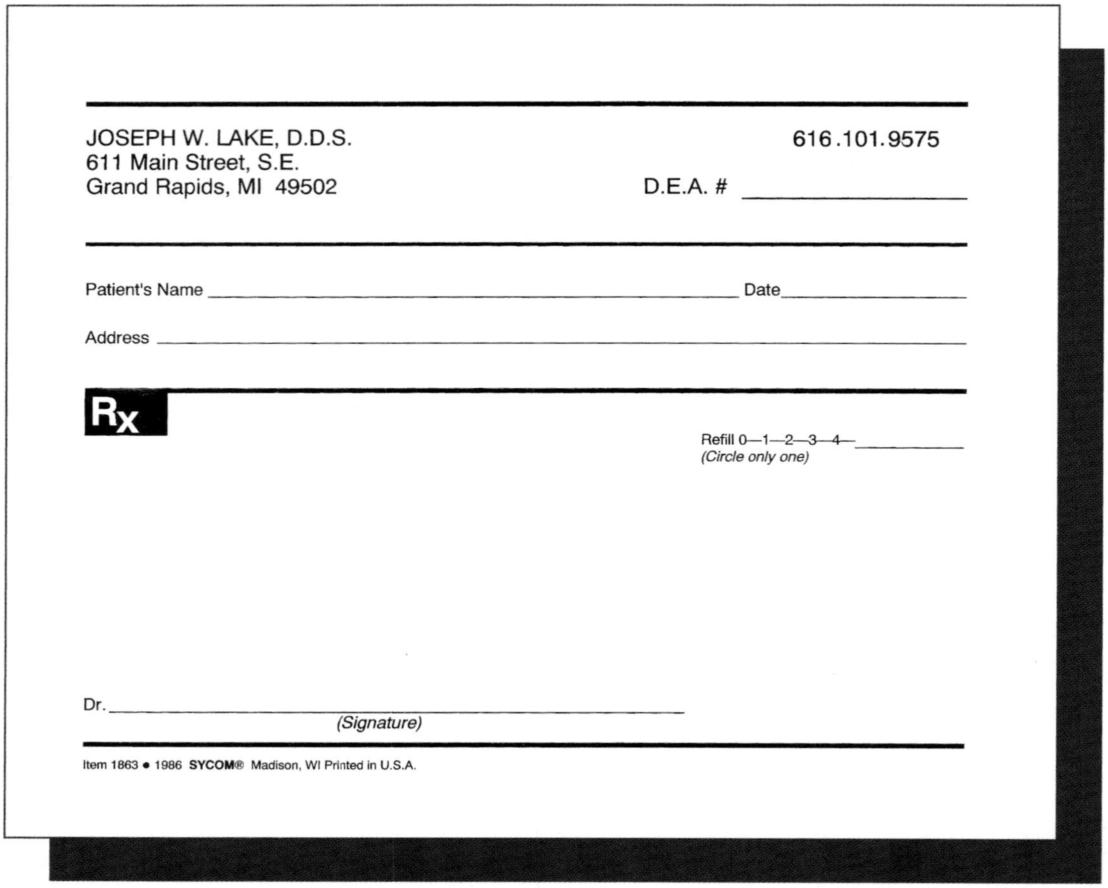

```
JOSEPH W. LAKE, D.D.S.                          616.101.9575
611 Main Street, S.E.
Grand Rapids, MI  49502            D.E.A. # _____


Patient's Name _____ Date_____

Address _____

Rx
                                        Refill 0—1—2—3—4—_____
                                        (Circle only one)




Dr._____
                    (Signature)

Item 1863 ● 1986 SYCOM® Madison, WI Printed in U.S.A.
```

A

Figure 7-27 A, Prescription form. (Courtesy SYCOM, Madison, WI.)

LETTERS. Copies of all written communications sent to or concerning a patient should become part of the patient's clinical record. The fact that these documents may become evidence in a malpractice suit warrants caution in writing and retaining them.

POSTAL RECEIPTS. Radiographs or other records transferred to another dentist should be sent by certified mail with return receipt requested. The receipt verifies that the films were mailed and by whom the package was received.

RADIOGRAPHIC FILMS. The radiographic films stored in a patient's record should be labeled with the patient's full name, the date of exposure, the number and type of films, and the dentist's name. If radiographs are copied and transferred to another practitioner, the name and date of transfer should be noted on the clinical chart. In addition, a signed request from the patient and a letter of transmittal must be retained in the file envelope.

Entering Data on a Clinical Chart

Several types of data are entered in the various components of a patient's record, such as charting of existing conditions, which is done with a variety of symbols and codes; recording of treatment procedures on progress notes, written in clear, concise detail using codes; treatment plans; and discussions

Rx/MEDICATION HISTORY

NAME _____ AGE _____ DATE _____ ACCT# _____
ALLERGIES _____ MEDICAL ALERT _____

Date _____ Medication _____
Rx/Dosage _____ ☐ Dispense as Written   Qty _____ Freq _____
                                                                          ☐ Substitute Permitted
_____ Refill (s), Instructions _____
☐ Rx to Patient / ☐ Rx to Pharmacy _____
Start: _____ Stop: _____ Disc: _____ Initials _____

Date _____ Medication _____
Rx/Dosage _____ ☐ Dispense as Written   Qty _____ Freq _____
                                                                          ☐ Substitute Permitted
_____ Refill (s), Instructions _____
☐ Rx to Patient / ☐ Rx to Pharmacy _____
Start: _____ Stop: _____ Disc: _____ Initials _____

Date _____ Medication _____
Rx/Dosage _____ ☐ Dispense as Written   Qty _____ Freq _____
                                                                          ☐ Substitute Permitted
_____ Refill (s), Instructions _____
☐ Rx to Patient / ☐ Rx to Pharmacy _____
Start: _____ Stop: _____ Disc: _____ Initials _____

Date _____ Medication _____
Rx/Dosage _____ ☐ Dispense as Written   Qty _____ Freq _____
                                                                          ☐ Substitute Permitted
_____ Refill (s), Instructions _____
☐ Rx to Patient / ☐ Rx to Pharmacy _____
Start: _____ Stop: _____ Disc: _____ Initials _____

Date _____ Medication _____
Rx/Dosage _____ ☐ Dispense as Written   Qty _____ Freq _____
                                                                          ☐ Substitute Permitted
_____ Refill (s), Instructions _____
☐ Rx to Patient / ☐ Rx to Pharmacy _____
Start: _____ Stop: _____ Disc: _____ Initials _____

Date _____ Medication _____
Rx/Dosage _____ ☐ Dispense as Written   Qty _____ Freq _____
                                                                          ☐ Substitute Permitted
_____ Refill (s), Instructions _____
☐ Rx to Patient / ☐ Rx to Pharmacy _____
Start: _____ Stop: _____ Disc: _____ Initials _____

Date _____ Medication _____
Rx/Dosage _____ ☐ Dispense as Written   Qty _____ Freq _____
                                                                          ☐ Substitute Permitted
_____ Refill (s), Instructions _____
☐ Rx to Patient / ☐ Rx to Pharmacy _____
Start: _____ Stop: _____ Disc: _____ Initials _____

Item 1862 • 3/93 SYCOM ® 1-800-356-8141

B

Figure 7-27, cont'd B, Medication history form (Courtesy Colwell, a Division of Patterson Companies, Inc., Champaign, IL.)

Include adequate time for return of lab case to be examined by the dentist before the patient's appointment.

Complete information is needed, including the full name of the dentist to avoid confusion with dentists who have a similar name.

Specific instructions about the case must be detailed here.

Details about the type of dental materials to be used in the case are recorded, including a shade button is helpful.

Signature stamp may be used. Verification must be filed with the laboratory.

Crown and Bridge

RX DATE _____

CASE # _____

DATE WANTED

DOCTOR INFORMATION

Name _____

Address _____

Telephone _____

PATIENT INFORMATION

Name _____

Sex _____ Age _____

○ Diagnostic wax up ○ pour temps (provisionals)
○ Call me (before proceeding with case)

Rx

HAVE YOU INCLUDED THE FOLLOWING?
○ Impression
○ Bite
○ Opposing
○ Shade
○ Pre-op model
○ Photos
○ Model of temps
○ Bite stick
○ Face bow

PLEASE SEND
○ Prescription forms
○ Plastic bags
○ Case boxes

RETURN FOR
○ Die Trim
○ Metal try in
○ Finish
○ Evaluation
○ Wax check
○ Bisque bake try in

IF INSUFFICIENT ROOM
○ Reduce and mark
○ Metal occlusion
○ Reduction coping
○ Please call

IF CASE WILL NOT DRAW
○ Make reduction copings
○ Please call

experience peace of mind

dti Ward Dental Laboratory

1319 Highland Road   T 810 632 6688
Hartland, MI 48353 USA   F 800 833 3865
    F 810 632 5009

SHADE _____   STUMP _____

AMOUNT OF TRANSLUCENCY
○ Light ○ Medium ○ Heavy

VALUE
○ Bright ○ Medium ○ Low

MIDLINE SHIFT
R ____ MM   L ____ MM
Length of centrals from cervical margin ____ MM

CIRCLE TEETH NUMBERS
1 2 3 4 5 6 7 8 9 10 11 12 13 14 15 16
32 31 30 29 28 27 26 25 24 23 22 21 20 19 18 17

METAL
○ High gold ○ Gold
○ Semi-precious ○ Non-precious

OCCLUSION
○ Metal ○ Porcelain

LATERAL EXCURSION
○ Cuspid guidance ○ Group function

LABIAL MARGIN
○ Fine metal collar on tooth # ____ ○ Show no metal standard on # ____
○ Show no metal 360° on tooth # ____ ○ Porcelain Butt margin on tooth # ____

CONTACTS
○ Broad ○ Normal ○ Point

OCCLUSAL CLEARANCE
○ Positive Contact ○ Cusp Fossa ○ Out of Occlusion
○ Foil Relief ○ Surgical Stent

OCCLUSAL STAINING
○ None
○ Light
○ Medium
○ Dark
○ Hypo-calcification
○ Shade tab enclosed

MOLD OF CROWN DESIRED
○ Follow study model
○ Match existing
○ Make ideal

SURFACE ANATOMY
○ Smooth
○ Textured
○ Mamelon development
○ Match existing
○ Close Diastema

PONTIC DESIGN
Harmony Ridge Lap Ovate
Cone Hygenic

PONTIC TISSUE RELIEF
○ Yes ○ No ____ mm deep

Doctor's Signature _____   License # _____

White – Lab Copy   Yellow – Lab Copy   Blue – Doctor's Copy

Figure 7-28 Laboratory requisition/prescription forms. **A,** Crown and bridge.

Figure 7-28, cont'd B, Removable prosthetics. (Courtesy Ward Dental Laboratory, Hartland, MI.)

Include adequate time for return of lab case to be examined by the dentist before the patient's appointment.

Complete information is needed, including the full name of the dentist to avoid confusion with dentists who have a similar name.

Specific instructions about the case must be detailed here.

Note specifics of prosthesis design here.

Details about the type of dental materials to be used in the case are recorded, including a shade button is helpful.

Signature stamp may be used. Verification must be filed with the laboratory.

Dalbert W. Fear Jr., D.D.S., M.S.
Roger P. Hitchcock, D.D.S., M.S.
William D. Baxter, Jr., D.D.S., M.S.

Oral and maxillofacial surgery

Consent for oral surgery

1. I hereby authorize Dr._____ , and such assistants as may be selected by him, to treat the condition(s) described below:

_____

_____

_____

2. The procedure(s) necessary to treat the condition(s) have been explained to me, and I understand the nature of the procedure(s) to be:

_____

_____

_____

3. I have been informed of possible alternative methods of treatment (if any).

4. I understand that this is an elective procedure, and that other forms of treatment, or even no treatment at all, are choices that I have, and that the treatment described in paragraph 2 above is (in my doctor's opinion), the most appropriate in the present situation.

5. The doctor has explained to me that there are certain inherent and potential risks in any treatment plan or procedure, and that in this specific instance such operative risks include, but are not limited to, the following:

_____ A. Adverse reaction to the local anesthetic agent.
_____ B. Postoperative discomfort and swelling, that may necessitate several days of home recuperation.
_____ C. Bleeding, which may be heavy or prolonged, and which may require additional treatment to control.
_____ D. Injury to adjacent teeth or fillings.
_____ E. Postoperative infection requiring additional treatment.
_____ F. Stretching of the corners of the mouth, with resultant cracking and bruising.
_____ G. Restricted mouth opening of several days or weeks.
_____ H. Decision to leave a small piece of root in the jaw if its removal would require extensive additional surgery
_____ I. Breakage of the jaw.
_____ J. Injury to the nerve underlying the lower teeth, resulting in numbness or tingling of the chin, lip, cheek, gums, and/or tongue on the side of the surgery; this may persist for several weeks, months, or in remote instances, permanently.
_____ K. Opening into the mouth of the sinus present above the upper teeth, which may require additional medication or surgery to close.
_____ L. Damage to the jaw joint, which may require treatment or surgery.
_____ M. Postoperative loss of the blood clot (dry socket), which would require treatment.

6. It has been explained to me that, during the course of the procedure(s) unforeseen conditions may be revealed that necessitate an extension of the original procedure(s), or different procedures than those set forth in paragraph 2 above. I, therefore, authorize and request that the person(s) described in paragraph 1 above perform such procedures as are necessary and desirable in the exercise of professional judgement. The authority granted under this paragraph 6 shall extend to the treatment of all conditions that require treatment and are not known at the time the original procedure is begun.

A

Figure 7-29 A, Consent for oral surgery.

7. I consent to the administration of local anesthetic and anti-inflammatory medications in connection with the procedure(s) referred to above, by any of the persons described in paragraph 1, and to the use of whichever such agents chosen by my doctor with the exception of: _____ , to which i have said i am allergic.

8. Medications, drugs, anesthetics and prescriptions may cause drowsiness and lack of awareness and coordination, which can be increased by the use of alcohol or other drugs; thus, I have been advised not to operate any vehicle, automobile or hazardous devices, or work, while taking such medications and/or drugs; or until fully recovered from the effects of these medications or drugs. I also agree not to consume any alcohol or other drug of which my doctor is unaware, while under the effect of medication given or prescribed to me by my doctor.

9. It has been explained to me, and I understand and accept, that a perfect result is not guaranteed or warranted, and in fact can not be guaranteed or warranted.

10. I certify that i read, write, and understand English and that I have read and fully understand this consent for surgery. All blanks requiring insertion or completion have been filled in. Inapplicable paragraphs, if any, were stricken before I signed. I understand that I should now ask my doctor any questions that I may still have concerning this consent form.

_____   _____
Patients signature   Date

_____   _____
Patients or Legal Guardian (if under 18)   Date

_____   _____
Witness   Date

_____   _____
A Surgeon   Date

Figure 7-29, cont'd A, Consent for oral surgery.

with the patient about recommended treatment. Some clinical charts provide space for data entry on the back of the form. As entries are made and the form becomes complete, or as a separate form, many dentists opt to use a progress sheet to enter clinical data. All data entered in a patient's clinical chart or progress note should be dated, accurate and complete, and initialed by the treating dentist and assistant (Figure 7-30). One of the major concerns in legal action is the incompleteness of data on a patient record. All action should be recorded in the clinical record. If a patient declines treatment, this notation should be entered on the record, dated, and signed. Failure to document any activity completely and accurately may prove costly in a lawsuit. Box 7-1 lists several rules for entering data, beginning with creation of the record.

Types of Clinical Data Entries

Entering information on the patient's clinical chart or progress notes involves the use of tooth numbering systems and an assortment of abbreviations and symbols. The administrative assistant must understand each of these systems, as well as the basic descriptions of the oral cavity. For example, there are two arches, the maxilla, or maxillary arch (upper jaw), and the mandible, or mandibular arch (lower jaw). There are four quadrants, maxillary right and left and mandibular right and left. There are six segments: the maxillary and mandibular right and left segments, which include the molars and premolars, and the two anterior segments, which include all anterior teeth on the right and left in both arches from canine to canine.

> Failure to document any activity completely and accurately may prove costly in a lawsuit.

JOSEPH W. LAKE, D.D.S.
611 Main Street, S.E.
Grand Rapids, MI 49502
616. 101. 9575

PARTIAL DENTURES

I have recommended a removable partial denture as part of the treatment plan devised for your dental needs. While this denture will not function as well as your natural teeth or a fixed bridge, it can offer you many years of reasonable service and function.

The bottom or base of your partial denture looks something like an upside down "U' and will rest on top of your gum tissue. The partial denture will be held in place by one or more of the following devices: clasps, rests, keyways, lingual bars and the like. I have explained which of these devices will be used in your denture.

Due to the situation created by the loss of teeth, partial dentures involve some problems which usually cannot be avoided. You may experience some soreness under the base where the denture rests on the gum tissue. This may be alleviated by adjustments to the denture and tissue treatment. If this is your first denture it may take you a while to become accustomed to its feel. Even experienced denture wearers need some time to adjust to a new denture. However, any continuing pain or discomfort should be brought to my attention.

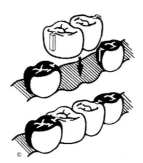

Because your partial denture may, for purposes of stability, rely in part upon a connection or attachment to your remaining teeth, there is a chance that over time these teeth may be weakened or compromised sooner than if they hadn't been so employed.

Even though your partial denture cannot itself decay, it will trap food particles. Without thorough and regular brushing and cleansing of the denture you may encourage decay to adjacent natural teeth, create or exacerbate periodontal disease in those adjacent teeth and promote bad breath.

I invite your questions concerning the risks discussed and contained in this document. By signing below you acknowledge that you have read this document, understand the information presented and have had all your questions answered satisfactorily.

Additional comments: _____   Signatures: Date:

_____   Patient _____

_____   Doctor _____

_____   Witness _____

_____

_____

_____

_____

Item 4287 © 07/93 **SYCOM**® 1-800-356-8141

B

Figure 7-29, cont'd B, Partial dentures. (Courtesy SYCOM, Madison, WI.)

JOSEPH W. LAKE, D.D.S.
611 Main Street, S.E.
Grand Rapids, MI 49502
616. 101. 9575

FULL DENTURES

I have recommended a full or complete denture (upper, lower or both) as part of the treatment plan devised for your dental needs. A full denture is used when <u>all</u> of the natural teeth are missing from a dental arch (upper or lower jaw).

While this substitute for your natural teeth will not function as well as your natural teeth, it can offer years of reasonable service and function.

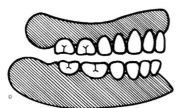

The denture is constructed so that it rests on top of your gum tissue and all of the chewing forces must be born by your gum tissue. As a consequence, you may experience some soreness or discomfort under the denture base. This may be alleviated by adjustments and tissue treatment. In some cases it takes several appointments before the denture can be made comfortable.

If this is your first denture it may take you awhile to become accustomed to its feel. Initially, the denture may stimulate your gag reflex, feel very large in your mouth or simply feel foreign. Even experienced denture wearers need some time to adjust to a new denture. However, any continuing pain, discomfort or difficulty in adapting to your denture should be brought to my immediate attention.

If you discontinue wearing your denture for any extended period of time you may find that it doesn't fit when you attempt to wear it again. This is due to the fact the gum tissue will change its shape over time if the denture base isn't resting upon it. If this occurs I will need to re-adjust the base to fit the tissue. In extreme cases a new base may need to be fashioned.

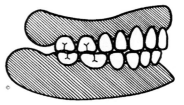

I invite your questions concerning the risks discussed and contained in this document. By signing below you acknowledge that you have read this document, understand the information presented and have had all your questions answered satisfactorily.

Additional comments: _____   Signatures: Date:

_____   Patient _____

_____   Doctor _____

_____   Witness _____

_____

_____

_____

_____

Item 4288 © 07/93 **SYCOM®** 1-800-356-8141

C

Figure 7-29, cont'd C, Full dentures. (Courtesy SYCOM, Madison, WI.)

JOSEPH W. LAKE, D.D.S.
611 Main Street, S.E.
Grand Rapids, MI 49502
616.101.9575

RESTORATIONS

I have recommended that one or more of your teeth needs a full or partial crown (cap), onlay or inlay. These restorations generally are used to repair teeth structurally compromised by decay or previous restorations, for cosmetic reasons, to change the way your teeth come together (occlusion) or to protect a tooth which has had a root canal. I have explained to you the specific reason of a cast restoration in your case.

I would like you to know what is involved in providing you with a cast restoration so you will have no surprises during the course of treatment.

Your tooth will need to be prepared to receive the restoration. This will require some of the tooth being removed with a high speed dental bur and water spray. A local anesthetic injection will prevent you from feeling any discomfort during the process. You should know that there is a chance your tooth may be sore or uncomfortable for a while after the preparation but this will pass after a short period of time. On occasion, the pulp (nerve and blood supply inside the tooth) may be irritated by the preparation process or by prior trauma or decay and may begin to cause you pain. If this persists, your tooth may need a root canal which may be an additional charge.

An impression will be taken of your teeth and mouth using a soft rubbery like material from which plaster casts will be made. These will be used by me or a laboratory to cast a restoration specifically made to fit your tooth. It usually takes one to two weeks for the restoration to be created and readied for placement on your tooth.

While you are waiting for your new crown to be made by the laboratory, I will have placed temporary crowns or restorations to protect the tooth and permit near normal chewing function. The temporary crown or restoration is designed to only last a short while. Wearing the temporary for longer than recommended may result in the loss of its protective integrity. Thus, it is important for you to return when scheduled to avoid decay, gum irritation and bite problems.

When the permanent cast restoration is placed, I will check with you to make sure the color and appearance are to your liking. After checking it for proper fit and harmony with your bite, it will be cemented on your tooth. I may have to make additional adjustments to your bite (occlusion) before you are completely comfortable. You may experience for a short while a sensation that the crown or restoration is "too tight" or "different" until you become accustomed to it.

Even though your crown or restoration is made of materials that cannot decay, you still must care for it as if it were a natural tooth by brushing and flossing regularly. This will minimize the chances of decay forming where the restoration meets the tooth or of gum disease around the tooth.

I invite your questions concerning the risks discussed and contained in this document. By signing below you acknowledge that you have read this document, understand the information presented and have had all your questions answered satisfactorily.

Additional comments: _____   Signatures: _____   Date: _____

_____   Patient _____

_____   Doctor _____

_____   Witness _____

_____

_____

_____

_____

Item 4285 © 07/93 SYCOM® 1-800-356-8141

D

Figure 7-29, cont'd D, Restorations.

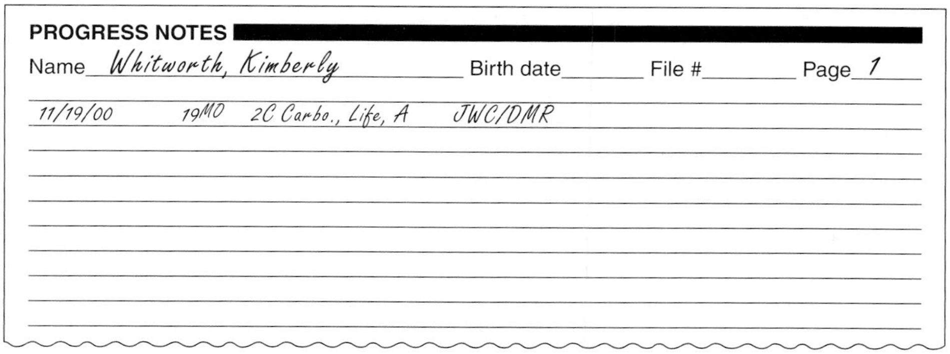

```
┌──────────────────────────────────────────────────────────────┐
│ PROGRESS NOTES ████████████████████                           │
│ Name  Whitworth, Kimberly          Birth date____ File #____ Page  1   │
│ ─────────────────────────────────────────────────────────     │
│ 11/19/00      19MO   2C Carbo., Life, A    JWC/DMR             │
│ ─────────────────────────────────────────────────────────     │
│ ─────────────────────────────────────────────────────────     │
│ ─────────────────────────────────────────────────────────     │
│ ─────────────────────────────────────────────────────────     │
│ ─────────────────────────────────────────────────────────     │
│ ─────────────────────────────────────────────────────────     │
│ ─────────────────────────────────────────────────────────     │
│ ─────────────────────────────────────────────────────────     │
└──────────────────────────────────────────────────────────────┘
```

Figure 7-30 Data entry on a clinical chart, initialed by the treating dentist and dental assistant.

TOOTH NOMENCLATURE. To begin with, the administrative assistant should be able to identify the names and numbers of teeth in both the primary and permanent dentition (Box 7-2). Mixed dentition (a combination of primary and permanent teeth) usually exists from approximately 6 to 12 years of age. Mixed dentition occurs when the permanent teeth begin to erupt while some of the primary teeth are still present. This is a common condition in a child of about 7 years of age. For example, the child may have lost the primary

---

Box 7-1
Rules for Entering Data on a Clinical Record

- Transfer the information from the registration and health history form to the dental chart completely and accurately.
- Enter general information about the patient neatly (the clinical record must be completed in ink, or it may be keyboarded).
- Underline in red any notation about a serious illness or allergies. Small, brightly colored labels (see Figure 7-31, A to D) also may be used to draw attention to special notations.
- The clinical assistant or dentist may make the entries for services rendered in the clinical record. Data can be entered on a barrier-protected keyboard in the treatment room or on a keyboard outside the treatment room. Both methods provide a neater record and, when properly implemented, can improve infection control in records management.
- Check information to ensure that it has been transferred or entered correctly.
- Place the record in the file envelope or folder with the patient's name visible on the record.
- After each patient has been treated, check each record carefully to determine if it has been completed for the day.
- Verify that the record has been initialed by the dentist and the clinical assistant who performed the treatment (see Figure 7-30). In offices with a large staff, this serves as a reference for follow-up and may be needed in case of a lawsuit.
- Ensure that all codes and charting techniques are consistent with the system used in the office. A list of these codes and symbols should be posted in each treatment room and available to all staff members.
- Never make a derogatory remark about a patient in the record that could prove damaging in a lawsuit.

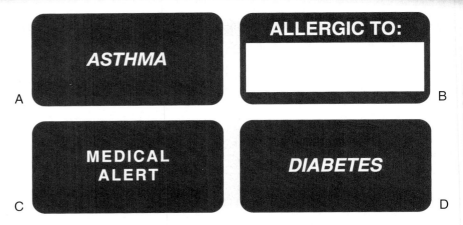

Figure 7-31 A to **D,** Colored chart labels draw attention to special medical conditions. (Courtesy SYCOM, Madison, WI.)

central incisors, and the first permanent molars may have erupted. Mixed dentition occasionally occurs in an adult when a primary tooth is retained and is not replaced by a permanent tooth.

Teeth present a good appearance and provide support for other structures. They also aid in swallowing, mastication, digestion, and the production of speech and phonetics. The primary dentition creates the framework for eruption of a healthy permanent dentition. Premature loss of the primary teeth can be directly related to future dental disease or other dental anomalies. Likewise the loss of a single permanent tooth, if not replaced, can be the start of serious dental impairment. The administrative assistant plays an important role in patient education and must take advantage of seminars promoting dental health, gaining knowledge that will make the assistant an ambassador for maintaining teeth for a lifetime.

Box 7-2
Primary and Permanent Dentition

Primary Dentition
2 central incisors
2 lateral incisors
2 cuspids (canines)
2 first molars
2 second molars
Total: 10 in each arch

Permanent Dentition
2 central incisors
2 lateral incisors
2 cuspids (canines)
2 first premolars
2 second premolars
2 first molars
2 second molars
2 third molars (may not develop)
Total: 16 in each arch (including third molars)

> **Box 7-3**
> **Categories of Tooth Identification**
>
> | **Dentition** | **Arch** |
> |---|---|
> | Primary | Maxillary |
> | Permanent | Mandibular |
> | | |
> | **Quadrant** | **Specific Tooth** |
> | Right | (e.g., first premolar, central incisor) |
> | Left | |

It is important to understand the correct identification of a tooth in the oral cavity and the sequence of terms used to identify it. Confusion in the order of identification can cause many communication problems. The correct sequence of identification is: the dentition, the arch, the quadrant, and the specific tooth (Box 7-3).

For example, in describing a patient's complaint, you would define the problem tooth as the permanent maxillary right first molar. This sequence of identification is commonly used in dental offices.

TOOTH NUMBERING SYSTEMS. Every dental office has a specific numbering system that is used in charting a patient's oral cavity or referring to dental treatment to be performed. There are several numbering systems, and the dentist and staff choose which will be used in the office. The objective of a numbering system is to name and code each tooth numerically or alphabetically. This number or letter provides an abbreviated form of tooth reference and aids in consistency in records management. The three most common numbering systems are the **Universal numbering system**, the **Palmer notation system**, and the **Federal Dentaire International (FDI) system.**

Universal numbering system. The most popular numbering system is the Universal numbering system. It uses the Arabic numerals from 1 to 32 for the permanent dentition and the letters *A* to *T* for the primary dentition.

The Universal system begins numbering the teeth with the most posterior tooth on the patient's maxillary right quadrant, the third molar (i.e., tooth #1), or the permanent maxillary right third molar. If the numbering is for the primary dentition, the tooth is labeled in an alpha code beginning with *A* for the primary maxillary right second molar. The numbering continues toward the anterior midline to the central incisor, or tooth #8 of the permanent dentition (tooth *#E* of the primary dentition). The numbering continues to the maxillary left quadrant, from the midline to the most posterior tooth, either #16 of the permanent dentition or *#J* of the primary dentition. The numbering then drops to the mandibular left quadrant to permanent tooth #17 (primary tooth *#K*) across the arch to the mandibular right most posterior tooth, #32 (or *#T*) (Figure 7-32).

Palmer notation system. The Palmer notation system assigns each of the four quadrants a bracket to designate the area of the mouth where the tooth is found. In Figure 7-32, *A*, the left side of the chart represents the patient's right side, and the right side of the chart represents the patient's left side. It might be depicted this way:

Maxillary right	Maxillary left
Mandibular right	Mandibular left

Each permanent tooth in any quadrant is assigned the same number with #1 beginning at the midline and increasing to #8 distally. For instance:

Maxillary right central incisor 1
Maxillary left central incisor 1
Mandibular left central incisor 1
Mandibular right central incisor 1

The direction of the bracket determines the arch, and the number within the bracket determines the tooth:

Maxillary right third molar 8
Maxillary left second molar 7
Mandibular right first premolar 4
Mandibular left lateral incisor 2

For the primary dentition, brackets are used to assign a quadrant, but the teeth are designated by the letters *A* to *E*. *A* specifies the central incisors, and *E* specifies the second molars (Figure 7-33, *B*).

Federal Dentaire International system. The Federal Dentaire International (FDI) system (Figure 7-34) assigns a two-digit number to each tooth in any quadrant. The first number indicates the quadrant in which the tooth is positioned, and the second number identifies the specific tooth. The numbers 1 to 4 are assigned to the permanent dentition, and 5 to 8 are

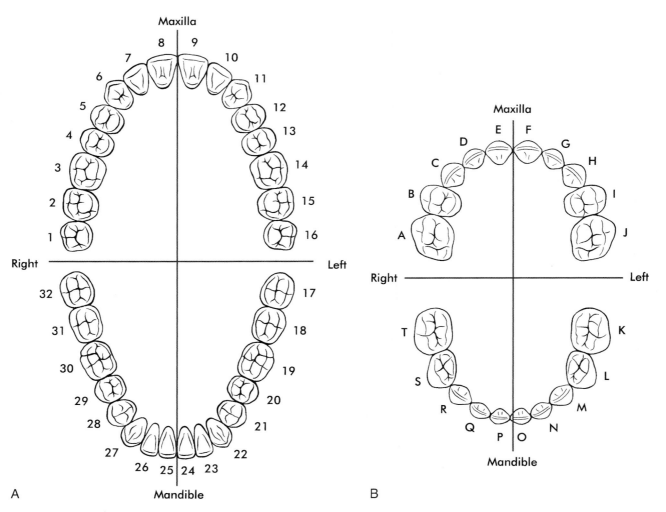

Figure 7-32 Universal numbering system. **A,** Permanent dentition. **B,** Primary dentition.

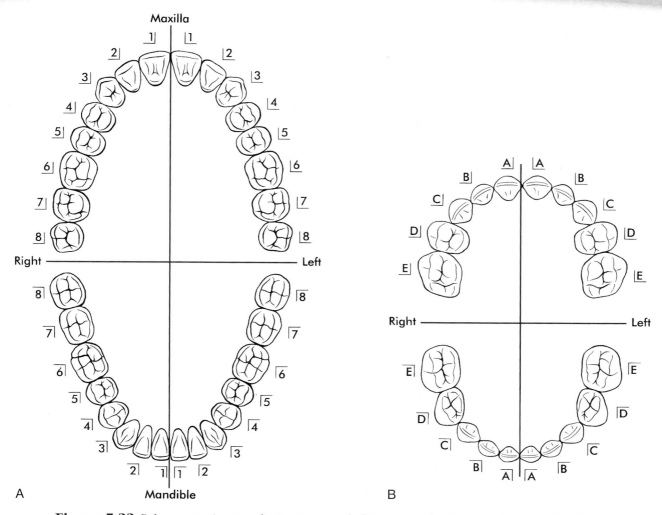

Figure 7-33 Palmer notation numbering system. **A,** Permanent dentition. **B,** Primary dentition.

assigned to the quadrants of the primary dentition. Therefore, the first number would be designated as follows:

Number	Quadrant
1	Permanent maxillary right
2	Permanent maxillary left
3	Permanent mandibular left
4	Permanent mandibular right
5	Primary maxillary right
6	Primary maxillary left
7	Primary mandibular left
8	Primary mandibular right

The second number identifies the specific tooth in the arch. The numbers 1 to 8 are assigned to the permanent dentition and 1 to 5 to the primary dentition. The #1 in both instances begins with the central incisors, and the numbering of the teeth proceeds posteriorly so that the last tooth in the quadrant is the highest number in the sequence. Some examples are:

Permanent maxillary right central incisor: #11 (which is read, "number one one")
Permanent maxillary left central incisor: #21 (number two one)
Permanent mandibular left central incisor: #31 (number three one)
Permanent mandibular right central incisor: #41 (number four one)

The primary dentition is handled in the same manner, but because there are only five teeth per quadrant, the numbers would range from 1 to 5 for each tooth and 5 to 8 for the quadrants. Therefore the primary maxillary right first molar is #54 (number five four) and the primary mandibular left lateral incisor is #72 (number seven two).

TOOTH SURFACES. During routine charting procedures, the chairside assistant uses various alpha codes for tooth surface annotation. Using tooth nomenclature and surface annotation makes it easy to identify a specific location on a tooth where there may be dental decay, a fracture, or a restoration. The administrative assistant must be familiar with this terminology to complete insurance forms and to consult with other dentists about patient treatment.

All crowns of the teeth are divided into surfaces, which are identified by their position in relation to the oral cavity. For example, the surfaces nearest the lips are referred to as the labial, or facial, surfaces. The posterior teeth (the premolars and molars) have five surfaces. The anterior teeth (the incisors and canines) have four surfaces with a ridge. Both anterior and posterior teeth have four axial surfaces. The **axial surface** runs vertically from the biting surface to the apex of a tooth. The posterior teeth have one additional surface, the **occlusal surface,** which is the horizontal surface that runs perpendicular to the other axial surfaces.

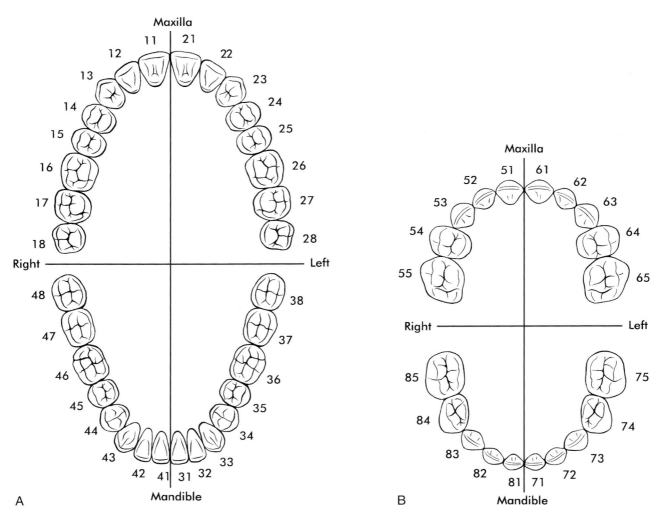

Figure 7-34 Federal Dentaire International (FDI) system. **A,** Permanent dentition. **B,** Primary dentition.

The surfaces of the teeth not only have names but are also identified by letters or numbers. This surface annotation is used to simplify charting notations and for all insurance reports. The letter or number is commonly placed as a superscript (above the print line) next to the tooth number. For example, using the Universal numbering system to describe a procedure involving the mesial surface of the permanent maxillary left first molar, the assistant would write: #14^M or #14^1. The surfaces of the teeth are as follows (Figure 7-35):

- The *mesial surface* (M or 1) is the axial surface closest to the midline of the mouth.
- The *distal surface* (D or 2) lies directly opposite the mesial surface and is the axial surface farthest from the midline.
- The *facial surface* (F or 3) faces the cheek and lips, or the exterior of the mouth.
- The *labial surface* (LA or 3) is the same as the facial surface but is found facing only the lips on the anterior teeth. This letter combination is not used frequently because it requires an extra space in data entry; the designation *facial* (F) is used more often.
- The *buccal surface* (B or 3) is the same as the facial surface but is found on posterior teeth only, facing the cheeks.
- The *lingual surface* (L or 4) is the surface closest to the tongue.
- The *occlusal surface* (O or 5) is found only on posterior teeth on a vertical plane, or the biting surface of the teeth.
- The *incisal ridge* (or *edge* or *surface*) (I or 5) is found only on anterior teeth that have a biting edge.
- The proximal areas or surfaces are the areas or surfaces where two teeth abut or face each other. Most teeth have two proximal surfaces, the mesial and the distal proximal surfaces. In the third molars, however, only the mesial surface may be considered a proximal surface.
- When more than one surface is involved (e.g., mesial, occlusal, and distal), the surface annotations are placed in order from mesial to distal: for example, #19^{MOD} instead of #19^{DOM} or #19^{ODM}. This standardization provides for uniform communication between dental professionals.

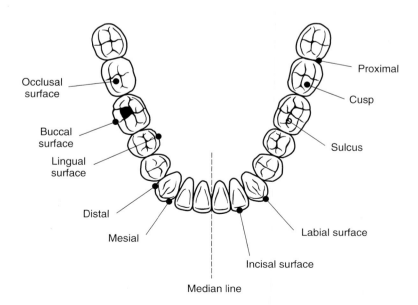

Figure 7-35 Tooth surface annotation.

Charting Symbols and Abbreviations

Charting symbols are a form of shorthand in the dental office. They allow the clinical assistant to quickly outline a condition on a graphic chart. The dentist later can use this information for the diagnosis, or the administrative assistant can quickly identify conditions in the patient's mouth without reading through a lengthy description. Figure 7-36 presents a variety of symbols commonly used in a dental office.

Clinical abbreviations are short versions of or initials for common clinical terminology. Table 7-1 is a detailed list of abbreviations commonly used for data entry on dental records.

Records Retention

The question often is asked, "How long should a patient's records be retained?" The answer seems awkward: The record should be retained for the period of time consistent with the statute of limitations within the state. The **statute of limitations,** the period within which a civil suit for alleged wrongdoing may be legally filed, varies from state to state. The average minimum for retention of a patient's records is approximately 6 years after performance of the last treatment, but it is better to retain the records longer than that. Chapter 8 offers suggestions for longer-term storage.

Records Transfer

Requests for transfer of records are made for many reasons such as (1) the patient wants to change dentists; (2) the patient is moving out of the area; (3) the dentist wants to consult with another dentist; and (4) the patient has been referred to another dentist.

Care must be taken in completing a request for transfer of a patient's records. By law, any information regarding a patient's care and treatment is confidential and privileged. This privilege belongs to the patient, not to the dentist. Therefore, for the dentist's protection, it is prudent to obtain a written consent signed by the patient or the patient's legal representative before transferring records to anyone other than the patient. Certain exceptions exist to this privilege prohibiting disclosure, such as legal action or court orders involving the dentist. In general, if the following suggestions are followed, record transfer can be handled efficiently and confidentially.

- Provide accurate and complete dental records.
- Never change dental records without maintaining the readability of the original entry; date any changes, and record the reason for the change.
- Obtain a signed consent form from the patient or the advice of legal counsel before providing copies of or allowing access to a patient's dental records to anyone other than the patient.
- Retain records in accordance with the state statute.
- Keep original records.
- Charge a reasonable clerical fee for furnishing records in accordance with local standards.
- Charge a reasonable professional fee for preparing and furnishing a narrative report for the patient.
- Require advance payment for clerical and preparation service in accordance with local standards.
- If records are mailed, send them certified mail with return receipt requested. The receipt will verify that the materials were received.

> By law, any information regarding a patient's care and treatment is confidential and privileged.

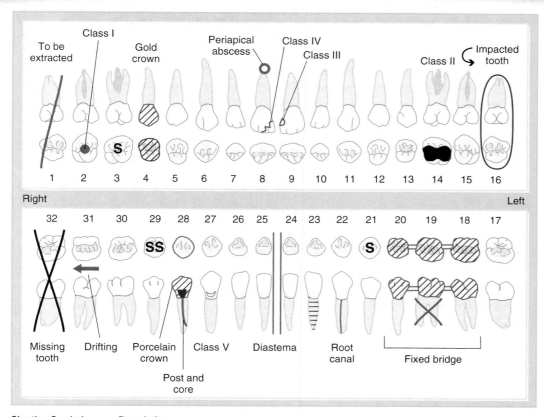

Charting Symbol	Description
Amalgam	Outline the surfaces that are involved (refer to teeth 2 and 14).
Composite	Outline the surfaces involved (refer to teeth 9 and 27).
Porcelain fused to metal (PFM)	Outline the tooth and draw diagonal lines on the occlusal or lingual surface where metal appears (refer to tooth 28).
Gold	Outline the crown of the tooth and place diagonal lines (refer to tooth 4).
Sealant	Place an "S" on the occlusal surface (refer to teeth 3 and 21).
Stainless steel crown	Outline crown of tooth and place "SS" on occlusal surface (refer to tooth 29).
To be extracted	Draw a red diagonal line through the tooth. An alternative method is to draw two red parallel lines through the tooth (refer to tooth 1).
Missing tooth	Draw a black or blue "X" through the tooth. It does not matter if the tooth was extracted or it never erupted, just as long as the tooth is not visible in the mouth. If a quadrant, or arch, is edentulous, make one "X" over all teeth (refer to tooth 32).
Impacted or unerupted	Draw a red circle around the whole tooth, including the root (refer to tooth 16).
Decay	Depending on the caries classification, outline and color the area for amalgam (refer to tooth 2), or outline the area for composite (refer to tooth 9).
Recurrent decay	Outline the existing restoration in red to indicate decay in the area (refer to tooth 14).
Root canal	Draw a line through the center of each root involved (refer to tooth 22).
Periapical abscess	Draw a red circle at the apex of the root to indicate infection (refer to tooth 8).
Post and core	Draw a line through the root that requires a post; then continue the line into the gingival one third of the crown, making a triangle shape (refer to tooth 6).
Rotated tooth	If a tooth has rotated in its position, indicate the direction the tooth has turned by placing a red arrow to the side of the tooth (refer to tooth 15).
Diastema	When there is more space than normal between two teeth, draw two red vertical lines between the areas (refer to teeth 24 and 25).
Fixed bridge	Draw an "X" through the roots of the missing tooth or teeth involved. Then draw a line to connect each of the teeth that make up the bridge. The type of material used to make the bridge will determine whether you outline the crown for porcelain, use diagonal lines for gold, or use a combination of the two (refer to teeth 18-20).
Full crown	Outline the complete crown if it is to be a porcelain crown, or outline and place diagonal lines if it will be a gold crown (refer to tooth 4).
Drifting	Place a red arrow pointing in the direction a tooth is drifting (refer to tooth 31).
Implant	In red, draw horizontal lines through the root or roots of a tooth (refer to tooth 23).
Bonded veneer	Veneers cover only the facial aspect of a tooth. Outline the facial portion only (refer to tooth 26).
Fractured tooth or root	If a tooth or a root is fractured, draw a red zigzag line where the fracture occurred (refer to tooth 8).

Figure 7-36 Example of an anatomic diagram for charting conditions of the mouth. (From Bird DL, Robinson DS: *Torres and Ehrlich's modern dental assisting*, ed 8, St. Louis, 2005, Elsevier.)

Table 7-1
Clinical Abbreviations

Abbreviation	Term
@	at
ac	before meals
ad	to, up to
a, ag, am	amalgam
AIDS	acquired immune deficiency syndrome
amp	ampule
amt	amount
anat	anatomy
anes	anesthesia
ant	anterior
appl	applicable, application, appliance
approx	approximate
BF	bone fragment
bid	twice a day
bio, boil	biological, biology
BP	blood pressure
Br	bridge
BW	bitewing radiograph
Bx	biopsy
c–	with
C	composite
caps	capsules
carbo	carbocaine
cav	cavity
CC	chief complaint
cm	centimeter
CM	cast metal
comp	compound, composite
conc	concentrate
cond	condition
CSX	complete series x-rays
cur	curettage
CV	cardiovascular
CVA	cerebrovascular accident
D	distal
DV	devital
dbl	double
DDS	Doctor of Dental Surgery/Science
DEF	defective
Dg or Dx	diagnosis
DM	diagnostic models
DMF	decayed, missing, and filled
DO	distoocclusal
DOB	date of birth
DR	doctor
dwt	pennyweight
emerg	emergency
EMT	emergency medical treatment
ENT	ears, nose, and throat
epith	epithelial
est	estimate, estimation
et	and
et al	and others
etc	and so on, and so forth
evac	evacuate, evacuation

Table 7-1
Clinical Abbreviations—cont'd

Abbreviation	Term
eval	evaluate, evaluation
ext	extract, external
F	Fahrenheit, female, field, formula
FB	foreign body
FBS	fasting blood sugar
FH	family history
FLD	full lower denture
FMS	full mouth series
FMX	full mouth x-ray
FR or frac	fracture
frag	fragment
freq	frequent, frequency
FUD	full upper denture
G	gold
GF	gold foil
GI	gold inlay
ging	gingiva, gingivectomy
GP	general practitioner
HBP	high blood pressure
Hdpc	handpiece
hosp	hospital
hr	hour
hs	hour of sleep
ht	height
Hx	history
I&D	incision and drainage
IA	incurred accidentally
IH	infectious hepatitis
IM	intramuscular
IMP	impacted
inc	incisal, incisive, incise
inf	infected, inferior, infusion
imp	impression
inj	injection, injury
inop	inoperable, inoperative
IV	intravenous
L	lingual
LA	labial
lab	laboratory
lac	laceration
lat	lateral
lig	ligament
ling	lingual
liq	liquid
LLQ	lower-left quadrant
LN	lymph node
LRQ	lower-right quadrant
lt	left
M, mes	mesial
mand	mandibular
max	maximum, maxillary
MDR	minimum daily requirement
med	medicine, medical
mg, mg, m	milligram

Continued

Table 7-1
Clinical Abbreviations—cont'd

Abbreviation	Term
micro	microscopic
ML	midline
MM	mucous membrane
mm	millimeter
MO	mesiocclusal
mo	month
MOD	mesiocclusodistal
MS	multiple sclerosis
narc	narcotic
nc	no change, no charge
NCP	not clinically present
neg	negative
nonrep	nonrepetitive
norm	normal
NPO	nothing by mouth
occ, occl	occlusal
OH	oral hygiene
OHI	oral hygiene instructions
opp	opposite
P	pulse
PA	periapical
Pan	panoramic oral examination
path	pathology
PDR	*Physicians' Desk Reference*
Ped	pediatrics
PLD	partial lower denture
PO, postop	postoperative
preop	preoperative
prep	preparation, prepare for treatment
prn	as needed
prog	prognosis
pt	patient
Px, Pro, Proph	prophylaxis
q	every
qd	every day
qh	every hour
q2h	every two hours
qid	four times a day
qn	every night
R	respiration
Rx, RX	prescribed
rad	radiograph
RC	root canal
RDA	Registered Dental Assistant
RDH	Registered Dental Hygienist
reg	regular
req	requisition
resp	respiration
RHD	rheumatic heart disease
ROA	received on account
SBE	subacute bacterial endocarditis
Sig	write on label
sol	solution
stat	immediately

Table 7-1
Clinical Abbreviations—cont'd

Abbreviation	Term
stim	stimulate, stimulator
strep	*Streptococcus pyogenes*
surg	surgery, surgeon
Sx	symptom
T	temperature
tab	tablet
TAT	tetanus antitoxin
TB	tuberculosis
TBI	toothbrush instructions
temp	temperature
tid	three times a day
TLC	tender loving care
TMJ	temporomandibular joint
TPR	temperature, pulse, respiration
Tr.P	treatment plan
U, u	unit
unk	unknown
ULQ	upper-left quadrant
URI	upper respiratory infection
URQ	upper-right quadrant
VD	venereal disease
wh	white
wnd	wound
x	times (e.g., 4×); x-ray
xyl, xylo	xylocaine
YOB	year of birth
yr	year

Record Maintenance

Financial records are as important as clinical records but must be maintained separately. A financial record protects the patient and the dentist, provides information for tax purposes, and verifies data for a business analysis. Inadequate or incomplete financial records can result in poor public relations and can create unnecessary legal problems with state and federal governments and third-party payers. Chapter 15 details the step-by-step procedure for creating and managing various financial records. At this point, suffice it to say that financial records differ from clinical records in that a ledger card can be used for a family unit or for a responsible party, whereas clinical records are created for each individual. Therefore if one person is responsible for payment for several dependents, all entries can be made on one ledger card.

Occupational Safety and Health Administration Records

Chapter 17 details the responsibility of the administrative assistant in disease prevention. Specific records must be maintained for OSHA. The *Regulatory Compliance Manual* (see Figure 17-2, *B*), developed by the American Dental Association, is an important source of samples and suggestions for developing the documents required by federal regulations.

Several **employee records** must be maintained in the office. These must be accurate and must be maintained with strict confidentiality. The administrative assistant is responsible for periodically updating these records. Many of the records relate to payroll, and these are discussed in Chapter 16.

Employee records are classified into various categories such as:

Employment forms
- Applications for employment (see Chapter 18)
- Employment agreements (see Chapter 18)
- Merit evaluation forms (see Chapter 18)
- Health forms and medical records (Figure 7-37)
- Federal Employment Eligibility Verification forms (Form I-9) (Figure 7-38)

Employment Tax Information forms (see Chapter 16)
- Employer identification number
- Amounts and dates of all wage, annuity, and pension payments
- Names, addresses, Social Security numbers, and documents of employees and recipients
- Periods for which employees and recipients are paid while absent due to sickness or injury, and the amount and weekly rate of payments made by the dentist or third-party payers
- Copies of employees' and recipients' income tax withholding allowance certificates
- Any employee copies of federal form W-2 that were returned as undeliverable
- Dates and copies of tax deposits made
- Copies of returns filed
- Record of fringe benefits provided including substantiation under the Internal Revenue Service (IRS) Code Section 274 and related regulations

OSHA records relating to each employee
- Medical records
- Copies of employee hepatitis B vaccination records
- Hepatitis B declination forms
- Exposure incident forms
- Follow-up documents for exposure incidents
- OSHA training records

Confidential employee medical record

Employee medical record
Employee name————————————————————————
Employee address————————————————————————
————————————————————————————————
————————————————————————————————
————————————————————————————————
————————————————————————————————

Employee social security number ———————————————
Employee starting date————————————————————
Employee termination date (if any) ——————————————
History of HBV vaccination———————————————————

(date received, or, if not received, a brief explanation of why not)
History of other immunizations ————————————————
————————————————————————————————

History of exposure incident(s) (dates, brief explanation, attachments)——————
————————————————————————————————
————————————————————————————————
————————————————————————————————
————————————————————————————————
————————————————————————————————

Results of medical exams and follow-up procedures regarding exposure incident or
hepatitis B immunity, including written opinion of healthcare professional
(dates, brief explanation, attachments)
————————————————————————————————
————————————————————————————————
————————————————————————————————
————————————————————————————————

Information provided to the health care professional regarding hepatitis B vaccination
and/or exposure incident(s)
(dates, brief explanation, attachments)
————————————————————————————————
————————————————————————————————
————————————————————————————————
————————————————————————————————

Attach pre-employment health records to this document.
Note: maintain the record for duration of employment plus 30 years

Figure 7-37 Employee health and medical records form. (Courtesy SYCOM, Madison, WI.)

U.S. Department of Justice
Immigration and Naturalization Service

OMB No. 1115-0136
Employment Eligibility Verification

Please read instructions carefully before completing this form. The instructions must be available during completion of this form. **ANTI-DISCRIMINATION NOTICE.** It is illegal to discriminate against work eligible individuals. Employers **CANNOT** specify which document(s) they will accept from an employee. The refusal to hire an individual because of a future expiration date may also constitute illegal discrimination.

Section 1.   Employee Information and Verification. To be completed and signed by employee at the time employment begins

Print Name: Last	First	Middle Initial	Maiden Name
Address (Street Name and Number)		Apt. #	Date of Birth (month/day/year)
City	State	Zip Code	Social Security #

I am aware that federal law provides for imprisonment and/or fines for false statements or use of false documents in connection with the completion of this form.	I attest, under penalty of perjury, that I am (check one of the following): ☐ A citizen or national of the United States ☐ A Lawful Permanent Resident (Alien # A_____) ☐ An alien authorized to work until____/____/____ (Alien # or Admission #_____)

Employee's Signature	Date (month/day/year)

Preparer and/or Translator Certification. *(To be completed and signed if Section 1 is prepared by a person other than the employee.) I attest, under penalty of perjury, that I have assisted in the completion of this form and that to the best of my knowledge the information is true and correct.*

Preparer's/Translator's Signature	Print Name
Address (Street Name and Number, City, State, Zip Code)	Date (month/day/year)

Section 2.   Employer Review and Verification. To be completed and signed by employer. **Examine one document from List A OR examine one document from List B and one from List C** as listed on the reverse of this form and record the title, number and expiration date, if any, of the document(s)

List A	OR	List B	AND	List C
Document title: _____		_____		_____
Issuing authority: _____		_____		_____
Document #: _____		_____		_____
Expiration Date (if any): ___/___/___		___/___/___		___/___/___
Document #: _____				
Expiration Date (if any): ___/___/___				

CERTIFICATION - I attest, under penalty of perjury, that I have examined the document(s) presented by the above-named employee, that the above-listed document(s) appear to be genuine and to relate to the employee named, that the employee began employment on *(month/day/year)* _____/_____/_____**and that to the best of my knowledge the employee is eligible to work in the United States. (State employment agencies may omit the date the employee began employment).**

Signature of Employer or Authorized Representative	Print Name	Title
Business or Organization Name	Address (Street Name and Number, City, State, Zip Code)	Date (month/day/year)

Section 3.   Updating and Reverification. To be completed and signed by employer

A. New Name (if applicable)	B. Date of rehire (month/day/year) (if applicable)

C. If employee's previous grant of work authorization has expired, provide the information below for the document that establishes current employment eligibility.

Document Title:_____   Document #:_____   Expiration Date (if any): ___/___/___

I attest, under penalty of perjury, that to the best of my knowledge, this employee is eligible to work in the United States, and if the employee presented document(s), the document(s) I have examined appear to be genuine and to relate to the individual.

Signature of Employer or Authorized Representative	Date (month/day/year)

Form I-9 (Rev. 11-21-91) N

Figure 7-38 Federal Employment Eligibility Verification form (Form I-9).

LISTS OF ACCEPTABLE DOCUMENTS

LIST A

Documents that Establish Both Identity and Employment Eligibility

1. U.S. Passport (unexpired or expired)

2. Certificate of U.S. Citizenship *(INS Form N-560 or N-561)*

3. Certificate of Naturalization *(INS Form N-550 or N-570)*

4. Unexpired foreign passport, with *I-551 stamp or* attached INS Form I-94 indicating unexpired employment authorization

5. Alien Registration Receipt Card with photograph *(INS Form I-151 or I-551)*

6. Unexpired Temporary Resident Card *(INS Form I-688)*

7. Unexpired Employment Authorization Card *(INS Form I-688A)*

8. Unexpired Reentry Permit *(INS Form I-327)*

9. Unexpired Refugee Travel Document *(INS Form I-571)*

10. Unexpired Employment Authorization Document issued by the INS which contains a photograph *(INS Form I-688B)*

OR

LIST B

Documents that Establish Identity

1. Driver's license or ID card issued by a state or outlying possession of the United States provided it contains a photograph or information such as name, date of birth, sex, height, eye color, and address

2. ID card issued by federal, state, or local government agencies or entities provided it contains a photograph or information such as name, date of birth, sex, height, eye color, and address

3. School ID card with a photograph

4. Voter's registration card

5. U.S. Military card or draft record

6. Military dependent's ID card

7. U.S. Coast Guard Merchant Mariner Card

8. Native American tribal document

9. Driver's license issued by a Canadian government authority

For persons under age 18 who are unable to present a document listed above:

10. School record or report card

11. Clinic, doctor, or hospital record

12. Day-care or nursery school record

AND

LIST C

Documents that Establish Employment Eligibility

1. U.S. social security card issued by the Social Security Administration *(other than a card stating it is not valid for employment)*

2. Certification of Birth Abroad issued by the Department of State *(Form FS-545 or Form DS-1350)*

3. Original or certified copy of a birth certificate issued by a state, county, municipal authority or outlying possession of the United States bearing an official seal

4. Native American tribal document

5. U.S. Citizen ID Card *(INS Form I-197)*

6. ID Card for use of Resident Citizen in the United States *(INS Form I-179)*

7. Unexpired employment authorization document issued by the INS *(other than those listed under List A)*

Illustrations of many of these documents appear in Part 8 of the Handbook for Employers (M-274)

Form I-9 (Rev. 11-21-91) N

Figure 7-38, cont'd

LEARNING ACTIVITIES

1. Describe the impact of HIPAA on a dental practice. Why is this important to you as a patient and healthcare professional?
2. List the various categories of records, and give examples of dental office documents that fit each category.
3. Explain why the clinical record is a vital record in the dental office.
4. Describe the parts of a clinical record.
5. Describe the retention and transfer of clinical records in the dental office.
6. Using a clinical chart obtained from the dental practice of an employer or instructor, transfer the information from a completed health questionnaire. This questionnaire may be completed in a classroom or obtained from a patient record in an office of employment.
7. Dr. Lake asks you to send a case to Parker Dental Laboratory. Complete a laboratory requisition that you obtain from an employer or instructor. Include information from below that was taken from the clinical chart:
   John W. Holmes, a male patient, age 36, is to have a porcelain-fused-to-metal crown on the maxillary right second premolar. The shade is C-3 Lumin. The occlusal is to be full porcelain. The final cementation appointment is scheduled for July 8 (today is June 20). Dr. Lake's license number is 7376, and the office address is 611 Main Street SE, Grand Rapids, MI 49502. The office telephone number is 616-101-9575.
8. Consider how one could save time using a computer charting system rather than a manual system with symbols. What would be the disadvantages of using a computer charting system? What would be the advantages to the office and the patient?

EXAMINE YOUR PROGRESS

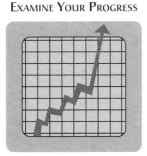

Practice by completing Working Forms 1, 2, and 3.

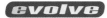

Key Terms

Axial surface The tooth surface that runs vertically from the biting surface to the apex of a tooth.

Charting symbols A type of shorthand in the dental office that is used to enter clinical data on tooth symbols on a patient chart.

Clinical abbreviations Initials or short terms used to explain a clinical condition in a patient's oral cavity.

Clinical record A collection of all information about a patient's dental treatment.

Consent form A form that is signed by the patient or by the parent or guardian of a pediatric patient, which grants permission for administration of an anesthetic and other specified procedures.

Federal Dentaire International (FDI) A tooth numbering system that assigns a two-digit number to each tooth in any quadrant. The first number indicates the quadrant in which the tooth is positioned, and the second number identifies the specific tooth.

Health history form A form that provides the patient's complete health history and is signed by the patient.

Health history update form This form should be completed periodically to keep both the health history and the personal information current. The patient should sign and date this form.

Health Portability and Accountability Act (HIPAA) Federal act that requires dental offices that transmit certain health information electronically to protect patient health information.

Important records Extremely valuable records for the office operation that are extremely valuable but not vital. They include accounts payable and receivable, invoices, canceled checks, inventory and payroll records, and other federal regulatory records.

Information management See *records management*.

Laboratory requisition A form that accompanies each case a dentist sends to a dental laboratory and includes information about the case.

Occlusal surface Biting surface

Palmer notation system A tooth numbering system that assigns each of the four quadrants a bracket to designate the area of the mouth where the tooth is found.

Records management The process of establishing a logical, functional system for storing and retrieving information. Also called *information management*.

Registration form A form containing general information such as addresses and phone numbers, as well as employment and insurance information. It may also be combined with a health history form.

Statute of limitations Period within which a civil suit for alleged wrongdoing may be legally filed.

Unimportant records Documents that lie around, have little importance, and take up space. They include such items as notes to you, reminders of meetings, outdated announcements, and pamphlets.

Universal numbering system The most popular numbering system. It uses Arabic numerals 1 to 32 for the permanent dentition, and the letters *A* to *T* for the primary dentition.

Useful records Records that include employment applications, expired insurance policies, petty cash vouchers, bank reconciliations, and general correspondence.

Vital records Essential documents that cannot be replaced, including patient clinical and financial records and the office's corporate charter and deed, mortgage, or bill of sale.

Bibliography

Fulton PJ: *General office procedures for colleges*, ed 12, Cincinnati, 2003, South-Western.
Furlong A: *Electronic claims filing made easy: New ADA tool shows dental community how*, ADA website, January 2005.
Mosley DC et al: *Supervisory management*, ed 6, Cincinnati, 2004, South-Western.

Recommended Websites

http://www.ada.org/goto/hipaa
http://www.hhs.gov/ocr/hipaa
http://www.hipaacomply.com/hipaafaq.htm
http://www.hipaadvisory.com
http://answers.hhs.gov/cgi-bin/hhs.cfg/php/enduser/std_alp.php

Chapter 8

Storage of Business Records

Chapter Outline

Learning Outcomes

Mastery of the content in this chapter will enable the reader to:

- Define key terms
- Identify and distinguish among the different storage systems
- Apply basic alphabetical indexing rules
- Determine the most efficient storage methods for various documents in a dental office
- Select supplies for the storage of records

Vast amounts of information are generated in the dental office each day. The idea of a paperless office sounds exciting, but reality dictates that traditional methods of record storage will be used for some time. In Chapter 7, disposition is identified as the final stage of a dental record—either destruction or storage. This chapter discusses records storage.

A dental office produces many kinds of information, including clinical and financial records, radiographs, diagnostic models, correspondence, employee records, Occupational Safety and Health Administration (OSHA) records, tax and insurance records, and accounts receivable and payable. Inability to find a document quickly is frustrating and can often delay a decision, diagnosis, or payment. Such delays can be costly and stressful. The administrative assistant is responsible for the storage of business records.

Although microfilm, microfiche, and computer storage are used frequently, many forms of information are still on paper and need to be filed manually. To many administrative assistants, filing is one of those dreaded, procrastinated, routine jobs done when the administrative assistant can "get around to it" or "has the time."

Anyone with office experience knows that records must be readily available. Wise planning can save a tremendous amount of time and effort. The heart of any professional office is its filing system. Business office files should not be a place to *put* materials, but rather a place to *find* materials. A systematic plan for storage, retrieval, transferring, protection, and retention must be established. When planning for the office files, consider ease in retrieval, confidentiality, and safety. The needs of the office, the size of the dental practice, and the space available for equipment are determining factors in establishing an efficient filing system.

> The heart of any professional office is its filing system.

PREPARING RECORDS FOR FILING

Certain routines should be followed in preparing materials for filing: (1) set aside some time each day or every few days for filing paper records; (2) keep papers or records to be filed in a basket marked *To Be Filed;* (3) file electronic records immediately as you input them on a floppy disk, hard drive, or network system. Make backup copies of all electronic files as you complete them.

Before mastering the different filing systems, it is necessary to learn and understand some basic steps, which are generally done in the order of inspecting, indexing, coding, sorting, and storing.

1. *Inspecting.* Review each record to determine if it is something that must be filed. If you are certain it can be disposed of (check the retention schedule or the originator of the form), dispose of it. If it is to be retained, continue to the next step.
2. *Indexing.* Determine under which caption or name an item is to be filed. Indexing is a mental process that requires you to make a decision. For instance, if the record is a receipt for a payment that was just made from the dentist's checking account, you must decide into which file to place the receipt. If files are organized by subject, you might file the receipt under the subject to which it pertains (e.g., a receipt for an electric bill might be filed under "utilities" or "electricity"). For a patient's clinical record, you would commonly use an alphabetical system and break down the name into first, second, and third units to consider for filing.

   Electronic records are indexed by determining on what disk and in what directory the file should be located and by following a uniform procedure for naming the files. Do not name electronic files with characters or words that do not identify the subject of the record.
3. *Coding.* Once you have determined the caption or title of the record, you must assign a code by highlighting, typing, or writing a caption on a paper record or by giving the electronic file a name. On an electronic record, this is done by creating a descriptive file name and including it on the document under the initials of the creator. If an electronic file also exists in paper form, the file name on the document allows for quick, easy retrieval. Examples of coding are shown in Figure 8-1.

The clinical record is coded with the patient's name, and the electronic document is coded with the name of the originator and other important information about the document.

4. *Sorting.* The records are arranged in the order in which they are to be placed in the file (e.g., if the file is alphabetical, put the records in alphabetical order). Electronic files are sorted as you save the files in the correct directory or on the correct disk. The system then sorts the files for you either alphabetically by file name, date, or by any other designation you make.

5. *Storing.* Put documents in folders and bulkier records in file drawers. Check and double-check that you are filing a document correctly. Also be sure to put floppy disks or other media, such as microfilm, in the correct place.

Two other aspects of document storage, cross-referencing and retrieval, deserve special consideration. **Cross-referencing** alerts staff members that a record normally kept in a specific location has been stored elsewhere. A cross-reference can be provided by making a copy of the record and filing it in the referenced file with a note that it is a copy, or a cross-reference sheet can be put in the file. A cross-reference sheet contains the name of the document, the date it was filed, a brief description of the subject of the record, and the places where the record could be found. This type of cross-referencing is often found in a library card catalog.

Retrieval is the removal of records from files using proper "charge-out" methods. When an entire file folder is removed, an out-folder is put in the place of the removed folder. The out-folder has the name of the individual or department that removed the folder and the date it was removed. Out-guides or substitution cards may be used instead of an out-folder.

Although it does not commonly happen with patient clinical charts during routine treatment, a record may need to be removed from a file and used in another location for consultation or study. In such cases, the out-folder should denote the area to which the record has been taken.

Retention of Records

It is not cost-effective to maintain unnecessary records and filing cabinets. Many records in the dental office are retained in accordance with state statutes. If the practice is large, a retention schedule may have been developed for various documents. If the office does not have a retention schedule, the administrative assistant should check with the dentist before deciding how documents should be transferred or destroyed. The National Archives and Records Service, a federal agency, has produced a helpful reference, *Guide to Record Retention Requirements*. It is available from the Superintendent of Documents, U.S. Government Printing Office, Washington, DC 20402.

Retention and destruction of files have taken on additional importance since the federal Revised Rule 26 of the Rules of Civil Procedure was approved in December 1993. This rule requires organizations to make available all relevant records that must be kept in compliance with prevailing statutes and regulations. Delay or failure to find information makes an office vulnerable to financial loss and adverse legal judgments.

CLASSIFICATION OF FILING SYSTEMS

The five basic classification systems of filing are the alphabetical system, the geographical system, the numerical system, the subject system, and the chronological system. All these methods except the chronological system basically apply alphabetical procedures. The method used in a dental office depends on the type of practice, but it is not uncommon to use several of these methods for various types of filing.

Check and double-check that you are filing a document correctly.

Cross-referencing alerts staff members that a record normally kept in a specific location has been stored elsewhere.

Delay or failure to find information makes an office vulnerable to financial loss and adverse legal judgments.

Selecting the Appropriate Filing System

ALPHABETICAL SYSTEM. In an **alphabetical filing system**, the arrangement of names appears in sequence from A to Z. The alphabetical filing system accounts for about 90 percent of the filing a person is likely to perform and can be applied to various captions. Standard rules exist for alphabetizing correctly. Box 8-1 illustrates alphabetical indexing rules applied to a variety of situations.

Box 8-1
Indexing Rules for the Alphabetical System

Names of individuals are indexed by units. The last name (surname) is the key unit, followed by the first name (given name), which is the second unit, and then by the middle name or initial, the third unit. Alphabetize names by comparing the first units of the names, letter by letter. Consider second units only when the first units are identical. Consider third units only if the first and second units are identical, and so on.

Name	1	2	3
Alice J. Gooding	Gooding	Alice	J.
Alice Marie Goodman	Goodman	Alice	Marie
William Grafton	Grafton	William	

If the last names are the same, consider the second indexing unit.

Name	1	2	3
Frank Martin	Martin	Frank	
George Martin	Martin	George	
George C. Martin	Martin	George	C.

If the last names are the same but vary in spelling, consider each letter.

Name	1	2	3
Joy Read	Read	Joy	
Janice Reed	Reed	Janice	
Phyllis J. Reid	Reid	Phyllis	J.

Initials are considered the same as a whole word and are filed before names beginning with the same initial. Names with no initial are filed before those with an initial ("nothing before something").

Name	1	2	3
Arthur Stone	Stone	Arthur	
C. Stone	Stone	C.	
Charles Stone	Stone	Charles	

If two people have the same name, they are indexed according to the alphabetical order of the city of residence, then by state. If two people have the same name and live in the same city, they are indexed according to street name.

Name	1	2	3
Richard Murphey (Grand Rapids)	Murphey	Richard	Grand Rapids
Richard Murphey (Grandville)	Murphey	Richard	Grandville

Box 8-1
Indexing Rules for the Alphabetical System—cont'd

Surname prefixes are considered part of the last name, not separate words. A hyphenated surname (e.g., Meyer-Schafer) is considered a single indexing unit. A compound personal name that is not hyphenated (e.g., Catherine Myers Schafer) is treated as separate indexing units.

Name	1	2	3
Connie MacDonald	MacDonald	Connie	
Connie McDonald	McDonald	Connie	
Alice Meyer-Schafer	Meyer-Schafer	Alice	
Martin O'Connor	O'Connor	Martin	
Frank M. O'Dell	O'Dell	Frank	M.
Catherine Myers Schafer	Schafer	Myers	Catherine

If the first word in a compound surname is one of the standard prefixes (St. in St. James), the surname is indexed as a single unit.

Name	1	2	3
Edward St. James	Saint James	Edward	
William. St. Johns	Saint Johns	William	
James. E. Sutton	Sutton	James	E.

Titles and degrees are disregarded but may be placed in parentheses after the names.

Name	1	2	3
Professor Joseph C. Kline	Kline	Joseph	C. (Prof.)
Father Patrick O'Reilly	O'Reilly	Patrick (Fr.)	
Capt. C. J. Walters	Walters	C.	J. (Capt.)

A seniority designation is not considered an indexing unit but is used as an identifying element to distinguish between identical names.

Name	1	2	3
Charles D. Flynn Jr.	Flynn	Charles	D. (Junior)
Charles D. Flynn Sr.	Flynn	Charles	D. (Senior)

Titles used without a complete name should be considered as the key indexing unit.

Name	1	2	3
Father Patrick	Father	Patrick	
Sister Mary Martha	Sister	Mary	Martha

Articles, conjunctions, and prepositions are disregarded in indexing.

Name	1	2	3
The Litton Dental Clinic	Litton	Dental	Clinic (The)

A firm or business name is indexed in the order written unless it contains an individual's name.

Name	1	2	3	4	5
The Harvey F. Andrew Dental Laboratory	Andrew	Harvey	F.	Dental	Laboratory (The)
Grand Rapids	Grand	Rapids	Dental Laboratory		

Box 8-1
Indexing Rules for the Alphabetical System—cont'd

Dental Laboratory
Horton Dental   Horton Dental   Ceramics
Ceramics

Agencies of the federal government are indexed under United States
    Government and then according to department, division, subdivision,
    and location for adequate differentiation.

Name	1	2	3	4	5	6
Federal Bureau of Investigation	United	States (Dept. of)	Govt. (Bur. of)	Justice	Federal	Investigation
Bureau of Labor	United	States (Dept. of)	Govt. (Bur. of)	Labor	Labor	Statistics

State, county, and city governments are indexed according to location and
    then by department, division, or subdivision.

Name	1	2	3
Park Department, Kent County	Kent	County	Park (Dept.)
Michigan State Department of Education	Michigan	State	Education (Dept. of)
Grandville Department of Health	Grandville	City	Health (Dept.)

Numbers spelled as words in business names are filed alphabetically.
    Numbers written in digit form are filed before letters or words.

Name	1	2	3	4
5-Cent Copy Center	5	Cent	Copy	Center
Four Seasons Health Spa	Four	Seasons	Health	Spa
Seventh Street Photo Center	Seventh	Street	Photo	Center

Names of schools are first indexed by the name of the city in which the
    school is located and then by the name of the school.
Local banking or other institutions with branch offices are indexed as the
    name is written; however, if banks from several cities are involved, the first
    indexing unit is the city where the bank is located, and the name of the
    bank follows.
Numbers, including Roman numerals, are filed before alphabetical information.
    However, all Arabic numerals come before Roman numerals.
Acronyms, abbreviations, and television and radio call letters are treated as
    one unit, and company names are filed as you see them.

GEOGRAPHICAL SYSTEM. In a **geographical filing system**, location is the
important factor of reference. The principle of geographical filing is essentially the same as alphabetical filing, except that geographical filing is done
by a territorial division (e.g., state, city, or street) rather than by name. Coding
should be done in a manner similar to that of the alphabetical system by
marking the caption under which the item will be filed (see Figure 8-1).

NUMERICAL SYSTEM. The **numerical filing system** uses a method of assigning numbers to each new patient or account. Numbers assigned are then

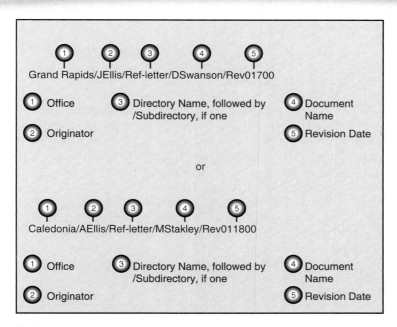

Figure 8-1 Electronic coding at the bottom of a document refers to the originator of the document, the directory name, the subdirectory (if used), and the document name.

recorded on an alphabetical card index or computer file for future reference. Additional papers relating to the same patient or account are subsequently filed according to the number originally allocated. In large clinics with access to computer centers, a numerical system can be used to great advantage because computers handle numerical data faster than alphabetical characters.

SUBJECT SYSTEM. The **subject filing system** is the alphabetical arrangement of papers according to the subject or topic of the papers. This system is used when it is more desirable to assemble information by topic than by name. For example, a subject file may be preferred if the dentist is involved in research or writing for publications. If a subject area is very broad, it can be broken down into smaller divisions by the use of secondary guides. This system is effective only if the administrative assistant is totally aware of the dentist's involvement in the relevant subject areas, or it may be used for filing receipts for the accounts payable.

CHRONOLOGICAL SYSTEM. The **chronological filing system** is a method of filing by date. It can be used within an alphabetical, geographical, subject, or numerical system by filing the most recent correspondence in the front of the file folder. This system can also be used for treatment records in a patient's clinical chart. The most current treatment data sheet would appear first, followed by past treatment records.

Tickler file. Another type of chronological classification system is a **tickler file,** or follow-up file. The most common type of tickler file contains the days of the month and the months of the year. The captions on a tickler file are most commonly the days of the month, from 1 to 31. Items to be completed are filed in the slot of the day you plan to complete the task. Take time each day to review the tickler file. Perform the task to be done on that day, or move the notation to the appropriate day if the activity has been rescheduled. Care should be taken to ensure that an activity is not placed on a weekend day or holiday on which you will not be in the office. The files for these days should be carefully checked in advance to ensure that the task is done before the weekend or holiday or that the task is placed in the slot of a later day.

ELECTRONIC FILES

Storage of electronic records requires a knowledge of computer systems and the storage of word processing, database, or spreadsheet files, as well as knowledge of tasks that require you to sort, search, retrieve, and print reports. As mentioned earlier, in a dental office you probably will most often use a manual filing system, but you may also use at least one type of electronic storage system: floppy disk, hard disk, compact disk, zip disk, tape cartridge, and jump drive. (These forms of storage are discussed in Chapter 5.)

In most dental offices where microcomputers are used, you will store all files from the hard drive on a removable disk or tape. One way to keep track of which files are on each storage unit is to label each storage unit with its own identifying number or code. A separate index stored in a database can list all the file names and the numbers or codes of the storage units on which they may be found. To retrieve a file, you can search your index for the file by file name; the index will show in what storage unit or directory the file is located.

Care of Diskettes

Special attention must be paid to the storage of diskettes to prevent damage and loss of data. Each manufacturer may recommend specific care for its products, but in general, disks should be protected from dust, magnetic fields, extreme temperatures, liquids, and vapors. Box 8-2 presents several suggestions for ensuring safe storage of data.

STORAGE EQUIPMENT

Once an appropriate filing system has been chosen, the administrative assistant must determine what types of supplies and equipment are necessary to maintain the system. The equipment should be practical for day-to-day use and for storage.

The term *filing equipment* refers to the actual structures that store files or records. Most manufacturers supply a variety of models in different colors with assorted features. Many practices still use vertical files, but open-shelf

---

Box 8-2
Diskette Care

- Never touch the internal disk; handle disks only by the protective outer cover.
- Do not expose disks to magnetic fields, such as those produced by telephones, radio speakers, or computer screens.
- Keep disks at temperatures of 50 to 140 degrees Fahrenheit (10 to 60 degrees Celsius); avoid extreme temperatures.
- Protect disks from dust and foreign particles.
- Do not expose disks to water or other liquids.
- If disks contain permanent information, use the *write protect* system to prevent data loss. (Write protect is a feature on a disk or tape that prevents writing over existing data.)

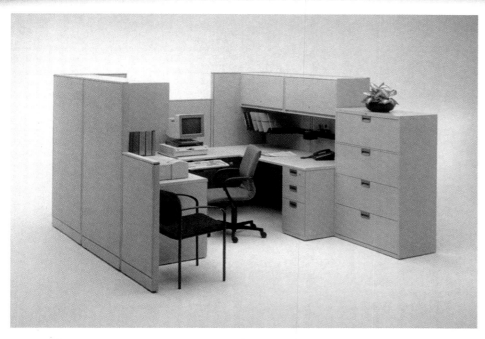

Figure 8-2 Lateral file. (Courtesy Steelcase, Inc., Grand Rapids, MI.)

or lateral filing has become very popular, especially if space is limited. A **vertical file** stores records in drawers; file folders are placed on the folder's edge and arranged according to the filing method selected. Vertical files are available in cabinets with one to five or more drawers and may accommodate either an 8½-by-11-inch (letter size) or 8½-by-14-inch (legal size) file. These are not the best file cabinets to use for saving space. You must allow room for the cabinet as well as the pull-out drawer space. This means you need approximately double the space of the vertical cabinet.

A **lateral file** (Figure 8-2) is similar to a vertical file, except that the longest side opens and the files are stored as if they were placed on a bookshelf. Lateral files have the added advantage of providing a countertop for reviewing files removed from the cabinet or for displaying books and other materials. Like vertical files, lateral files also are designed to accommodate letter- or legal-size files. Less actual floor space is needed because these cabinets can store more files and require less floor and pull-out drawer space.

Open-shelf filing is the most popular filing system among modern dental practices. This arrangement saves space and speeds filing and retrieval. The visibility and accessibility of open-shelf filing have proved to be two of the many advantages of this arrangement (Figure 8-3). Compared to a closed drawer filing system, open-shelf units hold twice as many files on half the floor space. The files give a visible sense of location and allow the users to take full advantage of index guides and color-coding techniques. Misfiled information becomes less of a problem. However, because the files are open, dirt and dust may accumulate if covers are not used.

> Open-shelf filing is the most popular filing system among modern dental practices.

A **card file** can be used to store small cards (3-by-5-inch, 4-by-6-inch, or larger) that are used for specialized systems. Such a system can also be used for a recall system. A card with the patient's name, telephone numbers, and other pertinent information may be set up in a metal or wooden box and used as a quick reference. These cards can then be set up in chronological order and used for patient recall.

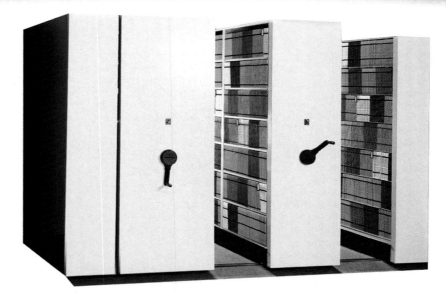

Figure 8-3 Open-shelf file. (Courtesy Kardex Systems, Marietta, OH.)

Another example of the card system that allows for quick reference to patients' names, addresses, telephone numbers, and special notations about the family is the rotary or Rolodex™ file (Figure 8-4). A second rotary file can be useful for addresses, e-mail addresses, telephone and fax numbers of dental suppliers, laboratories, and dental associates.

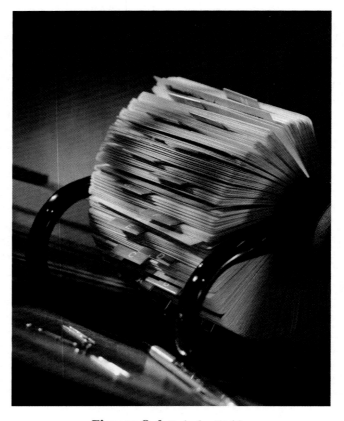

Figure 8-4 Rolodex™ file.

When selecting filing equipment for a dental office, the administrative assistant should also consider a fire-protection file. As a precaution against fire destruction, the patients' ledger cards, the appointment book, disk copies, and other vital records should be placed in the file at the end of each work-day. Many dentists buy an additional file for storing valuable records away from the office.

STORAGE SUPPLIES

Filing supplies for paper storage include file guides, file folders, folder labels (in a variety of colors for color-coding), cross-reference sheets, and out-guides.

File guides, usually heavy cardboard, divide the file drawer into separate sections. The division is indicated by a tab that extends above the guide. The guides divide the alphabet into sections, or they may show a division in a numerical sequence. The file drawer is marked on the outside to correspond with the division of the filing arrangement.

File folders are usually made of manila paper or another heavy type of material. Folders may be obtained in a variety of cuts. Using a variety of cuts allows the tabs to be arranged in a staggered fashion. The tabs may be on the far-left side, or they may be center-cut, one-third cut, or one-fifth cut.

Most dental practices prefer to use patient file folders or envelopes with labels that come in a variety of colors. This type of file and label guards against misplaced records (e.g., x-ray films) and provides space for the patient's name, address, and telephone number. Most file folders can be labeled with gummed labels, available in a variety of styles (rolls of labels, peel-off labels, and continuous folded strips) and colors that will make the folders easier to locate and refile (Figure 8-5). In a group practice, a different color may be used to designate the patients of each dentist. Color-codes may also be used for other pertinent patient information.

Points to remember when making the labels are (1) the labels should be keyed, not handwritten; (2) the keying should begin two or three spaces from the left edge of the label and at a uniform distance (usually one line space) from the top edge of the label; (3) the name may be keyed in all capital letters, or the first letter of each important word may be capitalized; and (4) the established format should be followed consistently.

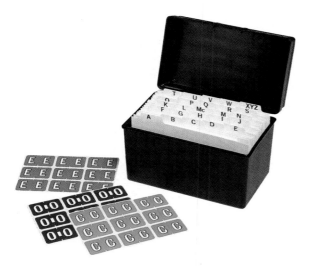

Figure 8-5 Label kit with assorted colored labels. (Courtesy SYCOM, Madison, WI.)

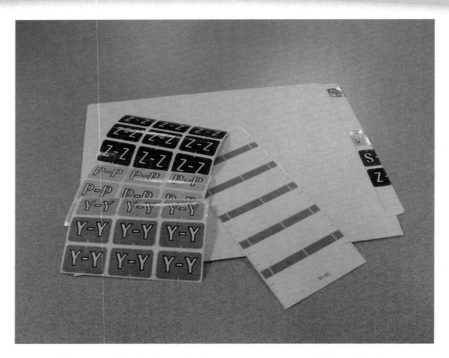

Figure 8-6 Patient file folders using colored filing labels.

Color-coding of file folders aids in fast retrieval and refiling. Figure 8-6 shows a typical open-shelf, end-tab filing system that uses colored filing labels on each file folder to translate the alphabetical rules discussed earlier into a color "code." The assignment of color to each alphabetical character has long been recognized by efficiency experts as a time and energy saver. When patient charts are filed alphabetically and when each letter in the alphabet has a different file label color, color block patterns begin to form in the open-shelf system—"block" patterns that immediately direct the eye toward the proper filing areas. This virtually eliminates the misfiling common in non–color-coded systems. By assigning a different color to each number, large filing systems that use the numerical system can also benefit from the added efficiency of color-coding.

Sometimes cross-referencing is necessary within the filing system. Cross-referencing helps the administrative assistant locate or file the information in its proper location. For example, if a letter is to be filed by the dental clinic name rather than by the name of the individual who has written the letter, you may look under the individual's name and find the cross-reference sheet, which will direct you to the name of the clinic (Figure 8-7).

The electronic supplies necessary for records management include specially designed storage units for disks or tapes. These may be small plastic or fabric units that hold one to five disks, plastic or wooden desktop boxes, rotary files, or ring binders with vinyl pages that have pockets. Similar boxes are available for compact disks. A tape backup system is necessary when large amounts of data stored on hard disks must be recorded. Some of these systems store the entire contents of a hard disk on a single minicassette.

MANAGING WORKSTATION RECORDS EFFECTIVELY

Regardless of the types of records or systems used in a dental office, organization of the workstation is an absolute necessity for successful records management. Almost all assistants spend some of their workday filing records of some type. Even if your filing duties are limited to organizing your own files, you need to develop and follow a simple system. The goal should be to

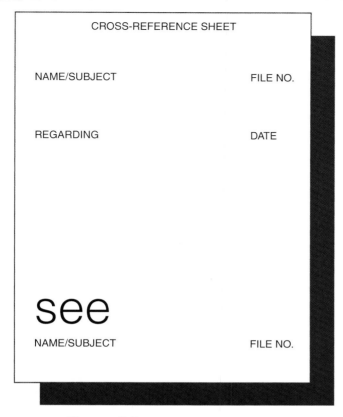

Figure 8-7 Cross-reference sheet.

establish a system that allows for easy retrieval. Successful retrieval means you will be able to find a record or document when needed in a minimal amount of time. As stated earlier, this type of efficiency eliminates time and motion and ultimately financial loss. Box 8-3 presents tips for successful records management.

Box 8-3
Tips for Successful Records Management

Paper Records
1. Organize incoming and outgoing papers in an In/Out box. Use a stackable style that has two or three trays. Label each tray In, Out, or Hold. The Hold tray is for papers that do not have to be acted upon immediately.
2. Use desk drawer files for personal records, forms, stationery, procedural handbooks, and other routinely used items.
3. Use logbooks to record recurring events or data, such as long distance telephone calls, petty cash, and appointment call lists.
4. Keep correspondence in a loose-leaf binder called a *correspondence* or *chronological file*, and date each folder for the year. This will provide a fingertip reference of all correspondence pertaining to any patient or given activity.
5. File copies of insurance claims in a loose-leaf binder in chronological or numerical order. Include a log sheet with an up-to-date reference on the status of each claim form. As forms are completed and paid, refile them in the patient record.

Box 8-3
Tips for Successful Records Management—cont'd

6. Plan a work schedule that includes filing as a daily routine.
7. When placing records in a folder, remove the folder from the file far enough so that the material can be placed completely in the folder and does not extend over the top edge of the folder or tab.
8. Be careful to place materials *in* a folder, not behind or in front of another folder.
9. Do not use paper clips on filed material. It is easy for other materials to attach themselves to the clips. Staples are better if materials must be held together, but remove the first staple before adding another.
10. To avoid filing errors, designate as few people as possible to file and retrieve records.
11. When searching for lost records, check transposition and alternate spellings of names.
12. Replace folders as they become worn out.
13. Avoid overuse of the *Miscellaneous* file. Be ready to begin a separate file for a patient or an associate.

Electronic Records
1. Store disks in a file box specifically designed for the disk style.
2. Label each disk with a general classification.
3. Print an index of the documents currently on disk each time a new document is added. The index can be folded and placed in the jacket or kept in a reference notebook.
4. When a disk becomes full and you want to use the same label for a new disk, number the disks in consecutive order (e.g., "Letters 1," "Letters 2"). Mark each new disk with the date it was first used.
5. Store documents in electronic folders named to represent the activity (e.g., "correspondence," "recall," "patient charts").

LEARNING ACTIVITIES

1. List four steps for preparing materials to be filed.
2. Define the five basic methods of filing.
3. Describe the use of the following filing equipment:
   a. Vertical file
   b. Open-shelf file
   c. Card file
   d. Rolodex™ file
   e. Tickler file
   f. Electronic file
      • Explain how color-coding can be used in dental office files.
      • List six helpful hints for more efficient filing.
4. Assume that the following list of names, with addresses, represents the accounts payable for the dental practice.
   a. Index each name by keying the name in proper indexing form.
   b. If using a manual system, arrange the cards in alphabetical order and prepare a list of alphabetical names.

LEARNING ACTIVITIES—cont'd

c. Using the same cards, rearrange them as they would appear in a geographical file in order by state, then by cities in the state. Then prepare a list of geographical names.

d. If using a computer, sort the names first in alphabetical order and second in a geographical file in order by state and then by cities in the state.

Apex Dental Supplies	Mark C. Sylvester
1816 S. Riverfront	2601 Beck Boulevard
Elgin, IL 26582	Albany, NY 30582
T. S. Davis	Telcom Credit Bureau
26058 S. State	914 E. Michigan
Chicago, IL 26528	Madison, WI 78034
Quality Instruments	C. V. Talbot
P.O. Box D-1	2247 Hamilton
Minneapolis, MN 48807	Charleston, WV 82506
J. P. T. Uniforms	Talbot & Associates
22803 Third Avenue	839 Frederick
Benton Harbor, MI 23062	Hampton, VA 26809
Davis & Davis Office Supplies	B B Waste Paper Co.
4800 N. Baseline	1308 Cadillac
Grand Rapids, MI 27501	Charlotte, NC 89045
M & M Creative Systems	Brian Baumgartner
11015 Orange Avenue	6262 Shield
Los Angeles, CA 90025	Jamestown, ND 45902
Albert D. Apple	Consumer Counseling
3668 N.W. Territorial	590 Bridge Street
Buffalo, NY 32506	Charleston, SC 78032
Quick Copy	E. S. Comstock
1108 Third Street	1255 Harbour Cove
Des Moines, IA 42106	Los Altos, CA 91256
QT Surgical Supplies	Community Pharmacy
1556 Eighth Street SW	2236 Stadium Drive
Dubuque, IA 42013	Kansas City, MO 64119
Robert S. Davis, C.P.A.	Krauss & Krauss Drugs, Inc.
90724 S. Hubbard	152 Barkber Boulevard
Gary, IN 30682	Kansas City, KS 78566

5. The following list of names (List A) represents patients' files.
   a. Prepare a list showing the first, second, third, and fourth indexing units.
   b. With the same list of names, prepare an alphabetical list as the names would appear in an alphabetical file.
   c. The patients' names also have an account number. Prepare another list (List B) by number as they would appear in a numerical file (number followed by name).
   d. Merge List B with List A, and prepare a new list of patients' names as they would appear in the alphabetic file.

List A			
		Phyllis Prestock	10005
Mary Martin	10002	Nora Nummy	10009
Donna Turnbolt	10044	Marian Goodman	10012
John Maxey Jr.	10046	Oahn Ho	10011

LEARNING ACTIVITIES—cont'd

Mary J. Martin	10026	G. R. Anderson	10006
Stanley Ferry	10021	Johnathan Reiker	10033
John Goodman	10031	Kathryn Geer	10007
Hong Viu	10035	G. Robert Andersen	10040
J. J. Goble	10047	J. T. Schmidt	10029
Jim Goble	10041	Andrea Herbert	10015
Philip Hansen	10014	Morris Edwards	10045
Patricia Dixon	10023		
Mark Hopkins	10020	**List B**	
Ralph Fletcher	10036	Henry Corrigan	10175
Nellie Trowbaum	10030	Mary Jane Fleming	10090
Amy Goble	10042	Michael Jensen	10190
Phil Hansen	10047	Mary Louise Puchaski	10116
Mary Richards	10003	Joseph Lind	10119
Richard Swartz	10019	Lacey Toogood	10097
Adam C. Fields	10001	Henry Strohs	10082
Gertrude Teiber	10010	Sally McBee	10114
Ralph Parker	10034	Jed Thompson	10046
Leonard Kuhn	10022	Tillie Chasteen	10074
Stephanie Carroll	10032	Sally Ferez	10192
Walter Busch	10008	Paul Douglas	10064
Dale Noeker	10050	Alice Thomas	10071
Frieda Graves	10028	Mary Jo Flemming	10068
Harold G. Hammond	10024	James LuNardelli	10143
Richard Schwartz	10016	Robert Lunde	10189
Tina Reese	10037	S. B. Porter	10092
Martin Reddick	10027	S. B. Darrett	10058
Susan Sasman	10043	Sam Barrett	10199
Debbie Jones	10049	Charles Saint John	10089
Fred Stanley	10025	Mark L. Puchaski	10074
Roger Nichols	10039	Brian S. Porter	10116
G. Harold Hamond	10038	Cliff McBride	10057
Phillip Rhodes	10017	Michele Janson	10096
Stephen Carole	10013	Charles St. Johns	10091

Key Terms

Alphabetical filing system Method of filing in which the arrangement of names appears in sequence from A to Z.

Card file A file that can be used to store small cards (3-by-5-inch, 4-by-6-inch, or larger) that are used for specialized systems.

Chronological filing system Method of filing by date. This system can be used within an alphabetical, geographical, subject, or numerical system by filing the most recent correspondence in front of the file folder.

Cross-referencing This system alerts staff members that a record normally kept in a specific location has been stored elsewhere.

Geographical filing system Method of filing in which location is the important factor of reference. The principle is essentially the same as alphabetical filing, except that it is done by territorial division (e.g., state, city, or street) rather than by name.

Lateral file A file that is similar to a vertical file, except that the longest side opens and the files are stored as if they were placed on a bookshelf.

Numerical filing system Method of filing that assigns a number to each new patient or account.

Open-shelf filing Method of filing that is similar to lateral filing but with no doors to close.

Retrieval Removal of records from files using proper "charge-out" methods.

Subject filing system Method of filing that uses an alphabetical arrangement of papers according to the subject or topic of the papers.

Tickler file A chronological method of filing that serves as a follow-up file and contains the days of the month and the months of the year to alert the administrative assistant to perform a task.

Vertical file A file that stores records in drawers. File folders are placed on the folder's edge and arranged according to the filing method selected.

Bibliography

Fulton PJ: *General office procedures for colleges,* ed 12, Cincinnati, 2003, South-Western.
Mosley DC et al: *Supervisory management,* ed 6, Cincinnati, 2004, South-Western.

Chapter

9

Written Communication

Chapter Outline

Preparing an Effective Letter
  Collecting Information
  Making an Outline
  Developing the Letter
  Selecting the Format
  Reviewing the Letter
  Producing the Final Letter
  Proofreading the Letter
  Distributing the Letter
  Storing the Document
Preparing the Envelope
  Address Format
  Punctuation on Address Labels
  Folding and Inserting the Letter
Electronic Mail (E-mail)
  E-mail Ethics and Etiquette
Other Types of Written Communication
  Postal Cards
  Interoffice Memoranda
  Manuscripts
  Dictation and Transcription
Managing Office Mail
  Processing Outgoing Mail
  Classification of Mail
    Postage Scale
    Postage Meter
    E-mail
    Facsimile
    Mailing Services
    Delivery Services
    Laboratory Services
  Processing Incoming Mail
  Managing Mail in the Dentist's Absence

Learning Outcomes

Mastery of the content in this chapter will enable the reader to:
- Describe the various types of written communication in a dental office
- Select stationery supplies
- Identify the characteristics of effective correspondence
- Identify the parts of a letter
- Review rules of punctuation and capitalization
- Describe the basic steps for preparing written communication
- Apply various formatting styles to written communication
- Describe standard procedures for preparing outgoing mail
- Observe ethical and legal obligations in written communication
- Explain the use of e-mail in the dental office

- Apply common business etiquette to the use of e-mail
- Identify the classifications of mail
- Identify special mail services
- Explain the function of a postage meter
- Discuss the process for packaging laboratory cases
- Explain the procedure for sorting incoming mail

Good business and professional writing should sound like a person talking to another person. Unfortunately, some of the writing produced in our professional lives today does not seem to be written by caring people.

Using an easy-to-read style makes the reader respond more positively to your ideas. You can make your writing easier to read in two ways. First, you can make individual sentences and paragraphs easy to read so the reader can easily skim the first paragraph or read the entire document in as short a time as possible. Second, you can make the document visually pleasant and structure signposts that lead the reader through the document.

Good business and professional writing is closer to a conversation and less formal than the style of writing that has traditionally earned high marks on college essays and term papers. However, many dental professionals also use professional papers that are easy to read and use good visual impact.

Most people have several styles of talking, which they vary instinctively depending on the audience. So it will be with your writing in the dental office. A letter to a dentist regarding a professional technique or a letter to a dental supplier demanding better service may be formal, whereas an e-mail to a colleague will be informal and perhaps even chatty.

In Chapter 7 you examined the various types of documents generated in the dental office. Now it is time to review the importance of other types of written communication in a dental practice, specifically the use of letters, forms, and newsletters. These documents are all created by the administrative assistant for a variety of reasons. This chapter discusses the creation and production of written communication, how it is distributed, and how incoming written communication is processed, both in the manual and electronic form.

LETTERS

A variety of written documents are generated in the dental office, but none are as important as the letters that seek to enhance public relations with patients and professional colleagues. These letters should be original and create a professional image. Most important, the letter should be one that you are proud to mail from the office.

With the increased use of word processing in the dental office, the dreaded task of creating an original letter each time one is needed can be eliminated. Today's administrative assistant can have a supply of sample letters stored as templates in an electronic file. When necessary, the assistant can transform the sample into an original letter that is professional and can be personalized within minutes.

The types of written communication most commonly sent from a dental office include thank-you notes for referral of patients, letters of appreciation, birthday or holiday greetings, congratulatory letters, sympathy messages, patient transfer letters or letters of consultation, recall notices, collection letters, order letters, and newsletters.

Thank You for Referral Letter

The dentist should be appreciative of the confidence expressed by a patient who refers a new patient to the office and should acknowledge such a referral with a personally signed letter. Although this letter should mention the name of the referred patient, it should not divulge any confidential information about the treatment. However, if this letter is to be sent to a physician or another dentist, a reference statement may be made about the patient's diagnosis and/or prognosis, if this was discussed in the initial referral. Several examples of this type of thank-you letter are shown in Figure 9-1. You will note that the differences in content vary according to the situation.

Letter of Appreciation to a Cooperative Patient

We often overlook a cooperative patient and think only of the patient who creates frustration. A dentist should acknowledge a patient who is prompt for appointments, maintains a regular payment plan, and cooperates with prescribed home care plans. This is an opportunity to give sincere compliments. When the opportunity presents itself, try writing a letter as in Figure 9-2 and see how appreciative your patients are. A letter of appreciation should be sincere, state the purpose briefly, and be written as though you were conversing with the patient in person.

Birthday Letter and Holiday Greetings

Patients, especially children and older adults, like to be recognized on their birthdays. These letters should be cheerful. Figure 9-3 shows a letter that could be sent to an older adult on a special birthday. Another method of handling this form of public relations is to send a birthday card. Many professional stationers provide appropriate greeting cards for all occasions and all dental specialties (Figure 9-4).

Congratulatory Letter

Through conversations with patients and via the daily newspaper, you can learn the outstanding achievements of patients. Such accomplishments should not go unnoticed by the dental office staff. A letter sent to congratulate a patient must be sent promptly. Include how you learned of the event and a sincere expression of congratulations (Figure 9-5). Congratulations can also be sent for the birth of a child, a wedding, or a graduation. A greeting card or brief letter is appropriate.

Referral for Consultation or Treatment

During the treatment of a patient, it is often necessary to call upon the services of a specialist. A series of letters may be sent between the two dental offices concerning the patient's treatment. A good example of such an experience is the transfer of a patient to an orthodontist for treatment (Figure 9-6). Figure 9-7 shows examples of several forms of communication that might be used during a patient's treatment. Note that the specialist's office has used a basic format that provides information about the patient's treatment. This letter can be stored electronically, or a pre-prepared form could be used in a specialty office, such as an orthodontics office, since there is a large patient volume and a similarity of basic treatment. Regardless of the type of form used, note that in each case the patient's name is referenced, the message is brief, and each tooth or condition is diagrammed or written out completely to avoid error in interpretation.

Dental Associates, PC
Joseph W. Lake, DDS – Ashley M. Lake, DDS

September 15, 20—

Mr. Carl Ladley
3567 Wines Drive
Wyoming, MI 49507

Dear Carl:

It was good of you to refer one of your employees, Raymone Hunchez, to me for treatment. My staff and I are always glad to be of assistance to you and your employees whenever possible.

You and your family have been valuable members of my dental practice. We hope that we will be able to provide Mr. Hunchez the same quality service that we have provided your family in the past.

Give my best regards to Mary and the boys.

Sincerely,

Ashley M. Lake, DDS

je

611 Main Street, SE – Grand Rapids, MI 49502   Phone: 616.101.9575 Fax: 616.101.9999
E-mail: office@dapc.com or Visit us at: www.Lakedental.com

B

Dental Associates, PC
Joseph W. Lake, DDS – Ashley M. Lake, DDS

April 17, 20—

Mr. Edward Aprill
347 North Wixom
Frankfort, MI 48223

Dear Mr. Aprill:

Your expression of confidence in referring Mr. Robert Smith to my office for treatment is greatly appreciated. It is always a pleasure to welcome new patients to our practice, especially when they are referred by another satisfied patient.

It gives my staff and me a sense of satisfaction that you have been pleased with the treatment we have rendered. We will make every effort to provide Mr. Smith with the same complete and thorough dentistry we have provided you during these past five years.

Thank you again for your confidence.

Sincerely,

Joseph W. Lake, DDS

je

611 Main Street, SE – Grand Rapids, MI 49502   Phone: 616.101.9575 Fax: 616.101.9999
E-mail: office@dapc.com or Visit us at: www.Lakedental.com

A

Figure 9-1 A, Thank-you-for-referral letter. **B,** Informal thank-you-for-referral letter to a patient who is a personal friend of the dentist.

Dental Associates, PC
Joseph W. Lake, DDS – Ashley M. Lake, DDS

December 19, 20—

Robert W. Wells, DDS
2146 Rochester Avenue
Grand Rapids, MI 49502

Dear Dr. Wells:

Mrs. Roger (Amy) Browne was in my office today for an examination. I confirmed your diagnosis of advanced periodontitis. We have set up a series of appointments for x-rays and beginning periodontal curettage.

The prognosis is favorable and Mrs. Browne was eager to begin treatment. Thank you for this referral and the kind remarks you made to her.

Sincerely,

Joseph W. Lake, DDS

je

611 Main Street, SE – Grand Rapids, MI 49502   Phone: 616.101.9575   Fax: 616.101.9999
E-mail: office@dapc.com or Visit us at: www.Lakedental.com

D

Dental Associates, PC
Joseph W. Lake, DDS – Ashley M. Lake, DDS

September 19, 20—

Ms. Angela Gualandi
2492 Plymouth Road
Comstock, MI 49829

Dear Ms. Gualandi:

I would like to take this opportunity to thank you for your confidence in referring your friend, Judy McKay, and her children, Debbie and Rick, to our office for treatment.

My staff and I are pleased to learn of your satisfaction. We will make every effort to justify the confidence you have shown in us during the treatment of Ms. McKay and her children.

Thank you again for your expression of confidence.

Sincerely,

Ashley M. Lake, DDS

je

611 Main Street, SE – Grand Rapids, MI 49502   Phone: 616.101.9575   Fax: 616.101.9999
E-mail: office@dapc.com or Visit us at: www.Lakedental.com

C

Figure 9-1 Cont'd C, General thank-you-for-referral letter. **D,** Thank-you-for-referral letter to a colleague.

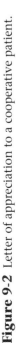

Dental Associates, PC

Joseph W. Lake, DDS – Ashley M. Lake, DDS

May 17, 20—

Mr. Michael Russo
1145 Collins Drive
Grand Rapids, MI 49502

Dear Mr. Russo:

My staff and I wish to send our best wishes for a happy birthday tomorrow. We hope you will enjoy your ninety-fifth birthday and reflect on your many accomplishments.

Your longevity may be attributed to your good health and heritage, but your continued personal contributions to the community are evidence of your unselfishness. We hope your example of good citizenship will impact the youth of this city.

Again, best wishes for a happy birthday and continued good health in the future.

Sincerely,

Ashley M. Lake, DDS

je

611 Main Street, SE – Grand Rapids, MI 49502   Phone: 616.101.9575 Fax: 616.101.9999
E-mail: office@dapc.com or Visit us at: www.Lakedental.com

Figure 9-3 Birthday letter to an older adult.

Dental Associates, PC

Joseph W. Lake, DDS – Ashley M. Lake, DDS

March 30, 20—

Mr. Ryan Hamlin
1334 Huron Road
Grandville, MI 49508

Dear Mr. Hamlin:

My staff and I would like to thank you for your cooperation during the treatment that we have just completed. A patient's cooperation and interest in his dental care is an integral part of our success.

Your cooperation in keeping your appointments, prompt payment of your account, and diligent home care has made our work much more enjoyable.

We look forward to seeing you for your oral examination in three months. We hope you continue to enjoy the wise investment you have made in your mouth.

Sincerely,

Joseph W. Lake, DDS

je

611 Main Street, SE – Grand Rapids, MI 49502   Phone: 616.101.9575 Fax: 616.101.9999
E-mail: office@dapc.com or Visit us at: www.Lakedental.com

Figure 9-2 Letter of appreciation to a cooperative patient.

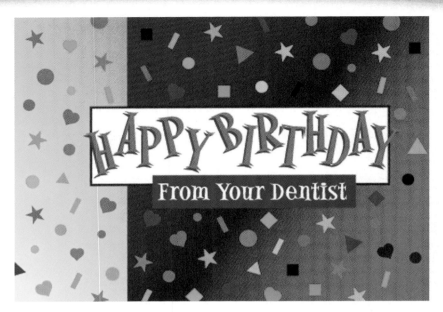

Figure 9-4 Birthday card. (Courtesy Colwell, a Division of Patterson Companies, Inc., Champaign, IL.)

Sympathy Message

Many people find it difficult to express sympathy in a letter. Therefore one of the best ways to handle this difficult situation is to send a sympathy card. It is the unexpected message that often means a great deal to family members in their time of grief.

Miscellaneous Letters

Many letters are not public relations letters and are not included in this chapter. Specific examples of recall, broken appointment, and collection letters are discussed in the chapters that specifically address each of these topics.

NEWSLETTERS AS MARKETING DEVICES

Today, as dentistry seeks to address the consumer market, marketing becomes part of the business of dentistry. If done ethically, with concern for the values of the community and the education of the public, marketing can be a valuable tool.

Automated systems in the dental office have made it easier to incorporate marketing procedures into the dental business. One of the products of automated systems is a patient newsletter. A newsletter can educate your patients about new ideas in dentistry, basic dental health concepts, community trends, and ideas your office is promoting.

Newsletters may be single- or multi-page (Figure 9-8) and should be mailed regularly—quarterly or biannually. Many offices use software packages to generate the original copy and then duplicate it at a discount printer. Others opt to have the entire newsletter generated and produced outside the office. Regardless of the method of production, it is important that the content originate from the dentist and the staff with their own philosophy and image affecting the final product.

Dental Associates, PC
Joseph W. Lake, DDS – Ashley M. Lake, DDS

September 25, 20—

Daniel R. Jacobsen, DDS, MS
2495 Packard Road SE
Grand Rapids, MI 49506

Dear Dr. Jacobsen:

I am referring Michael Moran, age 12, to you for an orthodontic evaluation. Mrs. Moran will be calling your office for an appointment. Michael appears to have a Class II malocclusion with crowding of the mandibular anterior teeth.

Enclosed you will find a complete series of radiographs that were taken on September 11, 20-- .

I will look forward to your diagnosis and assistance with this case.

Sincerely,

Joseph W. Lake, DDS

je

Enclosure:Full mouth series radiographs

611 Main Street, SE – Grand Rapids, MI 49502   Phone: 616.101.9575 Fax: 616.101.9999
E-mail: office@dapc.com or Visit us at: www.Lakedental.com

Figure 9-6 Referral of a patient to an orthodontist.

Dental Associates, PC
Joseph W. Lake, DDS – Ashley M. Lake, DDS

September 28, 20—

Mr. Jason Henkle
1135 Hollyhock Lane
Grand Rapids, MI 49503

Dear Mr. Henkle:

Last night the staff and I read in the *Grand Rapids News* about your promotion to Vice President of the Michigan Trust Company. We want to send our congratulations to you on this promotion.

It is a pleasure to learn of your advancement and I send my best wishes for success in this new position.I am certain this will be a challenging experience.

Again, my sincerest best wishes on your fine achievement.

Sincerely,

Ashley M. Lake, DDS

je

611 Main Street, SE – Grand Rapids, MI 49502   Phone: 616.101.9575 Fax: 616.101.9999
E-mail: office@dapc.com or Visit us at: www.Lakedental.com

Figure 9-5 Congratulatory letter.

John G. Clinthorne, D.D.S., M.S.
H. Ludia Kim, D.M.D., M.S.
Professional Corporation
Specialists in Orthodontics
1303 Packard
Ann Arbor, Michigan 48104
(734) 761-3116

«Todays_date_in_words»

«Responsible_party_name»
«Responsible_party_address»
«Responsible_party_city_state_zip»

Dear «Responsible_party_greeting»:

Welcome to our practice! My staff and I look forward to meeting you and «Patient_first_name» on «Next_appointment_date» at «Next_appointment_time». Be assured that «Patient_first_name possessive» first visit with us will be a pleasant and rewarding experience.

Please bring with you the enclosed information sheet as well as any insurance forms and information we may need to file with your insurance carrier.

At «Patient_first_name possessive» first visit to our office, we will proceed with an oral examination and discuss the findings with you. If a more thorough diagnosis is advisable, the following materials may be requested at an additional charge:

- Models of Teeth
- Panoramic X-ray
- Profile X-ray
- Diagnostic Photographs

After the above materials have been studied and the best course of therapy determined, the overall treatment plan will be discussed with you at a consultation appointment.

Sincerely,

John G. Clinthorne, D.D.S., M.S.
H. Ludia Kim, D.M.D., M.S.

Member American Association of **Orthodontists**

A

B

John G. Clinthorne, D.D.S., M.S.
H. Ludia Kim, D.M.D., M.S.
Professional Corporation
Specialists in Orthodontics
1303 Packard
Ann Arbor, Michigan 48104
(734) 761-3116

«Todays_date_in_words»

«Referring_party_name»
«Referring_party_address—line 1»
«Referring_party_address—line 2»«Referring_party_city_state_zip»

                                          RE: «Patient_full_name»   «Age: Patients_age»

Dear «Referring_party_greeting»:

DISPOSITION: ( ) Orthodontic treatment is indicated at this time and:
                    ( ) They intend to proceed with treatment.
                         Records and consultation appointments have been made.
                    ( ) They are to notify us if and when they wish to proceed.
                    ( ) They do not intend to proceed with treatment.

               ( ) «Patient_first_name» has been referred to your office for:
                    ( ) Dental examination and prophylaxis.
                    ( ) _____

               ( ) Orthodontic treatment may be indicated in the future and
                    «Patient_first_name» has been placed on recall
                    ( ) They prefer to call our office at a later date.

               ( ) Orthodontic treatment is not indicated.

REMARKS:

Member American Association of **Orthodontists**

Figure 9-7 A, Basic form letter from an orthodontist to welcome a new patient. Diagnosis text from the patient's record may be inserted. **B,** Basic form letter from an orthodontist to a referring dentist upon examination of a patient.

Figure 9-7 Cont'd **C**, Letter to a patient confirming consultation appointment and explaining the process. **D**, Final letter from an orthodontist to a referring dentist informing of completed treatment.

D

John G. Clinthorne, D.D.S., M.S.
H. Ludia Kim, D.M.D., M.S.
Professional Corporation
Specialists in Orthodontics
1303 Packard
Ann Arbor, Michigan 48104
(734) 761-3116

«Todays_date_in_words»

«Referring_party_name»
«Referring_party_address—line 1»
«Referring_party_city_state_zip»

Dear «Referring_party_greeting»:

I want to inform you that I have removed the fixed appliances on «Patient_full_name», age «Patients_age». The following summarizes this case to date:

TYPE OF TREATMENT:
( ) no extractions ( ) extraction of _____
( ) partial banding _____
( ) complete banding-duration _____

SEVERITY OF ORIGINAL PROBLEM:
Skeletal- ( ) very complex ( ) moderately complex ( ) routine
Dental- ( ) very complex ( ) moderately complex ( ) routine
Neuromuscular- ( ) very complex ( ) moderately complex ( ) routine

ORAL HYGIENE: ( ) outstanding ( ) good ( ) fair ( ) poor

COOPERATION: ( ) outstanding ( ) good ( ) fair ( ) poor

TYPE AND DURATION OF RETENTION: Approximate duration
( ) maxillary removable retainer _____
( ) mandibular removable retainer
( ) mandibular fixed strap

THE PATIENT HAS BEEN REFERRED TO YOUR OFFICE FOR:
( ) oral prophylaxis and dental examination

REMARKS:

Member American Association of **Orthodontists**

C

John G. Clinthorne, D.D.S., M.S.
H. Ludia Kim, D.M.D., M.S.
Professional Corporation
Specialists in Orthodontics
1303 Packard
Ann Arbor, Michigan 48104
(734) 761-3116

«Todays_date_in_words»

«Responsible_party_name»
«Responsible_party_address»
«Responsible_party_city_state_zip»

Dear «Responsible_party_greeting»:

The consultation appointment to discuss «Patient_first_name possessive» orthodontic treatment is scheduled for «Next_appointment_date» at «Next_appointment_time».

We shall present to you an outline of the treatment plan and our recommendations, the estimated length of treatment, cooperation requirements, and costs. We will answer any questions you may have, as well as discuss any particular problems, which bear on the success of the treatment. Both parents are encouraged to attend to gain a thorough understanding of our services. The patient is welcome but is not required to attend.

Thank you for giving us the opportunity to be of service to you and your child. We are delighted to have «Patient_first_name» as a new patient and we look forward to a continuing relationship.

Sincerely,

John G. Clinthorne, D.D.S., M.S.
H. Ludia Kim, D.M.D., M.S.

Member American Association of **Orthodontists**

JOHN G. CLINTHORNE, D.D.S., M.S.
H. LUDIA KIM, D.M.D., M.S.

ORTHODONTICS   1303 PACKARD, ANN ARBOR, MI. 48104   **734-761-3116**

DR. _____ PHONE _____

NAME _____ PHONE _____

_____

_____

_____

_____

_____

_____

_____

DATE _____ _____ D.D.S.

Extract Teeth Encircled

PERMANENT TEETH

UPPER

| 1 2 3 4 5 6 7 8 | 9 10 11 12 13 14 15 16 |

PATIENT'S RIGHT   PATIENT'S LEFT

| 32 31 30 29 28 27 26 25 | 24 23 22 21 20 19 18 17 |

LOWER

DECIDUOUS TEETH

UPPER

| A B C D E | F G H I J |

PATIENT'S RIGHT   PATIENT'S LEFT

| T S R Q P | O N M L K |

LOWER

☐ Enclosure - X-Rays
☐ Return Requested
☐ Please Keep For Your Records   If any questions ...... Please Telephone

E

Figure 9-7 Cont'd E, Requisition used by an orthodontist to refer a patient for extraction. (**A** to **E** Courtesy JG Clinthorne, D.D.S., and HL Kim, D.M.D., Ann Arbor, MI.)

BY Word of Mouth

Dental Health News for the Patients of: — No. 51

John W. Farah, D.D.S., Ph.D., Lori K. Brown, D.D.S., John Shamraj, D.D.S., Santine E. Anderson, D.D.S.

Crown Me!

For your smile to be your crowning glory, you need healthy, attractive teeth. Cracked, stained or damaged teeth will detract from your dental health as well as your appearance. To remedy these problems and make your smile radiant and white, the dentist will often suggest crowning a damaged tooth. Crowns replace large fillings that have very little tooth remaining. Crowns restore fractured teeth and protect them from cracking. Misaligned, poorly shaped or discolored teeth are masked and covered with crowns. Crowns are ideal for teeth with excessive wear from grinding or clenching and for strengthening teeth that have undergone root canal treatment. A crown restores a tooth to its normal size and shape and reinforces the tooth by covering or capping it.

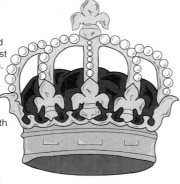

The dentist will have some valuable advice in choosing the best material for you.

Crowns are placed in two appointments. During the first visit, the dentist prepares your tooth by removing the outer portion to accommodate the thickness of the crown. Next, a temporary plastic crown is put in place, giving the laboratory a few weeks to handcraft a customized crown to fit your tooth. The second visit is quick and simple. The dentist removes the temporary crown and cements the permanent crown in place. Because the laboratory has custom-made the crown, the dentist will only have to make some minor adjustments.

Crowns are available in a couple of different types of material. The dentist will have some valuable advice in choosing the best material for you,

see CROWN, page 4

INSIDE

2 Beauty and the "Bad Breath" Beast

3 RECIPE CORNER: Fruit Baked Apples

3 Sweet Tooth Sabotage

Editors:
John W. Farah, D.D.S., Ph.D.
Jill G. Hutchinson, R.D.H., B.S.

Contributing Authors:
Jill G. Hutchinson, R.D.H., B.S.
Christina M. Pitzen, B.A.

Figure 9-8 Newsletter from a dental office to a patient. (Courtesy Farah and Associates, Ann Arbor, MI.)

SELECTING STATIONERY SUPPLIES

If you begin working in an established dental practice, the stationery supplies will already be available. However, you may have to choose business supplies yourself if you are asked to order them. Many of these supplies are listed in Chapter 6.

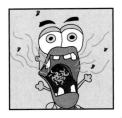

Beauty and the "Bad Breath" Beast

Suspicions of bad breath can certainly make one feel like a beast when talking to others in close proximity. Halitosis, commonly known as bad breath, can have an overwhelming effect on one's personal and professional life. While historically, halitosis has been a difficult problem to resolve, effective cleaning instruments and chemical solutions today makes even the worst cases manageable.

Many people are unaware that bad breath can originate orally or systemically. Bad breath can result from a mouth or tongue in need of a good brushing. Many halitosis cases originate specifically on the tongue, and very few people are aware of this. They try to fight it with breathmints or sprays that offer no real solution other than to temporarily mask the malodor. The surface of the tongue consists of many tiny crevices, which are perfect for collecting tiny bits of food and bacteria. By brushing your tongue, you can remove organisms that multiply on the back of the tongue, which emit sulfur gases or volatile sulfur compounds. *Oxygene* and *Enfresh* are products on the market that contain solutions of chlorine dioxide, which is said to eliminate the odor from volatile sulfur gases. Other products include tongue scrapers or brushes designed specifically to fight bad breath.

Bad breath may be a warning sign of a more serious problem in the mouth such as an oral infection, gum disease or poor oral hygiene. Dental appliances may also produce an odor indicating the need for cleaning and regular maintenance. If these conditions are eliminated and bad breath still persists, the malodor is most likely not of dental origin.

Many systematic factors may cause halitosis. Ulcers or gastrointestinal diseases may contribute to bad breath, as can maladies of the tonsils or sinuses. Medications may also have side effects, which can cause dry mouth and result in halitosis. Alcohol and tobacco use can greatly affect breath freshness systemically, as can odoriferous foods such as garlic, onions and some ethnic foods.

Wondering about your own breath? You're not alone. Americans spend over 500 million dollars a year on products to remedy oral malodor. To find out if you suffer from bad breath, the best way is to ask someone you trust to be honest with you. You can also blow into a balloon and breathe the air as you slowly deflate it. If you think you'd like fresher breath, talk to the dentist and staff about which products they recommend. Be sure to keep up-to-date with routine dental cleaning every 3-6 months so you can kiss bad breath goodbye once and for all!

Figure 9-8, cont'd

The office stationery (letterhead) is usually selected on the basis of simplicity, neatness, and quality. Bond paper, because of its quality, is often used. It can be made from all-cotton fiber (sometimes called rag), from all-sulfite (a wood pulp), or from any proportion of the two. High-cotton fiber bond indicates quality and prestige, and it ages without deterioration or chemical breakdown.

The following information may be used as a guide for future stationery needs.

Letterheads	Matching Envelopes
Standard office use: Business size 8½ by 11 inches	No. 10 (4⅛ by 9½ inches) Same weight and fiber content as letterhead
Usually 16# or 20# bond, 25% cotton fiber (rag)	
Executive use: Standard and Monarch size	No. 10 and No. 7 (3⅞ by 7½ inches) Same weight and fiber content as letterhead
(Monarch size: 7¼ by 10 inches) Usually 24# bond, 100% cotton-fiber	

A color theme for stationery items, such as letterheads, envelopes, appointment cards, prescription pads, medicine envelopes, and notepads, may be used. Color coordinates such as light and dark mauve or blue, or contrasting tones of grey with black print are attractive combinations. Most dental stationery supply houses have samples of stationery stock and logo designs from which you may select.

A popular alternative to purchasing stationery is to create the letterhead using appropriate computer software. A fine bond paper can be purchased. When a new letter is to be keyboarded, the letterhead is removed from the file where it is stored, the letter is prepared, and then it is printed on bond paper. This becomes less expensive and allows for more frequent changes and creativity. Clip art is available that makes it easy to create a professional letterhead that provides the office staff many options. Labels with the same clip art and office information can also be created in this manner. It is important that the labels selected are compatible with the office printer.

CHARACTERISTICS OF AN EFFECTIVE LETTER

Effective letters that generate good public relations have certain common elements. Keep in mind that direct, simple writing is easier to read. The best word depends on context: the situation, the purpose, the audience, and the words you have already used.

1. **Use words that are accurate, appropriate, and familiar.** Accurate words mean what you want to say. Appropriate words convey the attitudes you want to create and fit well with the other words in your document. Familiar words are easy to read and understand.
2. **Use technical terminology sparingly.** The exception to this rule is if you are communicating with another professional and need to describe a condition or treatment in technical terms. However, when communicating with patients or laypersons, it is wise to use a "plain English" equivalent instead of a technical term.
3. **Use active verbs most of the time.** This is common in writing for a job application or referring a patient to a specialist. If the verb describes something that the subject is doing, the verb is active. If the verb describes something that is being done to the grammatical subject, the verb is passive.

Active: *I recommend that the patient's third molar be removed.*

Passive: *It was recommended by me for the patient to have the third molar removed.*

Active: *I can expose digital radiographs.*
Passive: *Digital radiography is something I could do.*

4. **Tighten your writing.** Eliminate words that say nothing. Combine sentences to eliminate unnecessary words. Put the meaning of the sentence into the subject and verb. Cut words if the idea is already clear from other words in the sentence. Substitute single words for wordy phrases.

Wordy: *Keep this information in the patient's file for future reference.*
Tighter: *Keep this information for reference.*
Or: File this information.

Phrases beginning with *of, which,* and *that* can often be shortened.

Wordy: *The issue of most importance*
Tighter: *The most important issue.*
Wordy: *The estimate that is enclosed*
Tighter: *The enclosed estimate*
Wordy: *It is the case that Registered Dental Assistants are more qualified clinicians in the office.*
Tighter: *Registered Dental Assistants are more qualified clinicians in the office.*

Combine sentences to eliminate unnecessary words. In addition to saying words, combining sentences focuses the reader's attention on key points, makes your writing sound more sophisticated, and sharpens the relationship between ideas, thus making your writing more coherent.

Wordy: *I conducted a survey by telephone on Monday April 17th. I questioned 18 dental assistants, some Registered Dental Assistants and some Certified Dental Assistants, who according to the state directory were all currently working. The purpose of this survey was to find out how many of them were performing advanced functions that were delegated by the state. I also wanted to find out if there were any differences between their salaries.*
Tighter: *On Monday April 17th, I phoned Registered and Certified working dental assistants to determine (1) if they were performing the state delegated advanced functions, and (2) whether there was a distinction between salaries for these two credentials.*

5. **Vary sentence length and sentence structure.** A readable letter mixes sentence lengths and varies sentence structure. A really short sentence is under ten words and can add punch to your letter. Really long sentences of 30 to 40 words can raise a danger flag.

A simple sentence has one main clause:
We will open a new office this month.

A compound sentence has two main clauses joined with *and, but, or,* or another conjunction. Compound sentences are used best when the ideas in the two clauses are closely related.

We have hired three new dental assistants, and they will complete their orientation next week.

We hired a new intern, but he will be unable to begin work until the end of the month.

Complex sentences have one main and one subordinate clause; they are good for showing logical relationships.

When the new office opens, we will have an open house for local dentists and offer refreshments and door prizes.

Because we already have a strong patient base in Livingston County, we expect the new office will be as successful as the Ann Arbor office.

6. **Use parallel structure.** Parallel structure puts words, phrases, or clauses in the same grammatical and logical form. Clarity eliminates long, meaningless words and uses language that the reader will understand. Thus you can be certain each statement will not be misinterpreted.

Nonparallel: *The position is prestigious, challenging, and also offers good money.*
Parallel: *The position offers prestige, challenge, and money.*

Nonparallel: *The steps in the planning process include:*
                  Determining the objectives
                  An idea of who the reader is
                  A list of the facts
    Parallel: *Determine the objective*
                  Consider the reader
                  Gather the facts

7. **Put your readers in your sentences.** Use second person pronouns (you) rather than third person (he, she, one) or first person (I) to give your writing a greater team approach. The "you" approach to letter writing requires the writer to place the reader at the center of the message. When writing the letter, put yourself in place of the reader.

Third-person: *References for patients in this office are made by our office manager, and the patient will be contacted as soon as the appointment has been confirmed with the specialist.*

Second person: *Once you are referred to a specialist, you will receive a confirmation of your appointment from our office manager.*

In addition to the ideas presented above, the administrative assistant should review the basic characteristics of effective correspondence. These factors should be used in a review of the letter prior to it being sent. Remember that the letter sent from the dental office is representative of the quality of work or treatment produced in that practice.

- *Completeness.* Include all necessary data the reader needs to make a decision or take action.
- *Conciseness.* Requires you to be brief.
- *Confidentiality.* Release information only about the case that is relative to the contents of the letter and only after the patient has given consent to release specific information.
- *Courtesy.* Use good manners for good public relations. Don't make derogatory statements.
- *Accuracy.* All of the data are correct. Check details carefully. Use correct spelling and grammar.
- *Neatness.* Avoid smudges, tears, or wrinkles.
- *Use positive words that indicate you are helpful and caring* (Box 9-1).
- *Reader oriented.* Pronouns in letters should be "you-oriented"

> The "you" approach to letter writing requires the writer to place the reader at the center of the message.

BOX 9-1
Positive and Negative Words

Positive Words	Negative words
I will	I'm sorry
Congratulations	Complaint
Concern	Difficult
Pleasure	Unpleasant
Thank you	No
Satisfactory	Can't
I can	Careless
Welcome	Error
	Inconvenient
	Disappointed

PARTS OF A BUSINESS LETTER

A review of the parts of a business letter and the proper placement and purpose for each part is appropriate before you select a letter style or begin to create the letter. Most business letters contain the following parts:

- Date line
- Inside address (letter address)
- Salutation
- Body
- Complimentary close
- Keyboarded signature
- Reference initials
- Special notations such as attention line, subject line, or enclosures

When using most word processing software, many preformatted letter styles are available. Dates are automatic, and in most systems alignment and letter parts are already defined.

Date Line

The date line contains the date the letter is keyboarded. When using printed letterhead stationery, the date usually begins a double space below the lowest line of the letterhead. (The letterhead usually takes up about two inches, but this may vary depending on the style and design of the letterhead.) Many times the length of the letter determines whether the heading should be started lower on the paper; good judgment is needed. When keyboarding a personal business letter, the individual's return address is placed as the first two lines directly above the date line. The date line can be affected by the length of the letter. When using the computer, you may go to "Print Preview" to check the appearance of the letter. Then, necessary changes can be made before printing. General guidelines that relate to letter length are shown in Box 9-2.

Inside Address

The inside address provides all of the information for mailing the letter. The letter address should match the envelope address. When using word processing, the envelope often is addressed from the letter address by a minor key function on the computer. The information to be included is the recipient's name, the name of company (if appropriate), street number and name, city, and zip code. Three lines of space are left between the date and the first line of the letter address.

Use titles preceding the individual's name (Mr., Mrs., Ms., or Dr.). Do not use a double title, such as Dr. L. B. Crown, D.D.S.; this is redundant. An official title, such as President, may follow the name, for example, Ms. M. P. Coleman, President. The person's official title is often placed on the second line if it helps to balance the inside address lines. The city, state, and zip code

---

BOX 9-2
Placement of a Date Line

Letter Length	Side Margins	Top/Bottom Margins
Short (Less than 100 words)	2 inches	3 inches
Average (101 to 200 words)	1½ inches	2 inches
Long (201 to 300 words)	1 inch	1 inch

Note: Window envelopes require the date line to be placed on a line 2 inches below the top of the page.

are placed on the last line. The appropriate two-letter state abbreviation should be set in capital letters without a period. Leave two spaces following the abbreviation before entering the zip code.

Salutation

The salutation formally greets the reader. If the writer wishes the letter to be directed to an individual within a firm, it is acceptable to use an attention line (see p. 246). The salutation line should begin one double space below the letter address and should be even with the left margin. If you are writing to an individual, the most appropriate salutation is the individual's name. For example, if the letter is addressed to Mr. Ted Monroe, the salutation would be Dear Mr. Monroe. The salutation can be altered to be Dear Ted if the dentist is a close friend of the recipient. This change in formality should be recognized prior to keyboarding the letter. Special situations occur when the letter is to be sent to unknown individuals or to more than one person. Suggestions for salutations to be used in common situations are shown in Box 9-3, *A*. Addresses and salutations used for governmental and academic officials are shown in Box 9-3, *B*.

Body of the Letter

The body of the letter contains the message. It begins a double space after the salutation. The paragraphs within the body are single-spaced with double-spacing between paragraphs. Paragraphs may or may not be indented, depending on the format selected. Refer to Figures 9-2 to 9-7 for selection of the format. Many illustrations in this chapter demonstrate variations in format styles.

Complimentary Close

The complimentary close provides a courteous ending to the letter. It is keyboarded a double space after the last line of the body of the letter.

BOX 9-3, *A*
Appropriate Salutations for Various Situations

1. One person, sex unknown: Dear M.R. Rieger
2. One person, name unknown, title known: Dear Director of Surgical Technology
3. One woman, title unknown: Dear Ms. Hartwig
4. Two or more women, titles known: Dear Ms. Martin, Mrs. Leverett, and Ms. Grey
5. If all women are married: Dear Mrs. Franks, Mrs. Johnson, and Mrs. Sullens, or Dear Mesdames Franks, Johnson, and Sullens
6. If all women are unmarried: Dear Miss Franks, Miss Johnson, and Miss Sullens, or Dear Misses Franks, Johnson, and Sullens
7. If all recipients are women: Dear Ms. Franks, Johnson, and Sullens, or Dear Mses. or Mss. Franks, Johnson, and Sullens
8. A woman and a man: Dear Ms. Johnson and Mr. Ladley
9. A group or organization composed entirely of women: Ladies or Mesdames
10. A group or organization composed entirely of men: Gentlemen
11. A group composed of women and men: Ladies and Gentlemen

BOX 9-3, *B*
Addresses and Salutations for Government and Academic Officials

The following addresses and salutations are recommended in correspon–
  dence with governmental or academic officials. In each case, the proper
  ways to address letters are illustrated. On the left are addresses, and on
  the right, salutations. When one or more examples are given, they are
  arranged in order of decreasing formality.

Correspondence with government officials
The President

The President	Sir, Madam
The White House	Mr. (Mrs. or Ms.) President
Washington, DC 20500	Dear Mr. (Mrs. or Ms.) President
or	

The President of the United States
The White House
Washington, DC 20500

Chief Justice of the Supreme Court

The Chief Justice of the United States	Sir, Madam
Washington, DC 20543	Mr. or Madam Chief Justice
or	

The Honorable (full name)
United States Supreme Court
Washington, DC 20543

Associate Justice of the Supreme Court

The Honorable (full name)	Sir, Madam
Associate Justice of the Supreme Court	Mr. or Madam Justice
Washington, DC 20543	My dear Justice (surname)
	Dear Justice (surname)

Cabinet member

The Honorable (full name)	Sir, Madam
Secretary of State	Dear Sir, Madam
Washington, DC 20520	My dear Mr. or Madam Secretary
or	Dear Mr. or Madam Secretary

The Secretary of State
Washington, DC 20520

Senator

The Honorable (full name)	Sir, Madam
The United States Senate	Dear Sir, Madam
Washington, DC 20510	My dear Mr. or Madam Senator
or	My dear Senator (surname)
Senator (full name)	Dear Senator (surname)

The United States Senate
Washington, DC 20510

Representative

The Honorable (full name)	Sir, Madam
The House of Representatives	Dear Sir, Madam
Washington, DC 20515	My dear Representative (surname)
or	Dear Representative (surname)

BOX 9-3, *B*
Addresses and Salutations for Government and Academic Officials—cont'd

Representative (full name)
The House of Representatives
Washington, DC 20515

Chief, Director, or Commissioner of a Government Bureau
Mr., Ms., Mrs., or Miss (full name)   Sir, Madam
Director of Public Information   Dear Sir, Madam
Department of Justice   My dear Mr., Ms., Mrs., or Miss (surname)
Washington, DC 20530   Dear Mr., Ms., Mrs., or Miss
or
Director of Public Information
Department of Justice
Washington, DC 20530

Governor
The Honorable (full name)   Sir, Madam
Governor of Ohio   Dear Sir, Madam
Columbus, OH 43215   My dear Governor (surname)
or   Dear Governor (surname)
The Governor of Ohio   Dear Governor
Columbus, OH 43215

State Senator
The Honorable (full name)   Sir, Madam
The State Senate   Dear Sir, Madam
Columbus, OH 43215   My dear Senator
or   My dear Senator (surname)
Senator (full name)   Dear Senator (surname)
The State Senate   My dear Mr., Ms., Mrs., or Miss (surname)
Columbus, OH 43215   Dear Mr., Ms., Mrs., or Miss

State Representative
The Honorable (full name)   Sir, Madam
House of Representatives   Dear Sir, Madam
Columbus, OH 43215   My dear Representative (surname)
or   Dear Representative (surname)
Representative (full name)   My dear Mr., Ms., Mrs., or Miss (surname)
House of Representatives   Dear Mr., Ms., Mrs., or Miss (surname)
Columbus, OH 43215

Mayor of a city
The Honorable (full name)   Sir, Madam
Mayor of the City of Ann Arbor   My dear Sir or Madam
City Hall   Dear Sir or Madam
Ann Arbor, MI 48105   Dear Mr. or Madam Mayor
                                   My dear Mayor (surname)
                                   Dear Mayor (surname)

Correspondence with educators
President (College or University)
Dr. (full name)   My dear Sir, Madam
or   Dear Sir, Madam
(full name), Ph.D.   My dear President (surname)
President   Dear President (surname)

> **BOX 9-3, B**
> **Addresses and Salutations for Government and Academic Officials—cont'd**
>
> Ohio University
> Athens, OH 45701
> Dean of a college
> Dean (full name)   My dear Sir, Madam
> College of Business Administration   Dear Sir, Madam
> University of Cincinnati   My dear Dean (surname)
> Cincinnati, OH 45221   Dear Dean (surname)
> or
> Dr. (full name)
> Dean of the College of Business Administration
> University of Cincinnati
> Cincinnati, OH 45221
> (If the individual has a doctorate degree, the salutation may be Dear
>   Dr. Wilson instead of Dear Dean Wilson.)
> Professor (College or University)
> (full name), Ph.D.   My dear Sir, Madam
> Dr. (full name)   Dear Sir, Madam
> Vanderbilt University   My dear Professor (surname)
> Nashville, TN 37203   Dear Dr. (surname)
> Dear Mrs. Mr. Ms., or Miss (surname)

The complimentary close is entered at the same point as the date line position if using the modified block style, or aligned with the left margin if using the block style. Only the first word of the complimentary close should be capitalized. The most common complimentary closes are "Very truly yours" and "Sincerely." Other acceptable closures are "Yours very truly" and "Sincerely yours."

Keyboarded Signature

The keyboarded signature appears four line spaces below the complimentary close. If the name and title of the individual are short, they may be placed on the same line and separated by a comma. If, however, the name and title are relatively long, the name is keyboarded on the first line and the title is placed on the second line. The comma is not placed after the name. You should attempt to make the lines as even as possible.

Reference Initials

Reference initials are the initials of the person who keyboards the letter and should appear in lowercase one double space after the keyboarded signature, even with the left margin. If it is policy to enter the dentist's initials in capital letters before the keyer's in lowercase, it appears as JWL:db or JWL/db.

Attention Line

You may wish to direct a letter to a particular individual or department within an organization. This can be done by using an attention line. The following example illustrates how an attention line is used if the letter has been addressed to a firm:

Apex Dental Laboratories
Attention Mr. W. W. Thomas, President
1616 W. Riverfront Street
Grand Rapids, MI 49502

The attention line indicates that the letter writer prefers that the letter be directed to a particular individual. The salutation should agree with the inside address, not the attention line.

Subject Line

The subject line clearly states what the letter is about. For example, if writing to a patient regarding the office policy on broken appointments, the subject line is written as follows—Subject: Broken Appointments. The subject line is entered a double space after the salutation and is followed by a double space before continuing with the body of the letter. The subject line may be centered, begun at paragraph point, or aligned with the left margin when using block style. The style of letter will often determine the best position for the subject line. The word *subject* or abbreviation RE may be entered in all capital letters or in capitals and lowercase, or it may be underlined. Acceptable methods using the subject line are illustrated as follows:

Dear Mrs. Calloway:
SUBJECT: Broken Appointments
    or
Dear Mrs. Calloway:
RE: BROKEN APPOINTMENTS
    or
Dear Mrs. Calloway:
RE: Broken Appointments

In place of a subject line, you may wish to use a reference number. For example, in a clinical situation, the patient's registration number will appear in the same position as the subject line and is preceded by "Reference" or "Re":
Dear Dr. Wilcox:
Reference: No. 06920

Enclosures

It is common to transfer radiographs with a letter to another dentist when requesting a consultation. When the letter has mentioned that an item is enclosed or attached, an enclosure notation should be made. This notation is keyboarded after double spacing below the reference initials, even with the left margin. Two acceptable methods are as follows:

je
Enclosure
    or
je
Enclosures 2

Copy Notation

When additional copies of the letter are made for distribution to various persons, reference to each recipient is commonly made in the copy notation. This informs the recipient to whom copies were sent. Several types of notations are possible, including mail, copy, blind copy, postscript, as well as second-page headings.

SPECIAL MAILING NOTATIONS. Notations such as REGISTERED MAIL, SPECIAL DELIVERY, or CERTIFIED are keyboarded in all capital letters between the date and inside address, aligned with the left margin. Other special notations, such as CONFIDENTIAL or PERSONAL, are entered in the same location.

TYPES OF COPY NOTATIONS. With the use of word processing in the office today, copies of correspondence are stored electronically; however, paper copies of all business correspondence should be available in the office. When additional copies are made for distribution, it is necessary for the addressee to know this. A notation is keyboarded a double space below the enclosure, if used, or below the reference initials if there is no enclosure. When more than one person is to receive a copy, list each person on a succeeding line, indenting three spaces from the left margin. Because not all copies are photocopies or computer copies, variations may be used as they apply to the various copy styles. The notation may be keyboarded as follows:

Copy to O.J. Fox, D.D.S.
   or
c O.J. Fox, D.D.S. (copy)
   or
cc O.J. Fox, D.D.S. (courtesy copy)
   or
cc O.J. Fox, D.D.S. (courtesy copies to multiple parties)
R.C. Campbell, D.D.S.
M.A. Reynolds, RDA

BLIND COPY. If the person who receives the original letter does not need to know that a copy is being sent to a particular person, then a blind copy notation can be made. To do this, the original copy is removed from the computer or machine, and the notation is keyboarded on the copy one inch from the top at the left margin, as in the following example:
   bc Barbara Rice

POSTSCRIPT. A postscript is often used to highlight a particular point. It is not necessarily an item that has been omitted in the body of the letter. If a postscript is used, it is the last line entered. It is not necessary to precede the postscript with P.S.; however, the postscript paragraph should be blocked or indented, depending on the style of letter used (Figure 9-9).

You were right, Daniel. The experience of working alongside my father in his practice has been invaluable. I only hope it has been as rewarding for him as it has been for me. Again, thank you for your continued interest in my success.

Very truly yours,

Ashley M Lake, DDS

je

Please make a note to join us for the Martinique Open on December 29th.

Figure 9-9 Letter with a postscript.

SECOND-PAGE HEADING. When writing a patient referral letter, it is some-times necessary to send a lengthy letter to provide adequate information about the patient. If a second page is necessary, the continuation is made on plain paper that is the same size, color, and quality as the letterhead. Leave a one-inch bottom margin on the first page. Include at least two lines of a paragraph at the bottom of the first page, and continue with at least two lines of the same paragraph on the succeeding page. A heading consisting of the addressee, page number, and date is single-spaced, one inch (line six) from the top of the sheet. The following are two acceptable arrangements for beginning the second page.

Block form (used when the letter is in block style):

Ms. Margaret Thompson
Page 2
October 27, 2005

Horizontal form (used when the letter is in modified block style):

Ms. Margaret Thompson   2   October 27, 2005
(triple space)

PUNCTUATION STYLES IN BUSINESS LETTERS

Two common styles of punctuation are used in business letters: open punc-tuation and mixed or standard punctuation. Open punctuation omits all punctuation (except periods after abbreviations) in the salutation and complimentary close lines. Mixed or standard punctuation requires a colon after the salutation and a comma after the complimentary close. Either style of punctuation may be used with any of the basic letter styles.

The administrative assistant will frequently use titles and academic degrees in writing. The traditional rule is to never omit the period after the element of an academic degree or religious order and never include internal spaces: B.S., Ph.D., LL.B., D.M.D., C.D.A., R.D.A., R.D.H., or Ed.D. This rule may need to be altered, however, in contemporary use when addressing envelopes or completing specialized federal, state, or insurance forms that limit space for computerization or scanning. Addressing envelopes is dis-cussed in greater detail later in this chapter.

Correct punctuation is based on certain accepted rules and principles rather than on the whim of the writer. Punctuation is also important so that the reader can correctly interpret the writer's thoughts. The summary of rules given in this chapter will be helpful in using correct punctuation. The common use of periods, commas, colons, and other types of punctuation is illustrated in Boxes 9-4 to 9-14.

CAPITALIZATION

In addition to understanding the rules for punctuation, it is necessary to review the rules for capitalizing various initials and words. A summary of the rules for capitalization is convenient for reference purposes and is listed in Box 9-15.

TELEPHONE NUMBERS

There are several ways of entering telephone numbers in a letter. The paren-theses method (734) 956-9800 is frequently used, but does not work well in text material when the telephone number as a whole has to be enclosed in parentheses. One reason it is suggested not to use the parentheses is because

Text continued on p. 256

BOX 9-4
The Period

1. The period indicates a full stop and is used at the end of a complete declarative or imperative sentence.
2. It is also used following an abbreviation, and after a single or double initial that represents a word (does not apply to addressing envelopes).

   acct.   etc.   Ph.D.
   U.S.   viz.   P.M.
   N.E.   i.e.   pp.

3. Some abbreviations that are made up of several initial letters do not require periods.

   FDIC (Federal Deposit Insurance Corporation)
   ADA (American Dental Association)
   AAA (American Automobile Association)
   YWCA (Young Women's Christian Association)

4. Insert a period between dollars and cents (period and cipher are not required when an amount in even dollars is expressed in numerals).

   $42.65 $1.47 $25

4. Insert a period to indicate a decimal.

   3.5 bushels   12.65 percent   6.25 feet

BOX 9-5
The Comma

The comma indicates a partial stop and is used in the following instances:

1. To separate coordinate clauses that are connected by conjunctions, such as *and, but, or, for, neither,* or *nor,* unless the clauses are short and closely connected.

We have a supply on hand, but I think we should order an additional quantity.
She had to work late, because the auditors were examining the books.

2. To set off a subordinate clause that precedes the main clause.

Assuming that there will be no changes, I suggest that you proceed with your instructions.

3. After an introductory phrase containing a verb form.

To finish his work, he remained at the office after hours.
After planning the program, she proceeded to put it into effect.

4. If an introductory phrase does not contain a verb, it usually is not followed by a comma.

After much deliberation the plan was revoked. Because of the vacation period we have been extremely busy.

5. To set off a nonrestrictive clause.

Our group, which had never lost a debate, won the grand prize.

6. To set off a nonrestrictive phrase.

The beacon, rising proudly toward the sky, guided the pilots safely home.

7. To separate from the rest of the sentence a word or a group of words that breaks the continuity of a sentence.

The business manager, even though his work was completed, was always willing to help others.

8. To separate parenthetical expressions from the rest of the sentence.

   We have, as you know, two persons who can handle the reorganization.

9. To set off names used in direct address or to set off explanatory phrases or clauses.

BOX 9-5
The Comma—cont'd

I think you, Mr. Bennett, will agree with the statement. Ms. Linda Tom, our vice-president, will be in your city soon.

10. To separate from the rest of the sentence expressions that might be interpreted incorrectly without punctuation.

Misleading: *Ever since we have filed our reports monthly.*

Better: *Ever since, we have filed our reports monthly.*

11. To separate words or groups of words when they are used in a series of three or more.

Most executives agree that dependability, trustworthiness, ambition, and judgment are required of their office workers.

Again I emphasize that factory organization, correlation of sales and production, and good office organization are all necessary for maximum results.

12. To set off short quotations from the rest of the sentence.

He said, "I shall be there." "The committees have agreed," he said, "to work together on the project."

13. To separate the name of a city from the name of a state.

Our southern branch is located in Atlanta, Georgia.

14. To separate abbreviations of titles from the name.

William R. Warner, Jr.

Ramona Sanchez, Ph.D.

BOX 9-6
The Semicolon

The semicolon is used in the following instances:

1. Between independent groups or clauses that are long or that contain parts that are separated by commas.

He was outstanding in his knowledge of word processing, database, spreadsheets, and related software applications; however, he was lacking in many desirable personal qualities.

2. Between the members of a compound sentence when the conjunction is omitted.

Many executives would rather dictate to a machine than to a secretary; the machine won't talk back.

3. To precede expressions used to introduce a clause, such as *namely, viz., e.g.,* and *i.e.*

We selected the machine for two reasons; namely, because it is as reasonable in price as any other and because it does better work than others.

There are several reasons for changing the routine of handling mail; i.e., to reduce postage, to conserve time, and to place responsibility.

4. In a series of well-defined units when special emphasis is desired.

Emphatic: The prudent secretary considers the future; he or she ensures that all requirements are obtained, and he or she uses his or her talents to attain the desired goal successfully.

Less emphatic: The prudent secretary considers the future, ensures that all requirements are obtained, and uses his or her talents to attain the desired goal successfully.

BOX 9-7
The Colon

The colon is used in the following instances:
1. After the salutation in a business letter, except when open punctuation is used.

Ladies and Gentlemen:

Dear Ms. Carroll:

2. Following introductory expressions, such as *the following, thus, as follows,* and other expressions that precede enumerations.

Please send the following by parcel post:

Officers were elected as follows: president, vice-president, and secretary-treasurer.

3. To separate hours and minutes when indicating time.

2:10 PM 4:45 PM 12:15 AM

4. To introduce a long quotation.

The agreement read: "We the undersigned hereby agree. ..."

5. To separate two independent groups having no connecting words between them and in which the second group explains or expands the statement in the first group.

We selected the machine for one reason: in competitive tests it surpassed all other machines.

BOX 9-8
The Question Mark

The question mark (interrogation point) is used in the following instances:
1. After each direct question.

When do you expect to arrive in Philadelphia?

2. An exception to the foregoing rule is a sentence that is phrased in the form of a question, merely as a matter of courtesy, when it is actually a request.

Will you please send us an up-to-date statement of our account.

3. After each question in a series of questions within one sentence.

What is your opinion of the IBM word processor? the Xerox? the CPT?

BOX 9-9
The Exclamation Point

The exclamation point is used ordinarily after words or groups of words that express command, strong feeling, emotion, or an exclamation.

Don't waste office supplies!

It can't be done!

Stop!

BOX 9-10
The Dash

The dash is used in the following instances:
1. To indicate an omission of letters or figures.
Dear Mr.—   Date the letter July 16, 20—
2. Sometimes in letters, especially sales letters, to cause a definite stop in reading the letter. Usually the dash is used in such cases for increased emphasis. One must be careful, however, not to overdo the use of the dash.
This book is not a revision of an old book—it is a brand new book.
3. To separate parenthetical expressions when unusual emphasis is desired on the parenthetical expression.
These sales arguments—and every one of them is important—should result in getting the order.

BOX 9-11
The Apostrophe

The apostrophe should be used in the following instances:
1. To indicate possession.
    the patient's record
    the dentist's coat
    the assistants' responsibilities
    the dentists' records.
2. To form the possessive singular, add 's to the noun.
    man's work
    bird's wing
    hostess's plans
3. An exception to this rule is made when the word following the possessive begins with an *s* sound.
    for goodness' sake
    for conscience' sake
4. To form the possessive of a plural noun ending in an *s* or *z* sound, add only the apostrophe to the plural noun.
    workers' rights
    hostesses' duties
5. If the plural noun does not end in an *s* or *z* sound, add 's to the plural noun.
    women's clothes
    alumni's donations
6. Proper names that end in an *s* sound form the possessive singular by adding 's.
    Williams's house
    Fox's automobile
7. Proper names ending in *s* form the possessive plural by adding the apostrophe only.
    The Walters' property faces the Jones' swimming pool.
8. To indicate the omission of a letter or letters in a contraction.
    it's (it is)
    you're (you are)
    we'll (we shall)
9. To indicate the plurals of letters, figures, words, and abbreviations.
    Don't forget to dot your i's and cross your t's.
    I can add easily by 2's and 4's, but I have difficulty with 6's and 8's.
    More direct letters can be written by using shorter sentences and by omitting and's and but's.
    Two of the speakers were Ph.D.'s.

BOX 9-12
Quotation Marks

The following basic rules should be followed when using quotation marks:
1. When a quotation mark is used with a comma or a period, the comma or period should be placed inside the quotation mark.

She said, "I plan to complete my program in college before seeking a position."

2. When a quotation mark is used with a semicolon or a colon, the semicolon or colon should be placed outside the quotation mark.

The treasurer said, "I plan to go by train"; others in the group stated that they would go by plane.

3. When more than one paragraph of quoted material is used, quotation marks should appear at the beginning of each paragraph and at the end of the last paragraph.

"_____

_____

_____

_____"

"_____

_____

_____"

Quotation marks are used in the following instances:
1. Before and after direct quotations.

The author states, "Too frequent use of certain words weakens the appeal."

2. To indicate a quotation within a quotation, use single quotation marks.

The author states, "Too frequent use of 'very' and 'most' weakens the appeal."

3. To indicate the title of a published article.

Have you read the article, "Automation in the Office?"

He asked, "Have you read 'Automation in the Office'?"

---

of the growing use of the mandatory area code where there is a shortage of numbers. In these areas, the use of the parentheses with the telephone number might suggest you would not need to use the area code. Three other methods of entering telephone numbers are 707-555-3998, 707 555 3998, and 707.555.3998. The latter system seems to be gaining popularity as it uses periods to separate the elements. This is because these periods resemble the dots in e-mail addresses.

Text continued on p. 258

BOX 9-13
Omission Marks or Ellipses

Ellipses marks (… or ***) are frequently used to denote the omission of letters or words in quoted material. If the material omitted ends in a period, four omission marks are used (….). If the material omitted is elsewhere in the quoted material, three omission marks are used (…).

He quoted the proverb, "A soft answer turneth away wrath: but … ."

She quoted Plato, "Nothing is more unworthy of a wise man … than to have allowed more time for trifling and useless things than they deserved."

BOX 9-14
Parentheses

Although parentheses are frequently used as a catch-all in writing, they are correctly used in the following instances:
1. When amounts expressed in words are followed by figures.
He agreed to pay twenty-five dollars ($25) as soon as possible.
2. Around words that are used as parenthetical expressions.
Our letter costs (excluding paper and postage) are much too high for this type of business.
3. To indicate technical references.
Sodium chloride (NaCl) is the chemical name for common table salt.
4. When enumerations are included in narrative form.
The reasons for his resignation were three: (1) advanced age, (2) failing health, and (3) a desire to travel.

BOX 9-15
Rules for Capitalization

Common usage
1. The following are examples of the most common usage of capitalization:
2. The first word of every sentence should be capitalized.
3. The first word of a complete direct quotation should be capitalized.
4. The first word of a salutation and all nouns used in the salutation should be capitalized.
The first word in a complimentary close should be capitalized.

Outline Form
Capitalize the first word in each section of an outline form.

First Word After a Colon
Capitalize the first word after a colon only when the colon introduces a complete passage or sentence having independent meaning. In conclusion I wish to say: "The survey shows that ..." If the material following a colon is dependent on the preceding clause, the first word after the colon is not capitalized.
I present the following three reasons for changing: the volume of business does not justify the expense; we are short of people; and the product is decreasing in popularity.

Names
1. Capitalize the names of associations, buildings, churches, hotels, streets, organizations, and clubs.
   * *The American Dental Association, Merchandise Mart, Central District Dental Society, Peabody Hotel, Seventh Avenue, Administrative Management Society, Chicago Chamber of Commerce*
2. Capitalize all proper names
Great Britain, John G. Hammitt, Mexico
3. Capitalize names that are derived from proper names.
American, Chinese
4. Do not, however, capitalize words that are derived from proper nouns and that have developed a special meaning.
pasteurized milk, china dishes, moroccan leather

> ### BOX 9-15
> ### Rules for Capitalization—cont'd
>
> 5. Capitalize special names for regions and localities.
> *North Central states, the Far East, the East Side, the Hoosier State*
> 6. Do not, however, capitalize adjectives derived from such names or localities that are used as directional parts of states and countries.
> *far eastern lands, the southern United States, southern Illinois*
> 7. Capitalize names of government boards, agencies, bureaus, departments, and commissions.
> *Civil Service Commission, Social Security Board, Bureau of Navigation*
> 8. Capitalize names of the deity (deities), the Bible, holy days, and religious denominations.
> *God, Easter, Yom Kippur, Genesis, Church of Christ*
> 9. Capitalize the names of holidays.
> *Memorial Day, Labor Day*
> 10. Capitalize words used before numbers and numerals, with the exception of the common word, such as *page, line,* and *verse*.
> *The reservation is Lower 6, Car 27.*
> *He found the material in Part 3 of Chapter X.*
>
> ### Titles used in business and professions
> The following are rules for capitalizing titles in business and professions.
> 1. Any title that signifies rank, honor, and respect, and that immediately precedes an individual's name should be capitalized.
> *She asked President Harry G. Sanders to preside.*
> *He was attended by Dr. Howard Richards.*
> 2. Academic degrees should be capitalized when they precede or follow an individual name.
> *Constance R. Collins, Ph.D., was invited to direct the program.*
> *Fred R. Bowling, Master of Arts*
> 3. Capitalize titles of high-ranking government officers when the title is used in place of the proper name in referring to a specific person.
> *Our Senator invited us to visit him in Washington.*
> *The President will return to Washington soon.*
> 4. Capitalize military titles signifying rank.
> *Captain Meyers, Lieutenant White, Lieutenant Commander Murphy*

From Fulton PJ: *General office procedures for colleges,* ed 11, Cincinnati, 1998, South-Western.

PREPARING AN EFFECTIVE LETTER

To prepare an effective letter, it is necessary to follow several basic steps:
1. Collect the information
2. Make an outline
3. Develop the letter
4. Select a format style
5. Review and revise the letter
6. Produce the letter
7. Proofread the letter
8. Distribute the letter
9. Store the document

Before beginning each step of letter writing, it is necessary to determine who will receive the letter and what the person knows about the subject you are writing. If a letter is to be written to another dentist about a patient, it will require using technical language. On the other hand, if a patient is to receive a letter about an unknown subject, the educational level of the person needs to be determined so the letter can be written in understandable language.

Collecting Information

Before you begin to write the letter, you need to gather the important facts to be included in the letter. In general you will need to gather the following information: to whom the letter is being sent, by whom the letter is being written, and the subject of the letter. If it is a letter of referral, the name of the patient and any necessary personal information for which consent has been given, the nature of the problem, any possible symptoms or diagnosis, enclosures if any, anticipated response, deadline dates, and how the patient will contact the office. If it is a letter of inquiry, the nature of the inquiry, product names if available, quantity or specifications of the product, and date of needed reply.

Making an Outline

You may ask yourself, "Why is it necessary to make an outline if I know what I want to say?" You may find after writing several letters that it is natural for you to be organized. If you are a beginner or someone who dislikes letter writing, making an outline will provide organization and a framework that forces you to get your thoughts on paper, and in the process you may discover that you do not have all the facts you need. An outline helps you to see relationships between topics and determine if your letter is written in a logical sequence.

Developing the Letter

It is often said that once the outline is completed, you are nearly finished with the letter. This is partially true, but you do need to give special attention to how each part of the letter is developed and determine its format. A variety of format styles are illustrated in this chapter.

As you begin to develop the letter, remember that the first paragraph is the most important paragraph of any letter. It should get the reader's attention and set the tone for the letter. This paragraph places the emphasis on the reader and uses the "you" approach. Review each paragraph in the letter to determine if it gets the reader's attention first and clearly states the purpose of the letter. Make a natural transition from one paragraph to the next. Special consideration should be given to factors such as data and confidentiality that are included in various types of letters. Box 9-16 includes several suggestions for writing various types of letters.

> An outline helps you to see relationships between topics and determine if your letter is written in a logical sequence.

Selecting the Format

The administrative assistant may select a template from the word processing software in the office, but the letter will still require decisions about punctuation styles. Letter style is a personal choice that relates to a particular practice and complements the office stationery most effectively.

Most word processing software provides several templates for a variety of letter styles, which can be modified to meet the dentist's preference and

---

BOX 9-16
Special Considerations for Letter Content

Order letter
- Indicate quantity
- Provide description of the material or product
- List the price
- Define method of payment
- Indicate shipping preference

Referral letter
- Provide complete and proper name of patient
- State the condition and expected type of consultation or examination
- Always write out tooth names or provide an illustration; avoid using tooth numbers only
- Refer to enclosures
- Indicate timeliness if necessary
- Maintain confidentiality and provide only information for which consent is given
- Extend courteous expression of appreciation

Inquiry letter
- *State the objective
- Give all the necessary facts
- Close with good will

Thank-you letter
- State the purpose
- Explain your appreciation
- Maintain confidentiality
- Close with a sincere expression of good will

---

saved in the letter file as a specialized template. Several basic styles are shown in Figure 9-10 *A* to *E*, including the block style with mixed punctuation, block style with open punctuation, modified block style with mixed punctuation, block style with attention line and enclosure, and the Administrative Management Society (AMS) simplified style. The first styles are self explanatory. The AMS simplified style can be put to good use when informing all patients about a policy change or announcing that an associate will be joining the practice. The style has two basic rules.

- The letter must have a subject line. The word *subject* is omitted, and the subject line is keyboarded in all capital letters with a triple space before and after the subject line.
- The writer's name and title are keyboarded in all capital letters at least four lines below the last line of the letter.

Reviewing the Letter

Once the letter has been written, you need to determine if the letter meets all of the criteria of an effective letter, as described in Box 9-1. If the letter does not meet most of these criteria, take time to modify it. If you are unsure about a letter, ask another person to review and evaluate it. Make the necessary changes until all criteria are met.

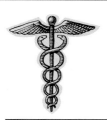

Dental Associates, PC
Joseph W. Lake, DDS – Ashley M. Lake, DDS

1–6 spaces depending
on length of letter

Line up
everything
with left
margin

September 16, 20—

1–1½"

Use first
name in
salutation
for
informal
greeting;
or title in
formal
greeting

Mr. Harry Wong
3489 W. Houghton Street
Grand Rapids, MI 49505

Dear Mr. Wong: Colon in mixed punctuation

After examination of your radiographs and oral examination taken on
September 11, 20—, I find it necessary to refer you to Dr. Ralph Murphey   ⅝–1"
for the extraction of the lower right third molar. At the same time, the small
cyst that is evident in the radiographs can be removed and examined.

Single
space in
paragraph

I will send Dr. Murphey your radiographs, along with a detailed report of
your recent examination. These should be in the mail later today.

Double
space
between
paragraphs
(one blank
line)

Please call Dr. Murphey's office at 616.429.7654 and make an appointment
as soon as possible. I know you will be pleased with the type of care he will
give you. Feel free to contact my office if you have any further questions.

1–2 spaces

Sincerely,

2–4
spaces

Joseph W. Lake, DDS

2 spaces

je

Leave bottom margin of
3–6 spaces

611 Main Street, SE – Grand Rapids, MI 49502   *Phone: 616.101.9575 Fax: 616.101.9999*
E-mail: office@dapc.com or Visit us at: www.Lakedental.com

Figure 9-10 A, Block style letter with mixed punctuation.

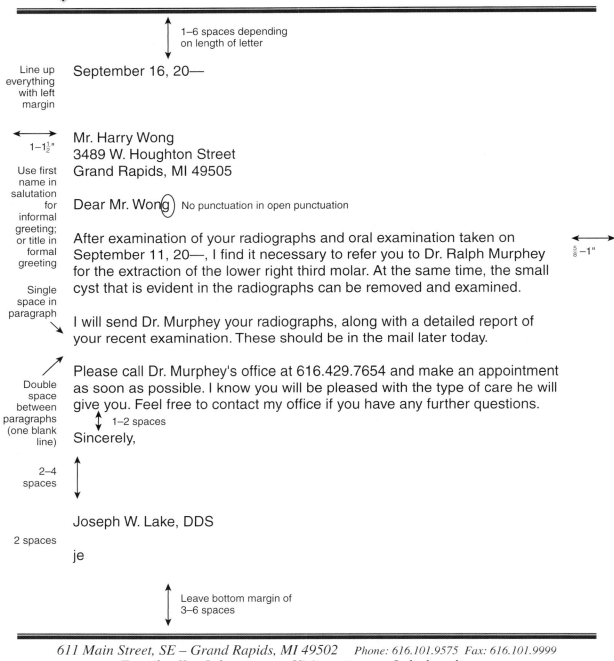

Dental Associates, PC

Joseph W. Lake, DDS – Ashley M. Lake, DDS

1–6 spaces depending
on length of letter

Line up
everything
with left
margin

September 16, 20—

1–1½"

Mr. Harry Wong
3489 W. Houghton Street
Grand Rapids, MI 49505

Use first
name in
salutation
for
informal
greeting;
or title in
formal
greeting

Dear Mr. Wong   No punctuation in open punctuation

After examination of your radiographs and oral examination taken on
September 11, 20—, I find it necessary to refer you to Dr. Ralph Murphey
for the extraction of the lower right third molar. At the same time, the small
cyst that is evident in the radiographs can be removed and examined.

⅝–1"

Single
space in
paragraph

I will send Dr. Murphey your radiographs, along with a detailed report of
your recent examination. These should be in the mail later today.

Double
space
between
paragraphs
(one blank
line)

Please call Dr. Murphey's office at 616.429.7654 and make an appointment
as soon as possible. I know you will be pleased with the type of care he will
give you. Feel free to contact my office if you have any further questions.

1–2 spaces

Sincerely,

2–4
spaces

Joseph W. Lake, DDS

2 spaces

je

Leave bottom margin of
3–6 spaces

611 Main Street, SE – Grand Rapids, MI 49502   Phone: 616.101.9575 Fax: 616.101.9999
E-mail: office@dapc.com or Visit us at: www.Lakedental.com

Figure 9-10, cont'd B, Block style letter with open punctuation.

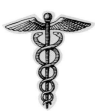

Dental Associates, PC
Joseph W. Lake, DDS – Ashley M. Lake, DDS

2–6 spaces depending on length of letter

September 16, 20—

Line up date with signature
block $\frac{1}{2}$ or $\frac{2}{3}$ of the way over
to the right

1–4 spaces

1–1½"

Mr. Harry Wong
3489 W. Houghton Street
Grand Rapids, MI 49505   Zip code on same line

Dear Mr. Wong: Colon in mixed punctuation

Indenting ¶
is optional
in modified
block

After examination of your radiographs and oral examination taken on
September 11, 20—, I find it necessary to refer you to Dr. Ralph Murphey
for the extraction of the lower right third molar. At the same time, the small
cyst that is evident in the radiographs can be removed and examined.

Single-
space
paragraphs

I will send Dr. Murphey your radiographs, along with a detailed report
of your recent examination. These should be in the mail later today.

Double
space
between
para-
graphs (one
blank line)

Please call Dr. Murphey's office at 616.429.7654 and make an
appointment as soon as possible. I know you will be pleased with the type
of care he will give you. Feel free to contact my office if you have any further
questions.

1–2 spaces

Sincerely,   Comma in mixed punctuation

Headings
are optional
in letters

2–4 spaces

Joseph W. Lake, DDS

Line up signature block with date

je

Leave at least 3–6 spaces at bottom
of page—more if letter is short

611 Main Street, SE – Grand Rapids, MI 49502   Phone: 616.101.9575 Fax: 616.101.9999
E-mail: office@dapc.com or Visit us at: www.Lakedental.com

Figure 9-10, cont'd C, Modified block style letter with mixed punctuation.

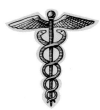

Dental Associates, PC
Joseph W. Lake, DDS – Ashley M. Lake, DDS

↕ 1–6 spaces depending on length of letter

Line up everything with left margin

September 16, 20—

Ralph Murphey, DDS, MS
1234 Highland Rd.
Grand Rapids, MI 49502

←→ 1–1½"

Use first name in salutation for informal greeting; or title in formal greeting

RE: Harry Wong   Attention line bolded

Dear Dr. Murphey: Colon in mixed punctuation

I am referring Mr. Harry Wong to you for the removal of the mandibular right third molar (#32). Enclosed you will find a periapical radiograph of this area.   ←→ ⅝–1"

Single space in paragraph

As you will note there appears to be a small cyst in this area. I have been able to palpate this area and want to have you examine the site also. I have indicated to Mr. Wong that you will likely recommend the removal of this small cyst at the time of the extraction. I will leave this decision up to you, however.

Double space between paragraphs (one blank line)

The patient will be contacting your office later this week to make an appointment. He has indicated he wishes to have a general anesthesia for this procedure.

Thank you so much for your assistance in this case. I will look forward to your diagnosis after seeing Mr. Wong.

↕ 1–2 spaces

Sincerely,

2–4 spaces

Joseph W. Lake, DDS

2 spaces

je

Enclosure: Periapical radiograph

↕ Leave bottom margin of 3–6 spaces

611 Main Street, SE – Grand Rapids, MI 49502   Phone: 616.101.9575 Fax: 616.101.9999
E-mail: office@dapc.com or Visit us at: www.Lakedental.com

Figure 9-10, cont'd D, Block style letter with attention line and enclosure.

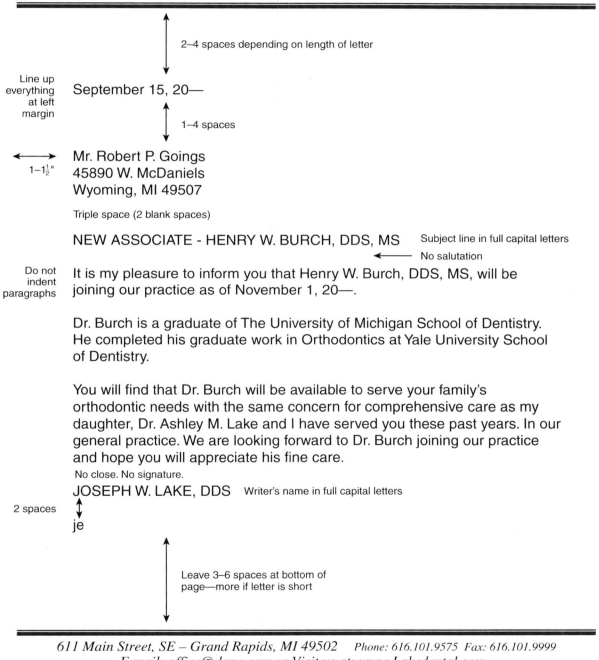

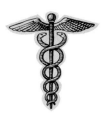

Dental Associates, PC

Joseph W. Lake, DDS – Ashley M. Lake, DDS

2–4 spaces depending on length of letter

Line up everything at left margin

September 15, 20—

1–4 spaces

1–1½"

Mr. Robert P. Goings
45890 W. McDaniels
Wyoming, MI 49507

Triple space (2 blank spaces)

NEW ASSOCIATE - HENRY W. BURCH, DDS, MS   Subject line in full capital letters

No salutation

Do not indent paragraphs

It is my pleasure to inform you that Henry W. Burch, DDS, MS, will be joining our practice as of November 1, 20—.

Dr. Burch is a graduate of The University of Michigan School of Dentistry. He completed his graduate work in Orthodontics at Yale University School of Dentistry.

You will find that Dr. Burch will be available to serve your family's orthodontic needs with the same concern for comprehensive care as my daughter, Dr. Ashley M. Lake and I have served you these past years. In our general practice. We are looking forward to Dr. Burch joining our practice and hope you will appreciate his fine care.

No close. No signature.

JOSEPH W. LAKE, DDS   Writer's name in full capital letters

2 spaces

je

Leave 3–6 spaces at bottom of page—more if letter is short

611 Main Street, SE – Grand Rapids, MI 49502   Phone: 616.101.9575 Fax: 616.101.9999
E-mail: office@dapc.com or Visit us at: www.Lakedental.com

Figure 9-10, cont'd E, Administrative Management Society (AMS) simplified style.

Producing the Final Letter

Prior to the final printing of the letter, use spell-check and grammar-check, if available. Whether the letter is created on a typewriter or electronically using word processing software, the letter needs to be produced on quality stationery that creates a professional image of the office.

Proofreading the Letter

> You cannot rely completely on an electronic system to proofread your letter.

You cannot rely completely on an electronic system to proofread your letter. Though software packages provide spell-check, many dental terms are not in the dictionary, unless you have inserted them. Likewise, English words are often misused, such as *there* or *their*. Both of these words will come up as correct, but you may have misused them. Not all word processing systems can be relied on for complete grammar accuracy. Therefore, make a final review of the letter to be certain the grammar, spelling, and punctuation are correct. Proofreading a letter is much like the final check of the margins on an amalgam restoration. It is your creation, and you want it to be perfect.

Distributing the Letter

There are several methods of distributing the letter: E-mail, traditional postal services, fax, or some form of specialized mail service. Each of these is explained in detail later in this chapter. Prior to creating the letter, you should be aware of the method of distribution to determine the type of envelope or mailing label necessary for production.

Storing the Document

If the letter is to be stored electronically, the procedure discussed in Chapter 8 should be followed. If not, a hard copy should be made and filed in the patient record or other location that is appropriate for the document. Remember, if you are striving for the paperless office you need to maximize the use of the electronic filing system.

PREPARING THE ENVELOPE

It is possible to prepare the envelope as part of the word processing procedure, or the envelope may be keyboarded on a typewriter. Larger mailing envelopes may require special labeling. In either case, it is necessary to prepare the envelope or package with a standardized delivery address. Most postal services use automatic sorting equipment, which begins an automatic sorting process with an optical character reader (OCR). A standardized address, readable by an OCR, contains the correct city name, state, and ZIP+4 code. To obtain zip codes for any address, visit the U.S. Postal Service website at www.usps.com, and select the zip code navigation bar. The address on the envelope should agree with the inside address of the letter, although the inside address may contain punctuation not recommended by the postal service for the envelope.

The address is should be single-spaced, even if the address is only two lines. In this case, the name of the individual or firm is on the first line, and the city, state, and zip code are on the second line. The two-letter state abbreviations, approved and recommended by the U.S. Postal Service, should be used. These abbreviations appear in Box 9-17. For further information,

BOX 9-17
Two-Letter Abbreviations for States

Alabama	AL	Montana	MT
Alaska	AK	Nebraska	NE
Arizona	AZ	Nevada	NV
Arkansas	AR	New Hampshire	NH
California	CA	New Jersey	NJ
Colorado	CO	New Mexico	NM
Connecticut	CT	New York	NY
Delaware	DE	North Carolina	NC
District of Columbia	DC	North Dakota	ND
Florida	FL	Ohio	OH
Georgia	GA	Oklahoma	OK
Hawaii	HI	Oregon	OR
Idaho	ID	Pennsylvania	PA
Illinois	IL	Rhode Island	RI
Indiana	IN	South Carolina	SC
Iowa	IA	South Dakota	SD
Kansas	KS	Tennessee	TN
Kentucky	KY	Texas	TX
Louisiana	LA	Utah	UT
Maine	ME	Vermont	VT
Maryland	MD	Virginia	VA
Massachusetts	MA	Washington	WA
Michigan	MI	West Virginia	WV
Minnesota	MN	Wisconsin	WI
Mississippi	MS	Wyoming	WY
Missouri	MO		

request Publication 28, Postal Addressing Standards, from your local Postal Business Center or by calling the National Address Information Center in Memphis, Tennessee, at 800-238-3150. Figure 9-11 illustrates how an address should be keyboarded on various business envelopes.

Other important elements of the address are suffixes, directionals, apartment or suite numbers, post office box numbers, and complete rural/highway contract route addresses with box numbers. All of these elements must be spelled correctly and clearly written. If the address is not electronically readable, the letter or package will be delayed for manual handling.

Address Format

Using the universal format for addresses expedites the processing capability of automated equipment at the post office. The format requires that you use a uniform left margin. Type the address in uppercase letters as follows:

MS MARY BALL
3347 MAPLE RD
ROCKFORD MI 48167-2345

A secondary address unit, such as an apartment (APT) or suite (STE) number, should be printed as part of the address. Always use APT or STE rather than the # (pound) sign. Common designations are APT, BLDG FLOOR

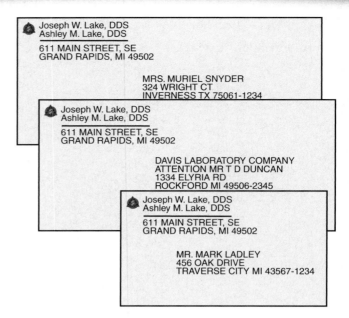

Figure 9-11 Address styles for different size envelopes. Note placement of attention line.

(FL), STE, UNIT, ROOM (RM), and DEPARTMENT (DEPT). Using this format, the address line might appear as follows:

    1334 RIVERSIDE APT 201
        or
    3745 KINSEY DR STE 301
        or
    845 KELSAY BLVD BLDG 5
        or
    1234 KELLOGG PL RM 136

If your letter or package is sent to the attention of an individual, that information precedes the line of the name of the firm or building. The attention line varies from the traditional format that many people have used. For example:

    ATTN: MS MARY CLINE
    ACME DENTAL COMPANY
    134 FLETCHER
    CUTLERVILLE MI 49504-2345

Avoid using dual addresses, even though you may have both a box number and street address available. Place the delivery address on the line immediately above the city, state, and ZIP+4 code.

Punctuation on Address Labels

The U.S. Postal Service prefers that you do not use punctuation, special characters, or multiple blanks in the address, with the exception of a hyphen in the ZIP+4 code or a hyphen that appears in the primary number of the delivery address, such as 51-234 HANCOCK ST. Spell out city names completely. If an abbreviation must be used because of labeling/space constraints, use existing abbreviations first for suffix or directional words. For instance:

    EAST MARKET becomes E MARKET
    JEFFERSON MOUNTAIN becomes JEFFERSON MT

The eight standard directionals can be abbreviated to one or two characters. For instance:

255 NW WASHINGTON ST

133 CHERRY DR S

If the first word in a street name is a directional word and no other directional is to the left of it, abbreviate it. For example:

NORTH CHERRY ST becomes N CHERRY ST

  or

LAKE DRIVE WEST becomes LAKE DRIVE W

When two directional words appear before the street name, the first one is abbreviated:

NORTH EAST SUGAR ST becomes N EAST SUGAR ST

Folding and Inserting the Letter

After all enclosures have been checked to be certain they correspond to the letter and that the items are correct, the letters must be signed and you must be sure that the right letter gets in the right envelope (letters get in the wrong envelopes surprisingly often). The letter is placed in the envelope so that the date and inside address are visible upon opening the letter. The reader should not be forced to turn the paper around to begin reading the letter. Figure 9-12 illustrates a step-by-step procedure for folding and inserting the letter in the proper size envelope.

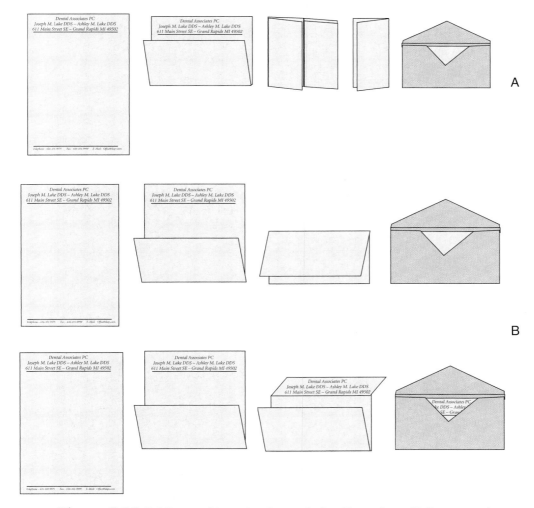

Figure 9-12 Folding and inserting letter. **A,** Small envelope. **B,** Large envelope.

ELECTRONIC MAIL (E-mail)

With the wide use of computers today, electronic mail (e-mail) has opened the doors to sending mail between computers within networked locations. E-mail within a large clinic or dental school has become the choice for sending memoranda to the staff. With more patients having e-mail, this becomes another source of communication with the office and patient. In fact, consideration should be given to including this on the personal questionnaire on admission. The patient's e-mail can be integrated into various software programs and may even be used to confirm appointments or act as a reminder for routine recalls. E-mail has many advantages as a communication tool.

- E-mail reaches its destination in a matter of seconds after it is sent, even if its destination is across the world.
- Multiple individuals may be sent the same message quickly, with all the recipients receiving the message instantly.
- Paper is saved. It is not necessary to make a hard copy of e-mail.
- E-mail may be filed electronically for later reference.
- E-mail may be forwarded to another party.
- E-mail may be destroyed immediately after it is read.
- E-mail takes less time to write than a paper letter. Only the receiver's name, the sender's name, and the body of the letter need to be entered. The date and time is entered automatically, and the letter or envelope does not need to be printed.
- Other documents and graphic images may be transferred as attachments through e-mail.
- The recipient is notified of the arrival of an e-mail by a message that appears at the bottom of the computer screen or by an audio signal that is emitted through the computer.
- A hard copy of the e-mail may be printed if necessary for retention in a manual file.
- Notations such as "confidential" and "urgent" can be made on the e-mail message.

As with any new system, a person often overlooks the need to follow basic protocol. E-mail should not become a quick system for communication with no concern given to punctuation or formatting.

Consider the following guidelines when using e-mail:

- Be certain you have thought about the purpose of the e-mail before you begin writing; in other words know what you are trying to achieve with your e-mail message.
- Be succinct. Before you send your e-mail, reread it. Delete unnecessary phrases, words, or sentences.
- Be polite. Think of your e-mail as a short letter, and follow etiquette rules. Use *please* and *thank you*.
- Be suitably formal when writing e-mail. The rule of thumb is to be almost as formal in e-mail as you are in standard memorandums to your employer, coworkers, or patients.
- Always capitalize the appropriate works, be specific about needs, and use proper closing.
- Use the subject line that is provided on the e-mail form. This line should be concise yet convey the purpose of the message to the reader.
- If you are replying to a message but are changing the subject of conversation, change the subject also.
- Edit and proofread carefully. Do not send an e-mail that contains inaccuracies or incorrect grammar.
- Use complete sentences.
- Capitalize and punctuate properly.

> E-mail should not become a quick system for communication with no concern given to punctuation or formatting.

- Do not run sentences together; it is difficult to read e-mail constructed in this manner.
- Insert the nature of the message on the subject line.
- Include a salutation.
- Use a colon after the salutation. A comma can be used in a nonbusiness application.
- Use complete sentences and paragraph structure.
- Check the letter for spelling and grammatical errors.
- Insert a blank line after each paragraph.
- Always include your name and title (if appropriate) when replying to an e-mail.
- Assume that any message you send is permanent. The message can be sitting in someone's private file or in a tape archive.

E-mail Ethics and Etiquette

There is a growing body of ethical issues in regard to e-mail. Some organizations have developed a code of ethics for using e-mail. This form of communication should follow the same ethical guidelines used in any form of written communication in the dental office.

- Do not send personal e-mail from your office computer.
- When people send you inappropriate e-mail, let them know politely that you cannot receive it.
- Do not use e-mail to berate or reprimand an employee.
- Do not use e-mail to send information that involves any type of legal action; third parties that should have no knowledge of the action may obtain the information.
- Do not forward junk mail or chain letters.
- Do not forward an e-mail unless you know it is true.
- Do not include credit card numbers.
- Do not forward confidential patient information.
- Do not criticize or insult third parties.
- Avoid using different types of fonts, colors, clip art and other graphics in e-mail. It clutters the message and may be difficult for the reader to view.
- Do not keyboard your message in all uppercase.
- Avoid sending messages when you are angry.
- Observe the Golden Rule in cyberspace; treat others as you would like to be treated.
- Act responsibly when sending e-mail or posting messages to a discussion group.
- Use a style and tone that are appropriate to the intended recipient(s).
- Before you reply to an e-mail, ask yourself if you really need to reply.
- Answer your e-mail promptly.

The contents of the letter can be retained as a permanent record, thus anything you do not want written documentation of should not be entered.

- Confidentiality must be maintained.
- Rules of courtesy should be followed.
- An appropriate closing should be included.

An alternative to dictation equipment that is discussed later in this chapter is the use of an attachment to e-mail. A dentist may wish to keyboard a document and not dictate it. This is often easier than handwriting. This could be done in word processing and sent to the administrative assistant via e-mail. The administrative assistant can download the document, print it, and store it in the appropriate file.

OTHER TYPES OF WRITTEN COMMUNICATION

Other types of written communication routinely prepared by the administrative assistant include postal cards, interoffice memoranda, and manuscripts. For many of these documents, there are templates available that aid in formatting and eliminate the steps of setting up the document.

Postal Cards

There will be times in a dental office when it is more practical to send a patient a postal card (e.g., for recall or confirmation of an appointment) rather than to write a letter. Figure 9-13 illustrates how a postal card should be addressed and the placement for the message.

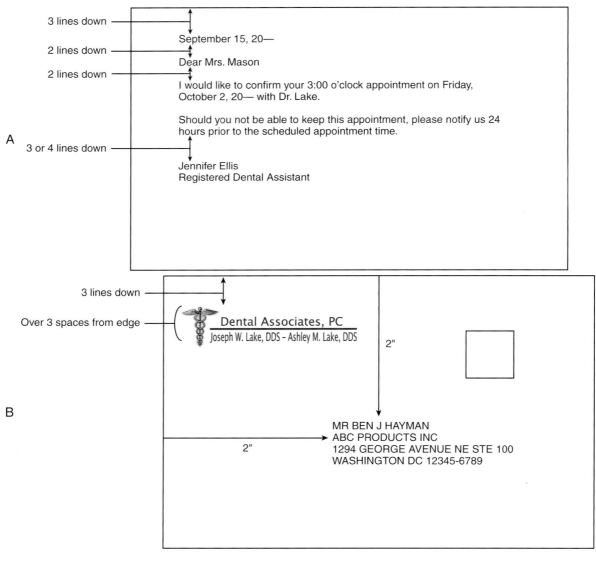

Figure 9-13 **A,** 5½-by-3½-inch postal card message. **B,** Postal card address.

Interoffice Memoranda

Although most office correspondence is keyboarded on office letterhead, the interoffice memorandum is a timesaving form and is entered on plain paper (Figure 9-14). This type of communication is often used within a clinic or group practice or within a professional building where several dental offices are located. The form provides space for the name of the department or individual(s) to whom the memorandum is being sent, the date, subject or reference line, and space for the sender's name. The memorandum should be brief, clearly stated, well-organized, and easy to read. A copy of the memorandum should be made for the office files. If several people are to receive the memorandum, their names are inserted in the space provided, or additional copies are made and the individual names entered on each memorandum.

Manuscripts

In the first part of this chapter, emphasis was placed on general correspondence. In both the academic and health environments, you may be asked to write a report or research paper for your employer. Such reports could range from a business proposal to a research paper. Whether you are writing a business report or an academic report, you should follow standard style when preparing it.

Many styles exist for manuscript preparation, depending on the nature of the report. Each style requires the same basic information. For example, one style may use the term *bibliography,* whereas another uses *references,* and a third prefers *works cited.* Although a publisher may provide the author with a format for a manuscript, a popular documentation style used today for research papers is presented by the Modern Language Association (MLA), as shown in Figure 9-15. When preparing a paper, you must adhere to some

INTEROFFICE MEMORANDUM

TO: Jennifer Ellis, RDA

FROM: Dr. Ashley Lake

SUBJECT: Reassignment to business manager position

DATE: October 19, 20--

For some time I have been thinking that we should promote you to the position of office manager. After our discussion last Friday, I would like to confirm this reassignment. Both my father and I feel that you have considerable expertise in patient management and have excelled in the recent courses in small business management in which you have been enrolled. Both of us would like to discuss this transition with you.

Let's meet on Friday, October 25, at 2 P.M. to discuss this matter. If this date is inconvenient for you, please let me know.

Figure 9-14 Interoffice memorandum.

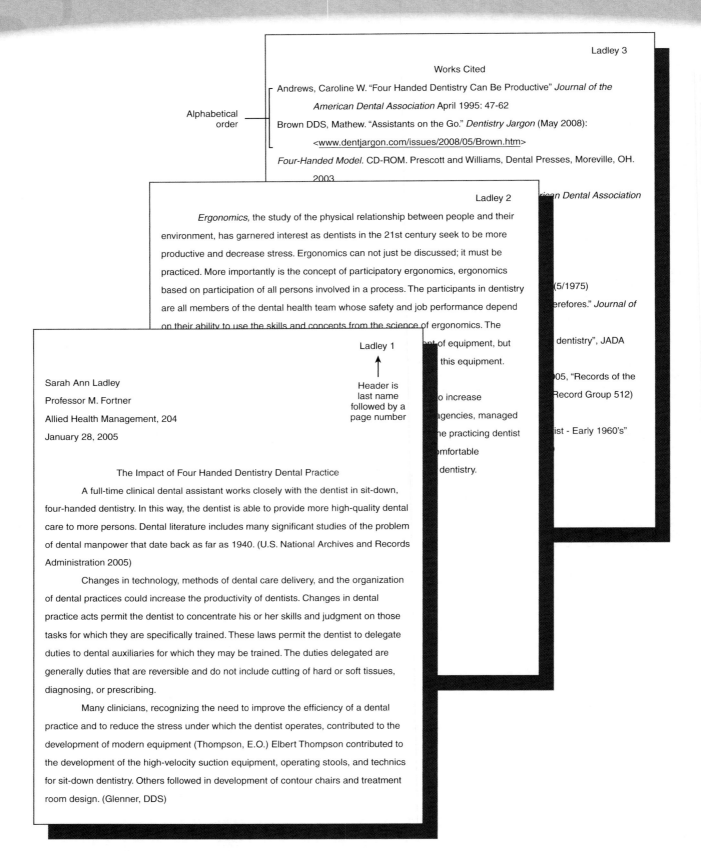

Figure 9-15 MLA manuscript format. Notice setup for first page, footnotes, and works cited page.

form of documentation style. Therefore, if none are given it is wise to select the MLA style, which includes the following:

- Use 8½ -by-11-inch paper
- Double-space all pages of the paper with 1-inch top, bottom, left, and right margins.
- Indent the first word of each paragraph ½ inch from the left margin.
- At the right margin of each page, place a page number ½ inch from the top margin and 1 inch from the right margin. Double-space between the header and the body. Only use Arabic numbers; do not use pp, p, or the # sign.
- On each page, precede the page number with the author's last name.
- When a quote contains less than six lines, set it off with quotation marks and keep it within the normal text, followed by the reference. When a quote contains six or more lines, set it off by indenting it one inch from the right and left margins. Check MLA sources for other requirements regarding longer quotes, special circumstances, and quotes within quotes.
- Each figure and table needs to be labeled and numbered. Place the words *figure* or *table* (and the number) a double space before the actual figure or table. Other materials, such as charts, photographs, and drawings, also need to be labeled and numbered, and should include a caption.
- No title page is required. Instead, on the first page only place the author's name on the first line and double space each successive line followed by the instructor's name, the course name and number, and the date. This should be in a block at the left margin beginning one inch from the top of the page.
- Center the title two double spaces below the date and other related information (e.g., the course number). The title's first, last and principal words should be capitalized. Do not underline, italicize, or use all caps in the title. Do not end with a period. A question or exclamation mark may be used if appropriate.
- Place author references in the body of the paper in parentheses with the page number(s) where the referenced information is located. These parenthetical citations are used instead of footnoting each source at the bottom of the page. Footnotes are used only for explanatory notes. In the body of the paper, use superscripts (raised numbers) to signal that an explanatory note exists. Explanatory notes are optional. If used, the note is placed either at the bottom of the page as a footnote or at the end of the paper as an endnote.
- MLA style uses the term *works cited* for bibliographic references. These are placed on a separate numbered page. Center the title (Works Cited) one inch from the top margin. List references in alphabetic order by each author's last name. Double-space all lines. Works cited from books, journals, magazines, newspapers, letters, online sites, and compact disks each have their own MLA reference style that should be followed.

Dictation and Transcription

Some dentists prefer to use dictation and transcription equipment as part of a written communication system. The use of dictation and transcription equipment (Figure 9-16) has become a vital link between the dentist and the administrative assistant. Studies show that machine dictation is six times faster than longhand and almost three times faster than shorthand. After considering the many advantages of dictation equipment, its importance in

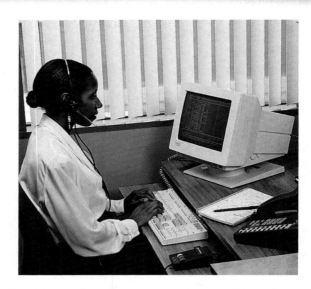

Figure 9-16 Dictation and transcription equipment. (From Young AP: *Kinn's the administrative medical assistant,* ed 5, St. Louis, 2003, WB Saunders.)

the word processing system can be easily recognized in the increase of both input and output.

At the conclusion of the workday or between patients, the dentist may use the dictation equipment for referral letters or for recording information to be transferred to clinical records, etc.

Effective dictation requires following a few guidelines:

- Indicate the message disposition to the transcriber before beginning to dictate the message: the number of copies to be made and to whom the copies are to be sent. If the material has priority over other dictation, this too should be indicated at the beginning. State what is being dictated (e.g., letter, memo, report). Also indicate whether the item is a rough draft or finished product, as well as spacing and margins.
- Spell out any words that might not be easily understood, as well as names, streets, and cities.
- Organize correspondence materials before beginning to dictate.
- Dictate clearly, at an easy pace, and in a conversational tone. Most dictation equipment provides for control of speed and volume, but the fewer adjustments you have to make, the faster the material will be transcribed.

The administrative assistant can schedule the daily work to include transcription periods to complete correspondence and reports on a priority basis. The following are some guidelines for effective transcription:

- Assemble all materials and necessary equipment.
- Use reference sources such as a dictionary, written communication reference book, spelling and grammar checker and thesaurus, and a name and address file.
- Listen to special instructions on the dictated material to determine priority. Some systems have audible indexing that gives a single tone signal to indicate the end of each document and double tones for

special instructions. Determine whether other materials are needed for enclosures or if there are special mailing procedures.
- If the dictation does not make sense or you have a question regarding the information, ask the dentist rather than transcribing incorrect information.
- Proofread the entire transcription before printing the document.

MANAGING OFFICE MAIL

With the increase in written communications in today's dental office, more demands for efficient processing and distribution of both incoming and outgoing mail must be met by the administrative assistant. Because of the constant flow of incoming and outgoing mail, the administrative assistant must know proper techniques for handling the mail.

Processing Outgoing Mail

Outgoing correspondence may be prepared earlier in the day but is often organized for mailing at the end of the day, as part of the daily routine.

Classification of Mail

Some of the outgoing mail will be sent as first-class mail, some as fourth class, some insured, and some special handling using the address guidelines in Figure 9-17. The administrative assistant must be aware of these various classes of mail and be able to select the best classification for the type of item being mailed.
- First-class mail consists of letters, government or private postcards, business reply mail, bills, and statements of accounts.
- Second-class mail includes newspapers and published periodicals.
- Third-class mail includes items such as books, circulars, catalogs, or miscellaneous printed material weighing less than 16 ounces.
- Fourth-class mail, often called parcel post, is for printed material and packages weighing more than 16 ounces. The rate of postage varies, depending on distance. The United States is divided into zones, and parcel post rates are figured accordingly.

Although mail will be classified in one of these four classifications, additional special services may be used.
- If sent first class, valuable or important items can be registered to provide protection and evidence that the article has been received. A special fee is charged for this service, and a receipt is furnished by the post office. The post office accepts the responsibility if the mail is lost and will pay the sender the insured amount. The fee for registered mail varies according to the declared value.
- Special delivery service is available for all classes of mail. The post office delivers special delivery mail as quickly as it reaches the post office of destination. Rates are determined by weight and destination.
- Certified mail is available for first-class mail; the sender is provided a receipt, and proof of delivery of the letter is recorded at the post office. No insurance coverage is available on certified mail.
- Insured mail service applies to third- and fourth-class mail; articles may be insured up to a value of $200 against damage, theft, or total loss. The fee for insured mail is determined by the amount of the insurance on the package contents.

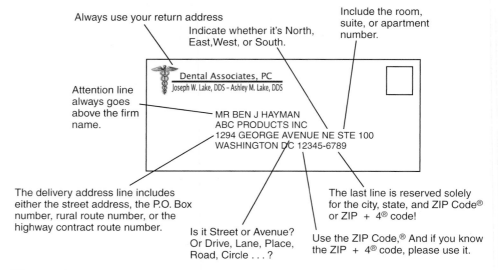

Follow these simple guidelines to help mail get where it's going faster.

Always use your return address

Indicate whether it's North, East, West, or South.

Include the room, suite, or apartment number.

Attention line always goes above the firm name.

Dental Associates, PC
Joseph W. Lake, DDS – Ashley M. Lake, DDS

MR BEN J HAYMAN
ABC PRODUCTS INC
1294 GEORGE AVENUE NE STE 100
WASHINGTON DC 12345-6789

The delivery address line includes either the street address, the P.O. Box number, rural route number, or the highway contract route number.

Is it Street or Avenue? Or Drive, Lane, Place, Road, Circle . . . ?

The last line is reserved solely for the city, state, and ZIP Code® or ZIP + 4® code!

Use the ZIP Code,® And if you know the ZIP + 4® code, please use it.

Figure 9-17 Guidelines recommended by the U.S. Postal Service for addressing mail correctly.

- Special handling service is available only for third- and fourth-class mail. If the mail is marked "special handling," it receives the fastest handling of third- and fourth-class mail, but it is not delivered by special messenger.
- Express mail service is provided by the U.S. Postal Service and provides delivery of mail within 24 hours. Express mail service is available 7 days a week, 365 days a year (weekend and holiday deliveries are no additional charge) for items up to 70 pounds in weight and 108 inches in combined length and girth.

Other questions that arise regarding outgoing mail can be answered by checking with the U.S. Postal Service. Manuals are available from the Superintendent of Documents, Government Printing Office, Washington, DC 20402\MDomestic Mail Manual, 19 and International Mail Manual, 14.

POSTAGE SCALE. A postage scale, to determine the weight of outgoing mail, is an asset in the dental business office. Mail sent with insufficient postage might be returned to the sender. This causes a delay in delivery of statements to patients and insurance forms to the carrier, thus delaying the return of money to the practice.

POSTAGE METER. A postage meter can be a timesaving device for the administrative assistant. Although various sizes of postage meters are available, a desk model is practical for a private practice. Group practices and clinics may need a larger meter that feeds envelopes through the machine automatically, both stamping and sealing them. The meters are purchased outright, but the meter mechanism is leased. A meter license is obtained from the U.S. Postal Service. With new electronic models, meter resetting is done by means of a telephone call. All that is needed is an active account with the Postage-By-Phone System and the appropriate meter. No special telephone hookups, computers, or software are required. The customer signs up for the system and then writes a check to put funds into an account to draw on as postage is ordered. Monthly reports listing the account activities are sent to the customer. In keeping with this new technology, postage scales are now available that weigh and automatically determine correct postage rates (Figure 9-18). The accuracy of electronic scales helps to eliminate overpayment in postage. The meter can also be set for the amount of postage required for packages. The amount is printed on a tape, which is then affixed to the package.

Outgoing mail that is addressed correctly, has the proper amount of postage, and is pre-postmarked goes through the post office faster and will arrive at its destination sooner.

E-MAIL. Dental practices often make use of e-mail through a computer network system. This is a type of message service (software) that allows users to communicate directly with other users by sending messages electronically over communication channels. E-mail can be used to leave messages for other staff members, and messages are safeguarded because the users must have their own identification code to access the messages. E-mail has gained wide use in processing insurance claim forms. Turnaround time has been greatly reduced, and the result is an increase in cash flow for the office.

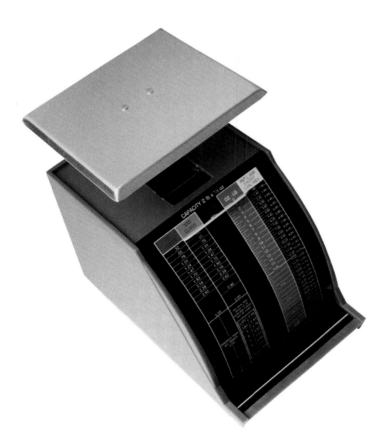

Figure 9-18 Postage meter.

FACSIMILE. Another electronic means of communication is the facsimile (fax) machine. A fax machine is a scanning device that transmits an image of a document over standard telephone lines and described in detail in Chapter 10. The dentist may find this method of transmitting written communication very effective when it is necessary to have an immediate response or if the information involves an emergency procedure. The use of such a transmission requires a transmission cover sheet and requires that transmitted information be maintained confidentially.

MAILING SERVICES. Mailing services are service enterprises that specialize in mail communications. A mailing service is an independent postal service that is a complete business center that processes metered and bulk mail, first-class mail, UPS, FedEx, air freight, and so on. Making use of such a service might be very useful for a dental practice with high-volume mailings. Some mailing services specialize in direct mail advertising, promotional sales, and billings. Other types of services available from a mailing service might include data entry, file maintenance, labels and listings, and personalized letters.

DELIVERY SERVICES. Delivery services, such as United Parcel Service (UPS), FedEx, Greyhound Package Express, Purolator Courier, and many others, are gaining popularity with businesses that wish letters or packages delivered the next day or need to send fourth-class material. When selecting this service, it is important to consider the cost, speed of delivery, and convenience. Most services will require the completion of a special form similar to the one shown in Figure 9-19 for use with FedEx.

The following list provides information about delivery services.
- Rates are determined by weight, distance within specified zones, and required time of delivery.
- Maximum weight varies with carrier.
- Each package may be insured against loss or damage.
- Most general commodities may be shipped.
- Packages to be shipped can be picked up at the dental office or place of business. Deliveries are made to the exact address indicated on the parcel.
- Deliveries are not made to post office boxes.
- Attempts are made for delivery at no additional charge.
- The sender is not charged for return of an undeliverable package.
- This service is available in most large cities; the address and telephone number of the nearest depot are listed in the telephone directory.

LABORATORY SERVICES. In areas where there is no local dental laboratory, cases must be shipped to the laboratory via the U.S. mail or commercial delivery services. The dental laboratory provides a dentist with a sturdy cardboard or plastic, insulated mail carton. All impressions or devices that have been placed in the patient's mouth must be disinfected in compliance with OSHA guidelines prior to packaging. The contents should be carefully wrapped. The case should be disassembled from articulators and each item wrapped separately to be reassembled when received by the laboratory. The laboratory requisition is enclosed in the box and a mailing label, supplied by the laboratory, is attached to the carton.

Processing Incoming Mail

The location of the dental practice may determine whether the mail is delivered to the office by a regular postal mail carrier or whether a post office box

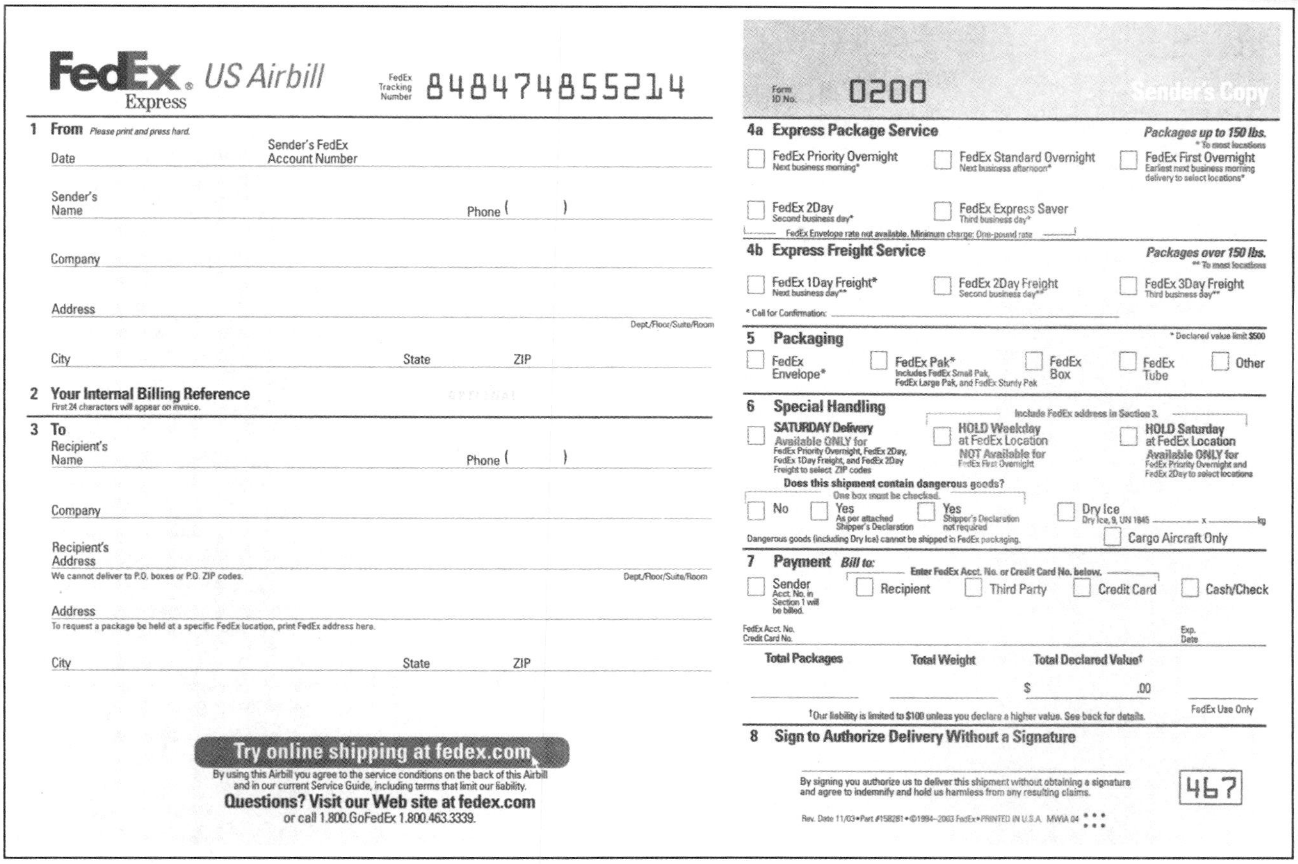
FedEx. US Airbill
Express
FedEx Tracking Number 848474855214
Form ID No. 0200
Sender's Copy

1 From Please print and press hard.
Date
Sender's FedEx Account Number
Sender's Name
Phone ( )
Company
Address
Dept./Floor/Suite/Room
City State ZIP

2 Your Internal Billing Reference
First 24 characters will appear on invoice.

3 To
Recipient's Name
Phone ( )
Company
Recipient's Address
We cannot deliver to P.O. boxes or P.O. ZIP codes.
Dept./Floor/Suite/Room
Address
To request a package be held at a specific FedEx location, print FedEx address here.
City State ZIP

Try online shipping at fedex.com
By using this Airbill you agree to the service conditions on the back of this Airbill and in our current Service Guide, including terms that limit our liability.
Questions? Visit our Web site at fedex.com
or call 1.800.GoFedEx 1.800.463.3339.

4a Express Package Service
Packages up to 150 lbs.
* To most locations
FedEx Priority Overnight — Next business morning*
FedEx Standard Overnight — Next business afternoon*
FedEx First Overnight — Earliest next business morning delivery to select locations*
FedEx 2Day — Second business day*
FedEx Express Saver — Third business day*
FedEx Envelope rate not available. Minimum charge: One-pound rate

4b Express Freight Service
Packages over 150 lbs.
** To most locations
FedEx 1Day Freight* — Next business day**
FedEx 2Day Freight — Second business day**
FedEx 3Day Freight — Third business day**
* Call for Confirmation:

5 Packaging
* Declared value limit $500
FedEx Envelope*
FedEx Pak* — Includes FedEx Small Pak, FedEx Large Pak, and FedEx Sturdy Pak
FedEx Box
FedEx Tube
Other

6 Special Handling
Include FedEx address in Section 3.
SATURDAY Delivery — Available ONLY for FedEx Priority Overnight, FedEx 2Day, FedEx 1Day Freight, and FedEx 2Day Freight to select ZIP codes
HOLD Weekday at FedEx Location — NOT Available for FedEx First Overnight
HOLD Saturday at FedEx Location — Available ONLY for FedEx Priority Overnight and FedEx 2Day to select locations
Does this shipment contain dangerous goods?
One box must be checked.
No
Yes — As per attached Shipper's Declaration
Yes — Shipper's Declaration not required
Dry Ice — Dry Ice, 9, UN 1845 ___ x ___ kg
Dangerous goods (including Dry Ice) cannot be shipped in FedEx packaging.
Cargo Aircraft Only

7 Payment Bill to:
Enter FedEx Acct. No. or Credit Card No. below.
Sender — Acct. No. in Section 1 will be billed.
Recipient
Third Party
Credit Card
Cash/Check
FedEx Acct. No. Credit Card No.
Exp. Date
Total Packages
Total Weight
Total Declared Value†
$ .00
†Our liability is limited to $100 unless you declare a higher value. See back for details.
FedEx Use Only

8 Sign to Authorize Delivery Without a Signature
By signing you authorize us to deliver this shipment without obtaining a signature and agree to indemnify and hold us harmless from any resulting claims.
Rev. Date 11/03•Part #158281•©1994–2003 FedEx•PRINTED IN U.S.A. MWIA 04
467

Figure 9-19 FedEx mailing label. (Courtesy FedEx, Ann Arbor, MI.)

is rented and the mail is picked up at the post office. For a clinic within an institution, mail may be routed from a central mailroom within the building. Whatever the situation, the administrative assistant will be responsible for proper sorting and distribution of the mail.

When the mail is first sorted, you will need to distinguish between the various types of mail received.

- First-class mail, including priority mail, personal mail, special delivery, registered or certified mail, payments, invoices, and general correspondence
- Printed matter, such as announcements of professional meetings, solicitations for contributions, collegiate newsletters, and other semiprofessional materials
- Magazines and newspapers for the reception room, as well as professional journals and periodicals
- Advertisements
- Samples of dental products and drugs
- Materials from laboratories
- Supplies ordered from a dental supply company

After the initial sorting, you will distribute the personal mail to the intended receiver and place it so that it will receive prompt attention.

When payments are received, attach the returned portion of the statement, or note on the envelope the amount of money received. Enclosures should be clipped to the letter, invoice, or statement, and all incoming correspondence should be stamped with the date and time received. Many offices find that an automated time-stamp machine, which stamps the date

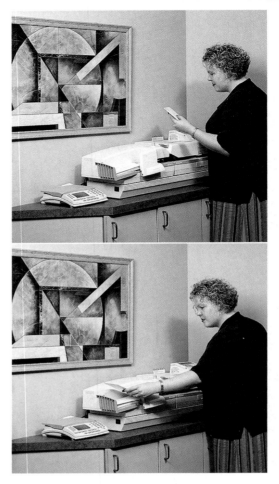

Figure 9-20 Automatic time-stamp machine. (From Young AP: *Kinn's the adminis-trative medical assistant,* ed 5, St. Louis, 2003, WB Saunders.)

and time received, is practical, especially if a question arises as to the time and date a particular item was received (Figure 9-20). If a time-stamp machine is not available, then the date and time the correspondence is received have to be written on the correspondence. Also, you may have the responsibility for opening and reading some first-class mail and highlighting the signifi-cant portions of the correspondence. When doing so, use a colored pen to make your notations. This procedure saves the dentist valuable time when he or she reads through important mail. If the incoming mail item makes reference to previous correspondence, copies of the latter can be attached or clinical records pulled and attached. This will save time when replying and also serves as a reminder of a previous conversation or correspondence. In a group practice or clinic, a routing slip may be used for a piece of correspon-dence when several people need to be informed of the contents (Figure 9-21). When discarding the envelopes of incoming mail, be sure the entire contents have been removed and all important data, such as company name, indi-vidual name, postmark date, and time if significant, have been recorded. You may even need to retain the envelope in some situations.

Some printed material such as meeting notices will be opened by the dentist and should be placed on his or her desk along with the personal mail. The magazines for the office should be distributed to the reception room and the older issues removed and recycled.

Dental Associates, PC

Joseph W. Lake, DDS - Ashley M. Lake, DDS

INTEROFFICE

ROUTING SLIP

Please read the attached _____
and record the date passed on to the persons indicated.

Refer to:	Date Received	Date Passed on
Dr. Austin	_____	_____
Dr. Baker	_____	_____
Dr. Downing	_____	_____
Dr. Green	_____	_____
Dr. Mann	_____	_____
Dr. Powers	_____	_____
Routed by:	_____	_____

Figure 9-21 Mail routing slip.

You may be asked to scan the professional magazines and make notes in the margins of special meetings and conferences that may be of interest to the dentist. This saves the dentist's time when reading the magazine.

The dental office receives many advertisements, and many of them are regarded as "junk" mail. It is the administrative assistant's responsibility to sort through the advertisements to determine which material should be examined by the dentist. The dentist will indicate the types of advertisements for review. If the advertisements are of no value, throw them away.

When dental supplies are received in the office through the mail, they need to be processed as soon as possible. This procedure is detailed in the inventory chapter, Chapter 12. Care should be taken, however, to ensure that any MSDSs that accompany the products remain with the products until the materials are checked in, stored, and appropriate labels and data entry are made.

Open any samples received in the mail, and place them on the dentist's desk. Most of these samples accompany literature that should remain with the product.

Extreme care should be taken when opening materials from dental laboratories. Follow appropriate disinfection procedures, inform the dentist of the arrival of a lab case, then confirm the patient's appointment.

Managing the Mail in the Dentist's Absence

When the dentist is away from the office, you will be responsible for handling all mail. Decisions will have to be made regarding the following:
- Contacting the dentist regarding any of the correspondence
- Forwarding mail to the dentist
- Answering mail and explaining that the dentist is away from the office
- Determining which correspondence can wait for an answer when the dentist returns

Before the dentist leaves the office for any length of time, a policy regarding handling of mail should be established.

Key Terms

Attention line - A line at the beginning of a letter that directs the letter to a particular individual or department within an organization.

Body - The main portion of a letter that include the message.

Complimentary close - A courteous ending to a letter, such as "Sincerely," "Yours truly," or "Sincerely yours."

Date line - The line that contains the date the letter is keyboarded. When using printed letterhead stationery, it usually begins a double space below the lowest line of the letterhead.

E-mail - Electronic mail used to communicate within the office and with external sources.

Inside address - The address that provides all information for mailing the letter and includes the recipient's name, the name of the company

(if appropriate), street number and name, city, and zip code.

Interoffice memorandum - Communication within the organization or office.

Keyboarded signature - The name and title of the person sending the letter or communication.

Mixed punctuation - The use of punctuation within a letter; a colon follows the salutation and a comma follows the close.

Open punctuation - The elimination of punctuation after the salutation and the close.

Reference initials - The initials of the person who produced the letter or memo if different than the signature.

Salutation - Formal greeting to the reader.

Subject line - A statement that concisely states what the letter is about.

LEARNING ACTIVITIES

1. List and explain the characteristics of an effective letter.
2. Explain the benefits a newsletter might have on a dental practice.
3. Outline the acceptable format for addressing envelopes.
4. Outline the procedures for sorting incoming mail.
5. List and define the four classifications of mail.
6. Discuss the special mail services that might be used by a dental office.
7. Explain the functions of a postage meter.
8. List the advantages of using a commercial delivery service.
9. Explain a situation that could be handled through a fax process.
10. On the computer, create and store in a file a letterhead for Joseph W. Lake, D.D.S. and Ashley M. Lake, D.D.S. Use the letterhead data found in this chapter for the dentists. If desired, add clip art as appropriate.
11. Using the letterhead created in #10, keyboard the following letters.
12. Keyboard the following letter in block style with mixed punctuation. Use the current date, and address a small envelope. Fold the letter to insert into a small envelope. Make a copy for the office files, or store it electronically.

Mrs. Jason Calloway, 2453 Prescott Avenue, Grandville, MI 49302 Dear Mrs. Calloway (P) We have written to Doctor Jack Notman as you requested. He is most interested in your case and will be expecting you to contact his office very soon. (P) When we first corresponded with Doctor Notman, we mailed him a complete set of radiographs. Also, we indicated to him at that time that you are a diabetic and have allergies to several drugs. (P) As soon as time is available for Doctor Notman to complete the work, I suggest you contact his office. If we can be of further assistance, do not hesitate to call us. Sincerely Joseph W. Lake, D.D.S. (reference initials)

LEARNING ACTIVITIES—cont'd

12. Keyboard the following letter in modified block style with open punctuation. Use the current date; address a large envelope. Fold the letter to insert into a large envelope. Make a copy for the office files, or store it electronically.

Reliance Dental Laboratory, 1600 Michigan Avenue, NE, Grand Rapids, MI 49502 Gentlemen (Subject line: Three-Unit Porcelain-Fused-to-Metal Bridge); (P) I am returning the three-unit porcelain-fused-to-metal bridge you constructed for our patient, Mr. H.B. Rider. There are open margins on teeth #9 on the mesial, #10 on the facial, and #11 on the distal. (P) I am mailing a new final impression that can be used for recasting of the bridge. I would like the bridge returned with the castings only soldered in place for a try-in. If the bridge is satisfactory, I will return the casting for final baking of the porcelain. (P) We appreciate your cooperation in this matter. Sincerely, Joseph W. Lake, D.D.S. (reference initials)

13. Keyboard the following letter in block style with mixed punctuation. Use the current date and an appropriate-size envelope. Make a copy for the office files, or store it electronically.

Mr. Robert Clay, 6690 Jefferson SW, Wyoming, MI 49507 Dear Mr. Clay (P) I know you have been pleased with the work our office has done for you and your wife. We have enjoyed having both of you as patients. (P) We feel sure you have misplaced the last two statements that we have sent to you, but we would appreciate it if you would stop by the office so we can make an arrangement to bring your account up-to-date. (P) Thank you for your cooperation in this matter. Sincerely, Jennifer Ellis, R.D.A.

14. Keyboard the following information as the continuation of a two-page letter (use blank stationery). The letter has been addressed to James Howard, D.D.S. Use modified block style and open punctuation. Make a copy for the office files, or store it electronically. Make an additional copy to be sent to O.J. Fox, D.D.S.

(P) To confirm an almost conclusive diagnosis, we are referring the patient to you for an incisional biopsy. The biopsy was not done in our office due to the potential hemorrhage problem. If my diagnosis of squamous cell carcinoma is confirmed, we recommend counseling to the patient so that treatment can begin immediately. (P) If we can be of further assistance, please feel free to contact our office. Sincerely, Joseph W. Lake, D.D.S. (reference initials)

15. Key the letter in #12 to the Reliance Dental Laboratory. Use the AMS simplified style. Address an envelope. Make a copy for the office files, or store it electronically.

16. The administrative assistant may write many letters using his or her own personal signature. The following note appears on your desk from Dr. Lake. Dr. Notman's address appears on your Rolodex as follows: Jack Notman, D.D.S., 255 W. Michigan, Grand Rapids, MI 49501.

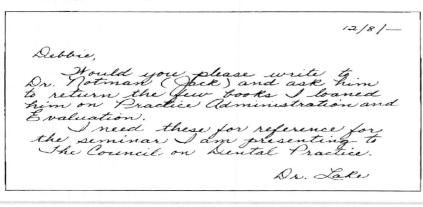

LEARNING ACTIVITIES—cont'd

17. The letter in Form 4 contains errors. Proofread the letter, and make corrections in spelling and punctuation. Rekey the letter using office stationery with block format and mixed punctuation, today's date. Address an appropriate envelope. Make a copy for the office files, or store it electronically.

18. The list of statements in Form 5 contains a variety of grammatical errors. Review each one, and in the space beneath each sentence make the corrections.

19. You are asked by Dr. Lake to keyboard a patient referral letter to Joseph E. Harrison, D.D.S., MS, 1718 West Stadium Boulevard, Ann Arbor, MI 48104. Compose a letter using the following information taken from the patient's clinical chart: The patient is Howard Phillips, age 37. Tooth #32 is to be removed. The patient prefers general anesthesia. His health history indicates that he has had rheumatic fever and is under the care of Mark Driscoll, M.D. at 211 Cutler Street SW, Grand Rapids, MI 49507. A periapical x-ray of this area is to be included. Keyboard the letter in modified block style, use the current date, make a copy, address an appropriate envelope, and have the letter available for Dr. Lake's signature.

20. Assume that the following list represents the morning incoming mail. How would you sort and handle each item?
    - Product advertisement and sample of a new alloy for Dr. Lake
    - Letter addressed to Dr. Lake marked "personal"
    - Letter addressed to the administrative assistant regarding overpayment of an account
    - Statement of account from Quick Copy
    - Check in the amount of $850 from Harold C. Hammond (a patient)
    - Two magazines, *The American Dental Association Journal* and *Reader's Digest*, addressed to Dr. Lake
    - Notice of a registered letter for Dr. Lake at the post office
    - OSHA *Update Newsletter* marked "Important Dated Material"
    - Concert tickets for Dr. Lake
    - Notice of Dental Assistant Advisory Committee meeting from Kent County Community College
    - Bill to Dr. Lake for Kent County District Dental Society dues
    - Letter to Dr. Lake from Rotary Club confirming a speaking engagement

21. The following list represents the outgoing mail for the office. Indicate how you would prepare each item for mailing. (Indicate any special handling or delivery services.)
    - Referral letter with two mounted periapical x-ray films enclosed
    - Letter and statement to a patient. (You want proof of its delivery.)
    - Pamphlet weighing 12 ounces
    - Completed insurance claim forms weighing 18 ounces
    - Recall notices to 30 patients
    - Package weighing 10 pounds, valued at $550
    - Package delivered to the office that Dr. Lake refuses to accept
    - Laboratory requisition with impressions and ancillary materials for a porcelain veneer crown that is to be sent to Nuva Dent Porcelain Laboratory, 819 West 43rd Street, New York, NY 67845
    - Mounted, complete series of radiographs with four bitewings mounted separately, to be mailed locally to a periodontist.
    - Videotape to be returned for credit to a distributor in Chicago, Illinois

EXAMINE YOUR PROGRESS

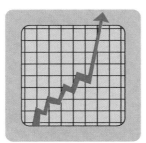

Practice by completing Working Forms 4 and 5.

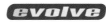

Bibliography

A guide for writing research papers based on modern language association (MLA) documentation, Hartford, Connecticut, 2004, http://www.ccc.commnet.edu/mla/index.shtml, Capital Community College.

FedExpress service guide, Memphis, 2004, FedEx Corporation.

Fulton PJ: *General office procedures for colleges,* ed 12, Cincinnati, 2003, South-Western.

Gibaldi J: *MLA handbook for writers of research papers,* ed 6, New York, 2003, Modern Language Association of America (for high school and undergraduate students).

Gibaldi J: *MLA style manual and guide to scholarly publishing,* ed 2, New York, 1998, Modern Language Association of America (for graduate students, scholars, and professional writers).

Locker KO: *Business and administrative communication,* ed 6, New York, 2003, McGraw Hill/Irwin.

Modern Language Association website, available at http://www.mla.org.

Netiquette tips: Keying in, *The Newsletter of the National Business Education Association,* 11:2. November 2000.

Sabin WA: *The Gregg reference manual,* ed 10, New York, 2004, McGraw Hill/Irwin.

U.S. Postal Service: *The postal manual,* Washington, DC, 2004, U.S. Government Printing Office.

Recommended Websites

http://www.mla.org
http://ww.mla.org/style

Chapter Outline

Learning Outcomes

Mastery of the content in this chapter will enable the reader to:
- Define key terms
- Define telecommunications

- Explain the application of telecommunications in a dental office
- Describe various types of telecommunication systems commonly used in a dental office
- Practice efficient telephone techniques
- Receive, transmit, and record telephone messages
- Plan and place outgoing telephone calls
- Use the features of special telephone equipment and services
- Describe the best way to manage telephone calls commonly encountered in the dental office

> The telephone is the most important piece of equipment in the office.

> For 90% of the patients in a dental office, the first contact is made by telephone.

The patient is the most important person in the dental office. The telephone is the most important piece of equipment in the office. It is the most common and most important communication device in the world because it is perhaps the fastest and easiest way to transmit messages.

Considerable attention is paid to choosing modern equipment for the dental treatment rooms, to hiring assistants highly skilled in business concepts or clinical procedures, and to using the latest technological advances in diagnosis. Yet the most important instrument in the office, the telephone, seldom receives much consideration.

For 90% of the patients in a dental office, the first contact is made by telephone. Like it or not, first impressions are lasting ones, and telephone management should not be entrusted to an inexperienced staff member. This responsibility should be delegated only to a person who has a broad knowledge of dentistry, possesses a high degree of self-confidence, is alert, is able to make decisions, and shows good verbal communication skills. Speaking with a smile in the voice, being enthusiastic, and having a cordial manner may not solve all problems automatically, but speaking with hostility or disinterest ensures that future communications with patients will be more difficult (Figure 10-1).

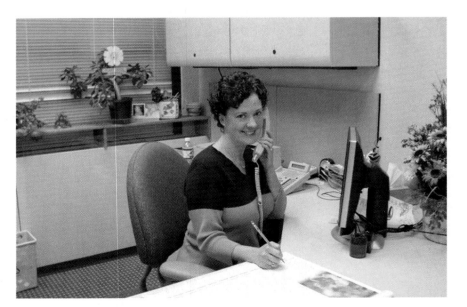

Figure 10-1 A voice that makes the caller feel as though a smile is coming through the receiver is a winning voice.

TELECOMMUNICATIONS IN DENTISTRY

The term **telecommunications** refers to the science and technology of communication by electronic transmission of impulses, as by telegraphy, cable, telephone, radio, or television. In a practical sense, telecommunications in a dental office refers to the different kinds of telephone systems and communication that result from the use of the telephone lines. In this chapter you will learn about the various types of telephone systems, such as key systems, cellular phones, hands-free telephones, conference calls, answering machines, and pagers. You will also learn how to manage communication using these systems.

Telephones

With the array of specialized telephone equipment now available, the dental staff can take advantage of state of the art equipment to become more efficient. For a modest price, dental business owners can buy sophisticated telephone systems that can improve the productivity and profitability of their enterprise. Telephone companies and agencies usually are very accommodating in helping businesses determine their needs for telephone equipment and in making recommendations. Various types of equipment also can be explored at product websites (e.g., www.lucent.com). The equipment and services listed below can be useful in the dental office.

- Integrated business communication systems offer features designed for a small business such as a dental practice. A system such as the one shown in Figure 10-2, *A,* automatically redials the last outside number dialed at the touch of a button; easily establishes a three-way conference call with the conference button; and, on most system phones, allows you to dial and

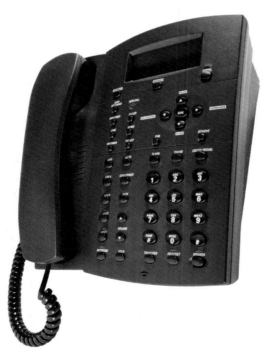

A

Figure 10-2 A, Basic, easy to use telephone systems for small businesses include features such as a built-in speakerphone for convenience and the ability to establish three-way conference calls.

Continued

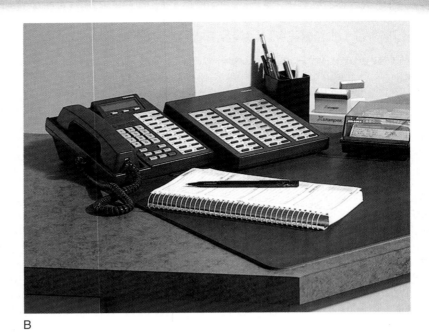

B

Figure 10-2 Cont'd B, A call assistant expands the capacity of a phone system.

talk without picking up the handset. It includes basic transfer and hold functions, as well as programming of multiple numbers to allow speed dialing of frequently called numbers. Information can be displayed in English, French, or Spanish. An expanded version of this system, shown in Figure 10-2, *B*, enables to administrative assistant to expand the capacity of the model with a call assistant. A dentist may feel that only a basic, traditional telephone is required; however, a versatile telephone system with the features described allows more efficient handling of the many telephone calls the office receives daily.

Communications can be improved from one area of the office or clinic to another through the paging and intercom features of this system. With single-button access, the person to be contacted can be reached quickly. Often the individual can answer intercom calls without touching the phone or interrupting work.

- "Plug-In" voicemail systems are fully integrated messaging systems residing on a plug-in circuit board that is used with the Partner Communications system. The voicemail system provides users in larger dental practices or clinics audio instructions on using personal speed dialing, conferencing, or group paging by dialing into the voicemail. It also offers callers a prompt connection to various departments or areas in a clinic and can record messages in the voicemail.
- PC-linked telecommunications systems let businesses manage incoming and outgoing calls, organize personal information, and store patient information (e.g., telephone numbers) in a database file that can be retrieved for autodialing. It also allows programming of phones from a personal computer (Figure 10-3).

With this type of computer-telephone integration, incoming calling information can be used to provide an automatic pop-up window on a personal computer that displays a caller's database file; this allows the administrative assistant to greet the caller by name and have detailed information readily available for answering questions. This system brings the efficiency and productivity of advanced telecommunications technology to small and medium-size businesses.

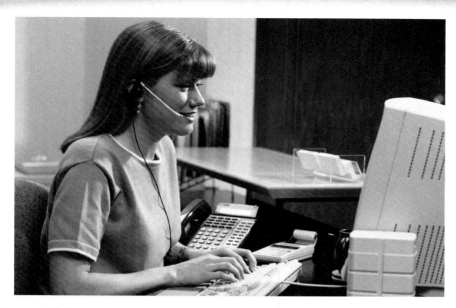

Figure 10-3 Telecommunications system linked to personal computers provide rapid access to patient data.

- Cordless telephone systems provide an extended mobility range in the office (Figure 10-4). This allows staff members to leave the base station and communicate with other areas without having to use answering machines or voicemail or play telephone tag.
- A cellular phone, or *cell phone,* is a portable communication device (Figure 10-5). When a dentist or staff member needs to maintain contact with a central location while driving from one place to another, **cellular technology** makes it possible to use a fully functional telephone. This technology breaks down a large service area into smaller areas, called *cells.*

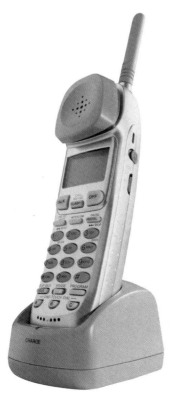

Figure 10-4 Cordless phone systems allow extended mobility in the dental office.

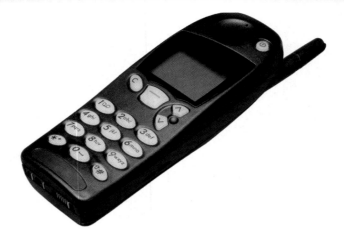

Figure 10-5 Cellular phones allow dentists and staff members to communicate while outside of the dental office. Some advanced cellular models include additional features such as multimedia access or the ability to capture and send or receive digital images.

Each cell is served by a low-powered receiver-transmitter. As the mobile caller moves from one cell to another, a switching office automatically moves the call in corresponding fashion. The mobile telephone switching office communicates with a land-based subscriber to complete mobile calls to fixed locations serviced by telephone lines.

- A still-image phone allows you the transmission of high-quality still images during a telephone discussion. This feature is useful for consultations when the specialist and general practitioner are in different locations. All health-care professionals can enjoy immediate voice and image transmission among all communication channels simply by pushing a button on the telephone to capture an image with a camera. This type of phone uses most industry-standard camcorders, document scanners, electronic cameras, and photo CD players to capture several types of images. Effective patient management requires seeing and discussing. If a patient in a remote area has a lesion that concerns the general practitioner, an image of the lesion can be transmitted to a specialist or dental school for review and examination. The cost of the transmission is the same as for a phone call. The image is free.

- A hands-free telephone allows the administrative assistant to work on the computer, access records, or perform some other task while talking on the telephone. This time-saving device is becoming very popular in clinics and private dental offices. The concept of a hands-free system can be carried into other methods of communication (e.g., pagers and walkie-talkie types of systems), allowing staff members to obtain messages from other areas of the office without using a keyboard or dialing system (Figure 10-6).

SELECTING A TELEPHONE SYSTEM. When a telephone service is selected for an office or when an existing service is changed, consultation with a telecommunications professional from the company responsible for service to the office may be required. Several factors should be considered in the purchase of a telephone system, including cost, flexibility, mobility, and future expansion. Before consulting with a telephone specialist, it is wise to do a task analysis to determine your present and future needs.

Cost generally is the primary factor in selecting a telephone system. The telephone market is cost competitive, but costs can vary considerably. Before selecting a system, examine the specifications carefully to determine the cost of the standard features and the cost of each of the optional features.

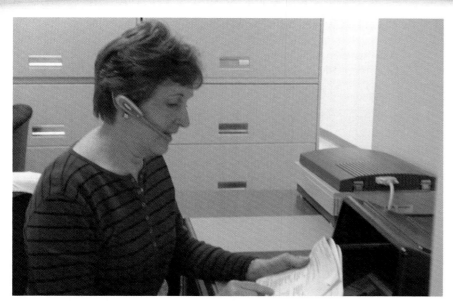

Figure 10-6 A hands-free telephone system allows the administrative assistant to perform other tasks while speaking on the telephone.

Also, be sure to consider the cost of operating and maintaining the system. A reliable system often saves money in future maintenance. In some areas suppliers provide maintenance contracts as insurance for multiple service calls.

Flexibility should also be a major consideration. Expansion or updating of the telephone system must be possible as the practice grows. The ability to move telephones between systems and facilities is also important.

Voice and data switching capabilities are an important consideration. A dental office staff must be sure that a telephone system can meet existing and future needs. For instance, a system equipped with data handling capabilities allows for data transmission and reception between users and equipment, such as computers linked to the system.

TELEPHONE FEATURES. As noted previously, telephones offer a multitude of features, from the very basic to the highly technical. The following sections describe some of the basic features.

Speakerphone. The dentist may find the hands-free speakerphone feature very convenient. With most systems, with just a push of a button the speaker's voice is picked up by a microphone and is heard anywhere in the office. The handset need not be picked up, and the volume of the loudspeaker is adjustable. The speakerphone function can be canceled, even in the middle of a conversation, by picking up the handset. Speakerphones are particularly valuable for group meetings.

Voicemail messaging. Voicemail messaging, or phone mail, uses advanced recording and routing functions to combine the features of a telephone, a computer, and a recording device. This feature can be learned quickly and is simple to use. The only equipment needed is a touch-tone telephone.

Users of **voicemail** can dial their voice mailboxes at any time, regardless of the location. A caller may hear previously recorded messages or may leave a message with such options as replaying the message, erasing it, adding to it, sending it by normal or urgent delivery, switching the call to another line, or having it directly recorded to a voice mailbox. Dental office applications include voice-recorded daily updates of office activities and directions to callers on ways to obtain emergency care.

The dentist usually decides which type of message service meets the particular needs of the practice. Alternatives to voicemail could include an answering machine or answering service. The stand-alone answering machine differs from voicemail in that it does not have the option of sending messages to various locations. However, callers can leave a message and receive information from the office.

An answering service with operator-answered calls can be used when patients call after office hours, on weekends, or on scheduled days off. The answering service operator informs the caller where the dentist can be reached for emergencies or takes the information from the caller and then notifies the dentist. This type of service is frequently used in an oral surgery practice, in which the likelihood of emergencies is greater than in a general practice.

Regardless of whether a voicemail system or a separate automatic answering device is used, some basic courtesies must be observed:

- If an answering machine is used, turn it on before leaving the office.
- In the outgoing message, indicate that the caller has reached an answering system.
- Give clear information about office hours or ways to contact the dentist.
- Make sure the caller has adequate time to record a message.
- Upon returning to the office, check the calls on the voicemail or recorder.
- Take care of any necessary follow-up to the recorded calls. Most systems allow the user to access the answering machine or voice mailbox to receive messages even when off site.
- Update the outgoing messages regularly.
- Avoid nonprofessional messages that are distracting to the caller.

Conference calls. If the dentist needs to talk to several people in various locations simultaneously, a **conference call** may be placed. Such a call is arranged through a conference call operator, who is given the names and telephone numbers of the individuals included in the call and the time the call should be made. With special equipment, several people can hear and participate in the call at each location.

Caller ID. The **caller ID** feature can help identify a caller before the telephone is answered by displaying the number of the telephone from which the person is calling. You may block your number from appearing by pressing a special key.

Call forwarding. A telephone call can be automatically forwarded to another telephone number with **call forwarding**.

Call holding. **Call holding** is frequently used in dental offices, which often receive calls in rapid succession. This feature allows you to answer a second call while the first caller "holds" on the line. Care should be taken to extend maximum courtesy to the caller asked to hold (Box 10-1).

Music on hold. The **music on hold** system provides the caller with music or a short narrative about treatment in the dental office while the person is on hold. The system can be personalized to address specific types of treatment in the office and then revert to music periodically. This feature tends to ease the caller's impatience and can offer short educational clips that may market certain aspects of the practice.

Automatic call back. A caller can give instructions to a busy station to call back as soon as the busy station is free.

Automatic call stacking. Calls that arrive at a busy station are automatically answered by a recorded wait message.

Speed dialing. Commonly called numbers can be stored in the telephone's memory, and the call can be made by keying in a one- or two-digit code. **Speed dialing** cuts down on the time the administrative assistant spends dialing other offices or laboratories that are contacted frequently.

Box 10-1
Using Call Holding

- Excuse yourself from the first caller before answering a second call.
- Greet the second caller with the standard office greeting.
- If the second caller requires only a short response, complete the call and return to the first caller.
- If the second caller appears to need more extensive assistance, explain that you are on another call, ask the caller if he or she can wait, and place the call on hold. If the caller does not want to wait, ask where the person can be reached and say that you will return the call. Always return the call promptly.
- In returning to the first caller, always thank the person for waiting before proceeding with the conversation.

Call timing. This feature is used in professional offices that charge clients by the time spent handling their business on the telephone. It is common in law and accounting firms and other professional offices that bill for consultation on the telephone.

Call restriction. Unauthorized long distance telephone calls can be eliminated with this feature. If an individual is authorized to make a long distance call, the call is given an authorization code that must be keyed into the telephone before the call can be processed. The telephone may also be programmed not to accept long distance calls.

Identified ringing. This feature provides distinctive ringing tones for different categories of calls. For example, internal calls may have one long ring, whereas outside calls may have two short rings.

Liquid crystal display. A **liquid crystal display (LCD)** allows the user to see the number dialed, prompts the user with instructions, and displays the number of minutes the individual remains on the telephone. When used for incoming calls, an LCD also displays the number of the caller.

Multiple lines or key telephones. Multiple lines are a standard feature on most telephones in a dental office. Special care must be taken when using them to ensure privacy and to avoid interfering with other calls in progress.

If multiple lines are available for receiving or placing calls, one of the lines often is for a number that is not listed in the telephone directory or printed on the business stationery; this line should be used for outgoing calls, leaving the other lines available for incoming calls.

A telephone system with multiple lines can be used for both inside and outside calls. This can be a very efficient system, but the administrative assistant must remember several key points, which are presented in Box 10-2.

Box 10-2
Using a Multiple-Line Telephone System

1. Determine which line is to be answered; this usually is indicated by a ring or buzz, and the button flashes until the line is answered. Depress the key to be answered before lifting the receiver.
2. If you are placing an outside call, determine which line is available (indicated by an unlighted button). Depress the key for that line and then dial the number. If you accidentally select a line that has been placed on hold, depress the hold key again to put the call back on hold.

Continued

Box 10-2
Using a Multiple-Line Telephone System—cont'd

3. If you place an incoming call on hold, indicate to the caller that you are doing so. Depress the hold key, which keeps the caller on the line (the hold key then returns to its normal position). The line key remains lighted, which indicates that the line is in use. Other calls then can be placed or received on another line.

4. Before transferring a call, be sure to inform the caller that you are doing so, because the person may not want the call transferred. Give the caller the extension number to which he or she is being transferred in case the call is disconnected. This allows the caller to call the person back directly.

    To transfer an outside call with the button system, you must first place the call on hold. Then push the button for local, which lights when in use (the local button is for in-office transfers only). Dial or buzz a number in the office telephone system; the telephone is answered on local in another office. Inform the dentist of a call on a particular line, and the dentist completes the call from that telephone. If you must return to the incoming line, remember which line your caller used. "Hold reminder" is a feature on advanced telephone systems that gives a reminder tone at various intervals to indicate that a caller is still waiting. Depress that button, which opens the line once more and allows you to complete the call.

Pagers

A **pager** is a telecommunication device that allows a person to receive accurate messages instantly. The pager can receive numeric messages, including phone numbers and special codes you have devised, or alphanumeric messages. Most pagers, such as the one shown in Figure 10-7, are easy to read, have various alert tones, display the date and time, offer various-size message slots, and retain messages in memory.

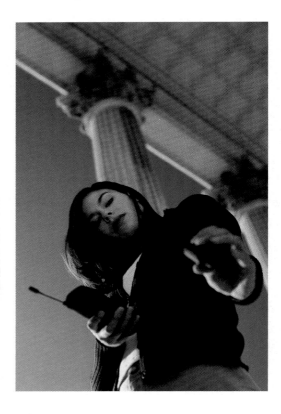

Figure 10-7 A dentist calls the office from a cellular phone after receiving a message from a portable pager.

The BlackBerry, a wireless, handheld personal digital assistant (PDA), allows the user to access mobile communication centers, reply to and forward voicemails, initiate conference calls, and access directories. Also, through Go.Web, users can access e-mail, corporate data, intranets, and the Internet. Such systems allow the dentist to access records and data while traveling or in satellite offices. New technology, such as the BlackBerry, continues to develop, and only the technologists can fathom where this element of the profession may go in the next decade.

Instant Messaging System

The intercom system was discussed in Chapter 6 as a method of interoffice, nonverbal communication by means of a light system. A more comprehensive messaging system can be established through the newest member of the DataTel family, DataTel Lite is an instant messaging program designed specifically for the small office. It provides secure, instant communication within the dental office. The result is a cost-effective, local area network (LAN) messaging program that delivers the benefits of larger, more expensive messaging systems. This system is easy to use and easy to administer and can support networks of up to 50 users.

HOW DOES IT WORK? While the dentist is at chairside, an important telephone call comes in. To let the dentist know who is calling, the administrative assistant uses DataTel (Figure 10-8) to type a message, such as "The patient is ready," and sends it to the dentist in the treatment room. The message instantly pops up on the computer screen in the treatment room. To reply, the dentist simply selects the desired response from the customizable message palette with a click of the mouse or by hitting the corresponding function key. The reply, such as "I'll be right there" or "I'll be just another 5 minutes," now appears on the administrative assistant's screen. This system prevents frantic waving, running back and forth, and cryptic hand signals about what to do with the call. The system is clear, crisp, and professional, and the keyboard and mouse can be protected with a barrier to prevent cross contamination.

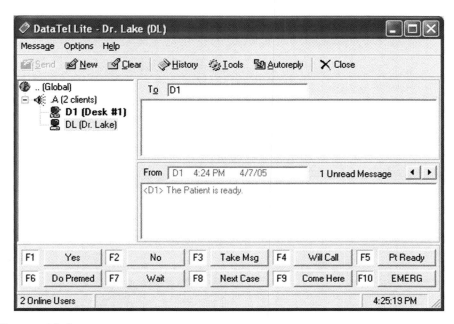

Figure 10-8 The DataTel screen indicates a message from the business office to the treatment room. (Courtesy RB Zack & Associates www.rbza.com.)

FEATURES. The DataTel Lite system has the following features:

- *Instant Messaging:* Unlike e-mail, DataTel Lite is designed to provide secure, instantaneous communication. Messages can be sent to one or more users, one or more groups, or to all on-line users.
- *Security:* Unlike many Internet-based instant messaging services currently available, DataTel Lite operates in the privacy of the dental office's computer network. The result is secure, private, internal communication between the dental staff without the risk of messages being viewed by outside parties.
- *Fast Responses:* A fully customizable 10-button message palette provides for quick, one-touch responses. Fast Responses can be sent with a single click of the mouse or a push of a button.
- *Visual and Audio Notification:* Pop-up windows and sounds are used to notify users of incoming communications. Both of these features can be turned on or off, depending on the user's preference.
- *AutoReply:* The system can be set to send a response automatically to any incoming message. For example, if the dentist, assistant, or hygienist expects to be involved in a procedure for a period of time and therefore unable to respond to messages, the AutoReply message "I cannot respond at this time" can be set, and this reply will be sent back for that person's incoming messages.
- *Message History:* The message history allows the user to view, delete, or print stored messages.
- *Customization:* Fast Responses, AutoReplies, sounds, and other features all can be customized to suit the needs of individual users.

Facsimile (FAX) Communication System

Another electronic means of communication is the **facsimile (FAX) machine** (Figure 10-9). A facsimile transmission machine is a scanning device that transmits an image of a document over standard telephone lines. The machine operates like a photocopy machine that sends an image by wire. At the receiving end, a similar machine receives the transmitted copy. The message may be a handwritten document (in ballpoint pen), a keyboarded page,

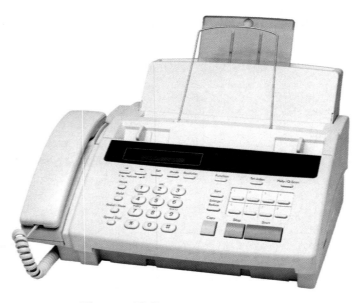

Figure 10-9 Facsimile (FAX) machine.

or a picture. The cost of transmitting a FAX message is the same as a telephone call because the message is transmitted through the telephone lines. Many dental offices prefer to have a dedicated telephone line for the FAX machine rather than using the business telephone number.

A FAX machine can be a stand-alone unit or may be incorporated into the office computer. The cost of the facsimile machine varies greatly, depending on added features.

In case of an emergency or for consultation purposes, the dentist might find FAX telecommunications very useful for transmitting a patient's clinical dental record either locally or out of town. Documents that require signatures can be transmitted via the FAX system, but most legal transactions require the signing parties eventually to sign the original document.

Long Distance Services

Because many businesses or other resources the dentist uses are more global than in the past, the administrative assistant may be responsible for placing long distance calls. Calls to other areas in the United States and abroad are not uncommon. Several types of services are available for long distance calling, including wide area telephone service (WATS), direct distance dialing (DDD), person to person or collect calls, calling cards, and 800/888 service.

WIDE AREA TELEPHONE SERVICE (WATS). In offices where many outgoing long distance calls are made, **wide area telephone service (WATS)** is often used. This service allows the subscriber to make telephone calls from the premises to telephones anywhere within a specified service area at a monthly rate rather than on a per-call basis. The calling area the customer wants determines the monthly charge for the WATS line.

DIRECT DISTANCE DIALING (DDD). With direct distance dialing, long distance numbers in other parts of the United States or in other countries can be dialed on a station to station basis. To use the DDD system, you must dial a 1 plus the area code when you are charging the call to the number from which you are calling and when you are willing to talk to anyone who answers. Therefore, if you were calling a party in St. Louis, Missouri, from Michigan, you would first check the front pages of the telephone directory to determine the area code and then do the following:

Key: 1 + 314 (or 636) + local number

To access a number in a foreign country, you would key the international access code (available from your long distance company) plus the country code, city code, and the local number of the company or person.

PERSON-TO-PERSON OR COLLECT CALLS. Person-to-person calls are more costly than direct-dial calls but in some cases may be necessary. The procedure for making this type of call may vary in certain areas of the country or with various long distance companies. Consult your local telephone directory for specific instructions. In most areas, the call can be made by keying 0, the area code, and the telephone number. If keying is complete, an operator will answer and ask for calling information. You then give the operator the name of the person you are calling.

A collect call, sometimes referred to as *"reversing the charges,"* can be made from a remote location. Again, when placing such a call, consult your local directory. Usually the same procedure as for placing a person-to-person call is followed. After you key the 0, area code, and the number, the operator will respond. You give your name and say that the call is being made collect. The person who answers the call must agree to accept the charges before the conversation can begin.

CALLING CARD CALLS. Many dentists and their administrative assistants now use calling cards. Calling cards allow calls that the person makes while traveling to be charged to the office. The procedure for making a calling card call is similar to that just described for the person to person call. You key 0, the area code, and then the telephone number. When the operator answers and requests your calling card number, you simply key in the number on your card.

800/888 SERVICE. An 800/888 number allows an individual to call a business toll free. Companies that use this service are listed in the telephone directory with an 800/888 number. If you know a company has such a number but it is not available in the local directory, it may be obtained through 800/888 information by keying 1-800-555-1212. As with most information services, a fee may be charged for this service.

Telephone Directories

The telephone directory is a vital tool in the business office. It is important that you look through it and become familiar with the type of information available so that you can use the directory as efficiently as possible. The telephone directory provides selected area codes for many cities in North America and foreign countries, as well as **time zones**. In addition, you may find the following information:
1. A community profile
   • Past and present
   • Community events
   • Things to do and see
   • Parks and recreation
   • Colleges and universities
   • Transportation services
2. Maps
   • Overview of the city
   • Area maps
   • Maps of nearby communities
3. Zip codes
4. Senior citizen information

In general, the front pages of the telephone directory provide important information, such as emergency phone numbers, including the police, fire, ambulance, suicide prevention, and poison control numbers. Page 1 of the front pages has a table of contents. Review this page so that you can quickly find other services listed in the directory.

The white pages of the telephone directory generally are divided into three sections: (1) the residence section, which is an alphabetical listing of the names, addresses, and telephone numbers of individuals; (2) the business white pages, which is an alphabetical listing of the names, addresses, and telephone numbers of businesses; and (3) the blue pages, a section that lists the names, addresses, and telephone numbers of local, state, and federal government offices.

The yellow pages list the names of particular businesses according to the type of service the business provides. For example, assume you are interested in obtaining laundry service for the office, but you are not familiar with companies in your area that provide such service. This category could be broken down as follows:

Laundries
Laundries—Self-service
Laundry—Equipment—Commercial

The companies specializing in each area are listed alphabetically. Because this section is used as a sales tool, it has additional advertisements and a variety of print styles.

DEVELOPING EFFECTIVE TELEPHONE ETIQUETTE

Most people take great care to exude a professional business appearance, but few people take as much pride in developing their telephone image. This is unfortunate if you are an administrative assistant who takes responsibility for telephone calls, because people spend more time listening to you than looking at you.

People often forget when using the telephone that the person on the other end of the line is a human being. Therefore you must take time to develop a professional telephone personality. To be effective on the telephone, you must keep a smile in your voice, answer calls promptly, be attentive and discreet, be cordial and responsive, ask questions tactfully, take messages courteously, speak distinctly, transfer calls carefully, place calls properly, avoid sexism, and be considerate to the caller. The techniques for successful telephone contact, which involves a voice-to-voice relationship, are somewhat different from those of successful personal contact, which involves a face-to-face relationship (Figure 10-10).

> To be effective on the telephone, you must keep a smile in your voice.

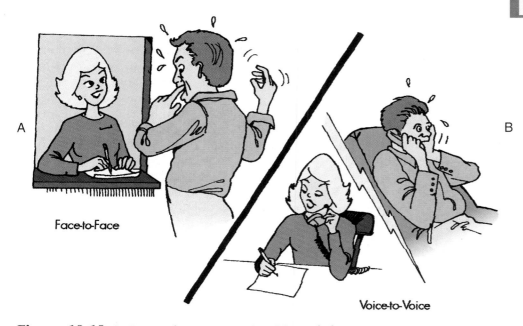

Face-to-Face

Voice-to-Voice

Figure 10-10 A, Face-to-face conversation. Nonverbal cues are apparent; a person smiles or gestures to make a point. Poise, interest, and sincerity provide observable feedback. Facial expressions help indicate the degree of understanding. Discussion is extemporaneous, and notes generally are not used. **B,** Voice-to-voice conversation. The impression of the person is acquired only through hearing. Interpretation comes only from the tone of voice. The degree of understanding is determined by questioning and by rephrasing statements. Notes are advantageous in this situation.

Your Speaking Voice

The speaking voice has four separate but interrelated components: loudness, pitch, rate, and quality.

Loudness refers to the volume of your voice. If you speak too loudly, the listener may be uncomfortable. Have you ever talked on the telephone with someone who spoke so loudly you had to hold the receiver away from your ear? If you have, then you know how unpleasant excessive volume is to the listener. The opposite situation can be equally unpleasant. If you lack confidence, your voice may be so quiet that people will ask you to repeat what you have said. If this happens, you should try to increase both your confidence and your volume.

The *rate* of speaking can determine how well another person understands you. When discussing familiar procedures with a patient, you may tend to speak rapidly, forgetting that this is new material to the patient. There is no ideal rate, but a general rule is to speak at a rate that does not detract from the clarity of your message and is easy and comfortable to listen to for an extended period.

Pitch is the tone of the voice. This is more difficult to change, because once it has been developed, persistent discipline is required to alter it. A low, gravelly voice or a high, squeaky voice may be unpleasant to listen to and are hard on your throat. Many exercises are available from the local telephone company and reference libraries for improving voice pitch.

The *quality* of your voice is a combination of physical and psychological factors. Changes in each of these alter the effectiveness of your speaking voice. Daily experiences affect this quality, and care should be taken to withhold depression, excitement, and anger from your voice when speaking on the dental office telephone.

To achieve a good telephone personality, you should develop the qualities of alertness, expressiveness, interest, naturalness, and distinctness.

A patient calling the dental office expects to have the call answered promptly. You should answer the phone within the first two rings. Everyone enjoys being recognized, and you should be attentive to the patient's identity and express this in your voice. When a patient calling the office identifies himself, the alert assistant replies, "Yes, Mr. Jones, how may I help you?"

Furthermore, when the patient presents a problem, don't stammer and stutter and say, "Yeah, well, uh, I don't know." Such a response indicates to the patient that you are inexperienced. "I will be glad to check your record" or "Let me check with the dentist and call you back within the next hour" is the type of response that indicates you have made a sincere effort to help and lets the patient know you are willing to seek an answer to the problem. Remember, if you promise a patient you will call back, do it at the time you promised. Offer to find an answer if you don't know; don't force the patient to ask you to seek the information.

Nothing is more boring than listening to a person who speaks in a monotone. Put expression into what you say. Add enthusiasm to your voice by using natural voice inflections. To create a smile in your voice, place a mirror in front of the telephone. This ensures that you put a smile on your face before you answer the telephone. Try it . . . it works! Act enthusiastic and you will be enthusiastic.

Patients calling the dental office have a definite purpose and expect you to be interested in their problems. Therefore give the patient your undivided attention. Don't interrupt or become preoccupied with another matter. You can show interest in the patient's problem by asking appropriate questions and by not rushing to terminate the conversation.

> Act enthusiastic and you will be enthusiastic.

> Give the patient your undivided attention.

To be natural, you must be yourself. Don't be a phony. An unnatural voice is easily detected. Keep the breathy "daaarhling," "sweetie," "honey," and "dear" words out of your vocabulary. Remember, "sugar and syrup" have no place in dentistry, so keep them out of your voice.

To speak distinctly, you must pronounce each syllable of the word completely. When using a handheld telephone, speak directly into the transmitter, which should be $\frac{1}{2}$ to 1 inch from your lips. Don't chew gum, bite on a pencil, or cover your mouth with your hand; these all create mumbled conversation and do not present a good image for the dental office. Avoid slang; it is neither businesslike nor in good taste. Some examples of what to say and what not to say include the following:

Avoid	Say
Bye-bye	Goodbye
Huh?	I do not understand.
	Would you please repeat that?
Uh-huh	Yes
	Of course
Yeah	Yes
	Certainly
	I agree
OK	Yes

> To be natural, you must be yourself.

Creating a Good Image

In addition to achieving good voice qualities, you must be able to choose the word or phrase that best communicates the message and makes the best impression. In general, to promote better understanding, you should use short, simple, descriptive words that are appropriate to the situation. When using technical dental terms, names, numbers, formulas, foreign words, or dictated material, the information should be given slowly and distinctly. Suggestions for identifying letters are presented in Box 10-3 and those for identifying numbers in Table 10-1.

A variety of words and phrases in the dental office can convey an unfavorable image to the patient (Figure 10-11). We call these *red flag phrases* and have suggested replacements for them that will create a more positive image (Table 10-2). Each time you speak on the telephone, think about what you're saying and ask yourself if that is what you really mean. Put yourself in the patient's position to decide whether you are communicating connotations that should be avoided.

Box 10-3
Using Words to Identify Letters

The following words might be used to identify letters for a caller:

A as in Alice	J as in Jack	S as in Susan
B as in Boy	K as in King	T as in Thomas
C as in Charles	L as in Lion	U as in Union
D as in Dog	M as in Mary	V as in Victory
E as in Edward	N as in Nancy	W as in William
F as in Frank	O as in Old	X as in X-ray
G as in George	P as in Peter	Y as in Young
H as in Hat	Q as in Queen	Z as in Zero
I as in Ida	R as in Robert	

Table 10-1
Pronouncing Numbers Clearly

Number	Sounds Like	Formation of the Sound
0	Zir-o	Well-sounded Z, short I, rolled R, long O
1	Wun	Strong W and N
2	Too	Strong T and OO
3	Th-r-ee	Single roll of the R, long EE
4	Fo-er	Long O, strong R
5	Fi-iv	I changes from long to short; strong V
6	Siks	Strong S and KS
7	Sev-en	Strong S and V, well-sounded EN
8	Ate	Long A, strong T
9	Ni-en	Strong N, well-sounded EN

> Each time you speak on the telephone, think about what you're saying and ask yourself if that is what you really mean.

Managing Incoming Calls

Although each call to and from the dental office presents a unique situation, most calls can be placed in specific categories and certain conditions will remain constant in each situation. As a result, you will be able to formulate certain questions and answers for each situation. Care should be exercised not to use these statements in a rote manner but to incorporate the ideas into your own words and develop a technique that fulfills the philosophy of the dental office. This is especially important when training new personnel who are unfamiliar with the common situations that may arise on the dental office telephone.

The following are examples of typical conversations that illustrate efficient management of the telephone in a dental office. Some suggestions for managing incoming calls are presented in Box 10-4.

The call: "I would like to make an appointment with the dentist to have my teeth cleaned."

The response: The caller has indicated the nature of the desired treatment, but you need to determine whether this is a new patient. You may ask, "When was the last time you were seen by Dr. Lake?" This indirectly determines whether this is a former patient (not an "old patient," please). If the patient has never seen Dr. Lake, further information should be obtained. First, obtain the person's name by asking, "How do I spell your name?" Then ask who referred the patient, the home and business telephone numbers, the home address, and the approximate date of the last dental treatment. Because the person has never been to the office, you should also ask if the caller knows where the office is located and, if not, give simple, explicit directions. Conclude the call by saying, "Thank you for calling, Mr. Jones. We look forward to meeting you on Thursday, February 8, at 1:30 PM." Wait for the patient to hang up before you do.

The call: An unidentified person calls and states, "I would like to speak to the dentist."

The response: This call may be simply to make an appointment, or it may be a personal call that the dentist wishes to receive. It may be someone the dentist does not know, and the person will not state the reason for the call. It is important that a policy be established by the dentist regarding the types of calls he or she will receive personally. Regardless of the form the call takes, you should follow up the person's initial request to speak to the dentist with, "Dr. Lake is with a patient; how may I help you?" The "how" is important; if you ask simply, "May I help you?" the caller may

> Don't hesitate to ask for the spelling of the caller's name.

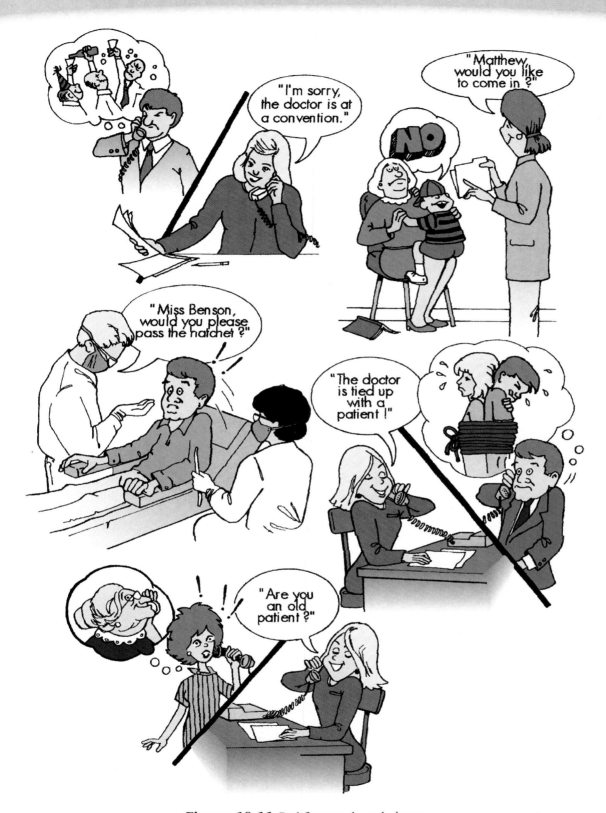

Figure 10-11 Red flag words and phrases.

Table 10-2
Red Flag Phrases

Red Flag Word or Phrase	Use Instead
Work	Dentistry
Plates	Dentures
Cancellation	Change in the schedule
Would you like to come in now?	Dr. Lake is ready to see you, Mrs. Ward
Waiting room	Reception room
Filling	Restoration
My girl	My assistant or hygienist
Thank you for calling (without use of name)	Thank you for calling, Mrs. Main
Cost	Investment
Pull	Remove or extract
Doctor is tied up; I'm sorry, Doctor is busy	Doctor is with a patient
Spit	Empty your mouth
Remind	Confirm
Check-up	Examination
Treatment filling	Treatment dressing
Grind the tooth; drill	Prepare the tooth
Case presentation	Consultation appointment
Rehabilitation	Complete dentistry
Hurt; pain	Uncomfortable
Old patient	Former patient
Operatory	Treatment room
Cost; price; charge	Fee
Bill	Account
Convention	Seminar
Hatchet; chisel	Instrument number
Doctor is running late.	Doctor has had an interruption in the schedule
When would you like to come in?	Do you prefer mornings or afternoons?
Shot	Injection
Joe; Doc; the doctor	Dr. Lake

Box 10-4
Telephone Etiquette for Incoming Calls

- Answer promptly.
- Identify yourself and the office.
- Speak distinctly, clearly, and slowly.
- Avoid slang.
- Listen attentively; do not interrupt.
- Do not talk to anyone else while speaking on the phone.
- Speak directly into the transmitter.
- Excuse yourself if you must attend to another call.
- Thank the caller if the person is asked to hold.
- Let the caller hang up first.

```
┌─────────────────────────────────────────┐
│ TO _____ │
│                                           │
│ DATE _____TIME _____   │
│                                           │
│        WHILE YOU WERE OUT                 │
│                                           │
│ M_____ │
│                                           │
│ of_____ │
│                                           │
│ Phone No._____  │
│ ┌─────────────────┬─────────────────────┐ │
│ │ TELEPHONED      │ PLEASE CALL         │ │
│ │                 │                     │ │
│ │ WAS IN TO SEE YOU│ WILL CALL BACK     │ │
│ │                 │                     │ │
│ │ WANTS TO SEE YOU│                     │ │
│ │                 │   URGENT            │ │
│ │ RETURNED YOUR CALL│                   │ │
│ └─────────────────┴─────────────────────┘ │
│ Message _____  │
│ _____  │
│ _____  │
│ _____  │
│ _____  │
│                                           │
│         Operator _____  │
└─────────────────────────────────────────┘
```

Figure 10-12 Message form. (Courtesy SYCOM, Madison, WI.)

respond, "No, I want to speak to the dentist." Furthermore, if the person refuses to give you his or her name, you may say, "The dentist has requested the name of the person calling so that he (or she) may return your call."

Fortunately, most people are cooperative at the outset of the conversation, and you may record any message on a message form (Figure 10-12) after asking, "May I have your name and phone number?" Don't hesitate to ask for the spelling of the caller's name. Then ask, "Is this call concerning dental treatment?" If so, the assistant should attach the message to the patient's clinical record before giving it to the dentist.

If the call is an emergency that you feel warrants the dentist's immediate attention, a short message may be written and given to him or her in the treatment room. Remember, do not discuss other patients or business in front of the person undergoing treatment.

The call: "Hello, this is Mrs. Harris, and I need to see the dentist today to have him look at a tooth that is bothering me."

The response: This type of call may or may not be an emergency. Therefore it is necessary to ask the patient, "How long has the tooth been bothering you?" "How severe is the discomfort?" "Is the tooth sensitive to extreme hot or cold?" These questions help you to determine whether an emergency exists. If the situation is an emergency, the patient should be seen immediately, during reserved buffer time. The patient should be informed that this appointment will be given to relieve the immediate discomfort and that if further treatment is necessary, you will schedule an additional appointment. (If this is not done, the patient may anticipate having all the treatment completed at the emergency appointment.)

If the existing condition is not an emergency, an appointment may be scheduled on another day in the near future.

The call: "This is Mrs. Frederick. My daughter, Stephanie, just fell off her bicycle and broke her front tooth. It's bleeding; what should I do?" (Caller is frantic.)

The response: Emergencies such as this should be seen immediately. The anxious mother should be told to bring the child into the office immediately. Remain calm and reassure the frantic mother by saying, "Place some cold compresses on the area." You should evaluate the situation further and, if the schedule is filled, call some of the later patients and detain them. Don't tell them you are "running late"; instead, inform them that there has been an unexpected emergency and ask them to come in a half hour later. Patients appreciate your consideration of their time.

The call: An unidentified person calls and asks, "How much does Dr. Lake charge for fillings?"

The response: Generally fees should not be quoted on the telephone. However, fees for basic treatment are often quoted. For major treatment the patient should come to the office for an examination to determine the extent of treatment needed, because diagnosis cannot be done on the telephone, nor can the dentist see the conditions in the patient's mouth. It should be remembered that the patient as a consumer has the right to know the basic fees before treatment, and in complex situations the patient should be given an estimate of fees. These factors must be considered when the dentist establishes a policy on quoting fees.

The call: "This is Mr. Huang, and I just received my statement. I think it is awfully high. You must have made a mistake."

The response: Two possibilities exist here: (1) the patient is right, and there is an error on his statement, and (2) there has been a lack of communication with the patient regarding the fee. Regardless of the reason, don't become defensive on the telephone. This always seems to be our first reaction when someone challenges us. Instead, reply, "I'm sorry, Mr. Huang, perhaps I can clarify the statement for you. What is your specific question?" This focuses on the particular problem. Don't make comments until you thoroughly understand the patient's concern. The patient may state, "I sent a check in the mail on the 28th and you didn't deduct it from the statement." To this you may respond, "Perhaps we didn't receive it before the billing date, Mr. Huang. If you will wait just a moment, I will be glad to get your record and check it for you." Depress the hold button and check the patient's record. In this case, you should check the patient's record, return to the telephone, thank him for waiting, and inform him whether you received the check. If an error has been made, tell the patient it will be corrected and you will send him a corrected statement in the mail immediately.

> Don't become defensive when dealing with callers.

However, if the statement is correct and the patient feels that the fee is too high, you should return the patient's call rather than keeping him on hold. Such calls are often the result of the dentist's failure to inform the patient of the fee before rendering the service. "Inform before you perform" is a rule that saves many hours on the telephone attempting to explain a patient's statement. Also, the patient may have been informed of the original treatment plan but because of a change in the plan, the fee was higher than originally quoted. It is also possible that the patient still does not understand the treatment plan. In any case, this type of problem is difficult to resolve on the telephone and is best managed by asking the patient to come into the office, where you can review the treatment plan once again in person.

Managing Outgoing Calls

As an administrative assistant, you will be placing many outgoing calls. The following tips are helpful for making such calls:

1. Plan ahead. Be sure to have the telephone numbers written correctly. If you are calling a patient, list the name with the telephone number; if you are calling another dentist's office or business, have that number written or easily accessible. Be sure to consult the telephone directory if you are in doubt about a correct telephone number. Names appear in the telephone directory in alphabetical order; however, some public services or governmental agencies may be listed differently. For example, state offices are listed under the state name first, then alphabetically according to office. County and city offices are also listed by county or city name first, then alphabetically according to the office. Federal offices are listed under United States Government first, then alphabetically according to the office. Parochial and other private schools are listed alphabetically by the name of the school.

   Another source for obtaining the correct telephone number for most businesses is the business white pages or yellow pages directory. If you know the name of the business, you can check in the business white pages in alphabetical order. If you do not know the name of a particular dental laboratory but know the location, you can find the number by consulting the yellow pages under "Dental Laboratories."

2. If the telephone you are using is a lighted push-button system, make sure the line is free before you place your call (the light signals when the line is in use). As the telephone receiver is lifted, make sure you hear the dial tone before starting to dial. When using a rotary telephone, use your index finger to dial the number, removing it from the dial opening on the return dial because the return of the dial determines what number you reach. When using a push button phone, press firmly but not too quickly.

3. When your call is answered, identify yourself and the name of the dentist for whom you are calling.

4. State your reason for calling. If you are changing a patient's appointment, have another appointment time available. Indicate why the change is being made, because it may cause a disruption in plans, and the patient may also have to adjust another appointment or work schedule.

5. The person who placed the call should also terminate it. It is discourteous to hang up without an indication that the conversation is finished. End the conversation with a courteous "goodbye" and then replace the receiver gently.

6. If you reach a wrong number, apologize for the inconvenience, verify that you dialed the number correctly, and recheck the number before redialing.
   Examples of common outgoing calls are given below:

> The person who placed the call should also terminate it.

The purpose: Confirmation of a patient's appointment for the following day.

The call: When the patient answers the telephone, identify yourself and state the reason for calling: "Hello, Mrs. Thompson, this is Ms. Benson from Dr. Lake's office." (Do not say, "This is Dr. Lake's office calling." Offices don't make calls—people do!) You may then continue with your message, stating it briefly and completely: "I would like to confirm (not "remind") your appointment for tomorrow at 1:30 PM with Dr. Lake." When the patient acknowledges it affirmatively, you may simply say, "We look forward to seeing you tomorrow at 1:30," and then conclude the call by saying, "Goodbye." Wait for the patient to hang up.

Sometimes patients send up a "trial balloon" and simply state, "I won't be able to keep the appointment tomorrow, and I'll call you later for another one." Although this may be a legitimate statement and the patient does plan to call you at a later date, you should pursue the conversation because it may be a signal that there has been a lack of communication with the patient. Instead of abruptly concluding the conversation, ask the patient, "Would it be possible to reschedule your appointment for a week from today?" If the patient continues to be negative, then asking, "I don't understand, is there something wrong?" will generally bring the patient to the point of explanation.

The purpose: To make plane and hotel reservations for the dentist for a dental meeting out of state.

The call: Before making calls for reservations, obtain information from the dentist about the desired arrival and departure times, type of service, airline preference (if a choice exists), name of the airport (if the city has more than one), name of the hotel, and type of accommodations. Once this preparation is done, you may call the appropriate airline and ask for "Reservations desk, please." Give the person who answers the necessary information: "I would like to make a reservation for Thursday, January 27, for a flight to Los Angeles, California, from Grand Rapids, Michigan, in the morning, returning on Tuesday, February 1, in the afternoon." Once the clerk has informed you of the available times, decide which flights will be agreeable to the dentist, then tell the clerk which ones you prefer. For example, "I would like to make a reservation in the first-class section for the flight leaving Grand Rapids at 8:20 AM and arriving at Los Angeles International Airport at 10:57 AM (California time), and returning on the nonstop flight leaving on Tuesday, February 1, at 3:30 PM and arriving at Grand Rapids at 12:35 AM. The reservation is made in the dentist's name. Obtain all flight numbers and details on where to pick up the tickets, and type a memo for the dentist, as shown in Box 10-5 (which includes the itinerary).

Many hotel reservations can be made through local offices or an 800 number. For instance, because Dr. Lake preferred to stay at an Ocean Inn, his assistant contacted a local Ocean Inn and made the reservation through them. Specific information should be given to the clerk regarding choice of accommodations, such as preference for a smoking or nonsmoking room or single or double occupancy. Once the reservation has been made and an identification number given to you, you should obtain information on the location of the facility. This information is included on the itinerary.

Long distance calls may have to be made when information is needed quickly and there isn't time for an exchange of letters.

The procedure for DDD calls was described earlier. However, several factors should be considered when making this type of call. First, when placing

---

Box 10-5
Travel Arrangements Memorandum

Departure
Leave: Grand Rapids, Thursday, January 27, Spirit Airlines—
   Flight #846—8:20 AM (nonstop)
Arrive: Los Angeles National Airport—10:57 AM
Hotel: Ocean Front Inn 2100 Wilshire Boulevard

Return
Leave: Los Angeles National Airport, Tuesday, February 1,
   Spirit Airlines—Flight #546—3:30 PM (nonstop)
Arrive: Grand Rapids—12:35 AM

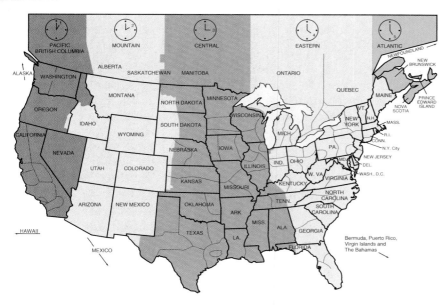

Figure 10-13 Time zones in the United States. (From Young AP: *Kinn's The administrative medical assistant*, ed 5, St. Louis, 2003, WB Saunders.)

a long distance call to different time zones, the time difference must be kept in mind. The United States is divided into four time zones: Eastern, Central, Mountain, and Pacific (Figure 10-13). For example, if it is 2 PM in Grand Rapids, Michigan (Eastern time zone), it is 1 PM in St. Louis, Missouri (Central time zone), 12 PM in Denver (Mountain time zone), and 11 AM in Los Angeles (Pacific time zone).

If you reach an incorrect number when dialing long distance, obtain the name of the city, the state, and the number you have reached and immediately notify the operator of the error so that no charge will be made for the call.

Taking Telephone Messages

Be prepared for incoming calls by keeping a pencil and message pad handy. Obtaining the correct information on messages is of utmost importance. Repeat the message, spelling of names, and the telephone number if the dentist is to return the call. Take sufficient time to obtain the correct information for the message. Be sure to date the message, indicate the time it was taken, and sign it with your name or initials. The message should always be signed by the person taking it in case questions arise later about the information. If the dentist must first find out who took the message, it takes extra time. Forms similar to the one shown in Figure 10-12 may be ordered from most stationery suppliers.

> Be prepared for incoming calls by keeping a pencil and message pad handy.

Personal Telephone Calls

The telephone in the dental office is installed as a service to the dental patients and should be maintained as a business telephone. Consequently, staff members should refrain from using the telephone for personal calls, and only emergency calls should be made.

Telegrams

Although the dentist and staff use letters and the telephone as the primary means of communication, the need to use a telegram may arise, such as to send an urgent message. You should be familiar with telegraph services and know how to prepare a telegram and count chargeable words and characters. One address and one signature are free, and there is no charge for punctuation marks. However, if such words as *stop, period,* or *quote* are used, they are considered chargeable words.

Before calling the Western Union office to relay the telegraph message, compose the message and type a copy of it for the office files. The charge for the telegram is included on the telephone bill. The three basic services are regular telegrams, overnight telegrams, and Mailgrams.

REGULAR TELEGRAM. A regular telegram can be sent at any time, and the message usually is delivered within 2 hours. The minimum rate is based on 15 words, exclusive of address and signature. An extra charge is made for each additional word.

OVERNIGHT TELEGRAM. Overnight telegrams may be sent at any time up to midnight for delivery the next morning. An overnight telegram is less expensive than a regular telegram. The minimum charge is based on 100 words.

MAILGRAM. A Mailgram is a combination of night telegram service and postal service. The message (up to 100 words) is wired to the office of the U.S. Postal Service nearest the recipient. The Mailgram is typed from a wired message, placed in a window Mailgram envelope, and delivered in the first mail delivery of the morning.

LEARNING ACTIVITIES

1. List and briefly explain five qualities of a good telephone service.
2. Explain the management of the following calls:
   a. Mr. Sanchez calls the office and tells you he has broken a tooth and needs to see the dentist right away.
   b. Mrs. Gross calls the office and states that she is new in town. She wants to make an appointment for her son, Jim, who needs to have his teeth cleaned.
   c. Mr. Hubbard calls and states that his daughter was just hit in the mouth with a softball bat and has some broken teeth. He asks, "What do I need to do?"
3. Replace the following statements with a statement that would create a better image.
   a. "I'm sorry, the dentist is tied up with a patient."
   b. "Johnny, would you like to come in now?"
   c. "Jennifer, this shot won't hurt much."
   d. "Doc, do you want the hatchet or chisel?"
   e. "I'm sorry, the dentist is running late."
4. Complete a message form using the following telephone conversation:
   Mr. Schultz from Pine Mutual Insurance Company calls the office and wants you to tell the dentist he will meet her at the Yacht Club at 4:30 PM today. If this isn't agreeable, Mr. Schultz can be reached at 495.8272.
5. List and briefly define four telephone systems or services available for use in a dental office.

Continued

LEARNING ACTIVITIES—cont'd

6. List and briefly describe various types of information that can be found in a telephone directory.
7. Locate telephone numbers for each of the following. Keyboard the names and telephone numbers in tabular format on a Rolodex-type form provided in the classroom or the office of employment.
   a. Internal Revenue Service
   b. Police Department
   c. U.S. Post Office
   d. State employment commission
8. Using the Yellow Pages, locate one company and telephone number for each of the following. Type the information on a Rolodex form provided in the classroom or the office of employment.
   a. Dental supply company
   b. Dental laboratory
   c. Computer repair service
   d. Pharmacy
9. You receive the following calls. Use telephone message forms to write down the appropriate message. Complete the information about each call and sign your name.
   a. Dr. Lake's wife calls at 10:30 AM and asks you to remind him he is to stop at Great Lake's Bank to pick up the mortgage forms on his way home today.
   b. Mr. Horace Schramm calls at 10:10 AM and reminds Dr. Lake that a special meeting of the Administration Council has been scheduled for 4 PM tomorrow.
   c. Mr. Daniel Rogers calls at 10:40 AM and wants to discuss the sale of some property. He will be leaving the office at noon and won't return until after 3 PM today. His number is 271.3364.
   d. Mrs. Tod Rae calls at 11 AM, upset about her account. She insists on talking to the dentist before he goes to lunch. She refuses to discuss the matter with you. Her phone number is 377.4721.
10. The dentist asks you to arrange her trip to the national meeting of the American Dental Association in San Francisco. She wants to travel by the most economical fare. She needs to arrive by noon on July 18 and must return home by early evening on July 23. In a narrative form, explain what you would do and type an itinerary for the trip.

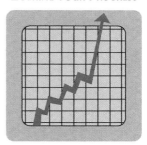

EXAMINE YOUR PROGRESS

Practice by completing Working Form 6.

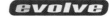

Key Terms

Call forwarding   A telephonic feature that automatically relays a call to another telephone number.

Call holding   A feature of many telephone systems that allows a second call to be answered while the first caller "holds" on the line.

Caller ID   A display that shows the number assigned to the telephone from which the person is calling.

Cellular technology   A mobile telephone system that breaks down a large service area into smaller areas, called cells. Each cell is served by a low-powered receiver-transmitter. As the caller moves from one cell to another, a switching office automatically moves the call in a corresponding fashion.

Conference call   A telephone call in which several people participate, often from a number of different locations. The call is arranged through a conference call operator, who is given the names and telephone numbers of the individuals to be included in the call and the time the call is to be made.

Facsimile (FAX) machine A facsimile transmission machine, which is a scanning device that transmits an image of a document over standard telephone lines.

Liquid crystal display (LCD) A device that allows the user to see the number dialed, prompts the user with instructions, and displays the number of minutes the individual remains on the telephone.

Multimedia messaging service (MMS) A system that provides several options for receiving messages, including text, visual, or voice mode.

Pager A telecommunication device that allows a person to receive accurate messages instantly or that alerts the person to return a call.

Speed dialing A feature that allows commonly called numbers to be stored in the telephone system's memory and subsequently dialed by keying in a one- or two-digit code.

Telecommunications The science and technology of communication by electronic transmission of impulses, as by telegraphy, cable, telephone, radio, or television.

Time zones Geographic regions in which the same standard time is used. The United States is divided into four time zones: Eastern, Central, Mountain, and Pacific.

Voicemail A telephone system that connects callers directly to an extension or a department and can record messages for that person or department.

Wide area telephone service (WATS) A telephone service that enables the subscriber to make calls from the premises to telephones anywhere within a specified service area at a monthly rate rather than on a per-call basis.

Bibliography

Fulton PJ: *General office procedures for colleges*, ed 12, Cincinnati, 2003, South-Western.
Rader MH, Kurth LA: *Business communication*, ed 2, Cincinnati, 1994, South-Western.
Roth M: Telephone on-hold-message-and-music systems, *Mich Med*, April 1993.

Recommended Website

www.dentamanagementu.com

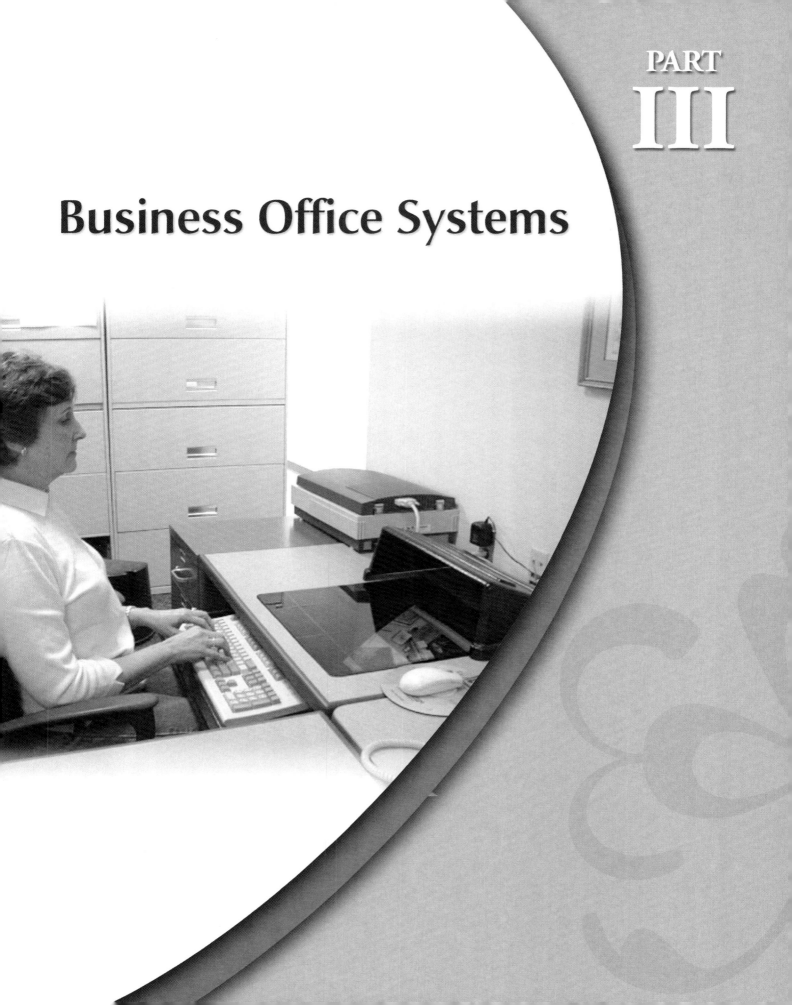

Business Office Systems

PART III

Appointment Management Systems

Chapter Outline

Learning Outcomes

Mastery of the content in this chapter will enable the reader to:
- Define glossary terms
- Describe appointment book styles
- Describe appointment software options

- Complete an appointment matrix
- Identify solutions to common appointment scheduling problems
- Make an appointment entry
- Design an appointment schedule list
- Identify common appointment book symbols
- Describe the use of a treatment plan
- Complete an appointment card
- Complete a daily schedule
- Describe a call list
- Explain advanced-function appointment scheduling

The appointment management system can take the form of a traditional **appointment book**, or software installed in the office computer can be used. Appointment management on the computer has been one of the last holdouts for many dentists. Some think that electronic appointment scheduling is time-consuming and makes checking future schedules difficult. This is not true. Box 11-1 lists the advantages of an electronic appointment book. The traditional appointment book is discussed in this text because it is still used by some practitioners.

The appointment system, which contains lists of all the scheduled patients and events for the dentist and staff, is the control center of the office and an important factor in the success or failure of a dental practice. The practice should be controlled through the appointment system, not by it. Whether an appointment book or an electronic system is used, poor management of appointments can result in mounting tension among staff members and can turn the reception room into a waiting room of discontented patients. Basic scheduling concepts (Box 11-2) are the same regardless of the type of system used. Only the process of data entry differs.

The staff of a dental office should analyze the practice and determine an organized system of appointment control that (1) maximizes productivity, (2) reduces staff tension, and (3) maintains concern for the patients' needs.

Because some dentists still feel strongly about having a hard copy of the appointment book to look at, both the electronic and traditional systems are addressed in this chapter. The concepts presented can be used either in an electronic or a manual system because they are the same for both.

> The practice should be controlled through the appointment system, not by it.

Box 11-1

Advantages of an Electronic Appointment System

- Treatment rooms can be color coded.
- Production goals can aid appointment scheduling.
- Production data are visible daily.
- Data entries are easier to read.
- Autoscheduling eliminates paging through the book.
- Various screen viewing modes are available.
- Cross-reference saves time and motion.
- Patient data are more likely to be accurate.
- Searching for appropriate appointment openings is easier.
- Procedures can be posted to several different records from one entry.
- Patient follow-up is easier.
- No manual record filing is necessary.

> **Box 11-2**
> **Tips for Efficient Appointment Management**
>
> 1. Put one person in charge of the appointment system.
> 2. In a traditional appointment book, make accurate, neat entries.
> 3. Accommodate the patient as much as possible but maintain control of the appointment schedule.
> 4. Avoid scheduling repetitive procedures over long periods.
> 5. Be aware of production goal criteria.
> 6. Be aware of scheduling in "power blocks."
> 7. Schedule the workload according to the staff member's body clock.
> 8. Assign clinical tasks only to legally qualified personnel.
> 9. Avoid leaving large blocks of time between appointments.
> 10. Establish guidelines for problem situations.
> 11. Make sure the practice is controlled through the appointment system, not by it.

SELECTION OF A TRADITIONAL APPOINTMENT BOOK

When an appointment book is used, the size and design of the book are determined by the needs of the dental practice. The administrative assistant should review the available styles to determine what is best for the office. Time and motion studies have indicated that the most efficient format for an appointment book is the week-at-a-glance style, in which all days of the week can be seen at one time; this allows the assistant to note openings in the schedule quickly (Figure 11-1).

The binding on the appointment book may have three to nine rings or may be spiral. Spiral-bound books appear to withstand a greater amount of use. The books may be printed with or without dates and may have one or more columns (Figure 11-2).

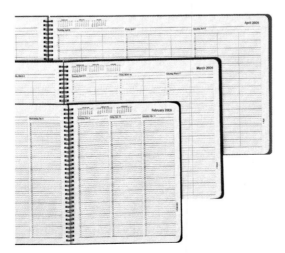

Figure 11-1 Week-at-a-glance appointment book in various sizes. (Courtesy SYCOM, Madison, WI.)

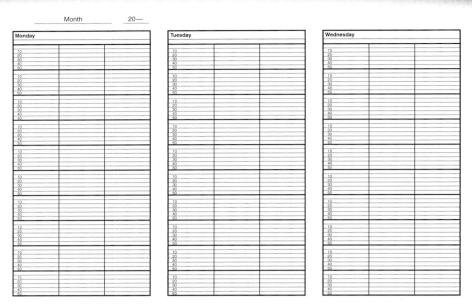

Figure 11-2 Undated multiple-column appointment book. (Courtesy SYCOM, Madison, WI.)

The individual days are divided into time increments. Some books provide 30-minute increments, others 10- or 15-minute increments. The smallest time increment is referred to as a **unit (u)**. The 15-minute unit has been widely used in dentistry with much success; the 10-minute unit has become generally accepted in advanced-function practices.

OPTIONS FOR THE ELECTRONIC APPOINTMENT BOOK

With the electronic appointment system, appointments can be entered, canceled, rescheduled, and moved easily with one keystroke. The benefits of the electronic system (see Box 11-1) set it apart from the traditional system. Electronic scheduling can be goal oriented, using state of the art technology to set production goals for the practice. With income a consideration, rather than just filling the book, the dentist can begin to maximize profits while controlling where and when certain procedures are performed.

Common electronic software scheduling packages generally have a number of components.

- *Goal scheduler:* This component takes into consideration fixed and variable overhead and the dentist's preset goals for the year. In this system a goal builder window indicates last year's goal and actual production for the same period last year. It then indicates this year's status.

- *Autoscheduler:* This feature allows the assistant to find an opening in a matter of seconds and even to post procedures right from the appointment card to the transaction file. Information can be viewed in several different formats. The daily appointment screen with a find window allows the assistant to find a date and time for a patient with minimal keystrokes.

- *Daily appointment screen:* Most systems allow the assistant to color code rooms. The daily appointment screen has two viewing modes. The regular view generally shows the treatment rooms in a column format with the patient's name, treatment information, and the resources needed for each time unit. The expanded view (Figure 11-3) shows details for a single treatment room and the procedural information for several others. The find option

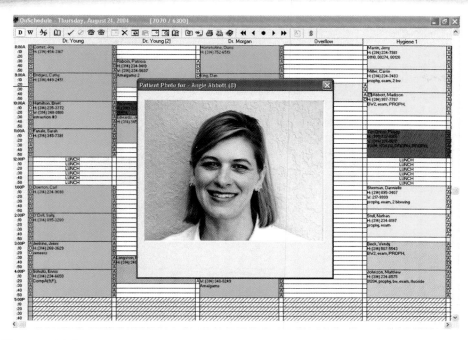

Figure 11-3 Daily appointment screen (expanded view). (Courtesy Patterson EagleSoft, Effingham, IL.)

brings up a calendar and lets the assistant go directly to any specified day or zoom out to the weekly or monthly screen (Figure 11-4).

• *Patient record:* The patient information screen (Figure 11-5) in most systems can be divided into different categories such as demographical, financial, insurance, recall, and appointments. Patient information that can be entered on this record includes the patient's complete name, marital status, gender,

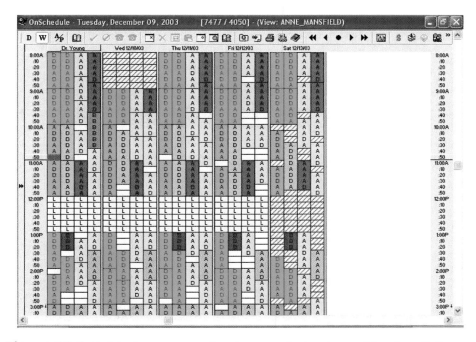

Figure 11-4 Quick-glance screen showing a week at a glance. (Courtesy Patterson EagleSoft, Effingham, IL.)

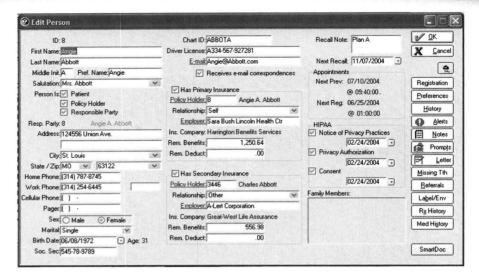

Figure 11-5 Patient information screen. (Courtesy Patterson EagleSoft, Effingham, IL.)

age, date of birth, Social Security number, work and home phone numbers, current balance, referrals, medical alerts, treatment completed, and appointment time preferences. Other information can be stored in other dialog boxes, such as pharmacy information and medication history, the patient's examination history, the treatment plan, or the account screen.

- *Goal screen.* The automated system provides a variety of analyses for the practice. The one shown in Figure 11-6 indicates the scheduled load versus the goals for the day.

DESIGNING THE APPOINTMENT BOOK MATRIX

An **appointment book matrix**, or outline of the appointment book, functions like the matrix of an amalgam restoration; it provides support. It is the framework around which appointments are made. A matrix should be completed before a new appointment book or electronic system is used. It should include the following elements.

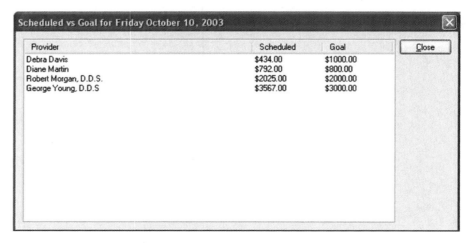

Figure 11-6 Schedule versus goals screen. (Courtesy Patterson EagleSoft, Effingham, IL.)

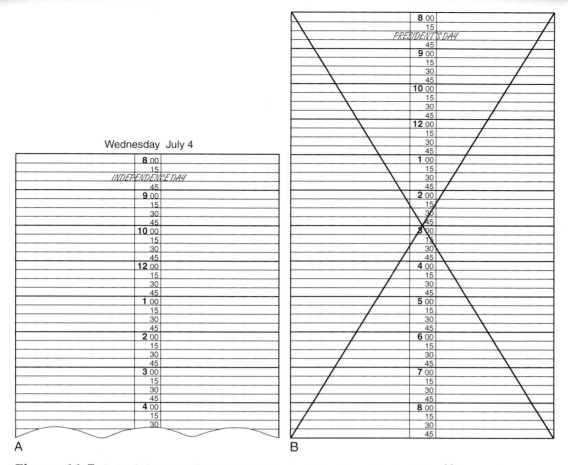

Figure 11-7 A, Holiday page from a traditional appointment book. **B,** An X drawn through a page from an appointment book to indicate a holiday or office closure.

- *Holidays.* In many traditional books, holidays are noted by the manufacturer (Figure 11-7, *A*). However, you may find it necessary to enter special holidays observed in your locale or office. This can be done by placing an X across the entire day and marking it with the name of the holiday (Figure 11-7, *B*).
- *Lunch hours.* Lines may be used to cross out lunch hours. However, a broad, yellow felt-tip marker accomplishes the same task and can be written over legibly (Figure 11-8). After you become experienced with the appointment book, it will be unnecessary to mark off these hours.
- *Buffer periods.* A **buffer period** is a small amount of time set aside to absorb the hectic workload of the day or to allow for emergencies. A 1-unit increment of time set aside in the morning and again in the afternoon

Figure 11-8 Lunch hour highlighted in a traditional appointment book with a felt-tip marker.

Tuesday, April 24

8	
15	
30	
45	
9	
15	
30	
45	
10	
15	
30	
45	
11	
15	
30	
45 JOHN FLETCHER FR #8	
12	
15	
30	
45	
1	
15	
30	
45	
2	
15	
30	
45	
3	
15	
30	

Figure 11-9 One-unit buffer highlighted in a traditional appointment book with a felt-tip marker.

allows time for unexpected emergencies or buffers an already hectic day. If this space is simply colored in with a yellow felt-tip pen, an entry can be made without erasing (Figure 11-9). The buffer period should not be inserted during the busiest periods of the day.

- *School calendar.* In some areas of the country the local dental society provides stick-on labels showing the local scheduled school closings and holidays (Figure 11-10). A school calendar may also be obtained from the local school system. Students and faculty members can then be scheduled for appointments when they are on vacation.
- *Professional meetings.* Some dental societies provide stickers for these dates; otherwise, a notation about the location and nature of the meeting can be made on the appropriate date, with an X blocking out the specified time (Figure 11-11).
- *Staff meetings.* Time should be set aside regularly, once or twice a month, for all members of the staff to meet and discuss goals for the office. This time should not be scheduled during the lunch period or after office hours but should be integrated into regular office hours (see Chapter 2 for suggestions on scheduling staff meetings).

IMPORTANT FACTORS IN SCHEDULING APPOINTMENTS

The administrative assistant must deal with a variety of situations in scheduling appointments. Management of the appointment book requires a

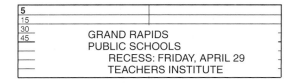

Figure 11-10 Label indicating school closing.

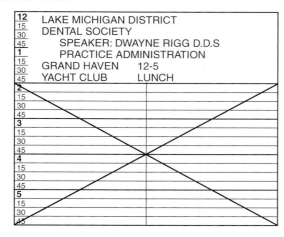

12	LAKE MICHIGAN DISTRICT
15	DENTAL SOCIETY
30	SPEAKER: DWAYNE RIGG D.D.S
45	PRACTICE ADMINISTRATION
1	
15	GRAND HAVEN 12-5
30	YACHT CLUB LUNCH

Figure 11-11 Label indicating meeting with an X.

well-defined treatment plan, an established appointment sequence, and an ability to maintain strict control over the appointment book while still meeting the needs of patients.

Several of these situations are common to all dental offices. For an assistant with several years of experience, managing such problems is fairly easy, but it may be more difficult for the inexperienced individual. The office staff should identify situations that commonly occur and develop a policy for managing appointments for these situations.

Emergency Patients

Patients who call the office for emergencies should be seen by the dentist during designated buffer periods. When a patient calls and requests an immediate appointment for a toothache, you must be alert to ask the patient the following questions: "How long has the tooth been bothering you?" "Which tooth is it?" "What type of discomfort are you experiencing—a sharp pain or a dull ache?" "Is it sensitive to hot, cold, or pressure?" At this point, determine whether it is a true emergency. It is prudent then to say, "The dentist's schedule is filled for the day, but Dr. Lake could see you to relieve the discomfort at 10:30 this morning. Then, if further treatment is necessary, we can schedule an additional appointment." This eliminates any preconceived idea that the dentist's schedule permits time for extensive treatment that has not been scheduled. If the patient finds it difficult to come in at the suggested time, it may be necessary to schedule the appointment at a later date.

A dentist should always be prepared to see patients of record for emergencies or to make provision for such coverage in his or her absence. Emergency treatment for new patients can become a lifeline for a dental practice. These patients often become excellent patients in the future. They appreciate being seen by the dentist on an emergency basis and often accept treatment plans willingly to avoid future emergencies.

Young Children

Young children should be scheduled at times that will not interfere with their nap periods or regularly scheduled activity times. For these reasons, early morning generally is considered a good time for young children's dental appointments. Have you ever encountered a cross child just before naptime, or have you ever had to call a child in from play to go to the dentist? Ask the mother about the child's daily routine and be considerate in your appointment scheduling.

Older Adults

Older patients often require special attention. Some, although they arise early, find rush hour traffic very disconcerting, whereas others find it difficult to rush about in the morning. Although many older patients need special consideration, remember not to embarrass them by calling attention to their age.

DENTIST'S BIOLOGICAL CLOCK

Difficult cases, such as crown and bridge work, are best scheduled at a time when the dentist is in a peak energy period. Not all people are at their best at all times of the day. Early morning generally has been considered the best time for extensive treatment. However, some dentists do not reach their peak period until 1 or 2 PM, when the early birds who were dynamic at 8 AM have begun to lose energy. This becomes an important factor in determining when certain types of treatment should be scheduled. As a rule, appointments for extensive operative and surgical treatment and management of difficult children should be made at the dentist's peak time.

Scheduling for Productivity

As mentioned earlier in this text, dentistry is a business, and one of the most effective ways to be profitable is to increase productivity. The dentist should focus on procedures that are most profitable while performing the routine tasks or delegating when at all legally possible. According to Theodore Schumann,[1] the typical practitioner in 2005 will produce about $300 to $500 per hour. It is not uncommon to produce even less than this if the scheduling system is not managed effectively. Over the year, if the dentist increased production by just $50 per hour, annual production could increase by $76,000, of which about $60,000 would be additional profit.

This is where the administrative assistant needs to "think outside the box" and modify the old ways of scheduling. To achieve this increased productivity, hourly production must increase. With this concept, considered in conjunction with the dentist's body clock, you can begin to modify the way scheduling is done. If "power blocks" of time are set aside for high productivity/high profit procedures, production will increase. Therefore, if the dentist's body clock is best from 10 AM to 2 PM, all high productivity procedures must be scheduled during that period and *no* other types of treatment. This time must be reserved for productive, profitable procedures, and all attempts to break into the "power blocks" must be forestalled. It takes time to make this system work, and it requires a different mind set at first, but after 6 months you will find this concept very effective, and the practice will begin to reap the profits.

Extended Office Hours

Many offices develop a schedule that includes extended office hours, which are hours beyond the traditional workday. These may include early morning, evening time, or weekend days. There is no significant difference in scheduling appointments for this type of practice, but it requires special attention in the selection of an appointment book and in designing the matrix. Care should be taken that the days identified for extended hours include times to cover all the hours the office will be open. This situation may require an unmarked appointment book that allows you to insert the days and times in accordance with the office schedule.

Management of Prime Time

Prime time is the time period most often requested by patients; in most offices it generally is the time after 3 PM. Obviously not all who request this time will receive it, therefore patients must be informed of the need to schedule this time on a rotating basis. Forms are available for students requesting that the patient be excused during class time (Figure 11-12).

Habitually Late Patients

A small number of patients persist in being late for their appointments. You should stress the importance of being on time for the appointment by explaining, "Mr. Campbell, the nature of your treatment requires all the time allotted, therefore we must ask your cooperation in being on time for your appointments." This should be done in a firm but pleasant manner. Another way of handling this situation is to enter an earlier time on the appointment card than is entered in the appointment book. But be careful; this could backfire!

Series Appointments

Care should be taken not to schedule too many appointments for a patient at one time. The patient who has a long series of appointments is likely to cancel more readily, thinking the appointment can be made up next week, when in reality the appointments may not be of the same length. This disrupts the treatment schedule. Make tentative appointments beyond 2 to 3 weeks, but do not list them on the appointment card until the patient has completed the first series.

Patient Who Arrives on the Wrong Day

No office would be complete without a patient who arrives on the wrong day or at the wrong time. The error may be the patient's, or the assistant may have written the wrong date on the appointment card. You should ask to see the appointment card and, if the patient has made the mistake, indicate the actual date and time of the appointment. Of course, if you or another staff member made the error, an apology is necessary and the patient should be seen by the dentist. You may be able to contact the scheduled patients,

JOSEPH W. LAKE, DDS-ASHLEY M. LAKE, DDS
611 Main Street, S.E. - Grand Rapids, MI 49502
616 - 101-9575

Date ____________

This is to certify that ______________________________

(has/had) an appointment at this office for professional attention on

date ____________________ at ______________ o'clock

Please excuse this absence.

Dr. ______________________

Figure 11-12 School excuse. (Courtesy SYCOM, Madison, WI.)

explain that an "unexpected change has occurred in the schedule," and delay their arrival. Regardless of who is responsible for the error, the assistant should remain tactful and helpful in correcting the mistake.

Drop-Ins

Nothing is more frustrating than to have a patient drop by the office and say, "I was just in the area and thought I'd drop in and see if Doc could do something to this tooth that's been bothering me" (probably for 6 months). Seeing a patient on this basis opens Pandora's box! Tactfully inform the patient that the dentist sees patients by appointment only and tell the person when the next appointment is available. If the drop-in patient has a legitimate emergency, try to accommodate the person.

This practice does not apply to the many walk-in (convenience) dental clinics established in the past few years. One of the prime objectives of these clinics is to accommodate patients without appointments.

Broken Appointments

At times a patient absolutely must cancel an appointment or is prevented from keeping the appointment by some unforeseen circumstance. Most patients respect the dentist's time, and the dentist should be understanding when a cancellation occurs. Other patients, unfortunately, seem always to find an excuse for breaking an appointment. Although most dentists' initial reaction is to charge for broken appointments, this becomes difficult to accomplish and results in poor public relations. Therefore the patient should be informed of the importance of keeping the appointment; for example, "Mr. Ward, since you failed to keep your 2-hour appointment, the treatment schedule has been delayed." You also should tactfully explain, "I can only reschedule such a lengthy appointment if we can be assured you will be here." Such cancellations should be noted on the patient's clinical chart (Figure 11-13).

If the patient continues to cancel appointments, he should be told, "Mr. Ward, we are unable to continue to make appointments for you because you have failed to cooperate with us." However, such a policy should be exercised only after it has been approved by the dentist.

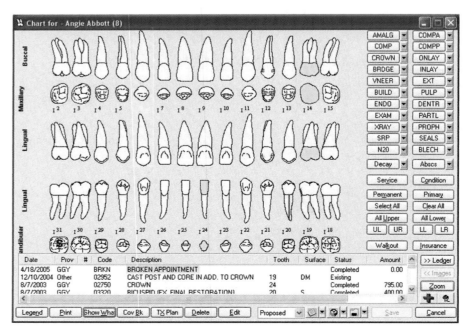

Figure 11-13 Clinical chart showing a broken appointment.

Figure 11-14 Dovetailing on an appointment page in a traditional appointment book.

Dovetailing

Minor types of treatment can easily be accomplished in less than 1 unit. **Dovetailing** means working a second patient into the schedule during another scheduled patient's treatment, for example, while the first patient waits for an anesthetic to take effect or an impression to set. The appointment page shown in Figure 11-14 has four places for dovetailing: at 8 AM, while waiting for anesthesia with Hazel Gates; at approximately 8:30 AM, while waiting for the final impression to set; at 8:45 AM, while waiting for anesthesia for John Monroe; and at 9 AM while waiting for John Monroe's final impression to set.

Many types of appointments can be dovetailed, such as denture adjustments, suture removal, healing check, amalgam polishing, or dressing changes. In an expanded-duties practice, many of these procedures are done by a dental auxiliary and must be dovetailed into the auxiliary's schedule.

Establishing an Appointment Time

To prevent conflicts with patients over appointment times, the assistant should avoid loaded questions. Don't ask, "What is the most convenient time for you?" "What is your day off?" or "When does Frank get out of school?" It is wiser to ask, "Is morning or afternoon better for you?" and then present two choices for the patient. You will lead the patient into making a choice realistically within your schedule, and you will not be forced to say "I'm sorry" to each of the patient's suggestions.

ENTERING APPOINTMENTS

One person should be in charge of the appointment system at all times. The dentist should never encourage friends or relatives to "drop by the office," but rather should direct everyone to contact the administrative assistant for an appointment.

An entry in the appointment book must be made in pencil. It must be accurate, complete, and legible and include the information shown in Box 11-3.

Box 11-3
Information to Include in an Appointment Book Entry

- Patient's full name, with cross-reference in case of duplication of names
- Home and business phone numbers to confirm the appointment or to reach the patient in case of an emergency
- Treatment to be done
- Age of patient (if a child)
- Length of the appointment, indicated with an arrow
- Special notations (e.g., new patient, premedication required, case at the laboratory)

Table 11-1
Symbols for Traditional Appointment Book Entries

Symbol	Meaning
N	New patient
*	Patient prefers an earlier appointment.
B	Business phone number
H	Home phone number
L	Case at the laboratory
Ⓛ	Case returned from the laboratory
PM	Premedicate (i.e., medicate before treatment)
÷	In red, denotes confirmed appointment
↓	Length of appointment

Because of the limited amount of space available for each entry, symbols must be used to make special notations about a patient. Table 11-1 lists several symbols commonly used in the appointment book. In the example in Figure 11-15, note that the two entries in the appointment book have been made using these symbols. Each entry was made in pencil and is accurate, complete, and legible. Here the assistant has used the special clinical codes used in Dr. Lake's office to indicate the treatment to be done. It is important to list the complete treatment, because this tells the assistant exactly what is to be done; also, the assistant can easily transfer this information to an appointment list later without referring to the clinical charts, thus saving time.

When appointments are made, the sequence normally followed in a dental office is initial examination and prophylaxis, radiographs, and diagnostic models (Figure 11-16). After the dentist has concluded the diagnosis and treatment plan, the patient returns for a consultation appointment. At this time, the patient accepts the original or modified treatment plan, and the assistant makes the necessary appointments.

Once treatment is complete, the patient is recalled periodically through the preventive recall system outlined in Chapter 12. An appointment sequence must be established, as mentioned previously, in coordination with the treatment plan. To do this, ask the dentist to establish the sequence and the amount of time needed for each appointment for all types of treatment. In a manual system, this list can be keyed and placed in a celluloid protective

10		
15		
30		
45		
11	MR. MARK RUSSELL	
15	SEAT #18 F.C. Ⓛ	
30	H-455-2466 B-459-2102 ↓	
45		
12		
15		
30		
45		
1		
15		
30	MARGARET UDELL (MICHEAL)	
45	GING, LRQ PM	
2	H-454-2370	
15		
30		
45		

Figure 11-15 Two appointment book entries using symbols in a traditional appointment book.

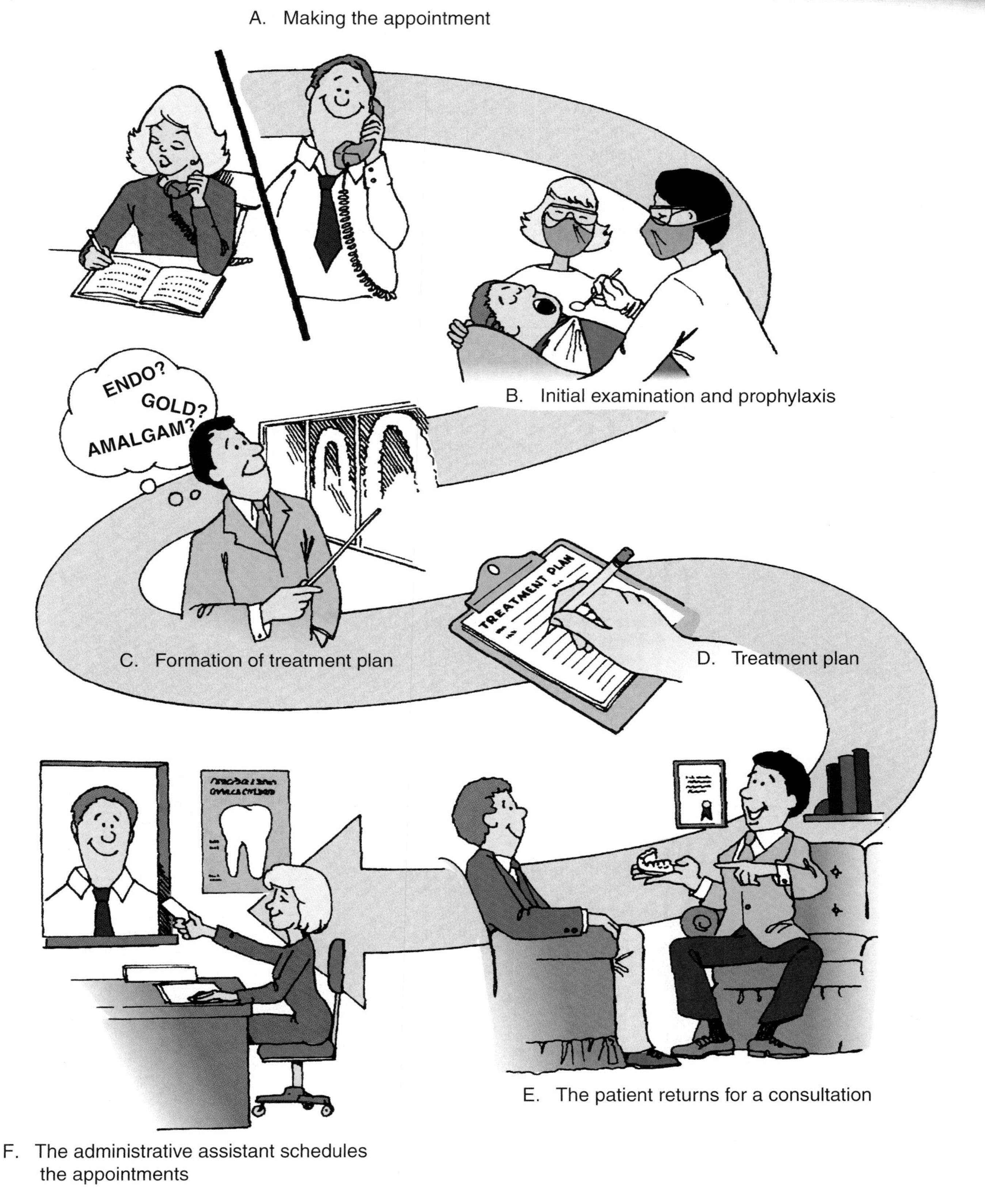

Figure 11-16 **A** to **F**, Appointment sequence.

cover for easy access. In an electronic system, the information is entered when the system is set up, and the appointment time is entered automatically. Table 11-2 shows a sample **appointment schedule list**. After a schedule for the office has been designed, you can stop guessing how much time is needed for each type of appointment. In a computer system, you can program the amount of time needed according to the type of treatment and thus eliminate any guessing.

Table 11-2
Appointment Schedule List

Treatment	Time Needed
Composite/Amalgam	
1 surface	1 u*
2 surfaces	2 u
3 surfaces	3 u
4 surfaces	4 u
5 surfaces	5 u
6 surfaces	6 u
Bonding	
1 tooth	2 u
2 teeth	3 u
3 teeth	4 u
Denture Construction	
Initial impression	2 u
Final impression—2-3 days later	3 u
Bite relationship—3-4 days later	3 u
Try in—4-5 days later	3 u
Insertion	
(If no changes in setup: 1 week later)	
Nonimmediate	2 u
Immediate if surgery done out of office	2 u
Immediate if surgery done in office	6 u
Denture check	1 u
Denture—Partial	
Consult with dentist for schedule.	

Denture Adjustment	Dovetail	
Endodontics	**Single Root**	**Multiple Root**
Single appointment	3 u	4 u
Multiple appointment treatment		
1st—Opening—filling	2 u	3 u
2nd—Open and remedicate	1 u	1 u
3rd—Final Point—sealing	1 u	3 u
Minimum of 48 hours between		
2nd and 3rd appts.		

Extractions	
"Uncomplicated" single	2 u
2 or 3 "uncomplicated" extractions	3 u
Quadrant	4 u
Removal of sutures	Dovetail

Continued

Table 11-2
Appointment Schedule List—cont'd

Treatment	Time Needed
Periodontal Treatment	
Quadrant	3 u
If surgical dressing placed—1 u 1 week later	
Cast Metal Restorations	
1-2 surface inlay	Prep—2 u
1 week to 10-day interval	Seat—2 u
3-4 week surface onlay	Prep—2 u
1 week to 10-day interval	Seat—2 u
¾ crown or full crown	Prep—3 u
1 week to 10-day interval	Seat—2 u
Fixed Bridge	
Consult with dentist.	
Porcelain Veneer Crowns	
1 tooth	Prep—3 u
2-week interval	Seat—2 u
Laminate	
1 tooth	
Preparation	2 u
Cementation	2 u
2 teeth	
Preparation	4 u
Cementation	3 u
Sealant	
4 or more teeth	2 u
Fewer or more teeth—schedule according to operator's recommendation.	
Bleaching	
Impression and consultation	2 u
Delivery, shade, and posttreatment instructions	2 u
Follow-up evaluation (optional)	2 u
Prophylaxis	
Adult with dentist	2 u
Adult with hygienist	4 u
Child with dentist	1 u
Child with hygienist	2 u
New patient—schedule with hygienist for prophylaxis and with dentist for examination.	2 u
Emergency	
Schedule according to nature; generally 2 u or use buffer as discussed.	

*1 u = 15 minutes.

After establishing the appointment sequence, you can refer to the patient's **treatment plan** to determine the treatment that must be done. The treatment plan is completed at the time of the diagnosis by the dentist and recorded on a treatment plan form (Figure 11-17). The same information is generated in either the manual or electronic treatment plan. The treatment plan in Figure 11-17 indicates that the first need of the patient is a full metal crown on tooth #30. By referring to the appointment list, you note the patient must have two appointments. The first is for preparation, 3 units; the second, at least 1 week later, is for cementation of the crown and requires 2 units. This system can be easily followed for all appointment scheduling.

At this point you are ready to determine the times for the appointments by using the suggestions made previously. Care should be taken to eliminate useless voids in the schedule by (1) always beginning to schedule appointments at the bottom or top of a large block of time, never in the middle, and (2) not leaving units of time (except for buffers) vacant between appointments.

APPOINTMENTS NECESSARY for DENTISTRY

SCHEDULE FOR _____CHARLES RUSSELL_____   TELEPHONE __112-4897__

TIME PREFERRED __EARLY A.M.__   DATE __2/81/—__

TIME NECESSARY	SERVICES PLANNED	DAYS BETWEEN APPTS	DATE & TIME APPOINTED	SERVICES NOT COMPLETED	TIME NECESSARY
3U/2U	FC #30	7-10	2/15-9:00 2/23-9:00		
2U	EXT #1	7	3/4-9:00		
	#30 MOD AMAL	—	3/11-9:00		
4U	#29 MO AMAL	—			
	#2 MO	—			

A

Figure 11-17 A, Traditional treatment plan.

Continued

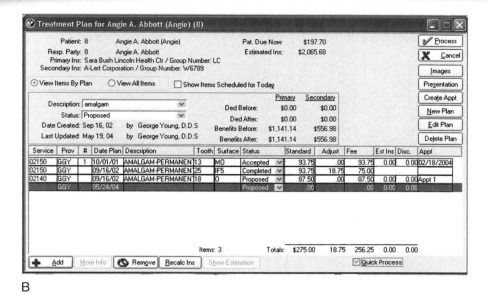

B

Figure 11-17, cont'd B, Electronic treatment plan screen. (**A** courtesy SYCOM, Madison, WI; **B** courtesy Patterson EagleSoft, Effingham, IL.)

Appointment Card

An **appointment card** is a written notification of the patient's appointment that the patient takes home. Once the entry has been made in the appointment book, transfer the information to the appointment card. It is entered directly from the appointment book in ink and should be easy to read. Recheck the appointment card before giving it to the patient to make sure the information in the book and on the card is the same.

A traditional appointment card generally is made of medium-weight or lightweight stock and measures about $2 \times 3\frac{1}{2}$ inches to fit easily into a wallet. Appointment cards usually are white with black print. However, many offices are now color coding cards, using matching or contrasting ink to carry out a color theme in the office. The information on the card includes the dentist's full name, degrees, address, and phone number and the office policy on broken appointments. Lines are provided for the patient's name and the day, date, and time of the appointment. Figure 11-18 shows a variety of appointment cards that can be used in the dental office. The cards shown in *A, B,* and *D* are for only one appointment; the card shown in *C* is a series-type appointment card, on which more than one appointment may be listed. The series card saves both the assistant's time and the cost of additional cards. In an electronic system, the appointment often is listed on the exit receipt.

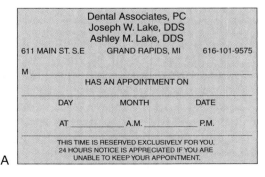

A

Figure 11-18 Appointment cards. **A** and **B,** Single appointment cards.

Dental Associates, PC
Joseph W. Lake, DDS
Ashley M. Lake, DDS

611 MAIN ST. S.E   GRAND RAPIDS, MI   616-101-9575

M _____

HAS AN APPOINTMENT ON

☐ MONDAY   THURSDAY ☐
☐ TUESDAY   FRIDAY ☐
☐ WEDNESDAY   SATURDAY ☐

DATE _____ TIME _____

A BROKEN APPOINTMENT IS A LOSS TO EVERYONE.
PLEASE INFORM US ONE DAY IN ADVANCE IF YOU
ARE UNABLE TO KEEP YOUR APPOINTMENT.

B

Dental Associates, PC
Joseph W. Lake, DDS
Ashley M. Lake, DDS

611 MAIN ST. S.E   GRAND RAPIDS, MI   616-101-9575

M _____

_____ AT ____   _____ AT ____
_____ AT ____   _____ AT ____
_____ AT ____   _____ AT ____

A BROKEN APPOINTMENT IS A LOSS TO EVERYONE.
PLEASE INFORM US ONE DAY IN ADVANCE IF YOU
ARE UNABLE TO KEEP YOUR APPOINTMENT.

C

Figure 11-18, cont'd C, Series style appointment card.

It also can be listed on a walk out statement, but many patients seem to like the security of a separate appointment card. The electronic system does eliminate the potential for error in writing on the appointment card.

DAILY APPOINTMENT SCHEDULE

Each day the administrative assistant pulls the clinical records for each of the next day's patients and completes a daily schedule. The **daily appointment schedule** is a chronological listing of the day's activities. This schedule is placed in the treatment rooms, the laboratory, and the dentist's private office. The information, transferred from the appointment book, may be written or typed onto the daily schedule or entered electronically (Figure 11-19). It should include the patient's name, the treatment to be done, and the time of the appointment. The schedule is placed for easy access by the staff; however, to protect confidentiality, it should not be in view to patients or other passersby. The administrative assistant should keep the schedule current if any changes take place during the day.

APPOINTMENT CALL LIST

Some refer to the **appointment call list** as a "will call," "contact," or "incomplete patient" list, although you may conclude it is easiest to refer to this list simply as the "call list." The appointment call list is a current list of patients who need appointments for a variety of reasons. It includes patients who want to be called if an earlier appointment becomes available, patients who did not make an appointment when they left the office, and patients who are waiting for healing to occur before completing their treatment. The patient's name and phone number and information about the treatment are listed in a notebook or at the back of the appointment book, or this data may be entered in a notes window on the computer software (Figure 11-20).

	MON.	TUES.	WED.	THURS.	FRI.	SAT.

DATE ___JANUARY 27___

	DR. LAKE	MS. CROWE	
	MR. EDWARD BROWN	MS. GENEVA HAHN	
8 15	29 MOD 30 0 A	15 P-4 BW	15
30	31 MO	30	30
45	↓	45 ↓	45
	MS. DOROTHY HILL	MR. DAVID SCHULTZ	
9 15	PREP. 30 F.C.	15 P-CSX	15
30	↓	30	30
45	MR. RICHARD BALL	45 ↓	45
	EXT. 29-32	MS. MARGARET TEAL	
10 15		15 P	15
30	↓	30	30
45	MS. JOY DE VRIES	45 ↓	45
	SEAT #28 PVC	MR. PHIL DYKSTRA	
11 15	SYLVIA DE HAAN	15 P-4 BW	15
30	↓ 29 MOA	30	30
45		45 ↓	45
12 15		15	15
30		30	30
45		45	45
1 15		15	15
30		30	30
45		45	45
2 15		15	15
30		30	30
45		45	45
3 15		15	15
30		30	30
45		45	45
4 15		15	15
30		30	30
45		45	45
5 15		15	15
30		30	30
45		45	45
15		15	15
30		30	30
45		45	45

A

Figure 11-19 A, Traditional daily schedule.

Continued

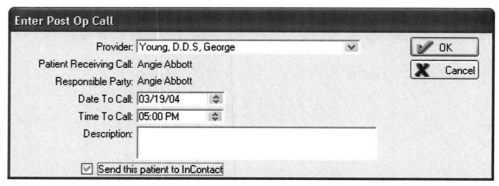

Figure 11-19, cont'd B, Electronic daily schedule. (Courtesy Patterson EagleSoft, Effingham, IL.)

			CALL LIST			
DATE	NAME	PHONE	SERVICES	TIME OF DAY	AMOUNT OF U	
1/16/—	MS. R. JOHNSON	112-9762	#30 ¾ CR PREP.	AFTER 4 P.M.	3 U	
1/20/—	MR. H. HAMMOND	112-6626	19 ᴰᴰ 20 ᴰᴰ	P.M.	3 U	
1/29/—	MR. J. WRIGHT	114-6729	MAND. GING.	AFTER EASTER	4 U	
1/29/—	MS. H. VANDERVEEN	118-7996	PRCL. DENT. IMP.	AFTER 3/11	2 U	

A

Figure 11-20 A, Call list. **B,** Electronic contact notes window. (Courtesy Patterson EagleSoft, Effingham, IL.)

SCHEDULING PATIENTS IN AN ADVANCED-FUNCTION PRACTICE

Scheduling of patients in an office that has an advanced- or expanded-function dental auxiliary requires a different time assignment concept. In such practices the patient does not see the dentist only. Depending on the state dental practice act and the qualifications of the various clinical staff members, time may also be assigned to the advanced-function assistant to perform various clinical tasks without the dentist needing to be assigned to the patient. A variety of tasks that can be assigned to the appropriately qualified assistant may include diagnostic impressions, dental radiographs, periodontal dressing placement or removal, placing or carving of amalgam, or various other specialty tasks.

It is vital that the administrative assistant understand the legal ramifications of assigning an unqualified or noncredentialed person to perform various clinical tasks. The administrative assistant must have a thorough understanding of the state law, and a clinical assistant's qualifications for a task must be verified before the individual is scheduled to treat patients.

Typically the units of time for the operator are modified but patient chair time remains the same in a specific room, because the advanced functions assistant performs intraoral tasks that in the past might have been performed by the dentist. It takes time on the part of the staff to determine how and by whom the intraoral duties will be performed, but once this is determined, the administrative assistant can plan on such treatment in the scheduling option of the appointment book.

Once you have become familiar with the techniques of appointment book management, it can be a very enjoyable part of the business office. Using time efficiently can make each day in the office more productive and can reduce tension while still meeting the patients' needs. If the rules in Box 11-2 are followed, the dental office can maintain efficiency.

LEARNING ACTIVITIES

1. Discuss the types of appointment systems available for use in the dental office.
2. Explain the advantages of an electronic appointment system.
3. Explain the components of an appointment matrix.
4. Explain the management of the following appointment scheduling situations:
   a. A mother calls the office, hysterical, because her child, age 8, has just fallen off his bicycle. She states that there is a great deal of bleeding and that his teeth are broken.
   b. A patient who has not been treated by the dentist in more than a year comes into the office about 2:30 PM. He states that he is having some discomfort around a bridge abutment and that he has severe bleeding when he brushes. The schedule for the remaining part of the day is filled.
   c. A patient appears on Monday, January 23, at 10 AM. You greet her, and she says she has a 10 o'clock appointment. On checking the appointment book, you do not find her name listed for that day.
   d. You confirmed a patient's appointment for 1 PM today. The patient does not show up for the appointment.

Continued

EXAMINE YOUR PROGRESS

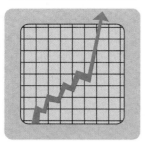

Practice by completing
Working Form 7.

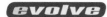

LEARNING ACTIVITIES—cont'd

5. List the information that should be entered in the appointment book when an appointment is made.
6. What information is included on the following forms?
   a. Appointment card
   b. Appointment daily schedule
   c. Call list
   d. Treatment plan
7. Explain how appointment scheduling in an advanced-function dental practice differs from scheduling in a traditional dental practice.
8. List four rules for efficient management of an appointment book.

SOFTWARE ACTIVITIES

1. Using the EagleSoft CD-ROM and the concepts discussed in the chapter, make appointments for the following patients, who are already patients of record on the CD-ROM.
   a. Patients are seen for treatment from 8:30 AM to 5 PM Monday through Friday. Lunches are taken from noon to 1 PM. Buffer periods are for 1 unit each to be scheduled in the late morning and midafternoon.
   b. The Lions Club meeting is on Thursday from noon to 1 PM. (It is a 15-minute drive each way to the meeting.)
   c. Staff meetings are scheduled on the first and third Fridays of every month. Other meetings during this month include
      • Dumont Study Club all day on the 9th
      • Von Trapp Study Club all day on the 14th
      • Western District Dental Society meeting all afternoon on the 20th; public school holiday on the 27th
2. The dentist has outlined the treatment necessary for Mr. John Abbott. He needs a full cast metal crown on #31. No preparation has been done on this tooth as of this date. He also needs #32 extracted, 30^{MOD} amalgam, 29MO composite, 2MO amalgam, and 12^{MOD} composite. You may enter the treatment plan electronically on the CD-ROM. After this has been done in a logical sequence, make the necessary appointments for Mr. Abbott, who prefers early morning appointments. His phone number is 251-215-4214.
3. Make appointments for the following patients as indicated.
   a. Two of Beth Burke's teeth, 18MO and 20DO, are to be restored with composite, because she has just taken a job as a television newscaster and wants to have an esthetic restoration. She prefers an appointment between 1 and 4 PM. Her telephone number is 217-895-2514.
   b. Glenn Davis has a roughness on a "back tooth" that he thinks he broke when he chewed on a piece of hard candy. Anytime is good for him. He can be reached at home at 217-857-4584. NOTE: The type of treatment needed hasn't yet been determined, therefore schedule an emergency oral examination.

Continued

SOFTWARE ACTIVITIES—cont'd

c. Karmen Little teaches, and she likes late afternoon appointments. Faculty meetings are at 3 PM on Mondays. She needs an appointment for preparation of #18 for a full porcelain fused to noble metal crown and an onlay on 19^{MOD} (cast metal). She can be reached at 217-459-5421.

d. Dennis Malone calls for an appointment for his prophylaxis. He can't come in on Mondays or Wednesdays. His telephone number is 217-923-5658.

e. James Burke needs labial veneers (porcelain laminates) on #8 and #9. He can be reached by calling his daughter, Rachael, at 217-895-2514.

f. Kathy Price needs endodontic treatment on #27. No treatment has begun. She prefers Tuesday shortly after lunch. Her phone number is 217-849-5684.

g. Kent Russell needs to have an only done on 3^{MOD} and an amalgam on 4DO. This patient likes late mornings. He can be reached at 217-347-5841.

h. Andrew Savage is to begin treatment for a root canal. No treatment has begun as of this date. Anytime is convenient. His phone number is 217-774-5623.

i. Lori Taylor is quite busy at the end of the first week of the schedule this month. If you make the appointment in the middle of the week, she could come in the late morning. She is to have an occlusal equilibration. She can be reached at 217-347-5841.

j. Michael Burke is to have composites placed on 7^{ML} and 8^{DL}. He likes to come on his lunch hour, about 1 PM. His phone number is 217-895-2514.

k. Vicki Davis has severe discomfort when chewing on the right side. She is too busy to come in this week, therefore make the appointment for the first of next week. Schedule her for an emergency oral examination. She can be reached at 217-857-4584.

l. Bob Price is to have a porcelain veneer crown prepared for the mandibular right first premolar. Because the dentist is concerned about the occlusion of this tooth, the patient needs an extra 1-unit appointment for a try-in before the cementation appointment. His phone number is 217-849-5684..

Key Terms

Appointment book The scheduling software or actual book into which patients and data are entered for appointment times.

Appointment book matrix An outline of various activities that routinely occur in the dental practice.

Appointment call list The current list of patients who need appointments for a variety of reasons.

Appointment card The form on which the patient's next appointment is scheduled; it includes the day, date, and time.

Appointment schedule list In a manual system, a list that can be keyed and placed in a celluloid protective cover for easy access. In an electronic system, the information is entered when the system is set up, and the appointment time is entered automatically.

Buffer period A small amount of time set aside to absorb the hectic workload of the day or to allow for emergencies.

Daily appointment schedule A chronological listing of the day's activities.

Dovetailing Working a second patient into the schedule during another scheduled patient's treatment.
Prime time The busiest time in the dental practice.
Treatment plan A sequential listing of the treatment to be completed for a patient.

Unit (u) A given amount of time, generally in 10- or 15-minute increments, into which each day of the appointment book is separated.

Bibliography

Schumann TC: Top five opportunities to improve your profit, *J Mich Dent Assoc* February 2005.

Chapter

12 Recall Systems

Chapter Outline

Learning Objectives

Mastery of the content in this chapter will enable the reader to:

- Define key terms
- Explain the purpose of a recall system
- Identify different types of recall systems
- Develop a recall system

A **recall system** notifies patients of the timing of routine dental care. It is an integral part of every modern dental practice and is essential to both the patient and the dentist. A recall system is the lifeline of the practice. It helps achieve one of the primary objectives of dentistry—helping patients maintain good oral health for a lifetime. The routine recall appointment generally is assigned to the dental hygienist, but each dental professional in the practice must assume a role in maintaining a successful recall system.

Patients are recalled to the office most often for oral prophylaxis and examination. However, a recall visit may be scheduled for a variety of other reasons:

- Examination of oral tissues after surgical procedures
- Examination of prosthetic devices (e.g., full or partial dentures or implants)

> A recall system is the lifeline of the practice. It helps achieve one of the primary objectives of dentistry—helping patients maintain good oral health for a lifetime.

- Determination of eruption patterns in children
- Determination of the status of orthodontic treatment
- Follow-up on endodontic treatment
- Follow-up for an implant
- Determination of periodontal tissue status

The success of a recall system depends on three factors: (1) dental health education, (2) motivation, and (3) consistent follow-up. As an administrative assistant, you must help patients develop a sense of responsibility toward their own dental health, even though such a behavioral change is not made quickly. In addition, the patient must be aware of how the practice's recall system operates. As Winston Churchill put it, "People love to learn but hate to be taught."

Motivation of patients, which is critical to the effectiveness of the recall system, is the responsibility of the dental staff. Once a patient has been educated and motivated to accept a recall system, the administrative assistant is responsible for maintaining the system efficiently. The importance of this step cannot be overemphasized. If an assistant ignores the recall system even for 1 month, the effect on the patient flow becomes noticeable within a short time, and patients begin to feel ignored.

> The success of a recall system depends on three factors: (1) dental health education, (2) motivation, and (3) consistent follow-up.

KEEPING PATIENTS INFORMED

Patients in the dental practice must understand the importance of recall regardless of the reason for the recall appointment. Much can be done through patient education to promote the recall system. Some practical and easy ways to keep patients informed about the dental procedures the office offers and the way the recall system works include the following:

- Updated practice brochures
- Newsletters
- Audiovisual materials in the reception room
- Intraoral cameras
- Before and after photographs
- Bulletin boards
- Follow-up e-mails

TYPES OF RECALL SYSTEMS

Any of several types of recall systems can be used. Most dentists find that no one system is perfect, therefore they often use more than one. The three most common recall systems are the advanced appointment system, the telephone recall system, and the mail recall system.

Advanced Appointment System

With the **advanced appointment system,** recall appointments are scheduled before the patient leaves the office. Traditionally, management experts have criticized this system because people cannot predict their schedules 6 months in advance. Chaos can result if the dentist or hygienist is absent from the office and misses a scheduled appointment or if patients are constantly canceling their appointments. Advocates of this system contend that most people know their routines and the appointment times that generally are best for them. The office staff should weigh the advantages and disadvantages listed in Box 12-1.

Box 12-1
Advanced Appointment System

Advantages
- No cost involved
- No time required of the administrative assistant
- Simple

Disadvantages
- Patients do not know what their future commitments might be.
- Hygienist's appointment book may be filled 6 months in advance, and then staff changes may occur.

Telephone Recall System

The **telephone recall system** allows the most immediate response, because the administrative assistant contacts each patient by telephone to schedule a recall appointment. This can be a good practice builder for a new practitioner, but it can be an exhausting and time-consuming task in a large, well-established practice.

When contacting a patient by telephone, you should use phrases that do not devalue the service. Eliminate such phrases as "for your check-up" or "for your cleaning." Some assistants find it cumbersome to use the words *prophylaxis* and *examination,* because they feel these terms are too technical; also, these words don't accurately convey the importance of the recall visit. This visit includes a complete dental examination, an examination of all oral tissues (to detect oral diseases early), and complete scaling and polishing of teeth. Take the time to inform your patients that this is an important preventive service or try using the phrase, *preventive recall appointment.*

Because many people have answering machines or voicemail, which allow you to leave messages, the telephone system can be an effective technique that provides personal contact with the patient. Box 12-2 lists a few suggestions

---

Box 12-2
Suggestions for Using the Telephone Recall System

1. Don't call too early in the morning.
2. Make sure your voice conveys a positive attitude; don't make calls if you're tired or grumpy.
3. Make the calls in private, out of hearing of other patients.
4. Don't pester patients. If they say they will call back, record it on the recall file cards and wait 2 to 3 weeks before contacting them again. If they do not respond after three calls, ask them if they wish to remain on your active recall program.
5. Have the patient's recall record in front of you so that you will be well informed.
6. Try calling on inclement days; patients are likely to be indoors on such days.
7. If you reach an answering machine, speak clearly and leave a complete message, including the reason for the call, the times the office will be open, the telephone number, and a cordial "Thank you."

---

for successfully using the telephone in a recall system. The advantages and disadvantages of the telephone system are listed in Box 12-3.

Mail Recall System

With the **mail recall system,** the patient is responsible for making the appointment. Patients receive a card that (1) asks them to contact the office to schedule a preventive recall appointment or (2) gives them an appointment time and asks them to confirm it (Figure 12-1). The card should emphasize the importance of the prophylaxis and should not use words such as *cleaning* or *check-up.* The office manager addresses the card or the patient addresses the card at the previous visit. The latter arrangement can be especially effective, because patients recognize their own handwriting when they receive the card, and this may confirm their interest in the recall system. Despite some drawbacks (Box 12-4), the mail recall system can be advantageous in a large practice.

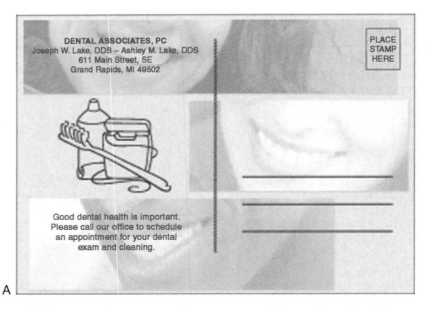

Figure 12-1 A, Recall notice to inform a patient of the need to schedule an appointment.

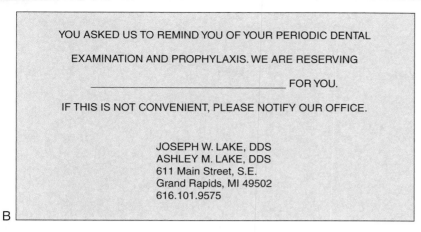

YOU ASKED US TO REMIND YOU OF YOUR PERIODIC DENTAL

EXAMINATION AND PROPHYLAXIS. WE ARE RESERVING

_____ FOR YOU.

IF THIS IS NOT CONVENIENT, PLEASE NOTIFY OUR OFFICE.

JOSEPH W. LAKE, DDS
ASHLEY M. LAKE, DDS
611 Main Street, S.E.
Grand Rapids, MI 49502
616.101.9575

B

Figure 12-1, cont'd B, Recall card sent to patient for confirmation. (Courtesy Colwell, a Division of Patterson Companies, Inc., Champaign, IL.)

Several types of recall messages can be used (Figure 12-2). Take care not to underestimate a child's maturity when deciding which type of message to send to pediatric patients.

ESTABLISHING A RECALL SYSTEM

Once the recall system has been determined, the administrative assistant should set up a recall file that is simple, efficient, and accurate. The most efficient recall system is managed electronically. In today's dental practice, this is simply too important a management tool to rely on a manual system.

Electronic Recall Files

The computer is a valuable component of recall management. With an electronic file, the software system generates a list of patients who need to be contacted (Figure 12-3). The computer also can produce the actual letter or card or create mailing labels for preprepared cards. If the office uses a telephone recall system, you can generate a master list of patients and their telephone numbers.

Follow-Up

As mentioned previously, it is vital that patients be recalled routinely. Patients need to be informed of how the recall system works and how they will be notified before they leave the office. The administrative assistant must maintain flawless records and manage the system so as to ensure that the patient returns to the office in a timely manner.

Box 12-4
Mail Recall System

Advantages
- Places responsibility on the patient
- Visible reminder

Disadvantages
- Possible to ignore notice
- Cost of postage
- Lack of immediate response

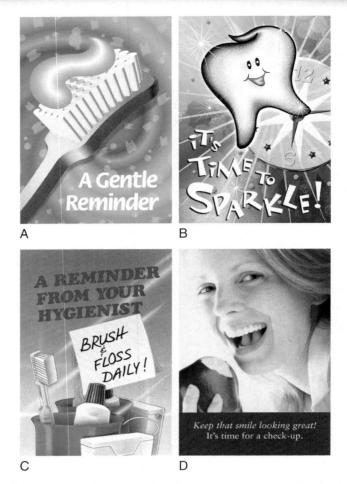

Figure 12-2 Four styles of recall cards. (Courtesy Colwell, a Division of Patterson Companies, Inc., Champaign, IL.)

Recalls to Process

Process	ID	Name	Recall Date	NPA	NRA
☑	19	Madison G. Abbott	1/30/2005		
☑	20	Mark Abbott	12/18/2004		
☑	25	Bryan Abernathy	12/18/2004		
☑	72	Bryan A. Abernathy	2/23/2005		
☑	43	Jeremy Adam	12/19/2004		
☑	42	Jedidah Adam	1/30/2005		
☑	45	Jesse Adam	1/30/2005		
☑	6	Scott Alexander	12/1/2004		
☑	32	Richard Ballard	12/18/2004		
☑	33	Megan Ballard	1/30/2005		
☑	68	Jim Carson	12/18/2004		
☑	61	Kelly Davies	12/1/2004		
☑	57	Matthew Dickson	1/30/2005		
☑	12	Jody Farkas	1/30/2005		
☑	23	Carl Malone	1/30/2005		
☑	50	Eugene Partridge	2/20/2005		
☑	67	Cole Walden	2/20/2005		

OK | Cancel | Mark All | Clear All

Patients to be processed: 17 E-mails to be processed: 0 Total Pages: 1

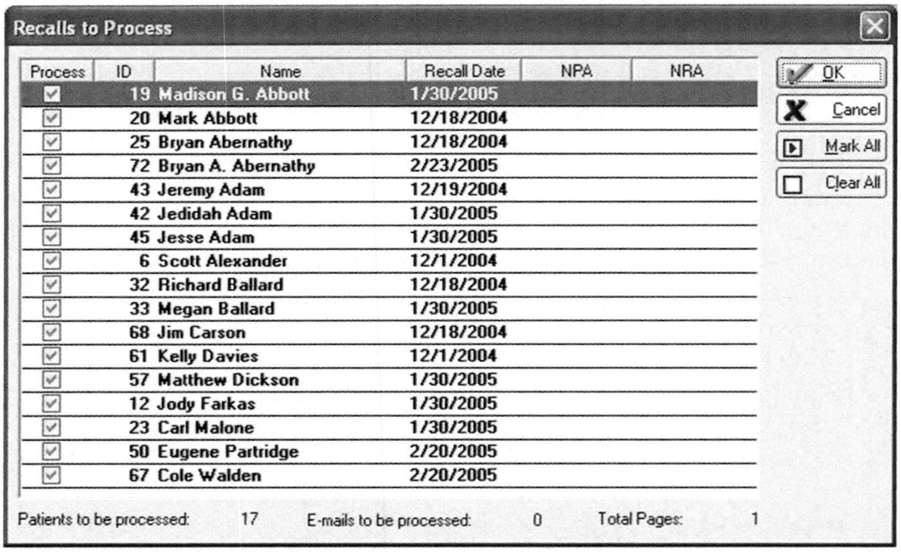

Figure 12-3 An electronic file generates a list of all patients due for recall in a specific month. (Courtesy Colwell, a Division of Patterson Companies, Inc., Champaign, IL.)

Purging the System

Periodically, as with any records management system, the recall records must be purged. This can be done electronically for patients who have not been in the practice recall system for a period of years. To avoid the possibility of litigation for negligence, the dental office should inform the patient that the record is being removed from the system. A letter should be sent to the patient (and included in the patient's record) informing the person that you are removing him or her from the recall system; this protects the practice and reminds the patient one last time of the importance of a preventive recall or follow-up appointment.

Key Terms

Advanced appointment system
A recall system in which appointments are scheduled at the time the patient leaves the office.

Mail recall system A recall system in which the patient receives a card that (1) asks the person to contact the office to make an appointment for a preventive recall visit or (2) gives the patient an appointment time and asks the individual to confirm the appointment.

Recall system A system by which patients are notified of the timing of routine dental care.

Telephone recall system A system in which the patient is contacted by telephone for a recall appointment.

LEARNING ACTIVITIES

1. Explain the value of a recall system to (a) a patient and (b) the dentist.
2. What determines the success of a recall system?
3. Explain the functions of the three basic recall systems.
4. Explain the advantages and disadvantages of each of the three basic recall systems.
5. What effect would a computer have on a recall system in a dental office?
6. Using the EagleSoft system for this textbook, review the procedure for entering a patient on recall for 4 months, 6 months, and 1 year.

EXAMINE YOUR PROGRESS

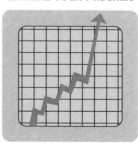

Practice by completing Working Form 8.

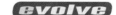

Bibliography

Salem G: The periodic exam: a vital key to practice success, *Dent Econ* May 2004.

Inventory Systems and Supply Ordering

Chapter Outline

Types of Supplies
    Selecting Supplies
Designing an Inventory System
    Capital Equipment Inventory Control
    Expendable and Nonexpendable Supplies Inventory Control
    Computerized Inventory Systems
    Manual Inventory Systems
    Card System
    Alphabetical List
Maintaining the Inventory System
    Identifying Reorder Points
    Determining Supply Quantity
    Receiving Supplies
    Receiving Credit
    Back-Ordered Supplies
    Purchase Orders
    Storage of Supplies
    Inventory Evaluation

Learning Objectives

Mastery of the content in this chapter will enable the reader to:
- Define key terms
- Identify three types of dental supplies
- Explain various types of inventory systems
- Establish an inventory system
- Explain factors determining supply quantity
- Describe a technique for receiving supplies
- Describe a computerized ordering system
- Identify common supply forms
- Explain the storage of hazardous materials

The administrative assistant may be responsible for maintaining the inventory system in the dental office. Whether at chairside, in the laboratory, or in the business office, dental professionals find it frustrating to reach for an item and find only an empty box. Only one person should be in charge of ordering, receiving, and storing supplies; managing hazardous waste; and maintaining **Material Safety Data Sheets (MSDSs)** (p. 365). Because the practice has both a business side and a clinical side, a business staff member may order all the business supplies, and a clinical staff member may be responsible for managing clinical supplies and hazardous materials. However, all staff members are responsible for noting whether supplies are low or exhausted as they perform their daily tasks.

Much of the efficiency of a dental office depends on a systematic and economical approach to ordering supplies. To ensure such efficiency, the administrative assistant must establish a simple inventory system that can be easily maintained. This system may be manual or computerized.

> Whether at chairside, in the laboratory, or in the business office, dental professionals find it frustrating to reach for an item and find only an empty box.

TYPES OF SUPPLIES

Supplies can be divided into three basic categories: expendable supplies, nonexpendable supplies, and capital supplies. **Expendable supplies** are single-use items such as dental cements, stationery, local anesthetics, and gypsum products. **Nonexpendable supplies** are reusable items that do not constitute a major expense; this category includes most dental instruments. **Capital supplies** are large, costly items that are seldom replaced, such as computers, sterilizers, and dental units.

Selecting Supplies

> Much of the efficiency of a dental office depends on a systematic and economical approach to ordering supplies.

Not all materials can be purchased from one supplier, and buying from several suppliers may be more economical. Shopping locally promotes good relations and stimulates the local economy, but for economic reasons a dentist may order supplies from a larger catalog or discount house.

A dental supply house can provide all the basic dental supplies, both brand name and generic. Purchasing from the dealers in your area is convenient, but many large wholesale supply houses provide quick service and special rates. Making use of toll-free telephone numbers also can speed up service. Make sure your vendor is reliable; the materials must be quality products and, where applicable, must meet American Dental Association (ADA) specifications.

Most dental supply houses send representatives to the office regularly, or they may contact the office by telephone or e-mail. Have the order ready when the salesperson contacts you. A manufacturer's representative who wants to see the dentist about a new product may accompany the supply person. If the dentist's schedule does not allow time to meet with the representative, obtain information about new products and relay the information to the dentist later.

Medicaments, which are not specifically a dental item, can be purchased from a local pharmacy. Surgical supply companies sell materials such as thermometers, surgical scissors, and hemostats.

Business materials are available from local business office supply stores or by mail order. Some supplies, such as cleaning materials, must be purchased at local businesses or specialty companies.

For convenience, you should list on the Rolodex the business addresses and telephone numbers of all the companies you patronize routinely (see Chapter 8).

DESIGNING AN INVENTORY SYSTEM

An *inventory system* is a list of the stock and assets in the dental office. This list is divided into two parts, capital equipment and expendable and nonexpendable supplies.

Capital Equipment Inventory Control

A spreadsheet or card file can be used to maintain an inventory of capital equipment. For a spreadsheet, a form such as Excel or Access can be used, and all the major categories of supplies can be listed as headings. The card shown in Figure 13-1 is filled out for each capital item and details important information about the item, including maintenance data. Both the card and spreadsheet systems can save much time and guesswork about the servicing of equipment and can be helpful to the accountant in determining depreciation. This information should be reviewed frequently for necessary preventive maintenance service. Such service is best scheduled when the dentist is out of the office.

Expendable and Nonexpendable Supplies Inventory Control

Dental offices generally do not keep a large stock of nonexpendable supplies on hand; however, a list may be included in an inventory system if the dentist wishes. Because the expendable supplies require more attention, an inventory of these items is important. The inventory can be automated on a computer or maintained manually.

Computerized Inventory Systems

A computerized inventory system can be created through a special software package or a database you create yourself. The system can be simple or complex. An automated inventory system set up in a centralized database allows the staff simply to enter the shipment data into the system and print new inventory reports. The system enters the inventory numbers in the accounts automatically, as long as the information is entered correctly. The computer program asks for the name of the person removing the stock, the type of stock removed, how many items are used, and the date. In this way the inventory count is adjusted as materials are taken from stock or as a requisition is generated. The inventory then is updated automatically.

PRODUCT: Transthorax unit w/fiberoptics		
MANUFACTURER: HSP		MODEL: T-3
SERIAL NUMBER: 00967-87534	PURCHASE DATE: 4/17/—	
SUPPLIER: HSP		COST: $4600.
COLOR: Taupe	WARRANTY EXPIRATION: 4/17/—	
DATE OF SERVICE	SERVICED BY	NATURE OF PROBLEM

Figure 13-1 Capital equipment inventory card.

+H49115864604K

Figure 13-2 Bar code used with a scanner for computerized inventory.

Another type of automated system uses bar codes as the main identification numbers (Figure 13-2). A light scanner reads the bar code, and the inventory is updated automatically when the item is scanned.

eMagine is one of the automated supply management software systems used in dentistry. It is a free service to Patterson Supply customers. With eMagine, merchandise orders are placed electronically. All special pricing and free goods are included, and many items have pictures and long descriptions. eMagine combines the benefits of a mail order catalog with the ease of ordering electronically. Customers' order and invoice histories are available, allowing them easily to track which products they ordered previously. Figure 13-3 shows an example of the screen image for this order technique.

The decision on whether to use any of these types of computer systems depends on the size and needs of the office. Regardless of the system selected, the inventory manager must decide ahead of time the desired minimum and maximum stock levels.

Another option for ordering is the Internet, because more dental supply houses are merchandising online. The administrative assistant finds the company's website, chooses the order screen, and checks off the items needed for the office. The order can be verified and then sent to the dental supplier. This automated system is efficient for the supplier and the dental office. Supply ordering is convenient and saves money for the supplier by eliminating the need for salespersons to visit the office. Product information and monthly or weekly specials are available. To personalize this system, the supplier and the dental office staff can e-mail inquiries to each other.

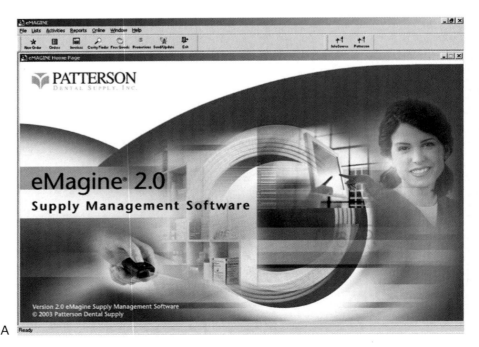

Figure 13-3 Screen views of eMagine ordering system. (Courtesy Patterson Dental Supply, St. Paul, MN.)

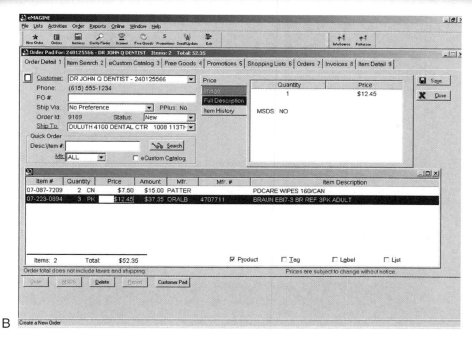

Figure 13-3 Cont'd

Manual Inventory Systems

Some dentists still find it difficult to hand over the supply ordering system to automation and may find that a manual systems is sufficient. If so, either a card system or an alphabetical list may suffice for an inventory system in many offices.

Card System

The card system requires a separate card for each product (Figure 13-4). The cards list complete information about each product and its supplier and are placed in alphabetical order according to the product name. They are

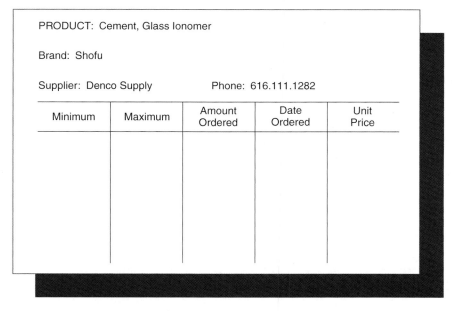

Figure 13-4 Inventory card.

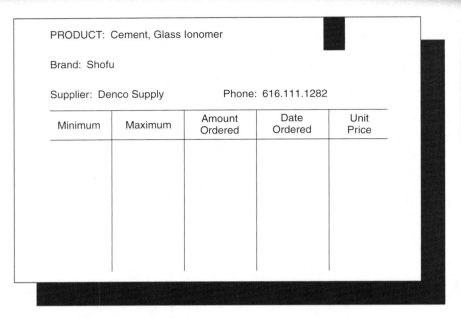

PRODUCT: Cement, Glass Ionomer

Brand: Shofu

Supplier: Denco Supply   Phone: 616.111.1282

Minimum	Maximum	Amount Ordered	Date Ordered	Unit Price

Figure 13-5 Colored tag on an inventory card.

kept in a file drawer or notebook. As it becomes necessary to order an item, the card is placed in a section of the file marked *To be ordered*. Once the item has been ordered, the card is moved to the *On order* section of the file. When the item arrives from the supplier, the card is replaced in its original alphabetical position in the file. If the item is currently out of stock and has been placed on back-order by the supplier, the card is placed in the *On back-order* section of the file.

A modification of this system leaves all the cards in the alphabetical section at all times, and the status of the item is indicated with a colored tag (Figure 13-5). A red label might indicate *To be ordered*; blue, *On order*; and yellow, *On back-order*. This system eliminates moving of the cards and the chance of misfiling and also indicates at a glance the status of the items.

Alphabetical List

Table 13-1 shows an example of an alphabetical list of materials for inventory. This master list includes a code number for each supplier, the name of each product, and columns for the maximum on-hand level and the minimum reorder point. This list is kept in a protective celluloid cover, and when the reorder point is reached, the assistant simply places a red check mark in the appropriate space with a waxed pencil. When visiting the office, the supply representative can review the list, find all the items checked off with the supplier's number, and complete the order. When the items are ordered, the red check marks are erased with a tissue.

MAINTAINING THE INVENTORY SYSTEM

Identifying Reorder Points

Several techniques can be used for reordering supplies. Colored tape may be used to indicate the reorder point on small items (Figure 13-6), or a tag can be placed on the item (Figure 13-7). For stationery supplies, a paper tab can be inserted into the stack of materials to indicate the reorder point (Figure 13-8).

Table 13-1
Example of a Master Supply List

Supplier Number	Product Name	Manufacturer	Maximum	Minimum Reorder Point
120	Aerosol spray	Regency	12 btls	3 btls
130	Alcohol, Misopropyl	Stock	2 gal	1 gal
110	Alginate, Jeltrate	Dentsply	250 pkgs	100 pkgs
110	Alloy, TYTIN 400 mg	Kerr	6 cns (500 caps)	10 cns (500 caps)
100	Alloy, TYTIN 800 mg	Kerr	6 cns (500 caps)	10 cns (500 caps)
100	Anesthetic, topical ointment	Schein	12 jars	4 jars
110	Anesthetic, mepivacaine 2% with	Surgimax	50 cns (50)	10 cns (50)
110	Anesthetic, mepivacaine 2% without	Surgimax	20 cns (50)	5 cns (50)
110	Bite blocks—foam	Strident	500	150
110	Burs—all	Kerr	25 of all sizes used	10 of all sizes used
110	Casting flux	Schein	2 btls	1 btl
110	Cotton rolls #2	Richmond	1000	250

Determining Supply Quantity

In deciding how to maintain an inventory system, you must decide the minimum and maximum amounts of each item you wish to keep in stock. Certain factors can help determine these amounts:

- *Rate of use:* Buying large quantities of infrequently used items is not cost efficient. However, buying bulk quantities of supplies used frequently

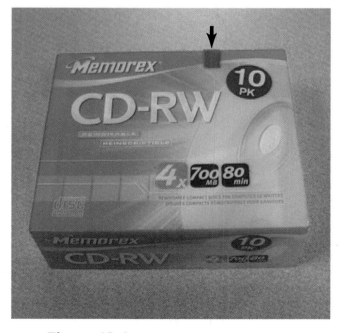

Figure 13-6 Colored tape on small items.

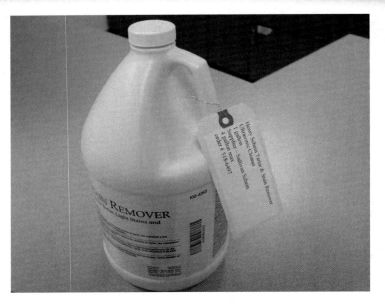

Figure 13-7 Tag on a bottle.

is economical. For example, buying paper products for the dental treatment room in large quantities is a good idea if storage space is available.

- *Shelf life:* Certain materials, such as x-ray film and some impression materials, begin to deteriorate after a certain period. Some manufacturers indicate an expiration date on the box. Do not purchase a large quantity of items that cannot be used before their expiration date.

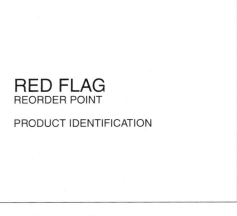

RED FLAG
REORDER POINT

PRODUCT IDENTIFICATION

Figure 13-8 Paper tab.

- *Amount of capital outlay:* In addition to prices, the amount of cash available often determines whether an item is purchased in bulk amounts.
- *Length of delivery time:* This factor affects the minimum quantity you wish to have in stock. If several days are required to receive an order for a frequently used item, you may wish to increase the minimum amount on hand.
- *Amount of storage space:* In some offices, storage space is a crucial factor, and lack of it prohibits the purchase of large supplies. Consequently, a large storage space is a benefit economically and increases your efficiency.
- *Manufacturer's special offers:* Manufacturers routinely offer special rates on various materials. However, a special price is not cost efficient if the item stays on the shelf and collects dust.

Receiving Supplies

All incoming materials should be handled and stored safely. Current regulations require that all manufacturers provide an MSDS with each hazardous material.

Every order that arrives in the office should have an invoice or a packing slip, or both. A **packing slip** is simply an enumeration of the enclosed items. An **invoice** (Figure 13-9) is a list of the contents of the package, the price of each item enclosed, and the total charge. Some companies use the invoice as a statement and indicate on the form that this is the statement from which you are to pay the account. Make sure that each item listed coincides with the original order, that each item on the invoice is in the package, and that the total amount listed on the invoice is accurate. Then put the invoice in the *To be paid* file.

At the end of the month, you will receive a statement, or a request for payment, from the supplier (Figure 13-10). Each invoice should be checked against the entries on the statement to ensure accuracy before payment is sent.

The check is made payable to the supplier (see Chapter 16). The check number is indicated on the retained portion of the statement, the invoices are attached, and these documents are filed in the appropriate subject file.

Receiving Credit

Sometimes supplies must be returned for credit. In such cases the dental supplier sends a **credit memo** (Figure 13-11), which indicates that the dentist's account has been credited for the cost of the returned item. This amount appears as a credit on the statement at the end of the month.

Back-Ordered Supplies

Sometimes an item ordered is not in stock at the supply house, and you will receive a **back-order memo**. The supplier notifies you that the article is back-ordered (see Figure 13-9), or this may be noted directly on the invoice. If you need the product immediately, you should attempt to obtain it from another supplier or make an alternative selection.

Purchase Orders

In large institutions supplies are ordered through a purchasing agent. All items are listed on a requisition, and the order is keyed into a **purchase order**, a standardized order form for supplies. Each purchase order is given a number and sent to the appropriate supplier, who in turn enters this number on all invoices when shipping the supplies.

PATTERSON
DENTAL

INVOICE#: 12345678910

SHIP TO   DENTAL ASSOCIATES, PC
JOSEPH W LAKE, DDS
611 MAIN STREET SE
GRAND RAPIDS MI 49502

Customer #: 555123456

Patterson Plus Level: Gold

SOLD BY   PATTERSON DENTAL SUPPLY
BRANCH 100
1031 MENDOTA HEIGHTS ROAD
ST. PAUL MN 55120

Telephone: (651) 555-0000
Representative: 100-70
Order #: 100/1234567
Submitted: 05/10/05   10:00 AM

Printed: 05/10/05   10:45 AM

CUSTOMER P.O.: 222-333
Account: REGULAR
Shipped from:
SOUTHEAST DISTRIBUTION CTR

Item#	Ordered	Shipped	Pkg	Mfr	MFR Catalog #	Item Description	Unit Price	Amount
07 111-2233	1	1	DZ	ACME	112233A	TOOTHBRUSH CROSS ACTION, 35 SOFT	18.00	18.00
07 111-4455	1	1	CA	ACME	445566B	TOOTHPASTE CAVT PROTECT .85 OZ	45.00	45.00

Sample only- Not Valid.

Buy 8 boxes Patterson brand gloves, receive 1 box FREE!
Offer valid 05/01/05 - 05/30/05
Contact your Patterson representative for details.
(Must be same item number on one invoice)

Subtotal		63.00
State Tax	6.5%	4.10

| Total | | | | 2 | 2 | | | |

Total		67.10

Payment Terms:
Payment due upon receipt of statement. Overdue balance is subject to service charge not to exceed 1.5% per month. To pay by invoice, send a copy of invoice(s) with remittance to: PATTERSON DENTAL SUPPLY INC., PO BOX 164, MINNEAPOLIS, MN 55440-0164

Page 1 of 1

Figure 13-9 Invoice. (Courtesy Dental Supply, St. Paul, MN.)

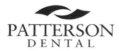

STATEMENT
Of Account

For questions regarding this billing please call 800.555.0000 or 651.555.0000.
Please retain this portion for your files.

Customer Information

Account Number 555123456

DENTAL ASSOCIATES, PC
JOSEPH W LAKE, DDS
611 MAIN STREET SE
GRAND RAPIDS MI 49502

Billing Summary

Statement Closing Date   5/30/2005

Total Due: $1,100.50

Current Billing Period Summary

Document Date	P.O. #	Document #	Original Amount	Payment/Credit #	Applied Amount	Document Balance
5/2/2005	334455	1234567891	108.50	1234567891	108.50	0.00
5/3/2005	667788	2345678912	550.00	2345678912	0.00	550.00
5/10/2005	991122	3456789123	250.50	3456789123	0.00	250.50
5/11/2005	112233	4567891234	300.00	4567891234	0.00	300.00

Sample only-
Not Valid.

A Service Charge not exceeding 1.50% per month may be applied to that portion of the
account balance not received by 6/30/05

Return this portion with your remittance

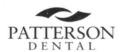

1031 Mendota Heights Rd
Mendota Heights MN 55120

Statement of Account
Statement Closing Date   05/30/2005
Account # 555123456
Total Due: $1,100.50
Please indicate
amount paid: _____

CORPORATE CUSTOMER SERVICE
1031 MENDOTA HEIGHTS RD
ST PAUL MN 55120-1419
||ᵤₙ|||||ᵤₙ|||ᵤₙ|||ₐₗₗₙ|||ᵤₙₙₙₙ|||ᵤₙₙₗ|ₐₗₐₗᵤₙₙ|||

111122223333444000

Patterson Dental Supply, Inc.
P.O. Box 1244
Minneapolis, MN 55440-1244
||ᵤₙ|||||ᵤₙₙ||||ᵤₙₙ|||ₐₗₗ|||ₐₗₗₙₙₙₙᵤₙₙₙₙₙ|||||ᵤₙₙₙ|||ᵤₙₙ|ₐₗₐₗₐₗᵤₙₙ||

Figure 13-10 Statement from a supplier. (Courtesy Dental Supply, St. Paul, MN.)

PATTERSON
DENTAL

CREDIT MEMO#: 987654321

SHIP TO DENTAL ASSOCIATES, PC
JOSEPH W LAKE, DDS
611 MAIN STREET SE
GRAND RAPIDS MI 49502

SOLD BY PATTERSON DENTAL SUPPLY
BRANCH 100
1031 MENDOTA HEIGHTS ROAD
ST. PAUL MN 55120

Printed: 05/11/05 11:00 AM

Customer #: 555123456

Telephone: (651) 555-0000
Representative: 100-70
Order #: 100/1234567
Submitted: 05/11/05 11:00 AM

CUSTOMER P.O.: 222-333
Account: REGULAR

Patterson Plus Level: Gold

Item#	Ordered	Shipped	Pkg	Mfr	MFR Catalog #	Item Description	Unit Price	Amount
07 111-2233	1		1 DZ	ACME	112233A	TOOTHBRUSH CROSS ACTION, 35 SOFT	(18.00)	(18.00)
07 111-4455	1		1 CA	ACME	445566B	TOOTHPASTE CAVT PROTECT .85 OZ	(45.00)	(45.00)

Total	2	2

Buy 8 boxes Patterson brand gloves, receive 1 box FREE!
Offer valid 05/01/05 - 05/30/05
Contact your Patterson representative for details.
(Must be same item number on one invoice)

**Sample only-
Not Valid.**

Subtotal	(63.00)
State Tax 6.5%	(4.10)
Total	(67.10)

Payment Terms:
Payment due upon receipt of statement. Overdue balance is subject to service charge not to exceed 1.5% per month. To pay by invoice, send a copy of invoice(s) with remittance to: PATTERSON DENTAL SUPPLY INC., PO BOX 164, MINNEAPOLIS, MN 55440-0164

Page 1 of 1

Figure 13-11 Credit memo. (Courtesy Dental Supply, St. Paul, MN.)

Material Safety Data Sheet
May be used to comply with
OSHA's Hazard Communication Standard,
29 CFR 1910.1200. Standard must be
consulted for specific requirements.

U.S. Department of Labor
Occupational Safety and Health Administration
(Non-Mandatory Form)
Form Approved
OMB No. 1218-0072

IDENTITY *(As Used on Label and List)*

Note: *Blank spaces are not permitted. If any item is not applicable, or no information is available, the space must be marked to indicate that.*

Section I

Manufacturer's Name	Emergency Telephone Number
Address *(Number, Street, City, State, and ZIP Code)*	Telephone Number for Information
	Date Prepared
	Signature of Preparer *(optional)*

Section II — Hazardous Ingredients/Identity Information

Hazardous Components (Specific Chemical Identity; Common Name(s))	OSHA PEL	ACGIH TLV	Other Limits Recommended	% *(optional)*

Section III — Physical/Chemical Characteristics

Boiling Point		Specific Gravity (H_2O = 1)	
Vapor Pressure (mm Hg.)		Melting Point	
Vapor Density (AIR = 1)		Evaporation Rate (Butyl Acetate = 1)	
Solubility in Water			
Appearance and Odor			

Section IV — Fire and Explosion Hazard Data

Flash Point (Method Used)	Flammable Limits	LEL	UEL
Extinguishing Media			
Special Fire Fighting Procedures			
Unusual Fire and Explosion Hazards			

(Reproduce locally)   OSHA 174, Sept. 1985

Figure 13-12 OSHA Material Safety Data Sheet (MSDS).

Section V — Reactivity Data

Stability	Unstable		Conditions to Avoid
	Stable		

Incompatibility (*Materials to Avoid*)

Hazardous Decomposition or Byproducts

Hazardous Polymerization	May Occur		Conditions to Avoid
	Will Not Occur		

Section VI — Health Hazard Data

Route(s) of Entry:	Inhalation?	Skin?	Ingestion?

Health Hazards (*Acute and Chronic*)

Carcinogenicity:	NTP?	IARC Monographs?	OSHA Regulated?

Signs and Symptoms of Exposure

Medical Conditions
Generally Aggravated by Exposure

Emergency and First Aid Procedures

Section VII — Precautions for Safe Handling and Use

Steps to Be Taken in Case Material Is Released or Spilled

Waste Disposal Method

Precautions to Be Taken in Handling and Storing

Other Precautions

Section VIII — Control Measures

Respiratory Protection (*Specify Type*)

Ventilation	Local Exhaust		Special
	Mechanical (*General*)		Other

Protective Gloves		Eye Protection	

Other Protective Clothing or Equipment

Work/Hygienic Practices

Page 2   ★ U.S.G.P.O.: 1986-491-529/45775

Figure 13-12 Cont'd.

> **Box 13-1**
> **Questions to Consider in Inventory Evaluation**
>
> 1. Does the system distinguish between expendable, nonexpendable, and capital items?
> 2. Is it simple to use?
> 3. Does everyone understand the system?
> 4. Can you identify supply sources for various materials?
> 5. Can you determine when an item has been ordered, back-ordered, and received?
> 6. Is stock always current?
> 7. Are supplies stored safely?

Storage of Supplies

All supplies should be stored in an organized manner that allows quick and easy retrieval. Certain materials require a cool, dry, or dark location. In addition, when new materials are received, they should be stocked behind older supplies so that the older supplies are used first.

The administrative assistant must be aware of the federal Occupational Safety and Health Administration (OSHA) guidelines regarding the use and storage of materials in the dental office. MSDSs provided by OSHA should be maintained on hazardous materials. The information on these sheets (Figure 13-12) includes the manufacturer's name, address, and emergency telephone numbers, as well as specific information about the ingredients of the product. Additional information should include storage instructions, health hazard data, spill or leak procedures, and special safety precautions (e.g., storage in a ventilated area). The dentist must make sure that such forms are made available to staff members. If hazardous materials are stored in the office, appropriate labeling must follow the guidelines given in Chapter 17.

When stationery supplies or large boxes are stored, a label describing the contents should be placed on the outside of each box.

Inventory Evaluation

Box 13-1 presents some useful questions to aid the evaluation of an inventory system in a dental office.

Key Terms

Back-order memo A form accompanying an order that notifies the purchaser that an item ordered is not currently in stock at the supply house and will be sent at a later date.

Capital supplies Large, costly items that are seldom replaced; they include equipment such as the computer, sterilizer, and dental unit.

Credit memo A form that indicates that the dentist's account has been credited for the cost of a returned item; the amount appears as a credit on the statement at the end of the month.

Expendable supplies Single-use items, such as dental cements, stationery, local anesthetics, and gypsum products.

Invoice A list of the contents of a package, the price of each item enclosed, and the total charge.

Material Safety Data Sheet (MSDS) A form supplied by the manufacturer that provides information about a hazardous material; these forms are required by the U.S. government.

Nonexpendable supplies Reusable items that do not constitute a major expense; this category generally includes most dental instruments.
Packing slip An enumeration of the items included in an order; it does not include the cost per item.

Purchase order A standardized form for ordering supplies.
Statement A request for payment submitted by the dental supplier.

LEARNING ACTIVITIES

1. Explain the following terms: expendable, nonexpendable, capital items, invoice, statement, credit slip, and back-order inventory.
2. Explain the processing of an item from the time it is ordered until it is received in the office and the statement is paid.
3. Describe the management of chemicals and hazardous materials in the dental office. What are OSHA guidelines and how do they affect the dental office?
4. Make a master supply list of 25 common expendable dental supplies and indicate the maximum and minimum levels, based on the factors that determine supply amounts discussed in this chapter. Identify the manufacturer and, if possible, the most cost-effective supplier of these products in your area.
5. The items below were purchased as capital equipment. Make out a card or enter into a database the following information:
   a. An Air Technique x-ray processor cleaner was purchased on October 17, 2005, from Apex Dental Supply for $7,700. It has a 12-month warranty from the date of purchase.
   b. A PCIV model sterilizer was purchased (model number PC 182-4/84923). It has a warranty of 6 months from the date of purchase.

EXAMINE YOUR PROGRESS

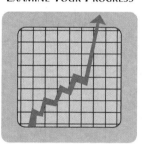

Practice by completing Working Form 9.

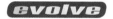

Dental Office Suppliers

Colwell/Patterson Professional Supplies
PO Box 9024
Champaign, IL 61826-9024
1-800-637-1140
www.colwellsystems.com

SYCOM Healthcare Products & Services
568 Grand Canyon Drive
Madison, WI 53719
1-800-356-8141
www.sycom.com

Chapter Outline

Dental Benefits Programs
  Indemnity
  Capitation
  Alternative Benefit Plans
Preparing Dental Claim Forms
  Paper Claim Form
  Electronic Claim Form
    Clearinghouse Method
    Direct to Carrier Method
  Code on Dental Procedures and Nomenclatures
Coordination of Benefits
  Determining the Order of Liability
Reviewing the Completed Claim Form
Payment Voucher and Check
Medicaid Claim Forms
Veterans Administration Claim Form
Guidelines for Preparing Claim Forms
Insurance Fraud

Learning Outcomes

Mastery of the content in this chapter will enable the reader to:
- Identify the four parties affected by dental benefit plans
- Differentiate among the different dental plan models
- Use the current American Dental Association (ADA) Code on Dental Procedures and Nomenclature and the *Code of Dental Terminology* (CDT) manual
- Complete an ADA form
- Submit Medicaid dental benefit claims
- Apply the rules for coordination of benefits
- Explain common dental benefit and claims terminology

In the early 20th century, **dental insurance** and dental benefits programs did not exist. Their emergence and rapid growth have helped to change the general perception of dentistry, transforming it in the public eye from a feared, undervalued profession into a regular and necessary part of healthcare, a vital part of the maintenance of overall quality of life.

As dental benefits became more available, oral health improved, and today the connection between oral health and overall general health is clear. In 1970 only 6% of Americans had dental coverage. Currently, nearly half of the nation's population is covered by employer-sponsored dental insurance. Because of the increasing availability of comprehensive dental care, more people are keeping their natural dentition throughout their lifetimes, and deadly diseases, such as diabetes, oral cancer, and acquired immunodeficiency syndrome (AIDS), can be detected through regular periodic examinations.

The process of dental insurance involves four parties: the patient, the group or program sponsor (e.g., employer, union, or business association), the dental benefits carrier, and the dentist.

1. *Patient.* In the past, most people sought dental treatment only when they were in pain or for emergencies. Now, individuals who were not motivated to seek treatment are going to the dentist because they have dental benefits, and they continue treatment once they learn how important regular dental care is to maintaining good overall health. Many patients see their dentist more often than their physician. NOTE: It is important to inform patients that, even though they are covered by a dental benefits program, they ultimately are liable for all treatment fees.

2. *Group* or *program sponsor (e.g., employer, union, or business association).* This group generally is represented by a benefits manager, who is responsible for purchasing the most comprehensive benefits plan at the lowest price.

3. *Dental benefits carrier.* This may be an **insurer, a third-party administrator (TPA), or a dental service corporation.** The group selects the benefits, levels of coverage, and payment model, and the carrier administers the program.

4. *Dentist.* Most dental offices work closely with carriers to help patients make the best use of their benefits. The dentist's primary commitment is to discuss and render necessary treatment, to establish and maintain the patient's oral health, and to adhere to the standards of care that prevail in the professional community.

For the process to succeed, a system of communication and information sharing must connect all four parties. The dental office administrative assistant is a key partner in this process. The administrative assistant communicates with the dentist regarding services, coding, and fees for treatment; with the patient to verify carrier information, benefits, and payment acceptance; and with the carrier for billing, payment, and benefit information. This job requires organization, perseverance, and strict attention to detail.

DENTAL BENEFITS PROGRAMS

The dental carrier's method of **reimbursement** depends on the dental plan design. The two basic models of benefits programs are indemnity and capitation, although many variations of each model exist.

Indemnity

Indemnity programs are most often referred to as *fee-for-service programs.* This type of program provides payment on a service-by-service basis, and reimbursement may be made to the enrollee or, by assignment, to the dentist. The following list presents types of fee-for-service programs.

- **Usual, customary, and reasonable (UCR) plan:** Payment for covered benefits is based on a combination of usual, customary, and reasonable fee criteria.
- **Reasonable and customary (R&C) plan:** Payment for covered benefits is based on reasonable and customary fee criteria.
- **Preferred provider organization (PPO) plan:** A participating dentist agrees to accept discounted fees for covered services rendered to plan enrollees.
- **Exclusive provider organization (EPO) plan:** Benefits are provided only if care is rendered by institutional and professional providers with whom the plan contracts. Some exceptions may be allowed for emergency and out-of-area services.
- **Point of service plan:** Benefits carrier reimbursement levels are determined by the participation status of the dentist rendering treatment.
- **Table of allowances plan:** Covered services have an assigned dollar amount that represents the total dollar amount payable for each service.
- **Open panel system:** Any licensed dentist may participate, enrollees may receive dental treatment from any licensed dentist, and benefits may be payable to either the enrollee or the dentist, and the dentist may accept or refuse any enrollee.
- **Closed panel system:** Enrollees can only receive benefits when services are provided by dentists who have signed an agreement with the benefit plan to provide treatment to eligible patients.

Capitation

Capitation is a benefits delivery system in which a dentist contracts with the program's sponsor or **administrator** to provide all or most of the dental services covered under the program in return for a fixed monthly payment per covered person (per capita). Such a program is also called a **dental health maintenance organization (DHMO),** and it typically is a closed panel system; that is, enrollees select a primary care dental office from a list of participating providers, and they go to that office for all their dental care unless the primary care dentist provides a written referral to a specialist. Generally some exceptions are made for emergency and out-of-area services. Enrollees usually have no out-of-pocket costs for routine services, although they may have a **copayment** for more extensive, expensive services, such as fixed bridges.

Many dental benefits carriers recruit dentists to participate in their programs. Although the dentist may be required to discount fees to enrollees, participation is a proven method of practice building and simplification of administration. Generally, when dentists sign a participation contract with a benefits carrier, they agree to certain terms and conditions of payment for services rendered to enrollees. Each carrier has a unique set of terms of participation, which may include accepting the carrier's fee table (no **balance billing** or unbundling of fees), receiving **assignment of benefits,** and filing claims for enrollees.

Alternative Benefit Plans

Employers or associations may elect to offer an **alternative benefit plan** for supplemental dental coverage. In most cases the enrollee pays the dentist directly. The following are examples of this type of plan.

- *Discount card.* Large employers or associations may contract with dentists or dental clinics to deliver dental services to their enrollees for a discounted rate.

The enrollee usually pays an enrollment fee and/or monthly fee and pays the dentist directly. With this program the dentist does not file claims, and the plan has no **exclusions, limitations,** or maximums.

- *Health savings account (HSA).* The federal government allows eligible employers to offer their employees a pretax salary savings account for payment assistance with healthcare-related expenses. The maximum amount employees can contribute is $4000 a year for eligible medical, dental, vision, and prescription expenses. Contributions to the account are made by payroll deduction, and employees save money because no federal or state taxes or Federal Insurance Contributions Act (FICA) withdrawals are taken out of their earnings. Patients with an HSA pay the dentist, submit a receipt to their employer, and receive reimbursement up to the limit they have selected for the HSA.
- **Direct reimbursement.** An employer or organization can set up a self-funded program for reimbursing covered individuals based on a percentage of the amount spent for dental care.

PREPARING DENTAL CLAIM FORMS

The administrative assistant or other clerical staff can prepare and submit a **claim form** either on paper or electronically. With both formats, the same information is required on all claim forms.

Paper Claim Form

Although some dental benefits carriers have their own claim form, most accept paper claims submitted on an ADA claim form. The ADA provides a standardized format for dental claim forms that includes comprehensive completion instructions (Figure 14-1). The form may be purchased from the ADA or through most dental supply vendors; it also can be provided by the patient or downloaded from most carriers' websites.

The administrative assistant can legibly print or type the information on the claim form or, if the office is computerized, generate and print the form from the software database. The assistant then batches the claim forms and mails them to the carriers. Some carriers require x-ray films or documentation for a limited number of services, such as fixed bridges or miscellaneous procedures. However, sending unnecessary films or documentation may slow down processing and payment. The assistant can check with the carrier to verify which procedure codes require x-ray films or documentation.

Electronic Claim Form

In computerized offices with access to the Internet, claim forms can be filed electronically. Under a provision of the **Health Insurance Portability and Accountability Act of 1996 (HIPAA),** effective October 2002, all healthcare providers, health plans, and healthcare clearinghouses that transmit data electronically must use a universal language and a standard format. The universal language is the ADA **Code on Dental Procedures and Nomenclature,** which is updated every 2 years (Figure 14-2) Most dental software companies have updated their programs to conform to this requirement. The claim form is also an ADA standardized electronic document. Attachments to the claim form, such as x-ray films, can also be submitted electronically, although special software and scanning equipment are required.

Claims can be filed electronically either through a clearinghouse or directly with the carrier.

ADA. Dental Claim Form

HEADER INFORMATION

1. Type of Transaction (Check all applicable boxes)

☐ Statement of Actual Services   ☐ Request for Predetermination / Preauthorization

☐ EPSDT / Title XIX

2. Predetermination / Preauthorization Number

PRIMARY PAYER INFORMATION

3. Name, Address, City, State, Zip Code

OTHER COVERAGE

4. Other Dental or Medical Coverage?   ☐ No (Skip 5-11)   ☐ Yes (Complete 5-11)

5. Other Insured's Name (Last, First, Middle Initial, Suffix)

6. Date of Birth (MM/DD/CCYY)   7. Gender ☐ M ☐ F   8. Subscriber Identifier (SSN or ID#)

9. Plan/Group Number   10. Patient's Relationship to Other Insured (Check applicable box) ☐ Self ☐ Spouse ☐ Dependent ☐ Other

11. Other Carrier Name, Address, City, State, Zip Code

PRIMARY INSURED INFORMATION

12. Name (Last, First, Middle Initial, Suffix), Address, City, State, Zip Code

13. Date of Birth (MM/DD/CCYY)   14. Gender ☐ M ☐ F   15. Subscriber Identifier (SSN or ID#)

16. Plan/Group Number   17. Employer Name

PATIENT INFORMATION

18. Relationship to Primary Insured (Check applicable box) ☐ Self ☐ Spouse ☐ Dependent Child ☐ Other   19. Student Status ☐ FTS ☐ PTS

20. Name (Last, First, Middle Initial, Suffix), Address, City, State, Zip Code

21. Date of Birth (MM/DD/CCYY)   22. Gender ☐ M ☐ F   23. Patient ID/Account # (Assigned by Dentist)

RECORD OF SERVICES PROVIDED

	24. Procedure Date (MM/DD/CCYY)	25. Area of Oral Cavity	26. Tooth System	27. Tooth Number(s) or Letter(s)	28. Tooth Surface	29. Procedure Code	30. Description	31. Fee
1								
2								
3								
4								
5								
6								
7								
8								
9								
10								

MISSING TEETH INFORMATION

34. (Place an 'X' on each missing tooth)

Permanent: 1 2 3 4 5 6 7 8 9 10 11 12 13 14 15 16 / 32 31 30 29 28 27 26 25 24 23 22 21 20 19 18 17

Primary: A B C D E F G H I J / T S R Q P O N M L K

32. Other Fee(s)

33. Total Fee

35. Remarks

AUTHORIZATIONS

36. I have been informed of the treatment plan and associated fees. I agree to be responsible for all charges for dental services and materials not paid by my dental benefit plan, unless prohibited by law, or the treating dentist or dental practice has a contractual agreement with my plan prohibiting all or a portion of such charges. To the extent permitted by law, I consent to your use and disclosure of my protected health information to carry out payment activities in connection with this claim.

X _____
Patient/Guardian signature   Date

37. I hereby authorize and direct payment of the dental benefits otherwise payable to me, directly to the below named dentist or dental entity.

X _____
Subscriber signature   Date

BILLING DENTIST OR DENTAL ENTITY (Leave blank if dentist or dental entity is not submitting claim on behalf of the patient or insured/subscriber)

48. Name, Address, City, State, Zip Code

49. Provider ID   50. License Number   51. SSN or TIN

52. Phone Number (   )   –

ANCILLARY CLAIM/TREATMENT INFORMATION

38. Place of Treatment (Check applicable box) ☐ Provider's Office ☐ Hospital ☐ ECF ☐ Other

39. Number of Enclosures (00 to 99) Radiograph(s) Oral Image(s) Model(s)

40. Is Treatment for Orthodontics? ☐ No (Skip 41-42) ☐ Yes (Complete 41-42)

41. Date Appliance Placed (MM/DD/CCYY)

42. Months of Treatment Remaining   43. Replacement of Prosthesis? ☐ No ☐ Yes (Complete 44)   44. Date Prior Placement (MM/DD/CCYY)

45. Treatment Resulting from (Check applicable box) ☐ Occupational illness/injury ☐ Auto accident ☐ Other accident

46. Date of Accident (MM/DD/CCYY)   47. Auto Accident State

TREATING DENTIST AND TREATMENT LOCATION INFORMATION

53. I hereby certify that the procedures as indicated by date are in progress (for procedures that require multiple visits) or have been completed and that the fees submitted are the actual fees I have charged and intend to collect for those procedures.

X _____
Signed (Treating Dentist)   Date

54. Provider ID   55. License Number

56. Address, City, State, Zip Code

57. Phone Number (   )   –   58. Treating Provider Specialty

©2002, 2004 American Dental Association
J515 (Same as ADA Dental Claim Form – J516, J517, J518, J519)

To Reorder call 1-800-947-4746
or go online at www.adacatalog.org

A

Figure 14-1 Front **(A)** and back **(B)** of an ADA dental claim form. (Courtesy American Dental Association, Chicago, IL.)

Comprehensive completion instructions for the ADA Dental Claim Form are found in Section 6 of the ADA Publication titled CDT-2005. Key extracts from that section of CDT-2005 follow:

GENERAL INSTRUCTIONS

    A. The form is designed so that the Primary Payer's (primary insurance company) name and address (Item 3) are visible in a standard #10 window envelope. Please fold the form using the 'tick-marks' printed in the margin.

    B. In the upper-right of the form, a blank space is provided for the convenience of the payer or insurance company, to allow the assignment of a claim or control number.

    C. All Items in the form must be completed unless it is noted on the form or in the comprehensive instructions that completion is not required.

    D. When a name and address field is required the full name of an individual or a business, address and zip code must be entered.

    E. All dates must include the four-digit year.

    F. If the number of procedures reported exceeds the number of lines available on one claim form, the remaining procedures must be listed on a separate, fully completed claim form.

COORDINATION OF BENEFITS (COB)

When a claim is being submitted to a secondary payer, complete the form in its entirety and attach the primary payers Explanation of Benefits (EOB) showing the amount paid by the primary payer. You may indicate the amount the primary carrier paid in the "Remarks" field (Item # 35).

ITEMS OF NOTE

    39. <u>Number of Enclosures (00 to 99)</u>: This item is completed whether or not radiographs, oral images, or study models are submitted with the claim. If no enclosures are submitted, enter 00 in each of the boxes to verify that nothing has been sent and therefore no possible attachments are missing.

        When supplementary material is sent with the claim, the number of each type is entered in the appropriate box, using two digits. If less than 10, use 0 in the first position. 'Oral Images' include digital radiographic images and photographs and are reported by the number of images.

    43. <u>Replacement of Prosthesis?</u>: This Item applies to Crowns and all Fixed or Removable Prostheses (e.g. bridges and dentures). Please review the following three situations in order to determine how to complete this Item.

        a) If the claim does not involve a prosthetic restoration check "NO" and proceed to Item 45.

        b) If the claim is for the initial placement of a crown, or a fixed or removable prosthesis, check "NO" and proceed to Item 45.

        c) If the patient has previously had these teeth replaced by a crown, or a fixed or removable prosthesis, or the claim is to replace an existing crown, check the "YES" field and complete section 44.

    53. <u>Certification</u>: Signature of the treating or rendering dentist and the date the form is signed. This is the dentist who performed, or is in the process of performing, procedures indicated by date for the patient. If the claim form is being used to obtain a pre-estimate or pre-authorization, it is not necessary for the dentist to sign the form. Dentists should be aware that they have an ethical and legal obligation to refund fees for services that are paid in advance but are not completed.

PROVIDER TAXONOMY CODES

    58. <u>Treating Provider Specialty</u>: Enter the code that indicates the type of dental professional who delivered the treatment. Available codes describing treating dentists are listed below. The general code listed as 'Dentist' may be used instead of any other dental practitioner code.

Category / Description Code	Code
Dentist / A dentist is a person qualified by a doctorate in dental surgery (D.D.S) or dental medicine (D.M.D.) licensed by the state to practice dentistry, and practicing within the scope of that license.	122300000X
General Practice / Many dentists are general practitioners who handle a wide variety of dental needs.	1223G0001X
Dental Specialty / Other dentists practice in one of the nine specialty areas recognized by the American Dental Association.	Various (see following list)
Dental Public Health	1223D0001X
Endodontics	1223E0200X
Orthodontics	1223X0400X
Pediatric Dentistry	1223P0221X
Periodontics	1223P0300X
Prosthodontics	1223P0700X
Oral & Maxillofacial Pathology	1223P0106X
Oral & Maxillofacial Radiology	1223D0008X
Oral & Maxillofacial Surgery	1223S0112X

Dental provider taxonomy codes listed above are a subset of the full code set that is posted at:
http://www.wpc-edi.com/codes/codes.asp

Any updates to ADA Dental Claim Form completion instructions
will be posted on the ADA's web site at:
www.ada.org/goto/dentalcode

ADA.

American Dental Association
www.ada.org

B

Figure 14-1 Cont'd

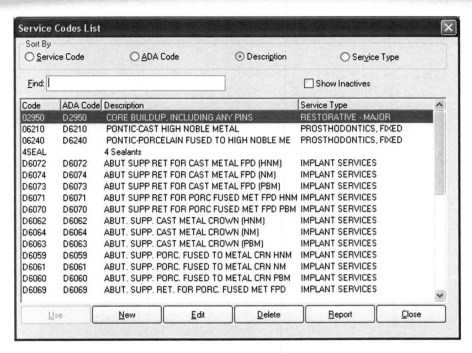

Figure 14-2 Pull-down screen of ADA service codes. (Courtesy Patterson-EagleSoft, Effingham, IL.)

CLEARINGHOUSE METHOD. With the clearinghouse method, batches of claims are transmitted to a clearinghouse, which scans the forms for errors or missing information and transmits error-free claims to the appropriate carrier. Claims with errors are electronically returned to the dental office for correction and resubmission. The clearinghouse prints and mails a paper claim for the few carriers unable to accept electronic claims. The advantages of using a clearinghouse are verification of claims and distribution of batches to multiple carriers. The disadvantage is the per-claim charge, which ranges from 25¢ to 75¢.

DIRECT TO CARRIER METHOD. With the direct to carrier method, the dental office staff sorts claims according to carrier and transmits the claims for each carrier separately. The carrier receives electronic claims the same day they are transmitted, and because the claims enter the carrier's processing system directly, turnaround time is reduced by an average of 2 to 4 days. Claim payment statements generally are available from the carrier's website, which can be accessed only by submitting the dentist's password. Many carriers also offer electronic funds transfer (direct deposit) of claim payments to the dental office's bank account. If both of these electronic systems are used, the benefit payment can reach the dental office's bank account within 24 to 48 hours of transmission of the claim.

Code on Dental Procedures and Nomenclature

As mentioned previously, the ADA's Code on Dental Procedures and Nomenclature (commonly known as *the Code*) is used to report dental services and procedures to dental benefits plans. These procedure codes identify and describe each specific dental treatment. The codes and the dentist's fees are used to report and bill treatment to the benefits carrier. Each procedure

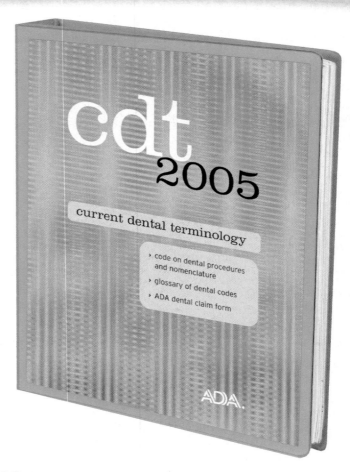

Figure 14-3 *Current Dental Terminology* (CDT), published by the American Dental Association. (Courtesy American Dental Association, Chicago, IL.)

code starts with a *D* followed by four numerals. The codes are categorized according to types of treatment:

Diagnostic	D0100–D0999
Preventive	D1000–D1999
Restorative	D2000–D2999
Endodontics	D3000–D3999
Periodontics	D4000–D4999
Prosthetics, removable	D5000–D5899
Maxillofacial prosthetics	D5900–D5999
Implant services	D6000–D6199
Prosthodontics, fixed	D6200–D6999
Oral surgery	D7000–D7999
Orthodontics	D8000–D8999
Adjunctive general services	D9000–D9999

Current Dental Terminology (CDT), which is published by the ADA, includes all the current dental procedure codes, their nomenclature and descriptors, changes in the code, an example and explanation of the ADA claim form, and a glossary of terms[1] (Figure 14-3). Every dental office should have a copy of the CDT, which can be ordered from the ADA by calling 800-947-4746 or through the association's website at www.ada.org.

COORDINATION OF BENEFITS

Coordination of benefits (COB) is the procedure used to pay healthcare expenses when a person is covered by more than one plan. Dental benefits carriers follow rules established by state law in deciding which plan pays first (i.e., the **primary carrier**) and how much the other plan or plans must pay. The objective is to provide the **maximum allowable benefit (MAB)** without exceeding the actual fee charged.

Some programs limit the scope of benefits coordination. For example, many contracts have a **nonduplication of benefits** clause, also called a *carve-out*. Reimbursement is limited to the higher amount allowed by the two contracts rather than a total of 100%. Other groups deny coordination of benefits to spouses who are both employees in the same group, although dual coverage of their **dependents** may be allowed. Spouses covered by employee-only programs do not have dual coverage.

Determining the Order of Liability

To identify the primary plan, the administrative assistant first must determine whether the patient is the subscriber or a dependent and whether the other plan has any special rules about coordination. The following sequence shows the order for identifying the primary plan.

1. *Employee/subscriber.* The plan covering the patient as an employee (subscriber) is always primary over a plan covering the person as a retiree, dependent, or COBRA-qualified beneficiary. If the patient is the subscriber for both plans, the plan covering the person as an active member is primary. If the subscriber is an active member under both plans, the plan that has covered the individual the longest is primary.

2. *Children/dependents.* Most carriers follow the **birthday rule;** that is, the plan of the parent with the first birthday in a calendar year is primary for the children. For example, if the mother's birthday is in January and the father's birthday is in March, the mother's plan is primary for all their children. Some plans may have a different coordination rule, such as the **gender rule,** under which the father's plan is always primary.

3. Children/dependents whose parents are divorced or legally separated. If a court decree makes one parent responsible for healthcare expenses, that parent's plan is primary. If a court decree does not mention healthcare, the following sequence applies for determining the order of liability:
   * Natural parent with custody
   * Spouse of natural parent with custody
   * Natural parent without custody
   * Spouse of natural parent without custody.

The primary carrier's claim is always filed first. If payment by the primary carrier leaves an unpaid balance, a claim can be submitted to the next liable, or secondary, carrier. A copy of the primary carrier's payment voucher should be attached, and the total amount paid by the primary carrier must be indicated in the field reserved for the primary carrier's payment (if any) or in the *Remarks* section.

REVIEWING THE COMPLETED CLAIM FORM

Figure 14-4, *A*, is an example of a claim form generated on a computer for a patient who was treated by Ashley Lake, DDS, and who is covered by Delta Dental Plan of Michigan. Entering the description is not necessary. This treatment plan includes the following information:

Tooth Number	Treatment	Procedure Number
	Periodic examination	D0120
	Complete series x-ray films	D0210
	Adult prophylaxis	D1110

Figure 14-4, *B,* is a claim for a patient of Dr. Lake who required restorative dentistry.

Tooth Number	Treatment	Procedure Number
3	High noble metal	D2790
4	High noble metal	D2790
13MO	Amalgam/two surfaces	D2150
14^{MOD}	Amalgam/three surfaces	D2160

A close look at these entries points up the importance of using and understanding the standardized codes. The codes for the two- and three-surface amalgam restorations are found in the list of restorative codes. The number of surfaces for the restoration determines the code number.

PAYMENT VOUCHER AND CHECK

Most carriers provide a voucher explaining the claim payment (Figure 14-5). However, a few do not send a voucher, which makes matching the payment with the patient's claim more difficult. The administrative assistant is responsible for recording this information accurately.

MEDICAID CLAIM FORMS

Medicaid is a federal assistance program established as Title XIX under the Social Security Act of 1965. It provides payment for healthcare for certain low-income individuals and families. The program is funded jointly by the federal and state governments and is administered by each state. Medicaid should not be confused with Medicare, which only subsidizes medical expenses for citizens 65 years of age or older.

Medicaid provides comprehensive dental benefits to low-income children and young adults under age 21 as required by federal law. Dental coverage for adults enrolled in Medicaid may be limited by the state. Eligibility for Medicaid programs is determined by the state and is generally limited to individuals receiving public financial assistance.

Because each state administers its own Medicaid program, rules and regulations governing covered dental services vary. Most programs have the following general conditions:

* The dentist agrees to accept the amount paid by the state (or any carrier designated by the state) as payment in full; there is no patient copayment.
* Any other third-party payer is primary.
* Reimbursement to the state is required if the patient or dentist receives payment from another third-party source.
* Records must be retained for a specified length of time and may be reviewed by an authorized state or federal official.
* Patients with Medicaid coverage may not be discriminated against for reasons of race, gender, color, creed, or financial status.
* Reimbursement is made only to dentists participating in the Medicaid program.
* All claims must be submitted within 12 months of the date of treatment.
* Prior authorization is required for certain treatments as outlined by the state.
* All patient records remain confidential.
* Handwritten forms are not accepted; forms must be typewritten, computer generated, or submitted electronically.

Medicaid offices of the federal government accept the standard ADA claim form, which may be submitted electronically to the nearest office. In some states the Medical Services Administration (MSA) has contracted with Delta

ATTENDING DENTIST'S STATEMENT
MAIL ORIGINAL TO:

△ **DELTA DENTAL**

P.O. Box 9085
Farmington Hills, Michigan 48333-9085

MARK (X) APPROPRIATE BOX

PLEASE TYPE ALL REQUIRED INFORMATION
SEE REVERSE FOR INSTRUCTIONS

| DENTIST'S STATEMENT OF ACTUAL SERVICES | X | DENTIST'S PRE-DETERMINATION REQUEST. | |

PATIENT & SUBSCRIBER INFORMATION

1. PATIENT NAME FIRST LAST MIDDLE INITIAL	2. PATIENT RELATIONSHIP TO SUBSCRIBER	3. PATIENT SEX	4. PATIENT BIRTHDATE
Rebecca Harris	SELF [X] SPOUSE CHILD OTHER	MALE FEMALE [X]	MM 03 DD 11 CC/YY 1963

5. SUBSCRIBER NUMBER	6. SUBSCRIBER BIRTHDATE	7. GROUP NUMBER	8. IF PATIENT IS A DEPENDENT OVER 19, PLEASE INDICATE STATUS
384-06-9122	MM 03 DD 11 CC/YY 1963	83300	FULL TIME STUDENT TOTALLY & PERM DISABLED IRS DEPENDENT SPONSORED DEPENDENT

9. SUBSCRIBER NAME FIRST LAST MIDDLE INITIAL	8a. ONLY FOR STATES ALLOWING ASSIGNMENT (SEE REVERSE): I HEREBY ASSIGN AND AUTHORIZE PAYMENT OF THE GROUP DENTAL BENEFITS OTHERWISE PAYABLE TO ME TO THE BELOW NAMED DENTIST, AND SIGN ON LINE 11 [X]
Rebecca Harris	

10. SUBSCRIBER MAILING ADDRESS	11. SUBSCRIBER SIGNATURE	DATE
421 Main	Signature on file	01/18/2005

12. CITY	STATE	ZIP CODE	13. EMPLOYER/COMPANY NAME
Grand Rapids	MI	49052	General Motors

IF PATIENT IS COVERED BY ANOTHER PLAN, COMPLETE ITEMS 14-24

14. SUBSCRIBER NAME FIRST LAST MIDDLE INITIAL	15. OTHER SUBSCRIBER NUMBER	16. BIRTHDATE MM DD CC/YY	17. GROUP NUMBER	18. AMOUNT OF PRIMARY PAYMENT $

19. MAILING ADDRESS	22. NAME OF OTHER CARRIER

20. CITY	STATE	ZIP CODE	23. CARRIER ADDRESS

21. NAME OF EMPLOYER	24. CITY	STATE	ZIP CODE

PROVIDER INFORMATION

IDENTIFY MISSING TEETH WITH "X"

25. PROVIDER BUSINESS NAME	26. PROVIDER TAX IDENTIFICATION NUMBER
Ashley Lake, D.D.S.	38-2546521

27. SERVICE OFFICE ADDRESS (NUMBER/STREET)	28. DDS LIC. NO.	29. STATE	30. SPEC. CD.
611 Main S.E.	53124	MI	

31. CITY	STATE	ZIP CODE	32. DENTIST PHONE NO.
Grand Rapids	MI	49052	(616) 101-9575

33. IS TREATMENT RESULT OF OCCUPATIONAL ILLNESS INJURY?	34. RADIOGRAPHS OR MODELS ENCLOSED?	HOW MANY?	35a. IS TREATMENT RELATED TO ORTHODONTICS?	35b. IF SERVICE ALREADY COMMENCED, DATE APPLIANCES PLACED MM DD CC/YY	35c. NUMBER OF ACTIVE MONTHS OF TREATMENT
No [X] Yes	No [X] Yes		No [X] Yes		

CAREFULLY FORM CHARACTERS AS SHOWN.   A B C D E F G H I J K L M N O P Q R S T U V W X Y Z 0 1 2 3 4 5 6 7 8 9

TOOTH NUMBER OR LETTER	SURFACE	DATE SERVICE PERFORMED MM DD YY	PROCEDURE NUMBER	FEE $ DOLLARS CENTS
		01 18 05	D 0 1 2 0	3 4 00
		01 18 05	D 0 2 1 0	1 1 0 00
		01 18 05	D 1 1 1 0	5 8 00

DO NOT TYPE IN SHADED AREA

REMARKS

I HEREBY CERTIFY THAT I HAVE PERFORMED THE PROCEDURES AS INDICATED BY DATE AND/OR WISH TO PREDETERMINE THE PROCEDURES WHICH ARE NOT DATED AND THE PROCEDURES WERE/ARE NECESSARY IN MY PROFESSIONAL JUDGEMENT.

SIGNED (DENTIST)	DATE	$ 202.00
Ashley Lake, D.D.S.	01/18/2005	TOTAL FEE CHARGED

241-02 (7-00)

COPYRIGHTED 1999

A

Figure 14-4 A, Computer-generated claim form. (Courtesy Delta Dental Plan of Michigan, Farmington Hills, MI.)

ATTENDING DENTIST'S STATEMENT
MAIL ORIGINAL TO:

△ DELTA DENTAL

P.O. Box 9085
Farmington Hills, Michigan 48333-9085

MARK (X) APPROPRIATE BOX

PLEASE TYPE ALL REQUIRED INFORMATION
SEE REVERSE FOR INSTRUCTIONS

| DENTIST'S STATEMENT OF ACTUAL SERVICES | X | DENTIST'S PRE-DETERMINATION REQUEST. | |

PATIENT & SUBSCRIBER INFORMATION

1. PATIENT NAME FIRST   LAST   MIDDLE INITIAL
Frederick Johnson

2. PATIENT RELATIONSHIP TO SUBSCRIBER: SELF | SPOUSE [X] | CHILD | OTHER

3. PATIENT SEX: MALE [X] | FEMALE

4. PATIENT BIRTHDATE MM DD CC/YY: **08 21 1971**

5. SUBSCRIBER NUMBER: **277-80-1219**

6. SUBSCRIBER BIRTHDATE MM DD CC/YY: **10 01 1973**

7. GROUP NUMBER: **12184**

8. IF PATIENT IS A DEPENDENT OVER 19, PLEASE INDICATE STATUS: FULL TIME STUDENT | TOTALLY & PERM DISABLED | IRS DEPENDENT | SPONSORED DEPENDENT

9. SUBSCRIBER NAME FIRST   LAST   MIDDLE INITIAL
Susan Reyes-Johnson

8a. ONLY FOR STATES ALLOWING ASSIGNMENT (SEE REVERSE): I HEREBY ASSIGN AND [X] AUTHORIZE PAYMENT OF THE GROUP DENTAL BENEFITS OTHERWISE PAYABLE TO ME TO THE BELOW NAMED DENTIST, AND SIGN ON LINE 11

10. SUBSCRIBER MAILING ADDRESS
881 Sunapple Drive

11. SUBSCRIBER SIGNATURE: **Signature on file**   DATE: **01/18/2005**

12. CITY: **Grand Rapids**   STATE: **MI**   ZIP CODE: **49055**

13. EMPLOYER/COMPANY NAME: **Grand Rapids Schools**

IF PATIENT IS COVERED BY ANOTHER PLAN, COMPLETE ITEMS 14-24
14. SUBSCRIBER NAME FIRST   LAST   MIDDLE INITIAL

15. OTHER SUBSCRIBER NUMBER

16. BIRTHDATE MM DD CC/YY

17. GROUP NUMBER

18. AMOUNT OF PRIMARY PAYMENT $

19. MAILING ADDRESS

22. NAME OF OTHER CARRIER

20. CITY   STATE   ZIP CODE

23. CARRIER ADDRESS

21. NAME OF EMPLOYER

24. CITY   STATE   ZIP CODE

PROVIDER INFORMATION

IDENTIFY MISSING TEETH WITH "X"

25. PROVIDER BUSINESS NAME: **Ashley Lake, D.D.S.**

26. PROVIDER TAX IDENTIFICATION NUMBER: **38-2546521**

27. SERVICE OFFICE ADDRESS (NUMBER/STREET): **611 Main S.E.**

28. DDS LIC. NO.: **53124**

29. STATE: **MI**

30. SPEC. CD.

31. CITY: **Grand Rapids**   STATE: **MI**   ZIP CODE: **49052**

32. DENTIST PHONE NO.: **(616) 101-9575**

33. IS TREATMENT RESULT OF OCCUPATIONAL ILLNESS INJURY? No [X] Yes

34. RADIOGRAPHS OR MODELS ENCLOSED? No Yes [X] HOW MANY? **2**

35a. IS TREATMENT RELATED TO ORTHODONTICS? No [X] Yes

35b. IF SERVICE ALREADY COMMENCED, DATE APPLIANCES PLACED MM DD CC/YY

35c. NUMBER OF ACTIVE MONTHS OF TREATMENT

CAREFULLY FORM CHARACTERS AS SHOWN. A B C D E F G H I J K L M N O P Q R S T U V W X Y Z 0 1 2 3 4 5 6 7 8 9

TOOTH NUMBER OR LETTER	SURFACE	DATE SERVICE PERFORMED MM DD YY	PROCEDURE NUMBER	FEE $ DOLLARS CENTS
0 3		0 1 1 8 0 5	D 2 7 9 0	6 0 0 0 0
0 4		0 1 1 8 0 5	D 2 7 5 0	6 5 0 0 0
1 3	M O	0 1 1 8 0 5	D 2 1 5 0	7 8 0 0
1 4	M O D	0 1 1 8 0 5	D 2 1 6 0	9 5 0 0

DO NOT TYPE IN SHADED AREA

REMARKS

I HEREBY CERTIFY THAT I HAVE PERFORMED THE PROCEDURES AS INDICATED BY DATE AND/OR WISH TO PREDETERMINE THE PROCEDURES WHICH ARE NOT DATED AND THE PROCEDURES WERE/ARE NECESSARY IN MY PROFESSIONAL JUDGEMENT.

SIGNED (DENTIST): **Ashley Lake, D.D.S.**

DATE: **01/18/2005**

$ **1423.00**
TOTAL FEE CHARGED

241-02 (7-00)

COPYRIGHTED 1999

B

Figure 14-4 Cont'd B, Claim form for more complex restorative treatment. (Courtesy Delta Dental Plan of Michigan, Farmington Hills, MI.)

△ DELTA DENTAL® Claim Payment Statement

Delta Dental Plan of Michigan
P.O. Box 30416
Lansing, MI 48909-7916

1-800-462-7283

Check No.: 000000123A
Issue Date: 12/17/2004

Patient Name: Jimmy Patient
Date of Birth: 02/14/1996
Relationship Code: 03
Subscriber Name: James Patient
Dentist: I.M. Gentle
License No.: 00217 MI
Provider TIN: 987654321
Specialty: 000

Receipt Date: 12/16/2004

Document No.: A234567892
Document Type: 1
DELTAPREMIER

IMPORTANT: Claims submitted with dates of service on or after January 1, 2005, should be submitted with CDT-5 Codes. Claims submitted on or after January 1, 2005, with 2004 dates of service should be submitted with CDT-4 Codes.

Pay To: P=Provider
S=Subscriber

Tooth Code	Surface	Date of Service	Procedure Code	Submitted Amount	Approved Amount	CD	Allowed Amount	CD	% Co-Pay	Patient Payment	Plan Payment	Pay To
GROUP	NO.:	0204033		SUBGROUP	NO.:	1000						
28		12/14/04	D1510	198.00	198.00	20	198.00	20	100	.00	198.00	P
30	O	12/14/04	D2140	73.00	73.00	20	73.00	20	100	.00	73.00	P
T	MOL	12/14/04	D2160	99.00	99.00	20	99.00	20	100	.00	99.00	P
S		12/14/04	D7140	96.00	95.00	20	95.00	20	100	.00	95.00	P

Payment for these services is determined in accordance with the specific terms of the member's dental plan and/or Delta Dental's agreements with its participating dentists.
ANTI-FRAUD TOLL-FREE HOTLINE 1-800-524-0147. Insurance fraud significantly increases the cost of health care. If you are aware of any false information submitted to Delta Dental, you can help us lower these costs by calling our toll-free hotline. You do not need to identify yourself. Only ANTI-FRAUD calls can be accepted on this line.

Ortho Maximum Used: .00   Class I, II and Maximum Used: 623.50

Totals:	.00	465.00	
Subscriber Deductible:	.00		

PAID TO SUBSCRIBER
Net Amount: .00

PAID TO PROVIDER
Gross Amount: 465.00
R & D Withhold: .00
Net Amount: 465.00

221104 12/2004

Gentle I.M.
32 Molar Drive
Lansing, MI 48910-1234

Figure 14-5 Check and voucher from the insurance company. (Courtesy Delta Dental Plan of Michigan, Farmington Hills, MI.)

Dental or other companies to partially administer dental benefits for children and young adults covered by Medicaid. A national model for expanding access to dental services for low-income individuals under age 21, Healthy Kids Dental (HKD), was established in Michigan and replaces Medicaid in 37 Michigan counties. The program has no special claim form, and claims, inquiries, and eligibility requests are addressed to Delta Dental. Some other states, such as Tennessee, Alabama, Connecticut, and Vermont, have public-private partnerships set up to improve access to care. A copy of State Innovations to Improve Dental Access for Low-Income Children: A Compendium Update is available at www.ada.org/goto/medicaid.

VETERANS ADMINISTRATION CLAIM FORM

Veterans of the U.S. armed forces may be eligible for limited dental benefits. Patients with this coverage receive a claim form from the Veterans Administration to give to the attending dentist, and the form includes all information necessary to assess benefits. Prior approval of treatment usually is required.

GUIDELINES FOR PREPARING CLAIM FORMS

As an administrative assistant, you know that proper handling of insurance forms and maintaining a constant awareness of the status of all claims are vital to the success of a dental practice. The following guidelines can help you achieve those goals.

- Document each subscriber's scope of coverage (excluding maximums, limitations, and any **deductible**) and obtain the complete mailing address and telephone number for claims and inquiries. Note any special information the carrier requires.
- Keep the above materials organized in a notebook or file.
- Inform each patient about his or her benefits and the amount for which the patient is responsible.
- Set aside a specific time to complete the claim forms or prepare each claim form at the completion of treatment.
- Keep a current file or computer record of outstanding claims and review it regularly.
- When required, request preauthorization for treatment.
- Regularly verify and update patients' general information.
- Maintain an adequate supply of claim forms.
- Be accurate and answer all questions on the claim form completely, providing details as required. If a question does not apply, leave it blank. Add comments only for codes that require documentation, such as miscellaneous codes (D2999, D6199). Use the CDT-2005 manual as a reference; the nomenclature will state "by report."
- Whenever possible, attend seminars presented by benefits carriers to keep current on billing practices.

INSURANCE FRAUD

It is illegal to misrepresent treatment or to inaccurately report fees and dates of service to benefits carriers. The following actions, whether deliberate or unintentional, constitute fraud:

- Billing the benefits carrier for higher fees than the patient is charged
- Billing before completion of service
- Predating or postdating services on claim forms
- Improperly reporting treatment (e.g., listing a bony extraction instead of a simple extraction)
- Billing for services not rendered

Accuracy and honesty are crucial. Administrative assistants who help defraud benefits carriers may be liable to legal prosecution.

Key Terms

Administrator The person who manages or directs a dental benefits program on behalf of the program's sponsor.

Allowed amount The maximum dollar amount the benefit carrier allows for each dental procedure; it is not always the same as the approved amount.

Alternative benefit plan A plan other than conventional dental benefits coverage for reimbursing a participating dentist for providing treatment to an enrolled group of patients.

Approved amount The amount used by the benefit carrier as the basis of payment for a submitted fee.

Approved services Services included in the patient's covered benefits. Payment for these services is subject to plan maximums, limitations, and deductibles.

Assignment of benefits Authorization by the enrollee/patient for the dental benefits administrator to forward payment for covered services directly to the treating dentist.

Attending dentist's statement A form developed by the ADA that the dentist uses to bill or predetermine dental procedures for a dental benefits carrier. Also known as the *ADA dental claim form*.

Balance billing The practice of charging the patient the difference between the dentist's actual fee and the amount reimbursed by the benefits carrier, in addition to any copayment, deductible, or maximum.

Benefit plan summary A description or synopsis of employee benefits, which employers are legally required to distribute to employees. Also called the *summary plan description*.

Birthday rule A method of determining the primary carrier for dependent children who are covered by more than one dental plan. With this method, the primary payer is the parent with the earlier date of birth by month and day, without regard to the year of birth.

Cafeteria plan A health coverage system under which employers offer eligible employees a list of options for health insurance benefits, which may include several carriers and levels of coverage. Participants may receive additional, taxable cash compensation if they select less expensive benefits.

Capitation A benefits delivery system in which a dentist contracts with the program's sponsor or administrator to provide all or most of the dental services covered under the program in return for a fixed monthly payment per covered person.

Claim audit An administrative or a professional review of the services reported on a claim to verify information, determine the appropriateness of treatment, or propose acceptable alternative treatment.

Claim form The form used to file for benefits under a dental benefits program (also see *attending dentist's statement*).

Claimant A person who files a claim for benefits.

Closed panel A dental benefits program in which enrollees can receive benefits only when services are provided by dentists who have signed an agreement with the benefit plan to provide treatment to eligible patients. Generally, only a small percentage of practicing dentists in a given geographical area are contracted by the plan to provide dental services.

Code on Dental Procedures and Nomenclature A list of codes (and their descriptions) used to report dental services and procedures; also called simply *the Code*. The Code is published by the ADA and is updated every 2 years.

Copayment The amount or percentage of the dentist's fee that the patient is obligated to pay.

Covered charges Charges for services rendered or supplies furnished by a dentist that qualify as covered services and are paid for in whole or in part by the dental benefits program. These charges may be subject to deductibles, copayments, coinsurance, and annual or lifetime maximums as specified by the terms of the contract.

Covered services   Services for which payment is provided under the terms of the dental benefits program.

Current Dental Terminology (CDT)   A reference manual developed by the ADA that includes the Code on Dental Procedures and Nomenclature and other instructional tools for reporting dental services to dental benefits plans and administrators.

Customary fee   The fee level determined by a dental benefits carrier based on actual submitted fees for a specific dental procedure; it is used to establish the maximum payable amount for that specific procedure (also see *usual fee* and *reasonable fee*).

Deductible   The amount of dental expense the patient must pay before the dental plan benefits begin. A deductible may be an annual or a one-time charge and can vary in amount. Individual deductibles are applied to one person; family deductibles are satisfied by combining the expenses of all covered family members.

Dental benefits carrier   A corporation or other business that contracts with groups of consumers to administer dental insurance.

Dental health maintenance organization (DHMO)   A dental capitation plan in which comprehensive care is provided to enrollees through participating providers. The dental provider receives a monthly payment for each enrollee accepted, and enrollees generally are required to remain in the program for a specific period.

Dental insurance   A plan that helps covered individuals pay for the prevention, treatment, and care of dental disease and for treatment of accidents involving teeth.

Dental service corporation   A legally constituted, nonprofit organization that negotiates and administers contracts for dental care.

Dependents   Individuals such as a spouse and children who are legally and contractually eligible for benefits under a subscriber's dental benefits contract.

Direct billing   A billing system in which the dentist bills the patient the full amount for services rendered.

Direct reimbursement   An employer's or organization's self-funded program for reimbursing covered individuals based on a percentage of the amount spent for dental care.

Effective date   The date an individual and/or dependents become eligible for benefits under a dental benefits contract; also called the *eligibility date*.

Eligible person   A person who is eligible for benefits under a dental benefits contract; also called *covered* or *insured individual, member, enrollee,* and *beneficiary*.

Exclusions   Dental services that are not covered under a dental benefits program.

Exclusive provider organization (EPO) plan   A dental benefits program in which benefits are provided only if care is rendered by institutional and professional providers with whom the plan contracts. Some exceptions may be allowed for emergency and out-of-area services. Any dental benefits model can be structured as an EPO.

Expiration date   The date on which the dental benefits contract expires or the date an individual ceases to be eligible for benefits.

Extension of benefits   An extension of eligibility designed to ensure completion of treatment started before the expiration date. The duration is limited and generally expressed in days.

Fee-for-service plan   A dental benefits program in which dentists are paid on a service by service basis.

Fee schedule   A list of charges established by or agreed to by a dentist for specific dental services.

Gender rule   A method of determining the primary carrier for dependent children who are covered by more than one dental plan. With this method, the primary payer is the plan that covers the father.

Health Insurance Portability and Accountability Act of 1996
(HIPAA) A federal law that requires all health plans, healthcare clearinghouses, and any dentist who transmits health information electronically to use a standard format and the ADA procedure codes. Paper transactions are not subject to this legislation.

Individual practice association
(IPA) A legal entity organized and operated on behalf of individual participating dentists for the primary purpose of collectively entering into contracts to provide dental services to enrolled populations. Dentists may practice in their own offices and provide care to patients not covered by the contract as well as to IPA patients.

Insurer An organization that bears the financial risk for the cost of defined categories or services for a defined group of beneficiaries.

Limitations Restrictions stated in a dental benefits contract that limit coverage of treatment; such restrictions may include age, waiting periods, and frequency of certain services.

Maximum allowable amount The highest dollar amount payable by a third-party payer for a covered dental treatment.

Maximum allowable benefit
(MAB) The highest total dollar amount a dental benefits program pays toward the cost of dental care incurred by an individual or family in a specified period, such as a calendar year, a contract year, or a lifetime.

Medicaid A federal assistance program, established as Title XIX under the Social Security Act of 1965, that provides payment for medical care for certain low-income individuals and families. The program is funded jointly by the state and federal governments and administered by the states.

Nonduplication of benefits An optional dental benefits contract provision that limits coordination of benefits. Reimbursement is limited to the greater level allowed by the two contracts, rather than a total of 100% of the charges. Also called a *carve-out*.

Nonparticipating dentist A dentist who does not have a contractual agreement with a dental benefits carrier to provide dental care to enrollees of a dental benefits program.

Open enrollment The annual period during which employees can select from a choice of dental benefits programs.

Open panel A dental benefits program in which any licensed dentist may participate; enrollees may receive dental treatment from any licensed dentist, and benefits may be payable to either the enrollee or the dentist. The dentist also may accept or refuse any enrollee.

Overcoding Reporting a more complex and/or more expensive procedure than was actually performed.

Participating dentist A dentist who has a contractual agreement with a dental benefits carrier to render care to eligible individuals.

Peer review A process by which licensed dentists review the care provided to a dental patient; disputes regarding fees; cases submitted by carriers, patients, or dentists; or quality of care and appropriateness of treatment. The review panel typically is organized by the state dental association.

Point of service plan A dental benefits program in which the level of payment is based on the participation status of the dentist rendering treatment. Benefit levels are higher with lower patient copayments for services rendered by providers who participate with the enrollee's dental program. Covered services provided by out-of-network providers are reimbursed on a lower fee scale, with higher out-of-pocket costs for the enrollee.

Predetermination Submission of a treatment plan of proposed services to a dental benefits carrier requesting an estimate of payment for covered services. Predetermination is not a guarantee of payment and is subject to eligibility, deductibles, and maximum used-to-date when services are rendered. Some programs require predetermination of services expected to exceed a specific amount, such as $200. Also called *precertification,* *preauthorization, pretreatment estimate,* and *prior authorization.*

Preexisting condition An oral health condition that existed before a person enrolled in a dental program.

Preferred provider organization (PPO) plan A dental benefits program in which participating dentists agree to accept discounted fees for services rendered to patients enrolled in the program.

Premium The amount charged by a dental benefits carrier for coverage of a level of benefits for a specified time.

Primary carrier The third-party payer determined to have initial responsibility for benefit payment when two or more payers have liability.

Reasonable and customary (R&C) plan A fee for service dental benefits program in which payment of benefits is based on reasonable and customary fee criteria (also see *customary fee* and *reasonable fee*).

Reasonable fee The fee charged for a specific dental procedure, which takes into consideration the nature and severity of the condition treated and any medical or dental complications or unusual circumstances that may affect treatment.

Reimbursement Payment made by a third-party payer to an enrollee or to a dentist on behalf of the enrollee as repayment of expenses incurred for a covered service.

Schedule of benefits A list of dental services covered by the dental benefits program.

Table of allowances plan A dental benefits program in which covered services have an assigned amount that represents the total amount payable for each service. The payable amount may not represent the dentist's full fee for that service. Also called a *schedule of allowances.*

Third-party administrator (TPA) A claims payer that administers health benefits plans without assuming any financial risk.

Unbundling of procedures The division of a dental procedure into component parts, with a separate charge for each, resulting in a cumulative charge that is higher than a single fee for the complete procedure.

Usual, customary, and reasonable (UCR) plan A dental benefits program in which payment for covered benefits is based on a combination of usual, customary, and reasonable fee criteria (see *usual fee, customary fee,* and *reasonable fee*).

Usual fee The fee a dentist most frequently charges for a given dental service.

Waiting period The period between employment or enrollment in a dental program and the date the enrollee becomes eligible for benefits.

LEARNING ACTIVITIES

Part A
Explain or identify the following:
1. The four parties affected by dental benefits and the roles of each
2. The types of dental benefits programs
3. Completion of a standard ADA claim form
4. The Code on Dental Procedures and Nomenclature and how it is used
5. The differences between using a paper claim form and an electronic claim form
6. The purpose of the claim payment voucher
7. Five actions that constitute dental benefits fraud
8. Procedure codes that require documentation

LEARNING ACTIVITIES—cont'd

Part B

Use the following information to complete the ADA claim form (Working Form 16).
Using the patient's benefits information, estimate the expected benefit payment and
   the patient's copayment. The patient has not used any maximum to date.

Subscriber's Information

Name:	Lisa Ryan
Social Security #:	301–16–2791
Birth date:	04/22/86
Address:	217 Chestnut, Lansing, MI 48933
Employer:	Ace Finishing, Inc.
	Lansing, MI 48910 (Group #1267)
Benefits carrier:	Delta Dental Plan of Michigan
	P.O. Box 9085
	Farmington Hills, MI 48333–9085
Program type:	DeltaPremier (fee for service)
Benefits level:	Class I: 80%
	Class II: 50%
	No deductible
	Annual maximum: $1,500

Patient's Information

Name:	James Ryan
Relationship to employee:	Spouse
Social Security #:	337–70–1278
Birth date:	07/14/79
Address:	Above

Dentist's Information

Name:	Jane R. Smith, DDS
Address:	2841 W. Saginaw
	Lansing, MI 48917
TIN #:	386–74–1234
License #:	10042
Telephone #:	517–482–3000

The following services have been completed for Mr. Ryan:

Periodic examination	10/12/04	$30
Prophy	10/12/04	$60
#2^{MOD} amalgam	10/12/04	$85
#18 Crown–full cast high noble metal	Prep: 10/21/04	$550
	Seating: 11/01/04	
#19 Pontic–cast high noble metal	Prep: 10/21/04	$550
	Seating: 11/01/04	
#20 Crownporcelain fused to high noble metal	Prep: 10/21/04	$600
	Seating: 11/01/04	

Additional Information

Treatment is not the result of illness or injury; the bridge initial placement.
   Tooth #19 was extracted in 1997. There is no coordination of benefits.

EXAMINE YOUR PROGRESS

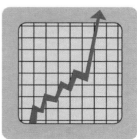

Practice by completing
Working Form 10.

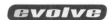

Reference

1. Council on Dental Benefit Programs: *Current dental terminology: CDT-4, CDT-2005,* Chicago, 1999, American Dental Association.

Bibliography

Delta Dental Plan of Michigan.
Michigan Department of Public Health, Bureau of Health Care Administration: *Dental services,* December 1994.

15 Bookkeeping Systems—Accounts Receivable

Chapter Outline

Learning Outcomes

Mastery of the content in this chapter will enable the reader to:

- Define key terms
- Define *bookkeeping*

- Define *accounting*
- Explain basic mathematical procedures
- Describe common bookkeeping systems in dentistry
- Explain the function of a computerized accounts receivable program
- Describe the components of a pegboard bookkeeping system
- Explain the procedures used in a pegboard bookkeeping system
- Explain the common systems of statement production
- Identify common payment and credit policies
- Describe the various laws affecting credit policies and collection procedures
- Identify common problems in maintaining a credit policy
- Identify the functions of a credit bureau
- Explain the function of a collection agency
- Compose collection letters

> The administrative assistant who maintains the business portion of the dental practice with a high degree of efficiency becomes a valuable asset.

Because dentistry is a business as well as a health profession, sound business practices must be integrated into the management of the dental office. Consequently, the administrative assistant who maintains the business portion of the dental practice with a high degree of efficiency becomes a valuable asset.

The two financial systems used in a dental business office are accounts receivable and accounts payable. The administrative assistant is responsible for both. The **accounts receivable** system includes all production; data are entered for treatment rendered and payments received, and new balances are calculated. After all computations have been made, the current accounts receivable amount, or the amount of money owed to the dentist (incoming money), is determined. **Accounts payable** refers to all the dentist's financial obligations, or money the dentist owes (outgoing money). This chapter discusses accounts receivable; Chapter 16 details accounts payable and other financial systems.

As mentioned in previous chapters, records management is a primary responsibility of the administrative assistant. Financial records are as important as clinical records but should be maintained separately. They provide (1) protection for both the dentist and the patient, (2) information for tax purposes, and (3) data for a business analysis. Inaccurate records result in poor public relations and may create unnecessary litigation with the state or federal government.

Bookkeeping, or the recording of financial transactions, is the responsibility of the administrative assistant. **Accounting,** which is the recording, classifying, and summarizing of financial and business records, generally is the job of the accountant. Most dentists have an accountant who audits the books and computes a variety of tax reports and financial statements.

UNDERSTANDING BASIC MATHEMATICAL COMPUTATIONS

Before you can become proficient at computing financial activity on various records, you must review some basic mathematical rules. Because computers are used to produce so many documents, it often is easy to forget how to perform basic calculations or compute percentages on insurance claim forms.

Although a computer can make the necessary calculations, you are responsible for entering the data in the appropriate fields to ensure that the final figures are accurate. You will often need to add and subtract figures with decimals and perform other business-related computations. Most people use manual or electronic calculators for these tasks; however, relying solely on technological devices without having an understanding of basic computation can result in embarrassment, patient dissatisfaction, and possibly loss of cash flow when errors are detected. The following descriptions cover basic mathematical procedures used for routine bookkeeping entries.

DECIMALS

Adding and Subtracting Decimals

Place the numbers to be added or subtracted in a vertical column, aligning the decimal points, before performing the addition or subtraction. To add columns of figures with decimals, add the numbers in each column, beginning with the column farthest to the right and working your way to the left:

$$
\begin{array}{r}
0.5 \\
2.8 \\
30.50 \\
67.945 \\
+\ 750.000 \\
\hline
851.745
\end{array}
$$

To subtract, follow the same procedure. Place the numbers to be subtracted in a vertical column, aligning the decimal points. Each amount must have the same number of decimals, therefore it may be necessary to add zeros before performing this procedure. For example, to subtract 1.75 from 3.876, add one zero at the end of the 1.75:

$$
\begin{array}{r}
3.876 \\
-1.750 \\
\hline
2.126
\end{array}
$$

Multiplying Decimals

To multiply decimals, perform the procedure as you would for all whole numbers, except the decimal point must be placed correctly in the answer. Count the number of digits to the right of the decimal point in the multiplicand and in the multiplier; then count the same number of places from right to left in the product and insert the decimal point:

600.75	2 decimals (multiplicand)
× .20	2 decimals (multiplier)
120.1500	2 + 2 = 4 decimals

or

$800.50	2 decimals
× .75	2 decimals
400250	
560350	
$600.3750	2 + 2 = 4 decimals

or

$800	0 decimals
× .75	2 decimals
$600.00	0 + 2 = 2 decimals

Percentages

Working with percentages is a common function of routine posting of accounts receivable. For example, if you are processing insurance claim forms manually, you must determine the subscriber and carrier percentages and any deductible amounts. In an automated system these figures are calculated for you, but again, you must understand this process to ensure accuracy. The following are examples of some very basic procedures.

To change a percent to a fraction, drop the percent sign, place the number over 100, and reduce the fraction to the lowest terms. If the numerator is a decimal, multiply both the numerator and denominator by an appropriate power of 10 to clear the decimal. For instance,

$$5\% = \frac{5}{100} = \frac{1}{20}$$

or

$$7.5\% = \frac{7.5}{100} = \frac{75}{1000} = \frac{3}{40}$$

To change a percent to a decimal, move the decimal point two places to the left and drop the percent sign.

$$15\% = 0.15$$
$$2\% = 0.02$$
$$110\% = 1.1$$

To find a certain percent of a number, convert the percent to a decimal and multiply by the number. For instance, the following computation shows how to calculate 80% of $670:

$$\$670$$
$$\times .80$$
$$\$536$$

TYPES OF BOOKKEEPING SYSTEMS

In the past, dentistry used a variety of bookkeeping systems, including the pegboard, or "write it once," system, which until the 1990s was the system most often used in dental offices. With the pegboard system, one notation provided an entry on the daily journal sheet, the ledger card, the **receipt,** and in some cases a statement. The system of choice now is a computer software program, which goes beyond the basic transactions of the pegboard system to provide all financial records, insurance claim forms, future appointments and recall management, and documents for practice analysis.

A computerized bookkeeping system can be integrated into total records management. In other words, you can make a clinical entry on a patient record that can then be transferred to a financial record. Using designated codes, you can transfer this information to a patient statement, and an insurance claim form can be generated from the original data entry. This type of system is more than just a mechanism for bookkeeping.

Components of a Computerized Bookkeeping System

Chapter 5 described the use of dental office management software. One component of most of these systems is the accounts receivable program. By entering data for a patient account, you can generate myriad reports, forms, or other types of information.

When a dentist purchases a software management program, some type of tutorial generally is provided, and you probably will be given some basic instruction in the use of the software. Once the software has been installed in the computer, you can begin entering basic patient clinical and financial data. To generate accounts receivable data, you generally follow specific steps outlined in the software package. The following description is an overview of some of the common steps in basic data entry. Although each software package has its own distinct features, most include these steps. Table 15-1 presents some common commands used in a variety of accounts receivable programs.

OPENING THE PROGRAM. When you open the program, you commonly are required to enter your name or your user name and a password. Generally, when you enter a password, the characters are not displayed on the screen as

Table 15-1
Common Commands in Accounts Receivable Software

Command	Meaning
ADD	Enter additional data; create a new record
APPOINTMENT/ SCHEDULER	Enter data for a patient appointment
DEL	Delete; to eliminate part or all of the data entry
EDIT	Alter or change data
ENTER	Insert data
ESC	Leave the screen
FILE	Open, close, print, or take action on files
INSURANCE	Make a data entry or obtain a hard copy of a claim form
LIST	Provides a screen view or hard copy of lists of patients, accounts, or other data
LOCATE	Find a patient, an account, or other data
N	No
PATIENT	Enter a field of patient records
POST	Enter data, financial or other
PRINT	Produce a hard copy of a document
RECALL	Enter data about a patient for recall
REPORTS	Obtain some form of report programmed into the system
SYSTEM	Change the system setting, log in, or password
TRANSACTION	Reference to financial activity
VIEW	Changes the format of the screen view
WINDOW	Allows a different configuration of the screen
WORD PROCESSOR	Program that allows letter writing
Y	Yes

you key them in. Most systems allow for reentry of your password in case you make an error, but after a specified number of entries, the program may abort.

LOCATING ACCOUNT INFORMATION. When you make a selection, such as Accounts, a drop-down screen opens; you then find a list, where you can click on Account, and a list of current accounts appears. A patient name can then be selected, and if the person is an existing patient, the account information window opens (Figure 15-1). If no account appears, one can be added by clicking on the Add icon and creating a new patient record (Figure 15-2). Certain basic account information is common to most systems, such as an ID number, dentist (the primary provider if an office has several dentists), user codes, name and address, personal data (e.g., telephone number or numbers, Social Security number, date of birth, gender, and age), insurance, employment, and special notes, such as last update, last payment, date of admission, and insurance numbers.

EDITING ACCOUNT INFORMATION. At times you will need to edit account information, such as when a patient's name or address changes. To do this, you enter the Account window and select Edit (*Edit* refers to the task of changing existing data).

ADDING OR DELETING A PATIENT. You may add patients to an account in the system shown by selecting ADD. This is commonly done to add a spouse or dependent to an account but also may be required in the case of marriage, divorce, or death or when older children are transferred to their own accounts. Likewise, you can delete a patient from the accounts by selecting DELETE while still in the account information screen. You will be asked to reply *Y* for yes or *N* for no to make sure you actually want to delete the account.

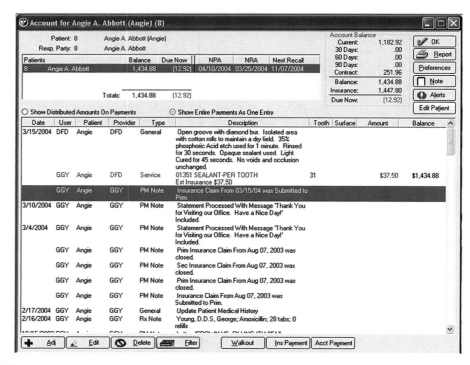

Figure 15-1 Account information screen. (Courtesy Patterson-EagleSoft, Effingham, IL.)

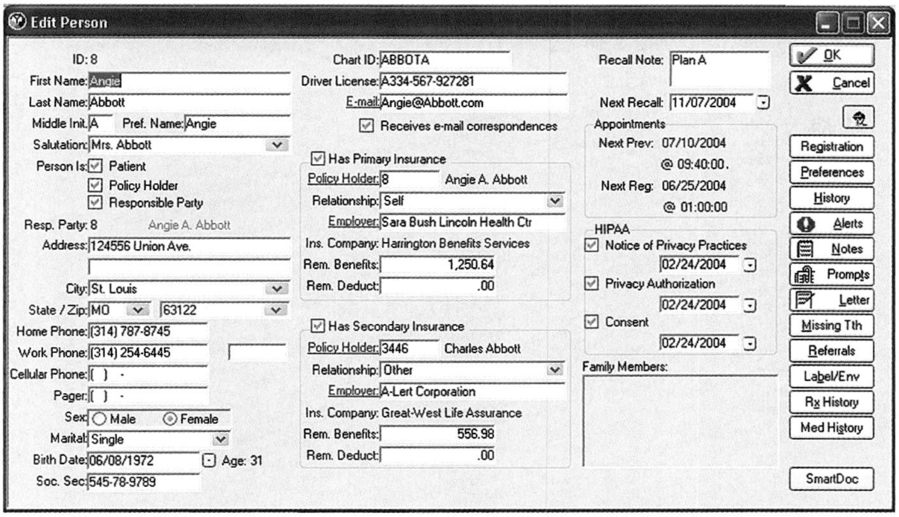

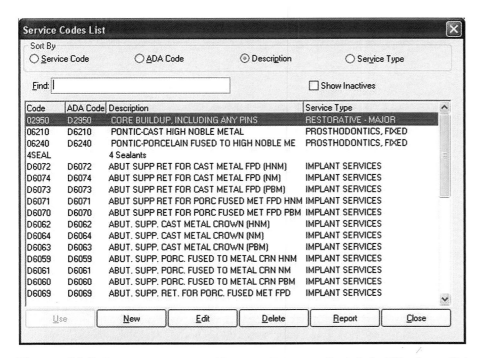

Figure 15-2 Patient information screen. (Courtesy Patterson-EagleSoft, Effingham, IL.)

POSTING TRANSACTIONS. Perhaps one of the most common daily activities in bookkeeping is entering transaction data. From the transaction screen (Figure 15-3), most systems are designed to allow you to enter clinical data about treatment, for which you may insert appropriate codes. When the data are entered, the program computes the financial activity and produces an account **balance.** Before these data are stored, you may be asked if an insurance claim form or other activity (e.g., recall or appointment scheduling) must be completed. Most programs ask you to respond with *Y* for yes or *N* for no to the series of questions. A walk out statement (Figure 15-4) and an insurance claim form can be generated after these data entries are complete.

Figure 15-3 Transaction screen. (Courtesy Patterson-EagleSoft, Effingham, IL.)

DENTAL ASSOCIATES, PC
Joseph W. Lake, DDS – Ashley M. Lake, DDS
611 Main Street, SE
Grand Rapids, MI 49502
(616) 101-9575

April 18, 2005

Account Aging	
Current	$55.00
30 Day	$0.00
60 Day	$0.00
90 Day	$0.00
Contract	$0.00
Balance Due	$55.00
Estimated Ins	$55.00
Balance Due Now	**$0.00**

Alice Patient
1234 Home Ave.
St. Charles, MO   63306

ID: 2886

Date	Provider	Transaction		Tth	Surface	Fee
04/18/05	Robert Morgan, D.D.S.	02150	AMALGAM-PERMANENT, 2 SURFACES	3	MO	93.75
			(Est Insurance $55.00)			
			Check Number 2335 for $38.75			
					Subtotal:	93.75

Tax:	0.00
Today's Charges:	93.75
- CheckToday's Payment:	38.75
+ Previous Balance:	0.00
Balance Due:	$55.00
- Estimated Insurance:	$55.00

Contract Balance	Estimated Insurance	Previous Balance	Charges Today	Payments Today	Adjustments Today	Balance Due Now
0.00	55.00	0.00	93.75	38.75	0.00	**0.00**

Future Family Appointments: None

THANK YOU FOR VISITING OUR OFFICE. HAVE A GREAT DAY!

Figure 15-4 Walk out statement. (Courtesy Patterson-EagleSoft, Effingham, IL.)

BACKING UP DATA. As mentioned earlier, maintaining all the practice data on a computer's hard drive is dangerous. Valuable information can be lost as the result of a power surge, computer crash, or misdirected ERASE or DEL command. For this reason, the hard drive must be backed up regularly. This can be done using a CD-ROM, DVD, or some other type of storage device. The office procedures manual must describe the backup procedure step by step, and a backup log must be maintained (Figure 15-5).

SPECIAL PROBLEMS

A day would not be complete without some unusual activity that cannot be recorded using the procedure exactly as listed previously. Several such situations and their solutions are presented in the following discussions.

A **credit balance** often occurs when payment is made in advance, as when a patient obtains a bank loan to pay for treatment. A credit balance of $50, for example, can be noted in three ways: (1) with the amount preceded by *CR* (CR$50); (2) with the amount preceded by a minus sign (–$50); and (3) with the amount, in color, enclosed in parentheses ($50) (Figure 15-6).

Each time treatment is rendered, charges are made against the credit balance, reducing it. Remember, the credit balance represents what is owed to the patient in services. Note that the credit balance is also shown when a patient pays on the account (Figure 15-7).

Nonsufficient funds (NSF) checks, or checks returned to the office for a lack of account funds, require some form of **adjustment** to the account. You may redeposit the check and not make an entry on the books. However, it may be necessary to charge the account with this returned check. Collection fees are paid to an agency for collecting a delinquent account, and these fees generally are deducted from the payment before it is sent to the dentist. Note that for the returned check in Figure 15-8, an NSF notation has been made and a service charge of $25 has been assessed to the account.

A courtesy discount is given when the dentist extends a professional courtesy to a patient. The courtesy discount is entered in the adjustment column (Figure 15-9).

STATEMENTS

A **statement** informs patients of their financial status with the dentist and indicates the charges, payments, and balances of their accounts for the month just concluded. The statement is also a request for payment. Statements may be sent on the first, fifteenth, or thirtieth day of the month or on a staggered basis according to the alphabet. The important factor is consistency; that is, be sure to send the statements at the same time each month.

A statement can be generated on the computer with an automated bookkeeping system (Figure 15-10). The itemized statement shows the dates of payments and the treatments for each member of the family during the month. With a computerized system, you can add special messages or aging columns to statements to enhance the collection process.

ESTABLISHING FINANCIAL ARRANGEMENTS

The adage, "Inform before you perform," still applies to the management of accounts in the dental office. A well-defined credit policy should be an integral part of the accounts receivable system. This policy must (1) conform to

BACKUP LOG

<u>Date</u>	<u>Disk/Tape</u>	<u>Initials</u>	<u>Storage Location</u>
_____	_____	_____	_____
_____	_____	_____	_____
_____	_____	_____	_____
_____	_____	_____	_____
_____	_____	_____	_____
_____	_____	_____	_____
_____	_____	_____	_____
_____	_____	_____	_____
_____	_____	_____	_____
_____	_____	_____	_____
_____	_____	_____	_____
_____	_____	_____	_____
_____	_____	_____	_____
_____	_____	_____	_____
_____	_____	_____	_____
_____	_____	_____	_____
_____	_____	_____	_____
_____	_____	_____	_____

Figure 15-5 Backup log.

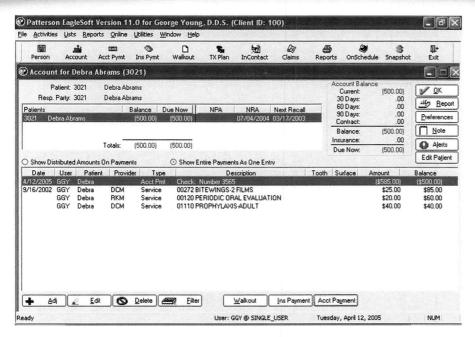

Figure 15-6 The current credit balance on the account is indicated in red and parentheses. (Courtesy Patterson-EagleSoft, Effingham, IL.)

community standards, (2) reflect the attitude of the dentist toward the patient's welfare, (3) represent sound business concepts, (4) be presented in written form to the patient, (5) provide options for the patient, and (6) be adhered to at all times. Many payment policies exist, therefore including this policy as part of the office policy is a wise move.

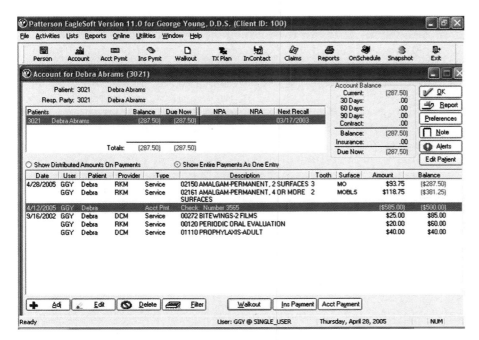

Figure 15-7 Credit is adjusted upon receipt of a payment by the patient. (Courtesy Patterson-EagleSoft, Effingham, IL.)

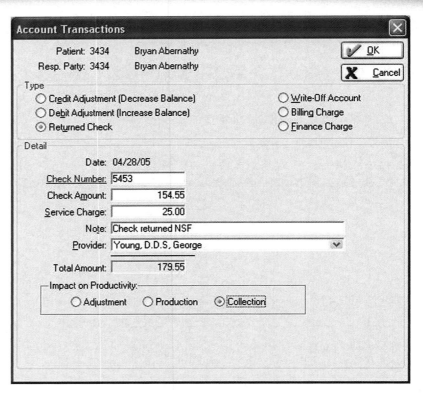

Figure 15-8 Account transaction screen indicates a nonsufficient funds (NSF) check with a service charge attached. (Courtesy Patterson-EagleSoft, Effingham, IL.)

Because financial arrangements generally are made by the administrative assistant, you must be well acquainted with the office credit policy. Furthermore, you must be firm yet polite in adhering to the policy and avoid becoming a victim of any of the following common situations.

1. The patient says he will take care of the bill in full when treatment has been completed. A patient having extensive restorative treatment should not be offended when you explain that office expenses and laboratory fees require some form of payment before completion of the treatment.
2. The patient becomes defensive or angry when you ask her about payment arrangements. Find out why she is irritated; patients with good intentions seldom become defensive when asked about payment.
3. The patient tells you he will pay the bill when his income tax refund or other windfall is received. You have no way of knowing whether he will actually receive the expected money or use it to pay his dental bills.
4. The patient makes promises and does not fulfill them. A consistent follow-up system must be initiated to eliminate such problems. Patients often become lax in their responsibility because the dental staff is not consistent.

Types of Payment Policies

Many payment policies are used in dentistry today, but a few are common to all practices.

CASH ONLY. The cash-only system obviously eliminates much paperwork in the business office, but it may place limitations on the dental practice.

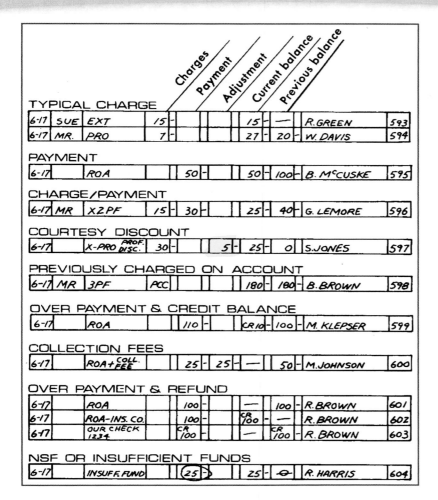

Figure 15-9 A courtesy discount is entered as credit to the account. (Courtesy Patterson-EagleSoft, Effingham, IL.)

PAYMENT OF STATEMENT IN FULL. Unless other arrangements have been made with the office, the patient is expected to pay in full within 10 days of receipt of the statement. Some form of notice, such as appropriate signage or a written policy statement, must be presented to the patient.

EXTENDED PAYMENT. Regulation 2 of the Truth in Lending Act requires that an agreement exist between the dentist and the patient if payment for services is to be made in more than four installments. Even if no finance charge is involved, the truth in lending form (Figure 15-11) must be completed to verify that such a payment agreement has been reached. In some areas this form has been modified to include an entry for insurance coverage. A payment booklet may be used to help the patient keep track of payments and to identify the payment when the slip is mailed with the check. This system is common in practices such as orthodontics.

USING A CREDIT BUREAU

Perhaps the best way to define a **credit bureau,** or *consumer reporting agency (CRA),* is to explain what it does not do: it does not lend money; it does not deny credit; and it is not a collection agency. A credit bureau reports specific information about a person's previous payment habits on deferred payment plans.

◼◼◼◼◼ MAKE CHECKS PAYABLE TO: ◼◼◼◼◼

DENTAL ASSOCIATES, PC
JOSEPH W. LAKE, DDS – ASHLEY M. LAKE, DDS
611 MAIN STREET, SE
GRAND RAPIDS, MI 49502

ADDRESS SERVICE REQUESTED

ACCOUNT NAME: JOHN Q. PATIENT
BILLING QUESTIONS, CALL: 000-000-0000

◼◼◼◼ ADDRESSEE: ◼◼◼◼

|ılıılıılllılıılllılılılılılılıııllıllıllıll|
JOHN Q. PATIENT
1234 STATE STREET
ANYTOWN, USA 12345-4321

IF PAYING BY MASTERCARD, DISCOVER, VISA OR AMERICAN EXPRESS, FILL OUT BELOW.
CHECK CARD USING FOR PAYMENT

☐ MASTERCARD   ☐ DISCOVER   ☐ VISA   ☐ AMERICAN EXPRESS

CARD NUMBER	AMOUNT
SIGNATURE	EXP. DATE

STATEMENT DATE	PAY THIS AMOUNT	ACCT. #
01/30/2005	$69.80	12345

PAGE NO. 1

SHOW AMOUNT PAID HERE	$

◼◼◼◼ REMIT TO: ◼◼◼◼

|ılıılıılllılıılllılılılılılılıııllıllıllıll|
DR. DENTIST D.D.S.
1234 STATE STREET
ANYTOWN, USA 12345-4321

PLEASE DETACH AND RETURN TOP PORTION WITH YOUR PAYMENT

STATEMENT

BALANCE FORWARD:

DATE	PATIENT	CODE	DESCRIPTION	AMOUNT
12/12/2004	JOHN Q. PATIENT	00130	PALLIATIVE EMERGENCY	$30.00
12/12/2004	JOHN Q. PATIENT	00220	INTRAORAL-PERIAPICAL FIRST FILM	$15.00
12/12/2004	JOHN Q. PATIENT	Acct. Paymnt	Check: Number 1443	-$45.00
12/13/2004	JOHN Q. PATIENT		Insurance Claim From 12/12/04 was Submitted to Prim.	
12/17/2004	JOHN Q. PATIENT	02386	RESIN-TWO SURFACES, POSTERIO-PERMANENT	$155.00
12/18/2004	JOHN Q. PATIENT		Insurance Claim From 12/17/04 was Submitted to Prim.	
01/13/2005	JOHN Q. PATIENT	Ins. Paymnt	Check: Number 2345 for claim from 12/17/04	-$15.20
01/14/2005	JOHN Q. PATIENT	Ins. Paymnt	Check: Number 5432 for claim from 12/12/04	-$30.00

Thank you for visiting our office.
Have a nice day.

TOTAL CHARGES:	**$109.80**
ESTIMATED INSURANCE PAYMENT:	**$ 40.00**
BALANCE DUE NOW:	$69.80

CURRENT	30 DAYS	60 DAYS	90 DAYS	EST. INSURANCE	ON CONTRACT	DUE DATE
$69.80				$ 40.00		02/15/2005

DR. DENTIST D.D.S.   108762

Figure 15-10 Computer-generated statement using ADA codes.

FINANCIAL AGREEMENT

For PROFESSIONAL SERVICES rendered or to be rendered to:

Patient ______________ Daytime Phone ______________

Parent if patient is a minor ______________

1. Cash price for services .... $ ______
2. Cash down payment .... $ ______
3. Charges covered by insurance service plan .... $ ______
4. Unpaid balance of cash price .... $ ______
5. Amount financed (the amount of credit provided to you) .... $ ______
6. **FINANCE CHARGE** (the dollar amount the credit will cost you). $ ______
7. **ANNUAL PERCENTAGE RATE** (the cost of credit as a yearly rate) .... ______ %
8. Total of payments (5 + 6 above-The amount you will have paid when you have made all scheduled payments) .... $ ______
9. Total sales price (1 + 6 above-Sum of cash price, financing charge and any other amounts financed by the creditor, not part of the finance charge) .... $ ______

You have the right at anytime to pay the unpaid balance due under this agreement without penality.
You have the right at this time to receive an itemization of the amount financed.
☐ **I want an itemization** ☐ **I do not want an itemization**

Total of payments (#8 above) is payable to Dr. ______________

in ______ monthly installments of $ ______ each and ______ installments of $ ______ each. The first installment being payable on ______ 19____ and subsequent installments on the same day of each consecutive month until paid in full.

NOTICE TO PATIENT

Do not sign this agreement if it contains any blank spaces. You are entitled to an exact copy of any agreement you sign. You have the right at any time to pay the unpaid balance due under this agreement.

The patient (parent or guardian) agrees to be and is fully responsible for total payment of services performed in this office including any amounts not covered by any health insurance or prepayment program the responsible party may have. See your contract documents for any additional information about nonpayment, default, any required prepayment in full before the scheduled date and prepayment refunds and penalties.

Signature of patient or one parent if patient is a minor:

X ______________

Doctor's Signature ______________

SCHEDULE OF PAYMENT

No.	Date Due	Amount of Installment	Date Paid	Amount Paid	Balance Owed
					Total Amount
D.P.					
1					
2					
3					
4					
5					
6					
7					
8					
9					
10					
11					
12					
13					
14					
15					
16					
17					
18					
19					
20					
21					
22					
23					

Figure 15-11 Truth in lending form. (Courtesy SYCOM, Madison, WI.)

It reports on accounts placed for collection and provides information of public interest, such as that regarding bankruptcies, judgments, and lawsuits.

The Fair Credit Reporting Act (FCRA) was passed in 1992 to promote accuracy, fairness, and privacy of information in the files of all CRAs. Most CRAs are credit bureaus that gather and sell information about a person (e.g., whether a person pays bills on time or has filed bankruptcy) to creditors, employers, landlords, and other businesses. The full text of this legislation is available on the Federal Trade Commission (FTC) website. Consumers may have additional rights under state law, and a state or local consumer protection agency or a state attorney general can provide that information.

CRAs charge a nominal fee for supplying information. When seeking information from a credit bureau, complete data should be given about the prospective creditor. This information should include the following information about the individual:

- Full name, including first and middle names. Accurate spelling is essential. The spouse's name should be used as a cross-reference for identification purposes only.
- Address or addresses for the past 3 years
- Place of employment for the past 3 years
- Names of stores and firms where credit has been established
- Name of bank or banks
- Social Security number

After this information has been given to the credit bureau, you will receive a credit report on the applicant. Care must be taken to record the

Table 15-2
Language Used in Consumer Credit Reports

Usual Manner of Payment	Symbol
Open account, 30 day account, 90 day account	0
Too new to rate; approved but not used	0-0
Pays (or paid) within 30 days of billing; pays 90-day accounts as agreed	0-1
Pays (or paid) in more than 30 days but not more than 60 days	0-2
Pays (or paid) in more than 60 days but not more than 90 days	0-3
Pays (or paid) in more than 90 days but not more than 120 days	0-4
Pays (or paid) in 120 days or more	0-5
Bad debt; placed for collection; suit; judgment; bankrupt; skip	0-9
Revolving or option account R or R $ _____*	*
Too new to rate; approved but not used	R-0
Pays (or paid) according to the terms agreed	R-1
Not paying (or paid) as agreed but not more than one payment past due	R-2
Not paying (or paid) as agreed and two payments past due	R-3
Not paying (or paid) as agreed and three payments past due	R-4
Bad debt; placed for collection; suit; judgment; bankrupt; skip	R-9
Installment account I or I $ _____*	*
Too new to rate; approved but not used	I-0
Pays (or paid) according to terms agreed	I-1
Not paying (or paid) as agreed but not more than one payment past due	I-2
Not paying (or paid) as agreed and two payments past due	I-3
Not paying (or paid) as agreed and three payments or more past due	I-4
Repossession	I-8
Bad debt; placed for collection; suit; judgment; bankrupt; skip	I-9

*When the monthly payment is known, it should be shown (e.g., R $20 or I $78).
Modified from the Associated Credit Bureau of America.

information accurately. The Associated Credit Bureaus of America have designed a common language, which incorporates symbols, for reporting this information (Table 15-2). The symbols should mean the same things throughout the consumer credit industry, such as *O* for open, *R* for revolving, and *I* for installment.

The dentist decides whether to extend credit to a patient. If the patient is denied credit, FCRA requires that the patient be informed of the reason for denial of credit and the name of the bureau from which a credit report was obtained. The dental office is not required to report the specific data obtained from the bureau; a patient who wants this information should contact the bureau personally.

COLLECTION PROCEDURES

Collecting fees in the dental office is an undesirable but crucial responsibility of the administrative assistant. Experience has shown that patients pay medical and dental bills last. People pay their rent for fear of eviction, their car payments for fear of repossession, and their utility bills for fear of losing service.

They even pay off loans before the dental bill because banks generally adhere to a stricter enforcement of collection procedures than the dentist does. Fortunately, only about 5% of patients become "uncollectable," but this 5% can be exasperating.

Aging Accounts

Each month the administrative assistant should age the accounts receivable. With a computer, this can be programmed into the system and an aging report of the accounts is automatically produced when desired. The dentist must determine a policy about aging accounts, and the administrative assistant must follow through with this policy routinely so that delinquent accounts do not become a drain on the practice.

Fair Debt Collection Practices Act

Collection procedures are regulated by the Fair Debt Collection Practices Act of 1996. This act was passed to protect the public from unethical collection procedures. The activities outlined specifically in the law are listed in Box 15-1.

Because these regulations generally apply to collection agencies, it is important that an agency verify its stringent adherence to them. These same regulations should be considered by the administrative assistant when performing collection procedures in the office.

Collection Letters

Letters may be sent at the discretion of the dentist. In offices that use a computer, a reminder notice can be included on the statement, and the first collection letter (Figure 15-12) is automatically generated when an account becomes past due. You may use a series of computer-generated reminder notices automatically sent at specified intervals (e.g., 30, 60, and 90 days past due) before assigning an account to a collector. Be responsible, however, in reviewing the list of delinquent accounts. One of these accounts might be a patient of long standing who, because of extenuating circumstances, was unable to pay the account. It is not wise to risk the loss of a well-established patient relationship by adding a message or sending an account to a collector without first checking to see if a reason exists for the oversight.

Generally the collection process should have four stages: reminder, inquiry/ discussion, urgency, and ultimatum. The previous discussion concerned the first stage, reminder, which is accomplished through a notice on the statement.

Box 15-1
Provisions of the Fair Debt Collection Practices Act

- Debtors may not be subjected to harassment, oppressive tactics, or abusive treatment. The law prohibits the collector from making any false statements to a debtor, such as claiming to be an attorney or a government agency.
- Debtors may not be called at work if the employer or the debtor objects and requests no calls.
- Debtors may not be called at inconvenient places or times, such as before 9 AM or after 9 PM.
- No one except the debtors themselves may be told they are behind on their bills.

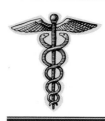

Dental Associates, PC
Joseph W. Lake, DDS – Ashley M. Lake, DDS

November 5, 20—

Mr. Marvin Beattie
1407 Colorado Street N.W.
Grand Rapids, MI 49505

Dear Mr. Beattie:

Your account of $565.00 is over 90 days past due. If you are unable to pay this account in full, perhaps we can help you in making arrangements to take care of this account.

Please contact us before November 15, 20—at 5:00 p.m.

Sincerely,

Jennifer Ellis, RDA
Administrative Assistant

611 Main Street, SE Ð Grand Rapids, MI 49502   *Phone: 616.101.9575 Fax: 616.101.9999*
E-mail: office@dapc.com or Visit us at: www.Lakedental.com

Figure 15-12 First collection letter.

In the second stage (inquiry), you personally contact the patient to determine the problem. The final two stages can be completed with letters. The letter of urgency must be more persuasive and urgent (Figure 15-13). An urgent phone call may be used as a follow-up as long as it does not result in harassment. In either situation you should be courteous, considerate, and helpful, yet firm.

The final stage, the ultimatum, arrives when a patient has failed to respond to all messages sent thus far. You must confront the patient with the ultimatum. Refrain from referring directly to lawsuits, attorneys, or collection agencies unless you intend to follow through. Send only one ultimatum letter with a deadline date (Figure 15-14). Send this letter by certified mail with a return receipt requested to prove that the debtor has received the letter. If payment is not received by the designated date, the account must be turned over immediately to an attorney or a collection agency.

The following rules can guide the composition of collection letters:
1. Keep the letter brief.
2. Make sure that data about the account are complete and accurate.
3. Use simple words and uncomplicated sentences.
4. Use phrases that will motivate the patient, such as "cooperation" or "maintenance of a good credit rating."
5. Don't make statements you don't intend to carry out. If you tell the patient that the account will be sent to a collection agency in 10 days, give a specific date and then follow through if necessary.
6. Set a specific date by which you expect payment, rather than saying "by the end of the month," or "in 10 days."
7. Be firm and polite.
8. Include a "thank you" in the letter closing because this, too, can be an important part of the collection procedure, and it is a valuable aid to public relations.

Telephone as a Collection Instrument

Many assistants find it difficult to use the telephone in collecting delinquent accounts. Experience should instill confidence in the assistant, but if not, another method of collection should be pursued. The telephone allows a more personal contact with a patient. When a patient who normally pays the account on time becomes delinquent, a phone call seems less formal than a letter and helps maintain a friendly relationship.

Specific rules should be followed when using the telephone for collections:
1. Do not call before 9 AM or after 9 PM.
2. Verify that you are speaking to the person whose account is overdue. Ask, "Is this Mr. Johnson?"
3. Identify yourself: "This is Miss Ellis, from Dr. Lake's office."
4. Ask whether it is a convenient time to talk. If not, ask when you may call back or find out when the patient will be able to call you. Do not give details to a third party or leave detailed messages on an answering machine or voicemail.
5. State the purpose of your call. Be friendly and display a helping attitude.
6. Be positive. Don't say, "I'm sorry to call you." Act as though you know the patient intends to pay and you are simply determining the arrangements for such a payment.
7. Have all of the information about the account in front of you.
8. Attempt to obtain a definite commitment; that is, the date and the amount of the payment. Follow up with written confirmation of the telephone discussion.
9. Make calls in a private area out of the hearing range of anyone in the reception room.

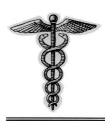

Dental Associates, PC
Joseph W. Lake, DDS – Ashley M. Lake, DDS

November 26, 20—

REGISTERED

Mr. Marvin Beattie
1407 Colorado Street N.W.
Grand Rapids, MI 49505

Dear Mr. Beattie:

Since we have not heard from you regarding your account of $565.00 from June 1, 20—, please be informed that it will be necessary to transfer this account to a collection agency.

This account must be paid in full by Friday, December 1, 20—to avoid such legal action.

Sincerely,

Jennifer Ellis, RDA
Administrative Assistant

611 Main Street, SE Đ Grand Rapids, MI 49502   Phone: 616.101.9575 Fax: 616.101.9999
E-mail: office@dapc.com or Visit us at: www.Lakedental.com

Figure 15-13 Urgent collection letter.

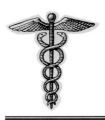

Dental Associates, PC

Joseph W. Lake, DDS – Ashley M. Lake, DDS

November 26, 20—

REGISTERED

Mr. Marvin Beattie
1407 Colorado Street N.W.
Grand Rapids, MI 49505

Dear Mr. Beattie:

Please be informed that your account of $565.00 from June 1, 20—, has been transferred to the Dunhill Collection Agency for collection.

Sincerely,

Ashley M. Lake, DDS

je

611 Main Street, SE – Grand Rapids, MI 49502   *Phone: 616.101.9575 Fax: 616.101.9999*
E-mail: office@dapc.com or Visit us at: www.Lakedental.com

Figure 15-14 Final collection letter.

10. Don't threaten the patient.
11. Follow up on the promises the patient makes.
12. Don't ever discuss the account with anyone else. If you call the patient at work and the person cannot talk with you, leave a message to "Call Miss Ellis at 101-9575." Don't leave the dentist's name; the patient may not return the call.

Collection Agency

After every attempt has been made to collect an account, it may be necessary to engage the services of a collection agency. These services are required when the patient fails to respond to a final collection letter or can no longer be located and becomes a "skip."

Delay in sending the account to a collection agency results in less chance of recovering a portion of the fee. Although the agency's fee reduces the portion recovered, continued unsuccessful attempts by the office are even less rewarding.

A collection agency should be selected that maintains high standards of professionalism. Investigate the agency thoroughly to determine its ethics and reliability.

1. Check the ownership of the agency through a banker, the local Chamber of Commerce, or the Better Business Bureau.
2. Contact the local dental society, National Retail Credit Association, or the Associated Credit Bureaus of America for information about the agency.
3. Find out whether the agency has contacts out of town to aid in collection of accounts.
4. Make sure the agency will not start legal action without the dentist's consent.
5. Make sure the agency understands a patient's needs and that you want reports on its activities.

Once the dentist has sought the services of an agency, the office should use these services routinely. To allow action to be taken promptly, complete data about each case should be given to the agency, including the following:

- Debtor's full name
- Last known address and phone number
- Total amount of account
- Date of last entry on account (credit or debit)
- Debtor's occupation
- Business address and phone number
- Any other pertinent information

When an account is turned over to a collection agency, the administrative assistant no longer pursues collection procedures on it. However, the dental office staff must cooperate with the agency. The staff should:

- Send no more statements.
- Indicate the transfer to the collection agency on the ledger card, giving the date of transfer.
- Refer the patient to the agency if the person contacts the office.
- Report the amount to the agency when payment is received in the office.
- Rely on the agency staff members to do the job (i.e., don't pester them with calls of inquiry about the account).

From the time the patient enters the office until final collection of the fee, the administrative assistant has many important duties in managing the accounts receivable. The importance of accuracy in each aspect cannot be overemphasized. If you can carry out this responsibility, your value to the office becomes immeasurable.

LEARNING ACTIVITIES

1. Explain the differences between accounting and bookkeeping.
2. List common types of bookkeeping systems used in dentistry.
3. List and explain the function of the components of a pegboard system.
4. List and explain the function of the components of a computer bookkeeping system.
5. What are the advantages of an electronic bookkeeping system versus a manual system?
6. Describe how monthly statements are prepared.
7. Identify the function of each of the following:
   a. Credit policy
   b. Credit bureau
   c. Collection agency
8. Explain the contents of an effective collection letter.

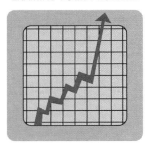

EXAMINE YOUR PROGRESS

Practice by completing Working Form 11.

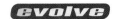

SOFTWARE ACTIVITIES

Use the EagleSoft CD-ROM in the back of the textbook to make entries for each of the patients and the activities listed. Please review the technique for using the CD-ROM before making the entries.

1. John Abbott
   827 Division St.
   Mattoon, IL 25134
   Balance, $1425
   19DO, 18MO amalgam
2. Beth Burke
   114 S. 4th St.
   Neoga, IL 62447
   Balance, $192
   Prophylaxis, examination, FMX w/4 BW
3. James Burke
   114 S. 4th St.
   Neoga, IL 62447
   Balance, 0
   Prep. crown #30—resin with high noble
4. Rachael Burke
   114 S. 4th St.
   Neoga, IL 62447
   Balance, $62.80
   Prep. crown #8—porcelain fused to high noble
5. Glenn Davis
   519 W. Walnut St.
   Teutopolis, IL 62467
   Balance, $97.50
   8^{D} & 9^{D} composite; 12DO, 14^{MOD} amalgam

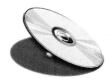

CHECK OUT THE CD

Continued

SOFTWARE ACTIVITIES—cont'd

6. Vicki Davis
   519 W. Walnut St.
   Teutopolis, IL 62467
   Balance, 0
   Adjust complete lower denture
7. Karmen Little
   2917 Richmond Ave.
   Windsor, IL 61957
   Balance, 0
   Prep. cast metal high noble crown #18
8. Dennis Malone
   1609 Marshall
   Greenup, IL 62428
   Balance, $116
   Labial veneer (porcelain laminate) #8 and #9
9. Bob Price
   1019 Arthur
   Toledo, IL 62468
   Balance, $138
   CSX, prophylaxis, and examination
10. Kathy Price
    1019 Arthur
    Toledo, IL 62468
    Balance, 0
    Prophylaxis, examination, and 2 BW x-ray films
11. Kent Russell
    3428 Willow Dr.
    Effingham, IL 62401
    Balance, $138
    Prep. crown #8—porcelain fused to high noble
12. Andrew Savage
    606 Maple Ave.
    Shelbyville, IL 62565
    Balance, 0
    Prophylaxis and examination

Checks Received Today

Beth Burke—$71 payment
Glenn Davis—$38 payment
Dennis Malone—$92.80 payment
Bob Price—$70.40 payment

Key Terms

Accounting The recording, classifying, and summarizing of financial and business records; this generally is the task of the accountant.

Accounts payable All the dentist's financial obligations, or money that the dentist owes (outgoing money).

Accounts receivable A category that includes all production; data are entered for treatment rendered and payments received, and new balances are calculated.

Adjustment Alteration of an account balance as a result of a courtesy discount, the return of a nonsufficient funds (NSF) check, or a payment.

Balance The credit or debit amount on an account.

Bookkeeping The process of recording of financial transactions.

Credit balance An amount owed to the patient for services for which the dentist has been paid in advance but that have not yet been performed.

Credit bureau An organization that reports specific information about a person's previous payment habits on deferred payment plans.

Debit balance An amount owed to the dentist for services rendered.

Nonsufficient funds (NSF) check A check returned unpaid to the payee because insufficient funds were available in the payer's account.

Previous balance The amount on an account, whether credit or debit, before activity was posted to the account.

Receipt A form given to the payer (patient) that acknowledges payment on an account.

Statement A document that informs patients of their financial status with the dentist; it indicates the charges, payments, and balances on an account for the month just concluded.

Chapter

16

Other Financial Systems

Chapter Outline

Learning Objectives

Mastery of the content in this chapter will enable the reader to:

- Explain the function of a budget
- Explain the use of electronic banking
- Identify the parts of a check
- Write a check and determine the correct balance on a checkbook register
- Identify various types of checks
- Prepare checks for deposit with correct endorsements and complete a deposit slip
- Reconcile a bank statement
- Explain the purpose of a monthly expense sheet
- Explain the purpose of a yearly summary
- Identify the purpose of payroll records
- Explain the purpose of the employee's earnings record
- Calculate gross and net wages
- Explain how withheld income tax and Social Security taxes are deposited
- Explain how federal unemployment taxes are deposited
- Describe how to complete a Form W-2
- Explain the importance of retaining payroll records
- Explain the use of an automated payroll system
- Use the Internet as a resource for financial forms and instructions

> In the processing of financial documents, accuracy is essential. Verification of data and attention to detail are necessary to ensure that the processed information is accurate.

All dental practices, regardless of size, have financial matters that need to be addressed by either internal or external accounting staff. As an administrative assistant, you can expect to perform many tasks in addition to the accounts receivable activities highlighted in the previous chapter. These tasks might include receiving and organizing statements, paying for materials and supplies, processing payroll or tax forms, recording and analyzing expenses, and other responsibilities. In a group practice or a larger organization, you may collect the data for these activities and support accounting personnel in the preparation of financial documents. Whether you do these tasks manually or use computer software, you must have a basic understanding of the systems involved.

In the processing of financial documents, accuracy is essential. Verification of data and attention to detail are necessary to ensure that the processed information is accurate. Incorrect data can mean improper cash flow analysis, inaccurate accounts receivable, erroneous claim form preparation, or inaccurate budget and expense figures. All of these can have very serious repercussions for the entire business.

As you become more skilled in the business office, your responsibilities probably will include completing many monthly and annual forms vital to the dental practice. This chapter presents the major types of financial systems and the data that must be processed and managed in a modern dental practice. You will learn how technology is applied to the financial operations of a practice to make it more productive. In addition, you will learn about the resources available through the Internet that can guide you in procuring and filling out many of the financial forms needed by the practice.

DETERMINING A BUDGET

A **budget** is a dental practice's financial plan of operation for a given period, usually 1 year. The purpose of the budget is to establish the practice's financial goals. To achieve an acceptable level of profit, **expenditures**, the amount of money spent to operate the practice, must be kept in balance with **revenue**, the amount of income received by the practice. Dentists can use spreadsheet software to develop a budget so that they can plan more thoroughly and in less time than with paper and pencil methods. Spreadsheets allow planners to see how a change in one calculation affects all the related calculations. A template of a business budget modified for a dental practice is shown in Figure 16-1.

BANK ACCOUNTS

One of the daily routine functions of the dental office administrative assistant is control of the *cash flow,* or the amounts of money received and the amounts disbursed. Therefore a good understanding of banking technology and procedures is necessary. Some of the administrative assistant's banking responsibilities are check writing, accepting checks from patients for payment of services, endorsing and depositing checks, keeping an accurate bank balance, and reconciling the bank statement.

> One of the daily routine functions of the dental office administrative assistant is control of the *cash flow,* or the amounts of money received and the amounts disbursed.

ELECTRONIC BANKING

For many dental offices, electronic banking means 24-hour access to cash through an automated teller machine or direct deposit of paychecks and accounts receivable into a checking or savings account. Electronic banking now involves many different types of transactions.

Electronic banking, also known as *electronic funds transfer (EFT),* uses a computer and electronic technology as a substitute for checks and other paper transactions. EFTs are initiated through devices such as cards or codes that let the dentist or those authorized by the dentist access an account. Many financial institutions use **automatic teller machines (ATMs)** or debit cards and personal identification numbers (PINs) for this purpose. Other institutions use devices such as debit cards or a signature or scan to access to an account. The federal Electronic Fund Transfer Act (EFT Act) covers some electronic consumer transactions.

ATMs, or 24-hour tellers, are electronic terminals that allow banking at almost any time. To withdraw money, make deposits, or transfer funds between accounts, an ATM card is inserted and a PIN number is entered. Generally, ATMs must indicate if a fee is charged and give the amount on or at the terminal screen before the transaction is completed.

Direct deposit enables a person to make a deposit to the account on a regular basis. In this system the dentist may preauthorize recurring bills to be paid automatically, such as insurance premiums, mortgages, and utility bills.

Pay by phone systems allow a person to call the financial institution with instructions to pay certain bills or to transfer funds between accounts. An agreement must exist between the institution and the company being paid that allows these funds to be transferred.

Personal computer banking allows the account to be accessed from a remote location, such as a personal computer. The account holder can view the account balance, request transfers between accounts, and pay bills electronically.

		DENTAL PRACTICE BUDGET			
			Month/Year:		
SUMMARY	**ACTUAL**	**BUDGETED**	**OVER BUDGET**	**UNDER BUDGET**	
Total income					
Total expenses					
Income less expenses:					
INCOME DETAILS	**ACTUAL**	**BUDGETED**	**OVER BUDGET**	**UNDER BUDGET**	**NOTES**
Fees					
Interest earned					
Rent					
Royalties					
Other					
Total income:					
EXPENSE DETAILS	**ACTUAL**	**BUDGETED**	**OVER BUDGET**	**UNDER BUDGET**	**NOTES**
Accounting					
Contributions					
Equipment purchases					
Insurance					
Legal					
Loans					
Office supplies					
Postage					
Professional Dues					
Rent & maintenance					
Salaries and wages					
Employee benefits					
Payroll taxes					
Telephone					
Travel					
Utilities					
Other					
Total expenses:					

Figure 16-1 Business budget modified for a dental practice.

The use of electronic transfers should be monitored carefully. The dentist and any other person responsible for electronic banking must read the documents you receive from the financial institution that issued the access device. No one should know the PIN except the responsible person or persons. In addition, before any electronic transfer system is used, the institution must provide the following information, which you should keep filed:

- A summary of the practice's liability for unauthorized transfers
- The telephone number and address of the person to be notified if an unauthorized transfer has been or may have been made, a statement of the institution's business days, and the number of days you have to report suspected unauthorized transfers
- The type of transfers that can be made, the fees for transfers, and any limits on the frequency and amount of transfers
- A summary of the right to receive documentation of transfers and to stop payment on a preauthorized transfer, as well as the procedures for stopping payment
- A summary of the institution's liability
- Privacy assurance

If problems arise in the use of the EFT, a complaint can be filed through the website for the state member banks of the Federal Reserve System at www.federalreserve.gov.

ESTABLISHING A CHECKING ACCOUNT

As a rule, the checking account for the dental practice will have been opened before you begin working for the practice. However, in opening the account, the dentist had to decide what type of an account would be used. The dentist also signed a signature card (Figure 16-2) that permitted him or her to write checks against the account. If another person is permitted to write checks against the account, that person's signature must also appear on a signature card for the account or on the same signature card that the dentist signed. However, if the administrative assistant is allowed to sign the checks, the bank may require that the assistant be given power of attorney (Figure 16-3).

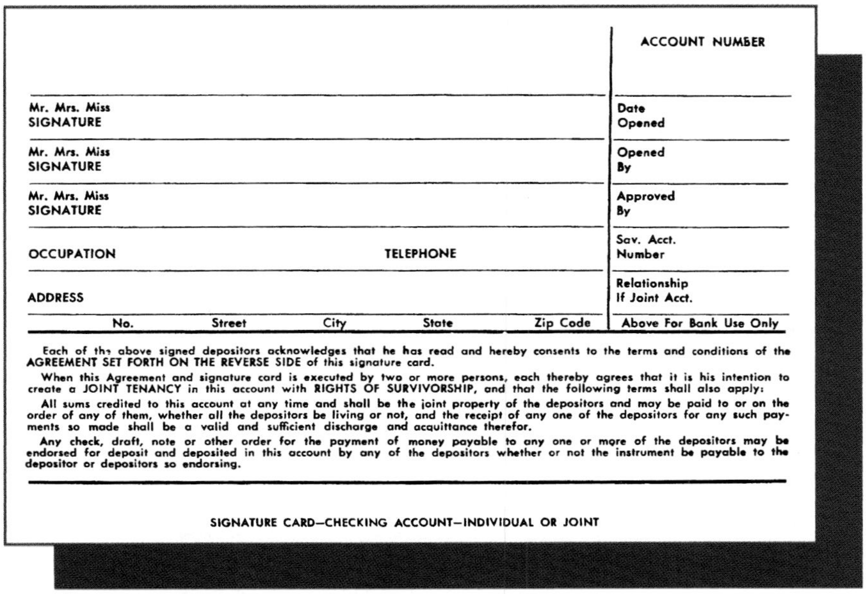
ACCOUNT NUMBER

Mr. Mrs. Miss
SIGNATURE
Date
Opened

Mr. Mrs. Miss
SIGNATURE
Opened
By

Mr. Mrs. Miss
SIGNATURE
Approved
By

OCCUPATION TELEPHONE
Sav. Acct.
Number

ADDRESS
Relationship
If Joint Acct.

No. Street City State Zip Code
Above For Bank Use Only

Each of th؛ above signed depositors acknowledges that he has read and hereby consents to the terms and conditions of the AGREEMENT SET FORTH ON THE REVERSE SIDE of this signature card.

When this Agreement and signature card is executed by two or more persons, each thereby agrees that it is his intention to create a JOINT TENANCY in this account with RIGHTS OF SURVIVORSHIP, and that the following terms shall also apply:

All sums credited to this account at any time and shall be the joint property of the depositors and may be paid to or on the order of any of them, whether all the depositors be living or not, and the receipt of any one of the depositors for any such payments so made shall be a valid and sufficient discharge and acquittance therefor.

Any check, draft, note or other order for the payment of money payable to any one or more of the depositors may be endorsed for deposit and deposited in this account by any of the depositors whether or not the instrument be payable to the depositor or depositors so endorsing.

SIGNATURE CARD—CHECKING ACCOUNT—INDIVIDUAL OR JOINT

Figure 16-2 Signature card.

```
┌─────────────────────────────────────────────────────────────┐
│                     POWER OF ATTORNEY                         │
│                                                               │
│                                    Date_____    │
│                                                               │
│   I/We_____, the undersigned,│
│                                                               │
│   hereby authorize _____ . │
│                                                               │
│   whose signature appears below, to sign checks against _____ │
│                                                               │
│   account in your bank as _____ attorney. │
│                                                               │
│   Signature of attorney _____ . │
│                                                               │
│   Signature _____ . │
│                                                               │
│   Signature _____ . │
│                                                               │
│   Cancelled _____ Date _____    │
│                                                               │
└─────────────────────────────────────────────────────────────┘
```

Figure 16-3 Power of attorney.

Checks

Checks are a means of ordering the bank to pay cash from the bank customer's account. In the past, checks accounted for more than 90% of all financial transactions in the United States. However, the use of debit cards rose from 39 percent in 1999 to 32 percent in 2003, and patients increasingly will use debit and cards, rather than cash or checks, to pay their bills. The percentage of consumers who use checks to pay recurring bills declined from 72 percent in 2001 to about 60 percent today. However, checks still constitute a major portion of the receipts for the dental practice.

Many parts of a check are self-explanatory; however, some parts need additional explanation. In Figure 16-4, part 3 is the American Bankers Association (ABA) bank identification number. Under this coding system, every bank is given its own number, which constitutes a numerical name

> More than 90% of all financial transactions in this country are done by check.

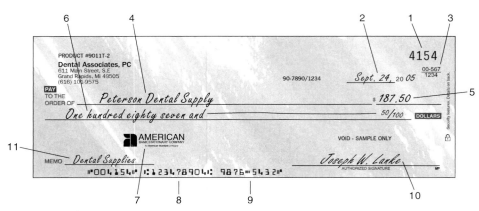

Figure 16-4 Parts of a check. *1*, Check number. *2*, Date of check. *3*, American Bankers Association (ABA) bank identification number. *4*, Payee, the person or company to be paid. *5*, Amount of check (in figures). *6*, Amount of check (in words). *7*, Drawee, the bank on which the check is drawn. *8*, Bank identification number magnetically printed for electronic processing. *9*, Customer account number magnetically printed for electronic processing. *10*, Signature of drawer. *11*, Reason the check was written. (Courtesy SYCOM, Madison, WI.)

for the bank. This number aids the sorting of checks for distribution to their proper destination. The ABA number is a fraction and usually is printed in the upper right corner of the check or slightly to the left of the check number. Part 4 of the check is the *payee,* the individual or company that will receive the money. Part 7, the *drawee,* is the bank that pays the check. Parts 8 and 9 are magnetic ink character recognition (MICR) numbers. These are encoded on all checks to facilitate high-speed handling by machine. The first number is the bank identification number (also found in the ABA identification number). The second number is the check writer's checking account number. These numbers can easily be read by people or by machine. Part 10 of the check is the signature of the *drawer* or check writer, the person who orders the bank to pay cash from the account.

WRITING CHECKS. The administrative assistant usually sets a time during the working day, as the schedule permits, to take care of check writing. This can be done manually or with the help of a computer system. The check stub or checkbook register should be completed before the check is written or printed. The stub or register provides a record of (1) the check number, (2) the date, (3) the payee, (4) the amount of the check, (5) the purpose of the check, and (6) the new balance brought forward after the amount of the check has been subtracted; or it provides the new balance if a deposit is to be added to the previous balance, as shown in the manual system (Figure 16-5).

Figure 16-6 presents a step-by-step procedure for writing a check. A similar procedure would be followed for entering checks in the one-step system (Figure 16-7) or for entering check information in a computerized bookkeeping system.

TYPES OF CHECKS. The following list describes a few of the types of checks the administrative assistant may receive.

• **Certified check.** A certified check is a guarantee that funds have been set aside to cover the amount of the check. The person goes to the bank and writes a personal check for the proper amount; the bank sets aside that amount from the customer's account, placing it in a special account, and then stamps *Certified* across the face of the check. Usually a nominal fee is charged for certifying a check.

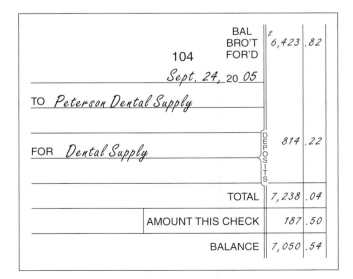

Figure 16-5 Check stub.

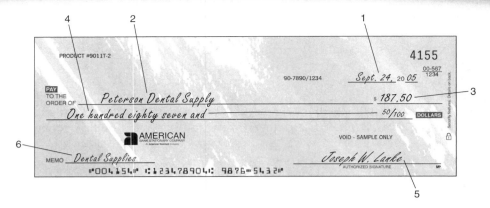

Figure 16-6 How to write a check. *1,* Date the check. *2,* Key or write the name of the person or firm to whom the check will be payable. *3,* Enter the amount of the check (in figures) opposite the dollar sign. *4,* Write the amount of the check (in words) under the "Pay to the order of" line. Start as far to the left margin as possible. *5,* The name on the signature line should be signed as it appears on the bank signature card. *6,* On the memo line, record the purpose of the payment. (Courtesy SYCOM, Madison, WI.)

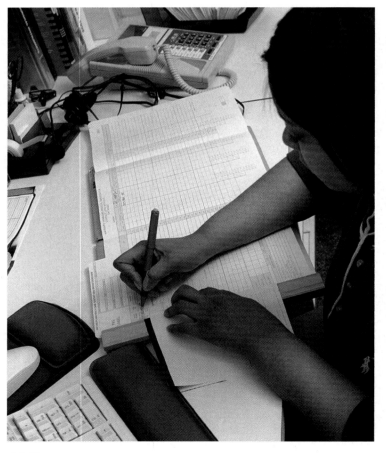

Figure 16-7 Pegboard check system. (From Young AP: *Kinn's the administrative medical assistant,* ed 5, St. Louis, 2003, WB Saunders.)

- **Cashier's check.** A cashier's check is the bank's own order to make payment out of the bank's funds. When a cashier's check is purchased, the person specifies to whom the bank makes the check payable and receives a carbon or stub of the check as a record. A fee is usually charged for this type of check.
- **Money order.** A money order is a means of transferring money without using cash or a personal check. People who do not maintain a personal checking account often use money orders to pay their creditors. The money order may be purchased in the form of a bank money order, a postal money order, or an express money order. The money order shows the name of the purchaser and the person who is to receive the payment (the payee). A fee is charged for this service.
- **Traveler's check.** Even though the **traveler's check** is designed as a payment device for a person who is away from home, it is not uncommon to receive a traveler's check in payment for dental services. Traveler's checks are purchased through a bank, American Express Company, or Railway Express Agency. The checks are preprinted in various denominations, usually $10, $20, $50, and $100. A small fee, determined by the amount purchased, is charged. When the checks are purchased, the individual signs his or her name in a designated place on each check. When the checks are used for payment or are cashed, they are *countersigned;* that is, the purchaser signs them again in the presence of the individual who cashes the check or accepts it for payment.
- **Bank draft.** A bank draft is a check drawn by the cashier of one bank on another bank where the first bank has available funds on deposit or credit. A bank draft is used if a person or company wants to send a sum of money and a personal check is not acceptable.
- **Voucher check.** A voucher check provides a detachable stub, which serves as an excellent accounting record for itemizing payment of invoices or any other type of itemization the payer would like as a reference.

ACCEPTING AND CASHING CHECKS. Many different types of checks may be used as payment for services. When you accept a check, make sure that it is (1) legibly written in ink or typewritten, (2) currently dated, (3) signed by the check writer, (4) drawn on a U.S. bank, (5) made payable in a certain sum of money (the amount in figures and the amount in words should agree), and (6) made payable to a payee or bearer.

At times you may be asked to accept a check for more than the charges. This may present a problem. For example, if the individual owes $100 and wants to pay $50 but writes a check for $100 and asks for $50 to be returned, a question may arise at a later date if the patient tries to use the canceled check as a receipt for full payment of the account. Another problem that may be encountered is the acceptance of payment for more than the balance and the return of the difference in cash to the patient. If the bank returns the patient's check for insufficient funds, you have paid cash out from the business, and the patient has the cash. To avoid problems of this nature, it is better to establish a firm policy of not accepting checks for more than the amount owed. This policy should be established by the dentist and enforced at all times.

Other Forms of Payment

As mentioned previously, credit or debit cards (e.g., MasterCard, VISA, Discover, and American Express) increasingly are being used to pay professional fees. The dentist makes arrangements through a bank, usually the one where the business account has been established, to use this banking service. The bank

> Credit cards such as MasterCard and VISA increasingly are being used to pay professional fees.

charges a fee for this service, generally 1 percent to 5 percent of the transactions handled. The bank supplies the user with the imprinter, merchant charge tickets, credit slips, and merchant batch headers. The merchant batch headers are used at the end of the working day to itemize payments made through the bank cards and are included on the deposit slips for the day (Figure 16-8).

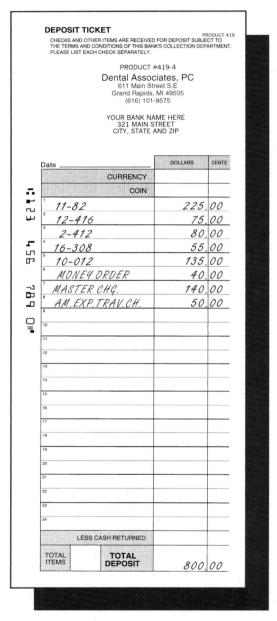

Figure 16-8 Deposit slip. *1,* Write or type the date on the front side. *2,* List currency and coins to be deposited. *3,* Identify checks to be deposited individually; if there are more than three, use the back side of the deposit slip. Checks should be listed on the deposit slip by the ABA numbers. However, you may prefer to list checks with the patient's name and number. If it is a money order, traveler's check, or MasterCard or VISA charge receipt, the total amount of money and the name of the item are listed. *4,* Enter the total from the back on the front side of the deposit slip. *5,* Total the entire deposit (net deposit). *6,* Optional: some deposit slips provide a line in case the depositor wants part of the deposit back in cash. The amount desired is entered on this line and subtracted from the total line above; the net deposit then is entered as in *5.*

A few precautions are necessary when patients use credit or debit cards for payment. Some cards have use restrictions and may not be acceptable for this kind of payment. The bank provides the practice with a list of stolen cards, and this list should be checked to make sure the patient's card is valid. Also, be sure to check the card's expiration date, and check the charge ticket to make sure the imprinter has printed the card information on all copies of the ticket. Some practices may be linked by telephone to the bank for credit verification or for debit transactions; with the latter, the amount is subtracted immediately from the customer's account.

Because some patients pay their accounts with cash, some cash must be kept in the office. However, large amounts of cash should not be routinely kept in the office, because it may end up being counted as part of the total cash receipts for the day. A separate cash balance can be maintained for petty cash (discussed later in the chapter).

DEPOSITS

Making a Deposit

Depositing money into the practice's checking account is usually a daily routine. A bank deposit represents the accumulation of money received for a single day or possibly a longer period. The bank provides checking account deposit slips, which have the dental practice's name and account number imprinted on them. Follow the step-by-step procedure presented in Figure 16-8 when completing the deposit form. A duplicate copy of the deposit form may be retained for office use to verify with the check register and bank statement at the end of the month.

Still another type of bank deposit slip might be used. In today's age of computers, software is being written specifically for the dental practice, and frequently the dental management software is written by a dentist. A common application on the computer is the management of the daily cash flow. At the end of the day, the bank deposit slip is generated from funds entered into the accounts receivable program (Figure 16-9).

DEPOSITS BY MAIL. Making deposits of the day's receipts by mail saves time for the administrative assistant. Mail deposit slips and envelopes are provided by the bank. Each check should be carefully endorsed on the back with a restrictive **endorsement** and the signature or stamp of the payee and then placed in the envelope with the deposit slip. The three most common types of endorsements are defined and illustrated in Figure 16-10. Currency and coins should not be sent through the mail unless sent by registered mail. Upon receipt of the deposit, the bank sends the customer a receipt of the deposit and another mail deposit slip and envelope.

NIGHT DEPOSITORY. Sometimes the practice receives large amounts of money after banking hours. The night depository is a means of depositing money in the bank vault when the bank is closed. Usually the deposit is completed the next business day by a bank teller; the depositor must go to the bank to pick up the deposit bag and receipt. However, if the depositor prefers, the deposit bag can remain locked until the person arrives at the bank to make the deposit personally.

AUTOMATIC TELLER MACHINE. As mentioned previously, in conjunction with the checking account, financial institutions offer special access cards that can be used to perform banking transactions virtually 24 hours a day, 7 days

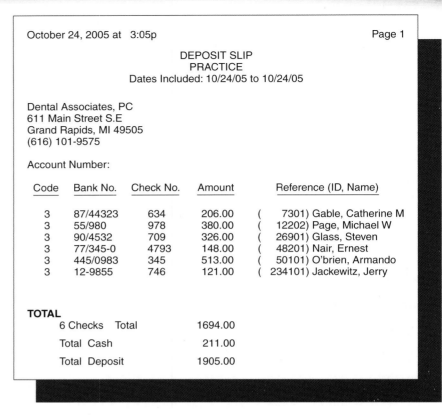

October 24, 2005 at   3:05p   Page 1

DEPOSIT SLIP
PRACTICE
Dates Included: 10/24/05 to 10/24/05

Dental Associates, PC
611 Main Street S.E
Grand Rapids, MI 49505
(616) 101-9575

Account Number:

Code	Bank No.	Check No.	Amount	Reference (ID, Name)
3	87/44323	634	206.00	(7301) Gable, Catherine M
3	55/980	978	380.00	(12202) Page, Michael W
3	90/4532	709	326.00	(26901) Glass, Steven
3	77/345-0	4793	148.00	(48201) Nair, Ernest
3	445/0983	345	513.00	(50101) O'brien, Armando
3	12-9855	746	121.00	(234101) Jackewitz, Jerry

TOTAL

6 Checks   Total   1694.00

Total Cash   211.00

Total Deposit   1905.00

Figure 16-9 Computer-generated deposit slip.

a week. The cards can be used at ATMs, which are computer workstations that electronically prompt the user through most routine banking activities. Deposits or withdrawals can be made, or funds can be transferred between accounts. However, some precautions must be taken when using an ATM (Box 16-1).

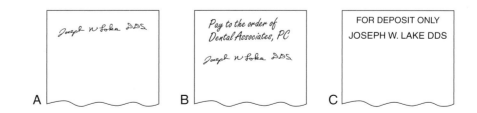

A   B   C

Figure 16-10 Check endorsements. **A,** *Blank endorsement*, which is an endorsement that consists of the signature of the payee. A blank endorsement makes the check payable to any holder. **B,** *Endorsement in full*, which is an endorsement that states to whom the check is to be paid and the signature of the payee. This endorsement specifies that the check can be cashed or transferred only on the order of the person, bank, or company named in the endorsement. **C,** *Restrictive endorsement*, which is an endorsement that includes special conditions or that limits the receiver of the check in the uses that can be made of it; this type of endorsement commonly is used when checks are prepared for deposit.

RECONCILING THE BANK STATEMENT

Although procedures may differ, most banks send a **bank statement** (Figure 16-11) to the depositor each month. The bank may return the *canceled checks* (checks that have been paid) along with the bank statement showing the balance of the account at the beginning of the month, deposits made during the month, checks drawn against the account, corrections or charges against the account (e.g., the service charge or stop payment charges), and the bank balance at the end of the month. To maintain an accurate record of the checking account, you should reconcile the bank statement as soon as the records are received from the bank.

You should use the following procedure to reconcile the bank statement.

1. Verify the amount of the canceled checks with the amounts on the bank statement (the canceled checks are usually returned in the order listed on the statement).
2. Arrange the canceled checks numerically.
3. Compare the amounts on the canceled checks and the deposits with the amounts written in the checkbook register. Check off (√) all canceled checks and deposits in the checkbook register.
4. List the *outstanding checks* (checks not yet returned to the bank), including the check number and the amount.
5. Total the outstanding checks. If a deposit has been made but does not appear on the bank statement, the deposit must be added to the bank statement balance before the outstanding checks are subtracted.
6. Look for charges other than checks that have been deducted from the account; for example, service charges (SC), debit memos (DM), and overdrafts (OD). These charges must be subtracted from the checkbook register.

In Figure 16-12, a reconciliation of the bank statement has been prepared for the practice of Dental Associates, PC (see Figure 16-11 for end of the month figures to determine how these computations were made).

Petty Cash

Although the cash receipts are deposited in the bank and invoices and miscellaneous items are paid by check, a small amount of cash should be kept on hand in the office. This should be established as a petty cash fund and controlled with the same accuracy as the checking account.

When it has been determined how much cash will be placed in the petty cash account, a check is written against the business account and cashed, and the cash is returned to the office and kept in a separate fund. To help eliminate errors in disbursements from the fund, one person in the office should have control over the petty cash. A voucher is completed each time money is taken from the fund. The voucher shows the date, voucher number, amount of payment, what the payment was for, to whom the payment was made, and the name of the person approving the payment (Figure 16-13).

Although the cash receipts are deposited in the bank and invoices and miscellaneous items are paid by check, a small amount of cash should be kept on hand in the office.

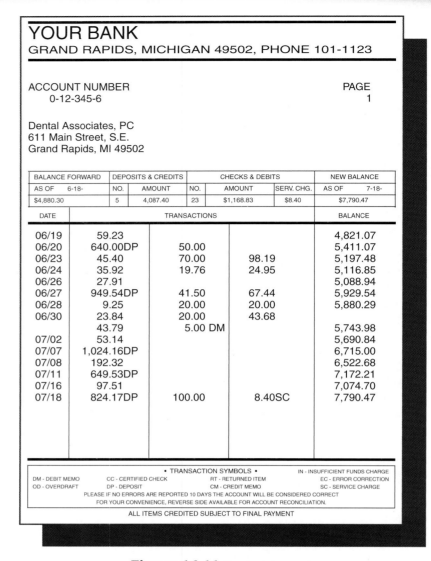

Figure 16-11 Bank statement.

Dental Associates, PC				
Bank Reconciliation				
July 25, 2005				
Balance per Bank Statement	$7,790.47	Balance per checkbook		$7,743.26
+ Deposit of 07-20- not		Subtract		
on statement	400.00	Debit memo	$5.00	
	$8,190.47	Service charge	8.40	13.40
Less Outstanding Checks				
No. 1102 - $50.00				
No. 1106 - 150.61				
No. 1110 - 75.00				
No. 1111 - 66.40				
No. 1112 - 118.60				
Total Outstanding checks	460.61			
Adjusted Bank Balance	$7,729.86	Adjusted Checkbook Balance		$7,729.86

Figure 16-12 Bank reconciliation.

Petty Cash Voucher

No.________ Date________

Paid to________________________________ Amount

For________________________________ ________

Charge to________________________________

________________________ ________________________

Approved by Payment received

Figure 16-13 Petty cash voucher.

After the voucher is completed, it is placed in the drawer as a reminder of the amount of cash taken from the fund. The vouchers and cash together should equal the original balance of petty cash.

A formal record of petty cash disbursements may also be used. This record shows all the disbursements in chronological order, the voucher number, and special columns for each expense item disbursed from the fund. It also provides a complete summary of how the money was disbursed. At the end of the month, the fund must be replenished. This involves writing another check for cash purposes and charging the various expense accounts for the amount used from the petty cash.

RECORDING BUSINESS EXPENSES

As invoices are processed, the expenditures represented on them need to be analyzed and verified for payment. A check is then made out to each supplier for payment of these statements. The administrative assistant records each item in an expense category. A monthly income and expense register provides a list of all the expenditures for the month, including the date of payment, the company to which the payment was made, the category of deduction, and the amount of payment. These totals are transferred to the annual summary. Figure 16-7 is an example of a one-step check writing and monthly expense sheet system. This combination checkbook and expense record provides space for deposit entries and checkbook balances, as well as itemization of each expenditure into specific categories. A software alternative would allow expenses to be recorded and checks printed using a computer system. Either of these systems can keep a running total of expenses or provide monthly and yearly totals.

MAINTAINING PAYROLL RECORDS

Various federal and state laws require that most businesses keep records to provide information about wages paid and to help in the preparation of required tax reports. Therefore the administrative assistant must have a good working knowledge of payroll and tax records.

Various federal and state laws require that most businesses keep records to provide information about wages paid and to help in the preparation of required tax reports.

INITIAL PAYROLL PROCEDURES

The dentist, as an employer, must apply for an **employer identification number**, a nine-digit number assigned to sole proprietors or corporations for filing and reporting payroll information. The application, **Form SS-4**, is available from the Internal Revenue Service (IRS) (Figure 16-14). Some states also require a state employer identification number.

The employer is required to have every employee complete an **Employee's Withholding Allowance Certificate (Form W-4)** (Figure 16-15). This form is needed to determine the status of each employee for income tax deductions from wages. Employees are required to complete a new Form W-4 when they change the number of withholding exemptions claimed.

EMPLOYEE EARNINGS RECORD

The employer must maintain employees' earnings records, including a summary of information for each employee (Figure 16-16). If the record has been properly designed, it provides the information needed for quarterly and annual reports. The employee's earnings record should contain the following information, which is used for various state and federal reports.

1. Name, address, Social Security number, rate of pay, withholding exemptions claimed, marital status, and special deductions (e.g., credit union account, bonds, United Fund)
2. The number of pay periods in a quarter and the date on which each pay period ends
3. Columns for regular earnings, overtime earnings, and total earnings (earnings records are available that provide columns for rate of pay and hours or days worked in a pay period)
4. A column for each deduction and for total deductions
5. A column for entering the net amount (net pay) received (*net pay* is the difference between total earnings and deductions)
6. A column for recording accumulated taxable earnings. This column provides the employer with information for taxable earnings, **Federal Insurance Contributions Act (FICA)** deductions (see the next section), and taxable wages for unemployment taxes.
7. Columns for quarterly and annual totals

Determining Employee Wages

> The dentist and employees must reach an agreement on an acceptable wage.

The dentist and employees must reach an agreement on an acceptable wage. This may be determined as an hourly rate, a weekly rate, or a monthly amount. After this rate has been established, the procedure must be decided for determining **net pay**. The administrative assistant often is responsible for figuring the payroll and preparing the checks for the dentist's signature.

1. The administrative assistant's hourly wage is $20 per hour.
2. If the workweek is based on 40 hours per week, the **gross wages** (amount earned before deductions) are $800 (40 hours × $20 per hour = $800).
3. Deductions are made from wages as follows:
   a. *FICA deduction (Social Security and Medicare taxes):* The amount to be withheld is determined by calculating at the combined 2000 rate (7.65% [or 0.0765] × $800 = $61.20). This tax rate is divided into two parts: the Social Security part, which is 6.2% on the first $76,200 earned in 2000, and the second part, for Medicare, which is 1.45% on all earnings, no ceiling. These tax rates are subject to change by Congress. The employer must keep track of such changes and make deductions according to the current rate. The *Employer's Tax Guide—Circular E,* available from the IRS, can be used to check the current tax rates.
   b. **Withholding** *(income tax deductions).* The amount withheld depends on the number of exemptions indicated on Form W-4. The tax amount withheld is determined from a table in the *Employer's Tax Guide—Circular E.*

Form SS-4
(Rev. December 2001)
Department of the Treasury
Internal Revenue Service

Application for Employer Identification Number
(For use by employers, corporations, partnerships, trusts, estates, churches, government agencies, Indian tribal entities, certain individuals, and others.)
See separate instructions for each line.   Keep a copy for your records.

EIN

OMB No. 1545-0003

Type or print clearly.

1   Legal name of entity (or individual) for whom the EIN is being requested

2   Trade name of business (if different from name on line 1)

3   Executor, trustee, "care of" name

4a   Mailing address (room, apt., suite no. and street, or P.O. box)

5a   Street address (if different) (Do not enter a P.O. box.)

4b   City, state, and ZIP code

5b   City, state, and ZIP code

6   County and state where principal business is located

7a   Name of principal officer, general partner, grantor, owner, or trustor

7b   SSN, ITIN, or EIN

8a   **Type of entity** (check only one box)
☐ Sole proprietor (SSN) _____
☐ Partnership
☐ Corporation (enter form number to be filed) _____
☐ Personal service corp.
☐ Church or church-controlled organization
☐ Other nonprofit organization (specify) _____
☐ Other (specify)

☐ Estate (SSN of decedent) _____
☐ Plan administrator (SSN) _____
☐ Trust (SSN of grantor) _____
☐ National Guard   ☐ State/local government
☐ Farmers' cooperative   ☐ Federal government/military
☐ REMIC   ☐ Indian tribal governments/enterprises
Group Exemption Number (GEN) _____

8b   If a corporation, name the state or foreign country (if applicable) where incorporated

State

Foreign country

9   **Reason for applying** (check only one box)
☐ Started new business (specify type) _____
☐ Hired employees (Check the box and see line 12.)
☐ Compliance with IRS withholding regulations
☐ Other (specify)

☐ Banking purpose (specify purpose) _____
☐ Changed type of organization (specify new type) _____
☐ Purchased going business
☐ Created a trust (specify type) _____
☐ Created a pension plan (specify type) _____

10   Date business started or acquired (month, day, year)

11   Closing month of accounting year

12   First date wages or annuities were paid or will be paid (month, day, year). **Note:** If applicant is a withholding agent, enter date income will first be paid to nonresident alien. (month, day, year)

13   Highest number of employees expected in the next 12 months. **Note:** If the applicant does not expect to have any employees during the period, enter "-0-."

Agricultural	Household	Other

14   Check **one** box that best describes the principal activity of your business.
☐ Construction   ☐ Rental & leasing   ☐ Transportation & warehousing
☐ Real estate   ☐ Manufacturing   ☐ Finance & insurance
☐ Health care & social assistance   ☐ Wholesale–agent/broker
☐ Accommodation & food service   ☐ Wholesale–other   ☐ Retail
☐ Other (specify)

15   Indicate principal line of merchandise sold; specific construction work done; products produced; or services provided.

16a   Has the applicant ever applied for an employer identification number for this or any other business?   ☐ Yes   ☐ No
Note: If "Yes," please complete lines 16b and 16c.

16b   If you checked "Yes" on line 16a, give applicant's legal name and trade name shown on prior application if different from line 1 or 2 above.
Legal name   Trade name

16c   Approximate date when, and city and state where, the application was filed. Enter previous employer identification number if known.
Approximate date when filed (mo., day, year)   City and state where filed   Previous EIN

Third Party Designee
Complete this section **only** if you want to authorize the named individual to receive the entity's EIN and answer questions about the completion of this form.
Designee's name
Address and ZIP code
Designee's telephone number (include area code)   (   )
Designee's fax number (include area code)   (   )

Under penalties of perjury, I declare that I have examined this application, and to the best of my knowledge and belief, it is true, correct, and complete.

Applicant's telephone number (include area code)   (   )

Name and title (type or print clearly)

Applicant's fax number (include area code)   (   )

Signature   Date

For Privacy Act and Paperwork Reduction Act Notice, see separate instructions.   Cat. No. 16055N   Form **SS-4** (Rev. 12-2001)

Figure 16-14 Application for employer identification number (Form SS-4).

Form W-4 (2005)

Purpose. Complete Form W-4 so that your employer can withhold the correct federal income tax from your pay. Because your tax situation may change, you may want to refigure your withholding each year.

Exemption from withholding. If you are exempt, complete only lines 1, 2, 3, 4, and 7 and sign the form to validate it. Your exemption for 2005 expires February 16, 2006. See Pub. 505, Tax Withholding and Estimated Tax.

Note. You cannot claim exemption from withholding if (a) your income exceeds $800 and includes more than $250 of unearned income (for example, interest and dividends) and (b) another person can claim you as a dependent on their tax return.

Basic instructions. If you are not exempt, complete the **Personal Allowances Worksheet** below. The worksheets on page 2 adjust your withholding allowances based on itemized deductions, certain credits, adjustments to income, or two-earner/two-job situations. Complete all worksheets that apply. However, you may claim fewer (or zero) allowances.

Head of household. Generally, you may claim head of household filing status on your tax return only if you are unmarried and pay more than 50% of the costs of keeping up a home for yourself and your dependent(s) or other qualifying individuals. See line **E** below.

Tax credits. You can take projected tax credits into account in figuring your allowable number of withholding allowances. Credits for child or dependent care expenses and the child tax credit may be claimed using the **Personal Allowances Worksheet** below. See Pub. 919, How Do I Adjust My Tax Withholding? for information on converting your other credits into withholding allowances.

Nonwage income. If you have a large amount of nonwage income, such as interest or dividends, consider making estimated tax payments using Form 1040-ES, Estimated Tax for Individuals. Otherwise, you may owe additional tax.

Two earners/two jobs. If you have a working spouse or more than one job, figure the total number of allowances you are entitled to claim on all jobs using worksheets from only one Form W-4. Your withholding usually will be most accurate when all allowances are claimed on the Form W-4 for the highest paying job and zero allowances are claimed on the others.

Nonresident alien. If you are a nonresident alien, see the Instructions for Form 8233 before completing this Form W-4.

Check your withholding. After your Form W-4 takes effect, use Pub. 919 to see how the dollar amount you are having withheld compares to your projected total tax for 2005. See Pub. 919, especially if your earnings exceed $125,000 (Single) or $175,000 (Married).

Recent name change? If your name on line 1 differs from that shown on your social security card, call 1-800-772-1213 to initiate a name change and obtain a social security card showing your correct name.

Personal Allowances Worksheet (Keep for your records.)

A Enter "1" for **yourself** if no one else can claim you as a dependent . . . . **A** _____

B Enter "1" if:
- You are single and have only one job; or
- You are married, have only one job, and your spouse does not work; or
- Your wages from a second job or your spouse's wages (or the total of both) are $1,000 or less.

       . . **B** _____

C Enter "1" for your **spouse.** But, you may choose to enter "-0-" if you are married and have either a working spouse or more than one job. (Entering "-0-" may help you avoid having too little tax withheld.) . . . . **C** _____

D Enter number of **dependents** (other than your spouse or yourself) you will claim on your tax return . . . . **D** _____

E Enter "1" if you will file as **head of household** on your tax return (see conditions under **Head of household** above) . **E** _____

F Enter "1" if you have at least $1,500 of **child or dependent care expenses** for which you plan to claim a credit . **F** _____

     (**Note.** Do **not** include child support payments. See **Pub. 503,** Child and Dependent Care Expenses, for details.)

G **Child Tax Credit** (including additional child tax credit):
- If your total income will be less than $54,000 ($79,000 if married), enter "2" for each eligible child.
- If your total income will be between $54,000 and $84,000 ($79,000 and $119,000 if married), enter "1" for each eligible child plus "1" **additional** if you have four or more eligible children. **G** _____

H Add lines A through G and enter total here. (**Note.** This may be different from the number of exemptions you claim on your tax return.) ▶ **H** _____

For accuracy, complete all worksheets that apply.
- If you plan to **itemize or claim adjustments to income** and want to reduce your withholding, see the **Deductions and Adjustments Worksheet** on page 2.
- If you have **more than one job** or are **married and you and your spouse both work** and the combined earnings from all jobs exceed $35,000 ($25,000 if married) see the **Two-Earner/Two-Job Worksheet** on page 2 to avoid having too little tax withheld.
- If **neither** of the above situations applies, **stop here** and enter the number from line H on line 5 of Form W-4 below.

- - - - - - - - - - - - - - - - **Cut here and give Form W-4 to your employer. Keep the top part for your records.** - - - - - - - - - - - - - - - - - -

Form **W-4**
Department of the Treasury
Internal Revenue Service

Employee's Withholding Allowance Certificate

▶ Whether you are entitled to claim a certain number of allowances or exemption from withholding is subject to review by the IRS. Your employer may be required to send a copy of this form to the IRS.

OMB No. 1545-0010

2005

1 Type or print your first name and middle initial	Last name	2 Your social security number

Home address (number and street or rural route)

3 ☐ Single ☐ Married ☐ Married, but withhold at higher Single rate.
Note. If married, but legally separated, or spouse is a nonresident alien, check the "Single" box.

City or town, state, and ZIP code

4 If your last name differs from that shown on your social security card, check here. You must call 1-800-772-1213 for a new card. ▶ ☐

5 Total number of allowances you are claiming (from line **H** above **or** from the applicable worksheet on page 2)   **5** ____

6 Additional amount, if any, you want withheld from each paycheck . . . . **6** $ ____

7 I claim exemption from withholding for 2005, and I certify that I meet **both** of the following conditions for exemption.
- Last year I had a right to a refund of **all** federal income tax withheld because I had **no** tax liability **and**
- This year I expect a refund of **all** federal income tax withheld because I expect to have **no** tax liability.

If you meet both conditions, write "Exempt" here . . . . ▶ **7** ____

Under penalties of perjury, I declare that I have examined this certificate and to the best of my knowledge and belief, it is true, correct, and complete.

Employee's signature
(Form is not valid unless you sign it.) ▶   **Date** ▶

8 Employer's name and address (Employer: Complete lines 8 and 10 only if sending to the IRS.)	9 Office code (optional)	10 Employer identification number (EIN)

For Privacy Act and Paperwork Reduction Act Notice, see page 2.   Cat. No. 10220Q   Form **W-4** (2005)

Figure 16-15 Employee's Withholding Allowance Certificate (Form W-4).

Form W-4 (2005) Page **2**

Deductions and Adjustments Worksheet

Note. Use this worksheet *only* if you plan to itemize deductions, claim certain credits, or claim adjustments to income on your 2005 tax return.

1	Enter an estimate of your 2005 itemized deductions. These include qualifying home mortgage interest, charitable contributions, state and local taxes, medical expenses in excess of 7.5% of your income, and miscellaneous deductions. (For 2005, you may have to reduce your itemized deductions if your income is over $145,950 ($72,975 if married filing separately). See *Worksheet 3* in Pub. 919 for details.)	**1**	$
2	Enter: { $10,000 if married filing jointly or qualifying widow(er) / $ 7,300 if head of household / $ 5,000 if single or married filing separately }	**2**	$
3	**Subtract** line 2 from line 1. If line 2 is greater than line 1, enter "-0-"	**3**	$
4	Enter an estimate of your 2005 adjustments to income, including alimony, deductible IRA contributions, and student loan interest	**4**	$
5	**Add** lines 3 and 4 and enter the total. (Include any amount for credits from *Worksheet 7* in Pub. 919)	**5**	$
6	Enter an estimate of your 2005 nonwage income (such as dividends or interest)	**6**	$
7	**Subtract** line 6 from line 5. Enter the result, but not less than "-0-"	**7**	$
8	**Divide** the amount on line 7 by $3,200 and enter the result here. Drop any fraction	**8**	
9	Enter the number from the **Personal Allowances Worksheet,** line H, page 1	**9**	
10	**Add** lines 8 and 9 and enter the total here. If you plan to use the **Two-Earner/Two-Job Worksheet,** also enter this total on line 1 below. Otherwise, **stop here** and enter this total on Form W-4, line 5, page 1	**10**	

Two-Earner/Two-Job Worksheet (See *Two earners/two jobs* on page 1.)

Note. Use this worksheet *only* if the instructions under line H on page 1 direct you here.

1	Enter the number from line H, page 1 (or from line 10 above if you used the **Deductions and Adjustments Worksheet**)	**1**	
2	Find the number in **Table 1** below that applies to the **LOWEST** paying job and enter it here	**2**	
3	If line 1 is **more than or equal to** line 2, subtract line 2 from line 1. Enter the result here (if zero, enter "-0-") and on Form W-4, line 5, page 1. **Do not** use the rest of this worksheet	**3**	

Note. If line 1 is *less than* line 2, enter "-0-" on Form W-4, line 5, page 1. Complete lines 4–9 below to calculate the additional withholding amount necessary to avoid a year-end tax bill.

4	Enter the number from line 2 of this worksheet	**4**	
5	Enter the number from line 1 of this worksheet	**5**	
6	**Subtract** line 5 from line 4	**6**	
7	Find the amount in **Table 2** below that applies to the **HIGHEST** paying job and enter it here	**7**	$
8	**Multiply** line 7 by line 6 and enter the result here. This is the additional annual withholding needed	**8**	$
9	Divide line 8 by the number of pay periods remaining in 2005. For example, divide by 26 if you are paid every two weeks and you complete this form in December 2004. Enter the result here and on Form W-4, line 6, page 1. This is the additional amount to be withheld from each paycheck	**9**	$

Table 1: Two-Earner/Two-Job Worksheet

Married Filing Jointly						All Others	
If wages from **HIGHEST** paying job are—	AND, wages from **LOWEST** paying job are—	Enter on line 2 above	If wages from **HIGHEST** paying job are—	AND, wages from **LOWEST** paying job are—	Enter on line 2 above	If wages from **LOWEST** paying job are—	Enter on line 2 above
$0 - $40,000	$0 - $4,000	0	$40,001 and over	30,001 - 36,000	6	$0 - $6,000	0
	4,001 - 8,000	1		36,001 - 45,000	7	6,001 - 12,000	1
	8,001 - 18,000	2		45,001 - 50,000	8	12,001 - 18,000	2
	18,001 and over	3		50,001 - 60,000	9	18,001 - 24,000	3
				60,001 - 65,000	10	24,001 - 31,000	4
$40,001 and over	$0 - $4,000	0		65,001 - 75,000	11	31,001 - 45,000	5
	4,001 - 8,000	1		75,001 - 90,000	12	45,001 - 60,000	6
	8,001 - 18,000	2		90,001 - 100,000	13	60,001 - 75,000	7
	18,001 - 22,000	3		100,001 - 115,000	14	75,001 - 80,000	8
	22,001 - 25,000	4		115,001 and over	15	80,001 - 100,000	9
	25,001 - 30,000	5				100,001 and over	10

Table 2: Two-Earner/Two-Job Worksheet

Married Filing Jointly		All Others	
If wages from **HIGHEST** paying job are—	Enter on line 7 above	If wages from **HIGHEST** paying job are—	Enter on line 7 above
$0 - $60,000	$480	$0 - $30,000	$480
60,001 - 110,000	800	30,001 - 70,000	800
110,001 - 160,000	900	70,001 - 140,000	900
160,001 - 280,000	1,060	140,001 - 320,000	1,060
280,001 and over	1,120	320,001 and over	1,120

 Printed on recycled paper

Figure 16-15 Cont'd

EMPLOYEE'S EARNINGS RECORD

Exemptions _____   Name _____

Date of Birth _____   Address _____

Date Employed _____   _____

Phone _____   Soc. Sec. No. _____

In Emergency Notify _____

REMARKS	DATE	CHECK NO.	GROSS SALARY	FEDERAL W.H. TAX	F.I.C.A.	STATE W.H. TAX	OTHER	OTHER	NET CHECK
THIRD QUARTER									
FOURTH QUARTER									
YEAR'S TOTALS									

Figure 16-16 Employee's earnings record. (Courtesy Sycom, Madison, WI.)

According to the table in Figure 16-17, the withholding tax on $800 for a married person claiming one exemption is $94.

c. *Local income tax.* Some cities and states have personal income taxes that must be deducted. Again, the employer must be familiar with the state and local laws regarding these taxes.

d. *Other deductions.* In addition to the standard deductions, the administrative assistant may have a weekly deduction of $60 for the credit union (noted on the earnings record).

4. The **net pay** (take-home pay), and the amount for which the paycheck is written, is $584.80.

Gross Wages	Minus Deductions	Deductions Total	Net Pay
$800	FICA: $61.20 Withholding tax: $94 Credit union: $60	$215.20	$584.80

The net pay for each member of the office staff must be calculated. After the amounts have been determined, the paychecks are written, the information is entered on each employee's earnings record, and a record is made on the expense sheet.

A pegboard system similar to the one described earlier, which uses a write it once method, can be a great time saver (see Figure 16-7). With this type of system, the employee's earnings are recorded on the earnings record and the monthly expense disbursement sheets when the check stubs are written. The columns on the check stubs, earnings records, and monthly expense disbursement sheet coincide. These systems have proved very popular with employers who have a number of employees.

Depositing Withheld Income Tax and Social Security Taxes

Generally, the employer must deposit withheld income tax, Social Security, and Medicare taxes in an authorized commercial bank or a Federal Reserve Bank. Since January 1, 2000, new coupon forms have been used for depositing taxes. The IRS sends the employer a Federal Tax Deposit (FTD) Coupon Book (Form 8109) containing 15 coupons for depositing all types of taxes. FTD forms are no longer mailed out periodically. If additional forms are needed, the FTD Reorder Form (Form 8109A) provided in the coupon book is used. If you do not have a coupon book, you may request one from the IRS district office.

The amount of taxes determines the frequency of deposits. These taxes are owed when the employer pays the wages (or makes the payments from which the taxes are withheld), not when the payroll period ends. To determine when the taxes are due and the amount on which they are based, the administrative assistant should check the instructions on the reverse side of the Employer's Quarterly Federal Tax Return (Form 941) (Figure 16-18).

Although the employer probably will make monthly deposits for the withholding taxes and FICA deductions, he or she must file a quarterly return on Form 941. The returns and tax payments are due on the following dates:

Quarter	Quarter Ending	Due Date
January to March	March 31	April 30
April to June	June 30	July 31
July to September	September 30	October 31
October to December	December 31	January 31

MARRIED Persons—WEEKLY Payroll Period
(For Wages Paid Through December 2004)

If the wages are—		And the number of withholding allowances claimed is—										
At least	But less than	0	1	2	3	4	5	6	7	8	9	10
		The amount of income tax to be withheld is—										
$0	$125	$0	$0	$0	$0	$0	$0	$0	$0	$0	$0	$0
125	130	0	0	0	0	0	0	0	0	0	0	0
130	135	0	0	0	0	0	0	0	0	0	0	0
135	140	0	0	0	0	0	0	0	0	0	0	0
140	145	0	0	0	0	0	0	0	0	0	0	0
145	150	0	0	0	0	0	0	0	0	0	0	0
150	155	0	0	0	0	0	0	0	0	0	0	0
155	160	0	0	0	0	0	0	0	0	0	0	0
160	165	1	0	0	0	0	0	0	0	0	0	0
165	170	1	0	0	0	0	0	0	0	0	0	0
170	175	2	0	0	0	0	0	0	0	0	0	0
175	180	2	0	0	0	0	0	0	0	0	0	0
180	185	3	0	0	0	0	0	0	0	0	0	0
185	190	3	0	0	0	0	0	0	0	0	0	0
190	195	4	0	0	0	0	0	0	0	0	0	0
195	200	4	0	0	0	0	0	0	0	0	0	0
200	210	5	0	0	0	0	0	0	0	0	0	0
210	220	6	0	0	0	0	0	0	0	0	0	0
220	230	7	1	0	0	0	0	0	0	0	0	0
230	240	8	2	0	0	0	0	0	0	0	0	0
240	250	9	3	0	0	0	0	0	0	0	0	0
250	260	10	4	0	0	0	0	0	0	0	0	0
260	270	11	5	0	0	0	0	0	0	0	0	0
270	280	12	6	0	0	0	0	0	0	0	0	0
280	290	13	7	1	0	0	0	0	0	0	0	0
290	300	14	8	2	0	0	0	0	0	0	0	0
300	310	15	9	3	0	0	0	0	0	0	0	0
310	320	16	10	4	0	0	0	0	0	0	0	0
320	330	17	11	5	0	0	0	0	0	0	0	0
330	340	18	12	6	0	0	0	0	0	0	0	0
340	350	19	13	7	1	0	0	0	0	0	0	0
350	360	20	14	8	2	0	0	0	0	0	0	0
360	370	21	15	9	3	0	0	0	0	0	0	0
370	380	22	16	10	4	0	0	0	0	0	0	0
380	390	23	17	11	5	0	0	0	0	0	0	0
390	400	24	18	12	6	0	0	0	0	0	0	0
400	410	25	19	13	7	1	0	0	0	0	0	0
410	420	26	20	14	8	2	0	0	0	0	0	0
420	430	27	21	15	9	3	0	0	0	0	0	0
430	440	28	22	16	10	4	0	0	0	0	0	0
440	450	30	23	17	11	5	0	0	0	0	0	0
450	460	31	24	18	12	6	0	0	0	0	0	0
460	470	33	25	19	13	7	1	0	0	0	0	0
470	480	34	26	20	14	8	2	0	0	0	0	0
480	490	36	27	21	15	9	3	0	0	0	0	0
490	500	37	28	22	16	10	4	0	0	0	0	0
500	510	39	30	23	17	11	5	0	0	0	0	0
510	520	40	31	24	18	12	6	0	0	0	0	0
520	530	42	33	25	19	13	7	1	0	0	0	0
530	540	43	34	26	20	14	8	2	0	0	0	0
540	550	45	36	27	21	15	9	3	0	0	0	0
550	560	46	37	29	22	16	10	4	0	0	0	0
560	570	48	39	30	23	17	11	5	0	0	0	0
570	580	49	40	32	24	18	12	6	0	0	0	0
580	590	51	42	33	25	19	13	7	1	0	0	0
590	600	52	43	35	26	20	14	8	2	0	0	0
600	610	54	45	36	27	21	15	9	3	0	0	0
610	620	55	46	38	29	22	16	10	4	0	0	0
620	630	57	48	39	30	23	17	11	5	0	0	0
630	640	58	49	41	32	24	18	12	6	0	0	0
640	650	60	51	42	33	25	19	13	7	1	0	0
650	660	61	52	44	35	26	20	14	8	2	0	0
660	670	63	54	45	36	27	21	15	9	3	0	0
670	680	64	55	47	38	29	22	16	10	4	0	0
680	690	66	57	48	39	30	23	17	11	5	0	0
690	700	67	58	50	41	32	24	18	12	6	0	0
700	710	69	60	51	42	33	25	19	13	7	1	0
710	720	70	61	53	44	35	26	20	14	8	2	0
720	730	72	63	54	45	36	27	21	15	9	3	0
730	740	73	64	56	47	38	29	22	16	10	4	0

Page 7

Figure 16-17 Withholding tax table.

Form **941 for 2005:** Employer's Quarterly Federal Tax Return

(Rev. January 2005)

Department of the Treasury — Internal Revenue Service

9901

OMB No. 1545-0029

Employer identification number

Name (not your trade name)

Trade name (if any)

Address

Number   Street   Suite or room number

City   State   ZIP code

Report for this Quarter ...
(Check one.)

☐ **1:** January, February, March

☐ **2:** April, May, June

☐ **3:** July, August, September

☐ **4:** October, November, December

Read the separate instructions before you fill out this form. Please type or print within the boxes.

Part 1: Answer these questions for this quarter.

1 Number of employees who received wages, tips, or other compensation for the pay period including: *Mar. 12* (Quarter 1), *June 12* (Quarter 2), *Sept. 12* (Quarter 3), *Dec. 12* (Quarter 4)   **1**

2 Wages, tips, and other compensation **2**

3 Total income tax withheld from wages, tips, and other compensation **3**

4 If no wages, tips, and other compensation are subject to social security or Medicare tax .   ☐ Check and go to line 6.

5 Taxable social security and Medicare wages and tips:

	Column 1			Column 2	
5a Taxable social security wages		.	× .124 =		.
5b Taxable social security tips		.	× .124 =		.
5c Taxable Medicare wages & tips		.	× .029 =		.

5d Total social security and Medicare taxes (*Column 2,* lines 5a + 5b + 5c = line 5d) .   **5d**

6 Total taxes before adjustments (lines 3 + 5d = line 6) **6**

7 Tax adjustments (If your answer is a negative number, write it in brackets.):

7a Current quarter's fractions of cents . . . .

7b Current quarter's sick pay . . . .

7c Current quarter's adjustments for tips and group-term life insurance

7d Current year's income tax withholding (Attach Form 941c) . .

7e Prior quarters' social security and Medicare taxes (Attach Form 941c)

7f Special additions to federal income tax (reserved use) . . .

7g Special additions to social security and Medicare (reserved use)

7h Total adjustments (Combine all amounts: lines 7a through 7g.) **7h**

8 Total taxes after adjustments (Combine lines 6 and 7h.) **8**

9 Advance earned income credit (EIC) payments made to employees **9**

10 Total taxes after adjustment for advance EIC (lines 8 – 9 = line 10) **10**

11 Total deposits for this quarter, including overpayment applied from a prior quarter . .   **11**

12 Balance due (lines 10 – 11 = line 12) Make checks payable to the *United States Treasury* .   **12**

13 Overpayment (If line 11 is more than line 10, write the difference here.)   Check one ☐ Apply to next return.
☐ Send a refund.

Next ➡

For Privacy Act and Paperwork Reduction Act Notice, see the back of the Payment Voucher.   Cat. No. 17001Z   Form **941** (Rev. 1-2005)

Figure 16-18 Employer's Quarterly Federal Tax Return (Form 941).

The employer completes Form 941 by entering the summarized payroll data for the quarter. Information about total wages and taxable FICA wages is obtained from the employee's earnings record. Further instructions are available in the IRS pamphlet instructions for Form 941.

Federal Unemployment Tax

The employer is subject to a federal unemployment tax under the provisions of the Federal Unemployment Tax Act (FUTA). This tax is 6.2% of wages paid and applies to the first $7,000 of wages paid during the calendar year. Generally, a credit may be taken against the federal unemployment tax for contributions to be paid into state unemployment funds. The federal unemployment tax is imposed on employers and must not be deducted from employees' wages. On or before January 31, the employer must file an unemployment tax return (i.e., Employers' Annual Federal Unemployment [FUTA] Tax Return [Form 940]) (Figure 16-19) and deposit or pay the balance of the tax in full. For deposit purposes, the employer must compute the federal unemployment tax on a quarterly basis. The deposit must be made on or before the last day of the first month after the close of the quarter.

To determine whether your employer must make a deposit for any of the first three quarters in a year, compute the total tax as follows:

1. Multiply the first $7,000 of each employee's annual wages paid during the quarter by 0.008.
2. If the amount subject to deposit (plus the amount subject to deposit but not deposited for any prior quarter) is more than $100, a deposit should be made during the first month after the quarter.

Wage and Tax Statement (Form W-2)

A federal **Wage and Tax Statement (Form W-2)** for a calendar year must be provided for each employee no later than January 31 of the following year (Figure 16-20). The Form W-2 is prepared in six parts and distributed in the following manner: one copy for IRS use; one copy to state, city, or local tax departments; three copies to the employee (one for filing federal tax returns, one for state or local tax purposes, and one for the employee's files); and one copy retained by the employer.

Form W-2 includes the following information:
* Employer's identification number, name, and address
* Employee's Social Security number, name, and address
* Federal income tax withheld
* Total sum of wages paid to the employee
* Total FICA employee tax withheld (Social Security and Medicare)
* Total wages paid that are subject to FICA
* State and local taxes withheld when applicable

To correct a Form W-2 after one has been issued to an employee, a corrected statement must be issued. The corrected statement must completely replace the original statement and be clearly marked as "CORRECTED RETURN" in capital letters directly above the title, Wage and Tax Statement. If a Form W-2 is lost or destroyed, the substitute copy issued to the employee is marked as "Reissued Return."

Report of Withheld Income Tax (Form W-3)

On or before February 28, copy A of all Form W-2s issued for the year and Form W-3, Transmittal of Wage and Tax Statements (Figure 16-21), must be sent to the IRS.

Form 940

Department of the Treasury
Internal Revenue Service (99)

**Employer's Annual Federal
Unemployment (FUTA) Tax Return**

▶ See the separate Instructions for Form 940 for information on completing this form.

OMB No. 1545-0028

2004

T		
FF		
FD		
FP		
I		
T		

**You must
complete
this section.** ▶

Name (as distinguished from trade name)   Calendar year

Trade name, if any   Employer identification number (EIN)

Address (number and street)   City, state, and ZIP code

A Are you required to pay unemployment contributions to only one state? (If "No," skip questions B and C.)   ☐ **Yes**   ☐ **No**

B Did you pay all state unemployment contributions by January 31, 2005? ((1) If you deposited your total FUTA tax when due, check "Yes" if you paid all state unemployment contributions by February 10, 2005. (2) If a 0% experience rate is granted, check "Yes." (3) If "No," skip question C.)   . . . .   ☐ **Yes**   ☐ **No**

C Were all wages that were taxable for FUTA tax also taxable for your state's unemployment tax?   . . .   ☐ **Yes**   ☐ **No**

D Did you pay all wages in a state other than New York? .   . . .   ☐ **Yes**   ☐ **No**

If you answered "No" to any of these questions, you must file Form 940. If you answered "Yes" to all the questions, you may file Form 940-EZ, which is a simplified version of Form 940. (Successor employers, see **Special credit for successor employers** in the separate instructions.) You can get Form 940-EZ by calling 1-800-TAX-FORM (1-800-829-3676) or from the IRS website at **www.irs.gov**.

If you will not have to file returns in the future, check here (see **Who Must File** in the separate instructions) **and complete and sign the return** . . . . ▶ ☐

If this is an Amended Return, check here (see **Amended Returns** in the separate instructions) . . . . . . ▶ ☐

Part I   **Computation of Taxable Wages**

1 Total payments (including payments shown on lines 2 and 3) during the calendar year for services of employees **1**

2 Exempt payments. (Explain all exempt payments, attaching additional sheets if necessary.) ▶ - **2**

3 Payments of more than $7,000 for services. Enter only amounts over the first $7,000 paid to each employee (see separate instructions). Do not include any exempt payments from line 2. The $7,000 amount is the federal wage base. Your state wage base may be different. **Do not use your state wage limitation** **3**

4 Add lines 2 and 3 . . . . **4**

5 **Total taxable wages** (subtract line 4 from line 1) . . . . ▶ **5**

6 Additional tax resulting from credit reduction for unpaid advances to the State of New York. Enter the wages included on line 5 for New York and multiply by .003. (See the separate Instructions for Form 940.) Enter the credit reduction amount here and in Part II, line 5:
New York wages _____ x .003 = ... ▶ **6**

Be sure to complete both sides of this form, and sign in the space provided on the back.

For Privacy Act and Paperwork Reduction Act Notice, see separate instructions.   ▼ **DETACH HERE** ▼   Cat. No. 11234O   Form **940** (2004)

- -

Form 940-V

Department of the Treasury
Internal Revenue Service

Payment Voucher

Use this voucher only when making a payment with your return.

OMB No. 1545-0028

2004

Complete boxes 1, 2, and 3. Do not send cash, and do not staple your payment to this voucher. Make your check or money order payable to the "United States Treasury." Be sure to enter your employer identification number (EIN), "Form 940," and "2004" on your payment.

1 Enter your employer identification number (EIN).

2 **Enter the amount of your payment.** ▶

Dollars	Cents

3 Enter your business name (individual name for sole proprietors).

Enter your address.

Enter your city, state, and ZIP code.

Figure 16-19 Employer's Annual Federal Unemployment (FUTA) Tax Return (Form 940).

Form 940 (2004)   Page **2**

Name

Employer identification number (EIN)

Part II **Tax Due or Refund**

1 Gross FUTA tax. (Multiply the wages from Part I, line 5, by .062) . . . . | **1**

2 Maximum credit. (Multiply the wages from Part I, line 5, by .054) . . | **2**

3 Computation of tentative credit (**Note:** *All taxpayers must complete the applicable columns.*)

(a) Name of state	(b) State reporting number(s) as shown on employer's state contribution returns	(c) Taxable payroll (as defined in state act)	(d) State experience rate period		(e) State experience rate	(f) Contributions if rate had been 5.4% (col. (c) x .054)	(g) Contributions payable at experience rate (col. (c) x col. (e))	(h) Additional credit (col. (f) minus col.(g)) If 0 or less, enter -0-.	(i) Contributions paid to state by 940 due date
			From	To					

3a Totals . . . . |

3b **Total tentative credit** (add line 3a, columns (h) and (i) only—for late payments, also see the instructions for Part II, line 4) . . . . ▶ **3b**

4 **Credit:** Enter the smaller of the amount from Part II, line 2 or line 3b; or the amount from the worksheet on page 7 of the separate instructions **4**

5 Enter the amount from Part I, line 6 . . . . **5**

6 **Credit allowable** (subtract line 5 from line 4). If zero or less, enter "-0-" **6**

7 **Total FUTA tax** (subtract line 6 from line 1). If the result is over $100, also complete Part III . **7**

8 Total FUTA tax deposited for the year, including any overpayment applied from a prior year . **8**

9 **Balance due** (subtract line 8 from line 7). Pay to the "United States Treasury." If you owe more than $100, see **Depositing FUTA Tax** on page 3 of the separate instructions . . . . . ▶ **9**

10 **Overpayment** (subtract line 7 from line 8). Check if it is to be: ☐ **Applied to next return** or ☐ **Refunded** . . . . ▶ **10**

Part III **Record of Quarterly Federal Unemployment Tax Liability** (Do not include state liability.) **Complete only if line 7 is over $100.** See page 7 of the separate instructions.

Quarter	First (Jan. 1–Mar. 31)	Second (Apr. 1–June 30)	Third (July 1–Sept. 30)	Fourth (Oct. 1–Dec. 31)	Total for year
Liability for quarter					

Third-Party Designee

Do you want to allow another person to discuss this return with the IRS (see separate instructions)? ☐ **Yes.** Complete the following. ☐ **No**

Designee's name ▶   Phone no. ▶ (   )   Personal identification number (PIN)

Under penalties of perjury, I declare that I have examined this return, including accompanying schedules and statements, and, to the best of my knowledge and belief, it is true, correct, and complete, and that no part of any payment made to a state unemployment fund claimed as a credit was, or is to be, deducted from the payments to employees.

Signature ▶   Title (Owner, etc.) ▶   Date ▶

Form **940** (2004)

Figure 16-19 Cont'd

Retention of Payroll and Tax Records

> The employer must keep all records pertaining to employment taxes available for inspection by the Internal Revenue Service.

The employer must keep all records pertaining to employment taxes available for inspection by the IRS. Although no form has been devised for such records, the employer must be able to supply the following information:

- Amounts and dates of all wages paid
- Names, addresses, and occupations of employees
- Periods of employees' employment
- Periods for which employees were paid while absent because of sickness
- Employees' Social Security numbers
- Employees' income tax withholding allowance certificates
- Employer's identification number
- Duplicate copies of returns filed and the dates and amounts of deposits made

These tax records should be kept for at least 4 years after the date the taxes to which they apply become due.

Employer's Responsibility for Tax Information

The *Employer's Tax Guide—Circular E,* mentioned previously, summarizes the employer's responsibilities for withholding, depositing, paying, and reporting

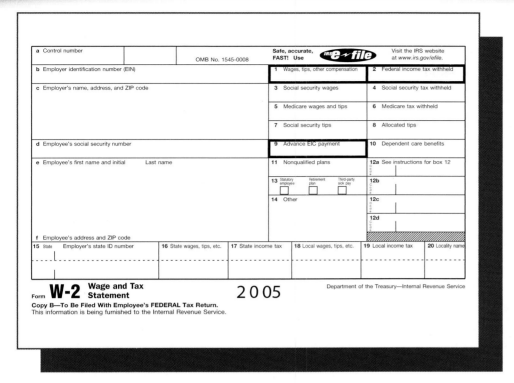

Figure 16-20 Wage and Tax Statement (Form W-2).

federal income tax, Social Security taxes, and federal unemployment tax. The circular is available to all employers and may be obtained from a local IRS office. Because tax rates increase so often, the administrative assistant would be wise to check with the IRS to make sure the most up-to-date forms and percentages are used for tax calculations. A Quick and Easy Access to Tax Help and Forms is shown in Figure 16-22. Additional information and help are available at the American Payroll Association website, www.apa.com.

ACCOUNTS PAYABLE SOFTWARE

Most dental office software packages do not provide a mechanism for writing checks and maintaining payroll records; therefore the dentist must rely on some form of commercial software to accomplish this task. QuickBooks Financial Software: 2005 gives small business owners the power to run their businesses more effectively. For small businesses with 1 to 20 employees, QuickBooks 2005 helps save time and increase productivity because it offers improvements to commonly used features and provides better help and learning tools to increase user knowledge and confidence. The software is available in a variety of editions, and the administrative assistant should review the needs of the office before making a selection. The benefits of such a package include the ability to

- Pay bills
- Print checks
- Create invoices and purchase orders
- Track business payments and expenses
- Manage payroll processing
- Direct deposit paychecks
- Create state and federal forms
- Track workers' compensation payments and easily calculate bonuses

DO NOT STAPLE OR FOLD

a Control number	33333	For Official Use Only ► OMB No. 1545-0008		

b Kind of Payer	941 ☐ Military ☐ 943 ☐ CT-1 ☐ Hshld. emp. ☐ Medicare govt. emp. ☐ Third-party sick pay ☐	1 Wages, tips, other compensation	2 Federal income tax withheld

	3 Social security wages	4 Social security tax withheld

c Total number of Forms W-2	Establishment number	5 Medicare wages and tips	6 Medicare tax withheld

e Employer identification number (EIN)	7 Social security tips	8 Allocated tips

f Employer's name	9 Advance EIC payments	10 Dependent care benefits

	11 Nonqualified plans	12 Deferred compensation

	13 For third-party sick pay use only

	14 Income tax withheld by payer of third-party sick pay

g Employer's address and ZIP code	
h Other EIN used this year	

15 State Employer's state ID number	16 State wages, tips, etc.	17 State income tax

	18 Local wages, tips, etc.	19 Local income tax

Contact person	Telephone number ( )	For Official Use Only
Email address	Fax number ( )	

Under penalties of perjury, I declare that I have examined this return and accompanying documents, and, to the best of my knowledge and belief, they are true, correct, and complete.

Signature ►   Title ►   Date ►

Form **W-3** Transmittal of Wage and Tax Statements   **2005**   Department of the Treasury
Internal Revenue Service

Send this entire page with the entire Copy A page of Form(s) W-2 to the Social Security Administration. Photocopies are not acceptable.

Do not send any payment (cash, checks, money orders, etc.) with Forms W-2 and W-3.

Reminder

Separate instructions. See the 2005 Instructions for Forms W-2 and W-3 for information on completing this form.

Purpose of Form

Use Form W-3 to transmit Copy A of Form(s) W-2, Wage and Tax Statement. Make a copy of Form W-3 and keep it with Copy D (For Employer) of Form(s) W-2 for your records. Use Form W-3 for the correct year. **File Form W-3 even if only one Form W-2 is being filed.** If you are filing Form(s) W-2 on magnetic media or electronically, **do not** file Form W-3.

When To File

File Form W-3 with Copy A of Form(s) W-2 by February 28, 2006.

Where To File

Send this entire page with the entire Copy A page of Form(s) W-2 to:

**Social Security Administration
Data Operations Center
Wilkes-Barre, PA 18769-0001**

Note. *If you use "Certified Mail" to file, change the ZIP code to "18769-0002." If you use an IRS-approved private delivery service, add "ATTN: W-2 Process, 1150 E. Mountain Dr." to the address and change the ZIP code to "18702-7997." See* **Publication 15** *(Circular E), Employer's Tax Guide, for a list of IRS-approved private delivery services.*

Do not send magnetic media to the address shown above.

For Privacy Act and Paperwork Reduction Act Notice, see back of Copy D of Form W-2.

Cat. No. 10159Y

Figure 16-21 Transmittal of Wage and Tax Statements (Form W-3).

Quick and Easy Access to IRS Tax Help and Tax Products

 Personal Computer

You can access the IRS website 24 hours a day, 7 days a week, at **www.irs.gov** to:

- Access commercial tax preparation and *e-file* services available for FREE to eligible taxpayers
- Check the status of your 2004 refund
- Download forms, instructions, and publications
- Order IRS products online
- See answers to frequently asked tax questions
- Search publications online by topic or keyword
- Figure your withholding allowances using our Withholding Calculator
- Send us comments or request help by email
- Sign up to receive local and national tax news by email

 Phone

Obtain forms, instructions, and publications by calling:

1-800-829-3676 to order current year forms, instructions, and publications and prior year forms and instructions. You should receive your order within 10 days.

 Walk-In

Pick up certain forms, instructions and publications at many post offices, libraries and IRS offices. Some grocery stores, copy centers, city and county government offices, credit unions and office supply stores have a collection of reproducible tax forms available to photocopy or print from a CD-ROM.

 Mail

Send your order for tax products to:

National Distribution Center
P.O. Box 8903
Bloomington, IL   61702-8903

You should receive your products within 10 days after we receive your order.

 CD-ROM

Order IRS Publication 1796, Federal Tax Products on CD-ROM, and obtain:

- Current tax forms, instructions, and publications
- Prior-year tax forms and instructions
- Popular tax forms which may be filled-in electronically, printed out for submission, and saved for recordkeeping
- Internal Revenue Bulletin

Purchase the CD-ROM via Internet at **http://www.irs.gov/cdorders** from the National Technical Information Service (NTIS) for $22 (no handling fee). Order by phone at 1-877-CDFORMS (1-877-233-6767) for $22 (plus $5 handling fee).

Availability: First release—early January
Final release—late February

Minimum System Requirements:

The 2004 Federal Tax Products CD-ROM can be used with the following operating systems (Windows 98SE, NT 4 (w/ SP 6), ME, 2000 (w/ SP 2), XP; Mac OS X v.10.2.2-10.3). It requires a minimum of 64 MB RAM, 128 MB RAM recommended; and a minimum of 120 MB available hard drive space. System requires either an Intel® Pentium® processor or PowerPC® G3 processor. Software is provided to view, search, **fill-in and save forms** using the free Adobe® Reader® 6.02. IRS applies document rights to their PDF forms so they can be filled in and saved locally using the free Adobe Reader. Some forms on the CD-ROM are intended as information only and may not be filled in and submitted as an official IRS form (e.g., Forms 1099, W-2, and W-3). **Additionally, this CD-ROM does not support electronic filing.**

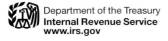 Department of the Treasury
Internal Revenue Service
www.irs.gov

Publication 2053A (4-2005)
Cat. No. 23267Z

Figure 16-22 A Quick and Easy Access to Tax Help and Forms.

LEARNING ACTIVITIES

1. Name and define the parts of a check.
2. List the necessary steps in writing a check.
3. Explain how a certified check and a cashier's check are different.
4. Describe the procedure for making a bank deposit.
5. Define the following:
   a. Blank endorsement
   b. Endorsement in full
   c. Restrictive endorsement
6. Describe the procedures for reconciling a bank statement.
7. Explain the function of a monthly expense sheet.
8. Explain the function of a yearly summary.
9. Why is it necessary to maintain accurate payroll records?
10. What is the purpose of an employee's earnings record?
11. Explain the difference between gross and net wages.
12. What is the purpose of Form 941 and when is the form prepared?
13. On what amount of the employee's wages must the employer pay unemployment taxes?
14. What information is included on Form W-2?
15. Explain the importance of payroll and tax record retention.
16. Using sample checks from the *Practice Management for the Dental Team* Evolve Learning Resources website or from an instructor, write the proper information on the check stubs and checks for Dental Associates, PC. The corporate name is imprinted on the checks. The bank's identification number and the corporate account number have been encoded on the checks for "reading" by the bank's electronic equipment. Prepare the check stubs and checks using the following information.

May 1, 20--
The balance in the checking account is $35,769.52. Record this balance on the first check stub (balance brought forward).

May 2, 20--
Number the first check #114. Make it payable to the American Dental Association (ADA), for a seminar, in the amount of $175.

May 4, 20--
Deposit $10,719.62 in the bank.

May 5, 20--
Issue check #115 for $4,325.60, payable to Cash, for the biweekly payroll.

May 8, 20--
Deposit $1,385.81 in the bank.

May 10, 20--
Issue check #116 for $2,416.85, payable to John T. Synder & Sons, for painting the office.

May 11, 20--
Deposit $5,667.16 in the bank.

May 14, 20--
Issue check #117 for $60.50, payable to the Magazine Clearinghouse, for three magazine subscriptions for the office.

May 17, 20--
Deposit $10,657.20 in the bank.

May 19, 20--
Issue check #118 for $4,325.60, payable to Cash, for the biweekly payroll.

Continued

LEARNING ACTIVITIES—cont'd

May 22, 20--

Issue check #119 for $2,500, payable to Health Science Dental Supply Co., as the balance of payment on a dental unit.

May 24, 20--

Deposit $6,225.50 in the bank.

May 24, 20--

Issue check #120 for $370.84, payable to Computer Depot, for a 4-inch scanner.

May 26, 20--

Deposit $4,308.20 in the bank.

May 26, 200--

Issue check #121 for $350.80, payable to Uniforms Unlimited.

May 28, 20--

Issue check #122 for $550, payable to Meyer Dental Co., for dental supplies.

May 28, 20--

Issue check #123 for $41.60, payable to Cash, to replenish the petty cash fund.

May 29, 20--

Deposit $13,179.40 in the bank.

May 29, 20--

Issue check #124 for $287.55, payable to Johnson Printing Co., for stationery and envelopes.

May 31, 20--

Deposit $924.16 in the bank.

17. Use the following information to complete a deposit slip. Deposit to the account of Dental Associates, PC, account no. 9876-5432.

   a. Currency: $100; Silver: 0.75

      Checks: ABA numbers 12-456, 03-471, 21-689, 31-82, 79-43, 66-101

      Amounts, respectively: $350, $140.75, $275, $45.80, $180.90, $320.10

      Cash returned: None

   b. Currency: $264; Silver: 0.85

      Money order: $60; Bank Americard: $313

      Checks: $260, $390, $189.59

      Cash returned: $50

18. On July 25 you received the bank statement for parts of the months of June and July (see Figure 16-11). After examining the transactions for the months, you note that a deposit for $500 made July 20 does not appear on the bank's statement. Also, checks no. 2008 ($1,100), 2014 ($256), and 2025 ($75) have not cleared the bank. Check no. 2005, incorrectly recorded on the check stubs as $76.20, should have been $67.20. The checkbook balance at this time is $8,027.80.

Reconcile the bank statement and checkbook to the adjusted balance.

19. Perform the following computations.

   A. Determine the weekly gross wages for the following four employees. Forty hours is the regular workweek. Overtime is paid at one and a half times the regular rate of pay for any hours over 40 during the week.

      (1) Mario Garcia: $782.50 weekly; married, 2 exemptions

      (2) Mary O'Brian: 41 hours, $14.50 per hour; married, 0 exemptions

      (3) Keith Sams: 48 hours, $16.50 per hour; married, 3 exemptions

      (4) Betty Todd: 43.5 hours, $18.50 per hour; married, 1 exemption

Continued

EXAMINE YOUR PROGRESS

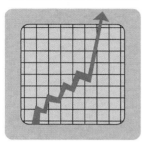

Practice by completing
Working Forms 12–14.

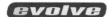

LEARNING ACTIVITIES—cont'd

B. Figure the weekly deductions using the following information:
   (1) FICA: 7.65%
   (2) Withholding tax: Use the table in Figure 16-18 or a current one from
       your office or classroom.
   (3) Credit union: $50 for O'Brian and Todd and $100 for Garcia.
   (4) Life insurance: $27.60 for each employee.
C. Determine the weekly net wages for each of the four employees.

20. Assume that Carla Simmons has earned $74,820 by November 15. She earns
    $1,627 weekly. (FICA is calculated at 7.65%, which is split between Social Security
    at 6.2% on the first $76,200 earned in the year and Medicare at 1.45% on all
    earnings with no yearly cap.) How much of her weekly earnings will be taxable
    for FICA? What amount of FICA tax will she pay?

21. With the following information, complete a W–2 form (obtained from www.
    IRS.gov, the office accountant, or classroom instructor) for Betty Todd, 2035
    East Maplewood, Grand Rapids, MI 49506, Social Security No. 833-43-7044.
    Employer Dental Associates, PC, 611 Main Street, SE, Grand Rapids, MI 49502,
    Tax No. 430038178. Total wages taxable for state, federal, and FICA were
    $32,240. Employee's deductions for the year were federal income tax, $4,056.00;
    state income tax, $626.20; and FICA, $2,466.36.

Key Terms

**American Banking
Association (ABA)** A national
organization of banks and holding
companies of all sizes that deals with
issues of importance to national
institutions.

Automatic teller machine (ATM)
A computer workstation that electronically prompts the user through most
routine banking activities.

Bank deposit Represents the accumulation of money received for a single
day or possibly a longer period.

Bank draft A check drawn by the
cashier of one bank on another bank in
which the first bank has available funds
on deposit or credit.

Bank statement A printed statement
from the bank showing the balance of
the account at the beginning of the
month, deposits made during the
month, checks drawn against the
account, corrections or charges against
the account (e.g., service charge or
stop payment charges), and the bank
balance at the end of the month.

Budget A financial plan of operation
for a given period, usually 1 year.

Cashier's check The bank's own
order to make payment out of the
bank's funds.

Certified check A check for which a
guarantee exists that funds have been
set aside to cover the amount of the
check.

Checks A means of ordering the bank
to pay cash from a bank customer's
account.

**Employee's Withholding Allowance
Certificate (Form W-4)** The federal
form used to determine the status of
each employee for income tax deductions from wages.

Employer identification number
A nine-digit number assigned to sole
proprietors or corporations for filing
and reporting payroll information.

Endorsement The signature or stamp
of the payee.

Expenditures The amount of
money spent to operate a business
or practice.

**Federal Insurance Contributions
Act (FICA)** A law that requires
deductions for Social Security and
Medicare taxes.

Form SS-4   The application form used to obtain an employer identification number.

Gross wages   The total amount of earnings before deductions.

Money order   A means of transferring money without using cash or a personal check.

Net pay   The total amount of earnings after deductions.

Petty cash   A small amount of cash kept on hand in the office to pay for small expenses.

Revenue   The amount of income received by a business or practice.

Traveler's check   A payment device purchased through a bank or other agency that serves as cash for a person who is away from home.

Voucher check   A check that provides a detachable stub, which can be used as an accounting record for itemizing payment of invoices or any type of itemization the payer would like as a reference.

Wage and Tax Statement (Form W-2)   A wage and tax statement for a calendar year must be provided for each employee no later than January 31 of the following year.

Withholding   The amount of money withheld for federal and/or state taxes.

Bibliography

Department of the Treasury, Internal Revenue Service: *Employer's tax guide*, pub no 15, circular E (revised), Washington, DC, 2005.

Fulton PJ: *General office procedures for colleges*, ed 12, Cincinnati, 2003, South-Western.

Hall J: *Consumers now favor credit and debit over cash and checks*, December 2003, American Banking Association, Washington, DC.

Recommended Websites

www.ftc.gov
http://americanbankassociation.com
www.federalreserve.gov
http://fdic.gov
http://www.irs.gov/publications
www.quickbooks.com/support (additional terms and conditions may apply)

Chapter
17
Infection Control Systems

Chapter Outline

Disease Transmission
   Types of Infections
   Routes of Infection Transmission
Infection Control in the Dental Office
   Health Protection Program for the Dental Staff
   Government Regulations
   Maintaining Regulatory Records
   Hazard Communication Program
   Equipment for Hazardous Situations
Infection Control Techniques
   Aseptic Technique
   Personal Protection
     Immunization
     Barrier Protection
   Instrument Sterilization
   Monitoring the Sterilization Process
   Disposables
   Laboratory Asepsis
Educating Patients About Infection Control Programs
Infectious Waste Disposal in the Dental Office

Learning Outcomes

Mastery of the content in this chapter will enable the reader to:
- List characteristics necessary for establishing relationships
- Define key terms
- Identify the importance to the administrative assistant of an understanding of disease transmission
- Identify the routes of disease transmission
- Describe basic infection control procedures
- Identify the various regulatory agencies that might affect the dental office
- Identify the various records required by the Occupational Safety and Health Administration that must be maintained in the business office
- Explain routine procedures that the administrative assistant might perform to maintain quality assurance in the office

As the administrative assistant, you generally have no direct patient contact. Nevertheless, you must understand both the risks and management of occupational exposures to **blood-borne pathogens.** Although your primary duties are in the business office, you may be called upon to perform some clinical task that could expose you to such a risk. Your assigned job, therefore, does not make it impossible for you to contract a **communicable disease.** The role of the administrative assistant in infection control is vital, because it involves the following responsibilities:

- Acquiring a thorough understanding of the routes of disease transmission
- Maintaining an adequate inventory of acceptable **disinfectants,** sterilants, and barrier covers
- Maintaining records verifying compliance with the requirements of the **Occupational Safety and Health Administration (OSHA)**
- Transmitting spore samples to the appropriate monitoring agencies for determination of sterilization effectiveness
- Attending training sessions
- Verifying employee compliance with OSHA
- Maintaining employee records
- Scheduling continuing education courses for the staff
- Verifying quality assurance
- Maintaining all Material Safety Data Sheets (MSDSs)
- Arranging for the disposal of **hazardous waste**
- Providing infection control training for new employees as designated by the employer
- Interacting with outside agencies

A variety of diseases can be transmitted by means of routine dental care. Fortunately, the dental profession, through the American Dental Association (ADA) and the **Centers for Disease Control and Prevention (CDC),** has worked vigorously to establish infection control and safety procedures for the **dental healthcare worker (DHCW)** to prevent the transmission of disease.

The CDC report, *Guidelines for Infection Control in Dental Health Care Settings,* was revised in 2003. Every dental office should have direct access to these guidelines through a link on the ADA's website (www.ada.org) or through the CDC website (www.cdc.gov). This report consolidates previous recommendations and adds new ones for infection control in dental settings. It provides recommendations on (1) educating and protecting dental healthcare personnel; (2) preventing the transmission of blood-borne pathogens; (3) hand hygiene; (4) **personal protective equipment (PPE);** (5) contact dermatitis and latex hypersensitivity; (6) **sterilization** and **disinfection** of patient care items; (7) environmental infection control; (8) dental unit water lines, biofilm, and water quality; and (9) special considerations (e.g., dental handpieces and other devices, radiology, parenteral medications, oral surgical procedures, and dental laboratories). These recommendations were developed in collaboration with and after review by authorities on infection control from the CDC and other public agencies, academia, and private and professional organizations.

> Infectious diseases can be transmitted by several media during dental treatment, including blood, saliva, nasal discharge, dust, hands, clothing, and hair.

DISEASE TRANSMISSION

Dental treatment involves several sources by which infectious diseases can be transmitted, including blood, saliva, nasal discharge, dust, hands, clothing, and hair. Any of these media can transmit a microbial or viral **infection.** Table 17-1 presents a list of several communicable diseases and their routes of transfer.

Table 17-1
Common Communicable Diseases and Routes of Transmission

Disease	Medium of Transmission	Route of Transmission
Acquired immunodeficiency syndrome (AIDS)	Blood, semen, or other body fluids, including breast milk	Inoculation by use of contaminated needles or by direct contact so that infected body fluids can enter the body
Gonococcal disease	Lesions, discharge from infected mucous membranes	Direct contact, as in sexual intercourse; towels, bathtubs, toilets; hands of infected individuals soiled with their own discharges; through breaks in hands of attendant
Hepatitis B, viral	Blood and serum-derived fluids, including semen and vaginal fluids	Contact with blood and body fluids
Measles (rubella)	Discharges from nose and throat	Direct contact, hands of health care worker, articles used by and about patient
Mumps	Discharges from infected glands and throat	Direct contact with affected person
Pneumonia	Sputum and discharges from nose and throat	Direct contact, hands of health care worker, articles used by and about the patient
Rubeola	Secretions from nose and throat	Through mouth and nose
Streptococcal sore throat	Discharges from nose and throat, skin lesions	Through mouth and nose
Syphilis	Infected tissues, lesions, blood, transfer though placenta to fetus	Direct contact, kissing or sexual intercourse, contaminated needles and syringes
Tuberculosis	Saliva, lesions, feces	Direct contact, droplet infection from a person coughing with mouth uncovered, saliva transferred from mouth to fingers and then to food and other articles

Types of Infections

Infections common to dental treatment generally can be divided into two categories, autogenous infections and cross infections. **Autogenous infections** are infections for which the patient is the source. For example, a patient who undergoes dental treatment, such as an extensive scaling procedure, may subsequently develop endocarditis; this condition can result from the introduction of virulent organisms (e.g., staphylococci or pneumococci) that live in the mouth and can be introduced into the bloodstream during the scaling procedure.

Cross infections are transferred from one patient or person to another. For example, when a child has an infection and coughs or sneezes, the caregiver may contract the infection through airborne or droplet transmission.

> With autogenous infections, the patient is the source of the infection.

> Cross infections are transferred from one patient or person to another.

Routes of Infection Transmission

Microbial transmission through dental-related secretions and exudates occurs by three general routes: (1) direct contact with a lesion, organisms, or debris during intraoral procedures; (2) indirect contact through contaminated dental instruments, equipment, or records; and (3) inhalation of micro-organisms aerosolized from a patient's blood or saliva during the use of high-speed or ultrasonic equipment, such as a high-speed handpiece or an ultrasonic scaler.

In many dental practices, treatment providers may not realize the dissemination potential of saliva and blood by these routes. Potential dangers often are missed, because much of the spatter from the patient's mouth is not readily noticeable. For example, **bioburden** (blood, saliva, exudate) may be transparent and may dry as a clear film on contaminated surfaces. Consequently, the administrative assistant must understand the potential risk of handling contaminated surfaces.

INFECTION CONTROL IN THE DENTAL OFFICE

Because patient care actually begins in the business office, it is important to identify the role of the administrative assistant as it relates to infection control in the clinical area. Every dental healthcare worker is responsible for breaking the cycle of **disease transmission** (Figure 17-1). Safe practice is based on the following principles:

- A complete and accurate patient history must be obtained and screening must be done.
- Aseptic techniques must be observed using personal protective equipment.
- Healthcare workers must strictly adhere to acceptable sterilization procedures.
- Acceptable disinfection procedures must be practiced.
- Equipment asepsis and dental laboratory asepsis must be practiced.

The administrative assistant is responsible for the first step in safe practice, obtaining complete and detailed information about the patient. The records discussed in Chapter 7 must be completed, dated, signed, and reviewed thoroughly by the dentist. During treatment procedures, the administrative assistant must make sure that protocols are followed and the necessary barrier materials are available for use. Finally, the administrative

> Every dental healthcare worker is responsible for breaking the cycle of disease transmission.

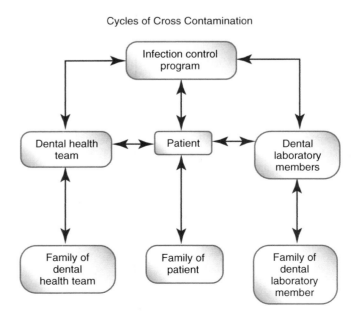

Cycles of Cross Contamination

Figure 17-1 Cycle of disease transmission.

assistant ensures that the records used during the treatment procedure are transferred safely from the clinical site to the business office without cross contamination.

Table 17-2 presents several situations that you, as the administrative assistant, may encounter in attempting to maintain safe practice in the office. You must be able to distinguish between right actions and wrong actions and must understand the consequences of a wrong action in infection control. Box 17-1 presents a self-assessing list of points you should live by when working in the dental office to make sure you are not promoting disease transmission.

Table 17-2
Recognizing Wrong from Right in Infection Control

Wrong	Effect	Right
Shaking hands while wearing contaminated gloves	Disease transmission may occur during cross-contamination.	Remove gloves and wash hands prior to leaving examination gloves treatment room; nod and speak greetings to the individual.
Pulling mask on and off	Contact with the face with contaminated gloves can expose unprotected tissues to disease. If mask is contaminated, contact with gloved or ungloved hands will also allow disease transmission.	Always leave mask in place; if movement for repositioning is necessary, either do it with clean gloves or slight readjustment may be made by using the upper arm or shoulder.
Wearing the same mask for more than one patient	Masks become moist field, allowing penetration of particles through the mask.	Always change masks between patients and use more than one mask if treatment procedure is lengthy.
Reusing same gloves	Most gloves have microscopic openings allowing penetration of microbes. Washing gloves increases the potential for disease transmission.	Gloves are always changed between patients; gloves may need to be changed during a treatment procedure that is lengthy.
Placing patient records in treatment room	Records may become exposed to aerosols or through handling; these records are transferred to the business office after treatment, thus exposing the business personnel to the potential for disease.	Records other than radiographs should be kept outside the treatment room to avoid contamination. If the records must be in the treatment room, they should be kept out of reach of aerosols and handled with clean hands or with overgloves rather than examination gloves.
Storing instruments in trays or drawers instead of sealed bags in treatment rooms	Instruments not individually bagged (if not part of a tray set-up) may be exposed to aerosols or other contact during treatment and may become contaminated.	All instruments processed through sterilization should be bagged to ensure their sterility when used. Instruments, even in closed drawers, may not remain sterile.
Eating in the laboratory or other contaminated site	Surfaces can become contaminated from instruments or materials exposed to patient aerosols or handling.	A staff lounge or eating area must be available in a site away from potentially contaminated materials.
Wearing a V-neck laboratory coat	Garments under lab coat can become contaminated. If wearing a V-neck shirt underneath, skin will be exposed.	Always wear high neck lab coat when working with patients or in the laboratory. These coats should be removed before leaving the workplace.
Wearing dangling earrings, piercings, necklaces, bracelets and/or ties	Items can become contaminated. They may hang in the patient's face or catch on something.	Minimize jewelry to only wearing wedding bands and small post earrings.

Box 17-1
Self-Assessment for the Administrative Assistant

If you can agree with each of the following statements, you probably can perform your duties safely and are free of potential risks. If you cannot agree with one of these statements, you may jeopardize your own health and the safety of others with whom you have contact.

1. I completely understand the Occupational Safety and Health Administration (OSHA) concepts and the need to perform my duties safely.
2. I understand the need for immunizations.
3. I am sure that the pencils, pens, and records with which I come in contact regularly are free of contamination.
4. I am never in contact with exposed surfaces, body fluids, or contaminated areas or involved with sterilization processes.
5. I never receive materials from the hands of a dental healthcare worker (DHCW) who is wearing contaminated examination gloves.
6. I never retrieve dental floss or toothbrushes that were used in a patient education treatment room.
7. I never subject myself to the potential for disease transmission by performing simple tasks such as removing armamentaria from a treatment room.
8. I will never be required to provide emergency care to patients or others without protective personal barriers.
9. I never come in contact with infectious waste or patient laboratory cases.
10. I have never encountered my colleagues wearing their clinical attire into a public area.
11. I never assume that because the patient is a family member or personal friend, he or she is not potentially contagious.

I understand that if I answered "no" to any of the preceding points, I must do so only if I strictly adhere to the appropriate barriers and protocols provided by the Centers for Disease Control and Prevention (CDC), OSHA, or the American Dental Association (ADA).

Health Protection Program for the Dental Staff

The administrative assistant plays a role in maintaining the health and safety of the patients and healthcare workers in the office. Although you may not be assigned the task of infection control coordinator, you should be familiar with the aspects of this process. After all, you are responsible for managing the office, and you must be able to access all records.

The office's personnel policy must include a health service program for the staff that covers the following:
- Education and training
- Immunizations
- Exposure prevention and postexposure management
- Medical conditions, work-related illness, and work restrictions
- Allergies or sensitivities to work-related materials, such as latex
- Records maintenance, data management, and confidentiality issue
- A referral arrangement with a medical physician who is available to treat staff members for emergencies and perform medical evaluation and treatment quickly and appropriately
- Confidential, up-to-date medical records for all workers, including documentation of immunizations and tests

You and the dentist must work together to maintain the safety of all staff members and patients. On your part, attention to records maintenance and continual education and training can ensure safe practice.

Government Regulations

All dental professionals are expected to comply with current guidelines and regulations governing infection control, hazard communication, and medical waste disposal. Several agencies are responsible for providing the dental professional with the current regulations affecting each of these areas. The employer is primarily responsible for maintaining current copies of all state and federal regulations that relate to the dental office. These guidelines must be reviewed, and their implementation in the office must be documented.

In 1986 OSHA established guidelines to protect workers from occupational exposure to blood-borne diseases. In 1988, employees in direct contact with blood or infectious materials and substances were required to use **standard precautions;** that is, all patients must be treated as if they are potentially infectious with the **human immunodeficiency virus (HIV),** the **hepatitis B virus (HBV),** or other infectious diseases. An overview of the latest required OSHA standards is presented in Box 17-2.

> All dental professionals are expected to comply with current guidelines and regulations governing infection control, hazard communications, and medical waste disposal.

Box 17-2
Overview of Standards Established by the Occupational Safety and Health Administration (OSHA)

- Employers must identify and train workers "reasonably anticipated" to be at risk of exposure. They also must reduce or eliminate exposure and offer medical care and counseling if exposure occurs.
- Employers must have written exposure control plans, identifying workers with occupational exposure to blood and other infectious materials and specifying ways to protect and train those workers.
- Employers must have a plan that includes protocols for **barrier techniques**, sterilization, disinfection, hepatitis B vaccination, and the handling of office accidents, including exposure to infectious materials. They must also have plans to protect and train employers; these plans must be reviewed and updated annually and must be available to employees at all times.
- The use of puncture-resistant containers, hand washing as gloves are changed, and proper personal protective equipment are required.
- Employers must provide laundering of protective clothing. Laundering of protective clothing at home is prohibited.
- Sharps must be recapped with a one-handed technique or a mechanical recapping device.
- Employees must wear gowns and gloves when a risk exists of exposure to or skin contact with blood, body fluids, or saliva.
- General work clothes are not considered protection against exposure to blood, body fluids, or saliva.
- Employees must wear masks, eyewear, or a face shield during exposure to splashes, spray, spatter, droplets of blood, body tissue, or saliva.
- Eyewear must have fixed side shields.

Continued

Box 17-2
1992 Overview of Standards Established by the Occupational Safety and Health Administration (OSHA)—cont'd

- Employers must provide personal protective equipment to be worn by all employees (i.e., gowns, gloves, masks, and eyewear) at no expense to employees.
- **Sharps containers** must be labeled and easily accessible to areas where sharps are used.
- Hepatitis B vaccinations must be offered to employees at no cost after training is completed but within 10 days of placement in a position that involves occupational exposure.
- If a worker declines the hepatitis B vaccination, access is still required if the employee has a change of mind.
- Employers must provide a training program during working hours for all employees in occupational exposure positions by June 4, 1992, and annually in subsequent years.
- Training records must be kept for 3 years after the training sessions.
- The following must be handled as infectious waste (i.e., placed in special, labeled containers): pathological waste sharps; blood and body fluid items that release blood, body fluid, or saliva when compressed; and items caked with dried blood, body fluid, or saliva if such contaminants can be released from the materials during handling.

From U.S. Department of Labor; Occupational Safety and Health Administration: *CP2-2.69; Exposure procedures for occupational exposure to bloodborne pathogens.*

When standard precautions are used, additional procedures are not necessary for treating a patient known to have an infectious disease. Under standard precautions, each workplace must

- Be hazard free
- Provide personal protective clothing and equipment
- Display poster no. 2203, a guide to OSHA regulations, in a prominent location

The **Environmental Protection Agency (EPA),** a federal regulatory agency, developed a program for overseeing the handling, tracking, transportation, and disposal of medical waste once it has left the dental office.

The CDC, a division of the U.S. Public Health Service, also provides recommendations for healthcare workers. It is responsible for investigating and controlling various diseases, such as dental caries, hepatitis, and tuberculosis, which currently is on the rise.

> If standard precautions are used, additional procedures are not necessary for treating a patient known to have an infectious disease.

Maintaining Regulatory Records

The dentist may assign the administrative assistant the job of maintaining the myriad records required to meet the various standards and regulations. To aid this process, many companies and organizations have provided brochures and manuals, such as the ADA's *Regulatory Compliance Manual* (Figure 17-2). A control form (Figure 17-3) can help ensure that all records are kept as required. Examples of all records should be included in the office procedures manual or the *Regulatory Compliance Manual.*

These records should be kept confidential and should include the following:

- Exposure determination forms (Figure 17-4), which describe the office infection control program and procedures

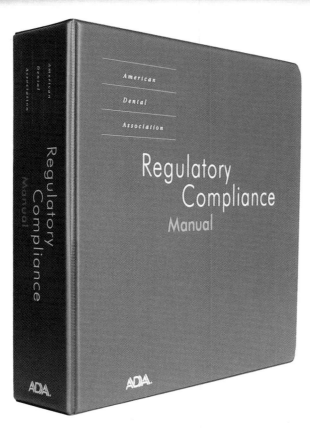

Figure 17-2 Regulatory Compliance Manual. (Courtesy of American Dental Association, Chicago, IL.)

- Employee training records (Figure 17-5), which describe HBV vaccination availability, requirements, and implementation
- Employee medical records (Figure 17-6)
- Informed refusal for hepatitis B vaccination (Figure 17-7)
- Postexposure evaluation and follow-up training
- Employee informed refusal of postexposure medical evaluation (Figure 17-8)
- Incident report of exposure to occupational illness (Figure 17-9)

Hazard Communication Program

OSHA's hazard communication standards require all dental professionals to develop and implement a program involving employee training, compilation of a list of hazardous chemicals, maintenance of MSDSs, and proper labeling of all chemicals in the office. This program must apply to all activities in which an individual may be exposed to hazardous chemicals under normal working conditions or during an emergency.

One individual (often the administrative assistant) is designated the hazard communication program coordinator. This person is responsible for
- Disseminating information about the program
- Recognizing the hazardous properties of chemicals found in the workplace
- Keeping up-to-date on procedures for safe handling of chemicals
- Implementing measures for protecting the office staff from hazardous chemicals

Text cont'd on pp 466

Implementation Records of OSHA Requirements

SECTION   **DATE**

Exposure determination   _____

Infection control program   _____

HBV vaccination   _____

Postexposure evaluation
and follow-up   _____

Training   _____

Recordkeeping   _____

Figure 17-3 Implementation control form.

Exposure determination form

All employees holding the following positions in my office have occupational exposure.

Position   Names

1. _____   1. _____

2. _____   2. _____

3. _____   3. _____

Some employees holding the following positions in my office have occupational exposure.
That is, they are occasionally called upon to perform tasks that may result in occupational
exposure.

Position   Names

1. _____   1. _____

2. _____   2. _____

3. _____   3. _____

This table contains tasks and procedures that might result in occupational exposure to
employees in job classifications in which only some employees have occupational exposure.

Position	Name	Tasks that may result in exposure
1. _____	1. _____	1. _____
		_____
		_____
		_____
2. _____	2. _____	2. _____
		_____
		_____
		_____

Positions listed below have no occupational exposure

Position   Names

1. _____   1. _____

2. _____   2. _____

The office of   _____

located at   _____

                     _____

Figure 17-4 Example of an exposure determination form.

Hazard Communication Training Record

This office facility has conducted a training session for individuals incorporating OSHA Hazard Communication Standard.

Name of Employer _____

Office Address _____

Date _____

Conducted by _____

Signature _____

Attended by _____

Signatures _____

_____

_____

_____

_____

_____

_____

_____

_____

_____

_____

_____

A

Figure 17-5 A, Employee training record.

Employee Comment Form

Please provide your view of the training program to the program coordinator.

Name of Employer _____

Office Address _____

Date of training session _____

What items did you find useful? _____

_____

_____

_____

What items would you like to be covered in more detail? _____

_____

_____

_____

_____

What suggestions can you offer for improvement in the training program? _____

_____

_____

B

Figure 17-5, Cont'd B, Employee evaluation form for training session.

Confidential employee medical record

Employee medical record
Employee name————————————————————————
Employee address————————————————————————

————————————————————————————————
————————————————————————————————
————————————————————————————————

Employee social security number ————————————————
Employee starting date————————————————————————
Employee termination date (if any) ——————————————
History of HBV vaccination (date received, or, if not received, a brief explanation of
why not) ——————————————————————————
————————————————————————————————

History of other immunizations ——————————————————

History of exposure incident(s) (dates, brief explanation, attachments)————————
————————————————————————————————
————————————————————————————————
————————————————————————————————
————————————————————————————————
————————————————————————————————

Results of medical exams and follow-up procedures regarding exposure incident or
hepatitis B immunity, including written opinion of healthcare professional
(dates, brief explanation, attachments)
————————————————————————————————
————————————————————————————————
————————————————————————————————
————————————————————————————————
————————————————————————————————

Information provided to the health care professional regarding hepatitis B vaccination
and/or exposure incident(s)
(dates, brief explanation, attachments)
————————————————————————————————
————————————————————————————————
————————————————————————————————
————————————————————————————————
————————————————————————————————

Attach pre-employment health records to this document.
Note: maintain the record for duration of employment plus 30 years

Figure 17-6 Employee medical record.

Informed Refusal for Hepatitis B Vaccination

I, _____ am employed as a dentist/dental assistant/ dental hygienist/laboratory technician in the office of _____ . I have been provided training regarding the hepatitis B vaccine. I understand the effectiveness of the vaccine, the risks of contracting hepatitis B in the dental office, and the importance of taking active steps to reduce the risk.

However, I, of my own free will and volition, and despite the urging of Dr. _____, have elected not to be vaccinated against hepatitis B. I have personal reasons for making the decision not to be vaccinated.

_____
Signature

_____   _____
Witness   Name

_____
Address

_____
City   State   Zip Code

_____
Date

Figure 17-7 Form for informed refusal of hepatitis B vaccination.

Employee Informed Refusal of Postexposure Medical Evaluation

I, _____ , am employed by _____ as a dentist, dental assistant, dental hygienist, or laboratory technician. Dr. _____ has provided training for me regarding infection control and the risk of disease transmission in this dental facility.

On_____ ,20__ , I was involved in an exposure incident when I

_____

_____

_____

_____

(describe details of needlestick, etc.)   I have been offered follow-up medical evaluation in order to ensure that I have full knowledge of whether I have been exposed to or contracted an infectious disease from this incident.

However, I, of my own free will and volition, and despite Dr. _____'s offer, have elected not to have a medical evaluation. I have personal reasons for making this decision.

_____
Signature

_____
Witness

_____
Name

_____
Address

_____
City　　　　　　　　　State　　　　Zip Code

_____
Date

Figure 17-8 Employee form for informed refusal of postexposure medical evaluation.

Bureau of Statistics
Supplementary Record of
Occupational Injuries and Illnesses

U.S. Department of Labor

This form is required by Public Law 91-596 and must be kept in the establishment for 5 years. Failure to maintain can result in the issuance of citations and assessment of penalties.	Case or File No.	Form approved O.M.B. No. 1220-0029

Employer

1. Name

2. Mail address (*No. and street, city or town, State, and zip code*)

3. Location, if different from mail address

Injured or Ill Employee

4. Name (*First, middle, and last*)   Social Security No.

5. Home address (*No. and street, city or town, State, and zip code*)

6. Age   7. Sex: (*Check one*)   Male ☐   Female ☐

8. Occupation (*Enter regular job title*, not *the specific activity he was performing at the time of injury.*)

9. Department (*Enter name of department or division in which the injured person is regularly employed, even though he may have been temporarily working in another department at the time of injury.*)

The Accident or Exposure to Occupational Illness

If accident or exposure occurred on employer's premises, give address of plant or establishment in which it occurred. Do not indicate department or division within the plant or establishment. If accident occurred outside employer's premises at an identifiable address, give that address. If it occurred on a public highway or at any other place which cannot be identified by number and street, please provide place references locating the place of injury as accurately as possible.

10. Place of accident or exposure (*No. and street, city or town, State, and zip code*)

11. Was place of accident or exposure on employer's premises?   Yes ☐   No ☐

12. What was the employee doing when injured? (*Be specific. If he was using tools or equipment or handling material, name them and tell what he was doing with them.*)

13. How did the accident occur? (*Describe fully the events which resulted in the injury or occupational illness. Tell what happened and how it happened. Name any objects or substances involved and tell how they were involved. Give full details on all factors which led or contributed to the accident. Use separate sheet for additional space.*)

Occupational Injury or Occupational Illness

14. Describe the injury or illness in detail and indicate the part of body affected. (*E.g., amputation of right index finger at second joint; fracture of ribs; lead poisoning; dermatitis of left hand, etc.*)

15. Name the object or substance which directly injured the employee. (*For example, the machine or thing he struck against or which struck him; the vapor or poison he inhaled or swallowed; the chemical or radiation which irritated his skin; or in cases of strains, hernias, etc., the thing he was lifting, pulling, etc.*)

16. Date of injury or initial diagnosis of occupational illness   17. Did employee die? (*Check one*)   Yes ☐   No ☐

Other

18. Name and address of physician

19. If hospitalized, name and address of hospital

Date of report	Prepared by	Official position

OSHA No. 101 (Feb. 1981)

Figure 17-9 Incident report of exposure to occupational illness.

MATERIAL SAFETY DATA SHEETS (MSDS). If you are assigned the job of hazard communication program coordinator, you should make and keep updated a list of all products in the office that contain hazardous chemicals (Figure 17-10). MSDSs, which are a government-approved or equivalent forms that provide specific information about chemicals purchased for use in a workplace, are an important part of the records. MSDSs for all products with hazardous potential are compiled and kept updated in a master list available to all individuals. An MSDS should include the manufacturer's name and address, the product name, the generic name (if applicable), potential routes of entry, the organs affected by the chemical, and means of protecting against or reducing the effects of chemical exposure (e.g., **eyewash**).

LABELING OF HAZARDOUS MATERIALS. The hazard communication program coordinator also is responsible for properly labeling hazardous chemicals and substances. Many products purchased from dental supply companies arrive with permanently affixed information about hazardous chemicals. When items are purchased in bulk and then transferred to smaller containers, hazard communication labels must be put on these containers. The label must show that the MSDS was obtained and must designate the chemical's hazard class, the routes of entry into the body, and the organs affected. Labeling kits (Figure 17-11) and informational materials are available from a variety of companies.

Equipment for Hazardous Situations

The administrative assistant may be responsible for ordering equipment and training office staff members in the use of a variety of materials during a hazardous situation. Spills of chemicals, gypsum products, and flammable materials may produce different reactions, depending on the hazardous chemical. Again, even though you may not work directly with hazardous materials, it becomes your responsibility to ensure that safe practice is implemented, to understand how to prevent accidents, and to know how to react in the event of an accident.

The following equipment should be kept readily available for use in preventing or dealing with a hazardous spill:
- Fire extinguisher
- Eyewash stations
- Amalgam spill kit
- Masks approved by the National Institute for Occupational Safety and Health (NIOSH)
- Protective clothing (long sleeves, high neck, fluid-impervious fabric)
- Kitty litter and broom and dustpan
- Protective nitral gloves and glasses
- Bags in which to seal spilled materials and contaminated objects
- Well-ventilated areas for work (which allow the ventilation to be turned off if an accident occurs)
- Scavenging system (for use with nitrous oxide)

INFECTION CONTROL TECHNIQUES

In the course of dental treatment, some bioburden contamination of equipment, surfaces, instruments, and other devices occurs; sometimes these items and areas simply are not clean. The goal of any infection control program must be to maintain sterile techniques and to prevent cross infection through aseptic technique.

Hazardous Chemicals and the Dental Products in Which They Are Found

CHEMICAL NAME	MAY BE FOUND IN:	CHEMICAL NAME	MAY BE FOUND IN:
acetic acid	photographic solutions	nickel (metal and soluble compounds)	nickel-based casting alloys, stainless steel orthodontic appliances
acetone	solvents		
aluminum oxide	polishing disks		
aluminum soluble salts	astringent agents	nitric acid	pickling solutions, some bleaching solutions
asbestos	some cast ring liners		
benzoyl peroxide	resin systems, denture resins	nitrous oxide	nitrous oxide
beryllium	nickle based casting alloys	oil mist, mineral	handpiece lubricants
calcium carbonate	polishing agents	petroleum distillates	solvents, waxes, jellies
carbon tetrachloride	solvents	phenol	disinfectants
chloroform	solvents	phosphoric acid	etching agents, phosphate cements
chromium	casting alloys		
cobalt	casting alloys	phthalic anhydride	resins
copper	amalgam, casting alloys	picric acid	pickling agents
cresol, all isomers	endodontic materials	platinum soluble salts	impression materials (addition silicones)
cyanide as CN	plating solutions		
dibutylphthalate	impression materials	platinum	casting alloys
ethyl acetate	solvents	propane	burners
ethyl acrylate	resins	rouge	polishing agents
ethyl alcohol	solvents, sterilizing agents	silica, amorphous including natural distomaceous earth	composite resins, materials
ethyl chloride	solvents, topical refrigerants		
ethyl silicate	silicate investments, impression materials (condensation silicones)	silica, crystalline (quartz)	composite resins, porcelain, investments
		silicon carbide	polishing disks, cutting wheels
ethylene oxide	sterilizing agents	silver (metal and soluble compounds)	amalgam, endodontic points, casting alloys, photographic solutions
fluoride dust	fluoride-containing composites		
formaldehyde	sterilizing agents		
glutaraldehyde	sterilizing agents	sulfuric acid	etchant for alloys, copper plating solutions
hydrochloric acid	pickling solutions, bleaching agents		
		talc, nonasbestos form	gloves
hydrogen fluoride	etching agents for porcelain	tantalum	nickel-chromium-cobalt alloys
hydroquinone	methacrylate and denture base resins, photographic solutions	tin, inorganic compounds	amalgam, polishing pastes
		tin, organic compounds	impression material (condensation silicones)
iodine	iodophor disinfectants and antimicrobial hand cleansers	titanium dioxide	porcelain, impression materials
isopropyl alcohol	solvents, wiping agents	toluene	solvents
lead/inorganic lead compounds	impression materials (some polysulfides)	trichloroethane	solvents
		uranium, insoluble compounds	porcelain
LPG (liquid petroleum gas)	burners		
mercury	amalgam	vinyl chloride	maxillofacial plastics, mouth guard trays
mercury/organic	topical antiseptics		
methyl acetate	solvents	xylene	solvents
methyl alcohol	denatured alcohol	zirconium compounds	porcelain, polishing pastes
methyl methacrylate	denture base resins		
methylene chloride	solvents		
molybdenum, insoluble compounds	casting alloys (chromium-cobalt alloys, stainless steel)		

Figure 17-10 List of common chemicals found in a dental office. (From Finkbeiner BL, Johnson CS: *Mosby's comprehensive dental assisting: a clinical approach,* St. Louis, 1995, Mosby.)

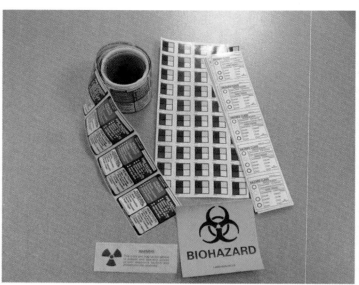

A

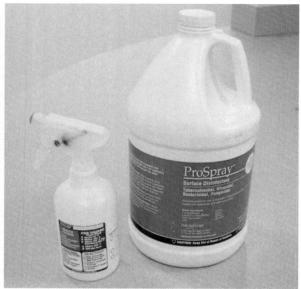

B

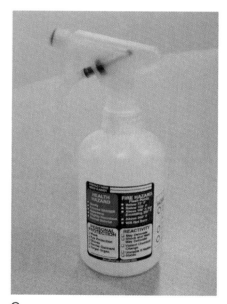

C

Figure 17-11 A, Supply kit for hazardous materials labeling. **B** and **C,** Hazardous labels affixed to containers.

Aseptic Technique

The term *aseptic technique,* or *asepsis,* refers to procedures that break the circle of infection and, ideally, eliminate cross contamination. With cross contamination, a previously sterile environment is exposed to harmful agents.

Procedures commonly used to maintain asepsis and prevent cross contamination include the following:

- Barrier coverings are used on surfaces that cannot be sterilized.
- Exposed surfaces are cleaned and disinfected.
- Sterile disposable items are used whenever possible.
- All contaminated reusable items are cleaned and sterilized.
- Contaminated gloved hands are not allowed to touch protective eyewear, masks, or the hair.

- Patients are asked to use a pretreatment antimicrobial mouth rinse.
- The hands are washed regularly throughout the day with an antimicrobial cleanser, such as before and after lunch and just before and immediately after the treatment of each patient.
- A complete and comprehensive health history is obtained for every patient.

    Under OSHA standards, employees are allowed access to a patient's health history information. This is especially important if an employee is exposed to blood-borne pathogens in the dental office. Such information is maintained as part of a confidential medical record for employees. OSHA requires that these records be kept for all employees at risk of blood-borne pathogen transmission in an occupational setting such as the dental office.

    All patients should be treated in the same manner, as potentially infectious for HBV, HIV, or other blood-borne pathogens or infectious diseases. Consistent adherence to these standard precautions is a primary professional standard of care and reduces the guesswork of determining a patient's infection status.

    The following sections describe techniques that can be used to minimize contamination during treatment procedures.

Personal Protection

Personal protection involves two basic considerations, immunological protection (immunization) and barrier protection.

IMMUNIZATION. *Immunization* is the process by which resistance to an infectious disease is induced or augmented. The human body can produce immunity to particular diseases or conditions. When no natural immunity exists for a disease, immunization may be provided through certain vaccinations.

    Immunization to prevent and control cross infection is an important aspect of healthcare for dental professionals. The HBV vaccine, for example, is effective and widely available. However, several other diseases may also

---

Box 17-3
Flowchart for Management of Occupational Exposures to Blood-Borne Pathogens

Before an Exposure Occurs...

Dental Worker	Employer/Infection Control Coordinator	Qualified Healthcare Provider
• Receives training in risks of occupational exposures, immediate reporting of injuries/exposures, and reporting procedures within the practice setting	• Establishes referral arrangements and protocol for employees to follow in the event of exposures to blood or saliva via puncture injury, mucous membrane, or non-intact skin • Trains occupationally exposed employees in postexposure protocols • Trains occupationally exposed employees in postexposure protocols • Makes available and pays for hepatitis B vaccine for workers at occupational risk	• Contracts with dentist–employer to provide medical evaluation, counseling, and follow-up care to dental office employees exposed to blood or other potentially infectious materials • Keeps current on public health guidelines for managing occupational exposure incidents and is aware of evaluating healthcare provider's responsibilities ethically and by law

Continued

Box 17-3
Flowchart for Management of Occupational Exposures to Blood-Borne Pathogens—cont'd

When an Exposure Incident Occurs...

Dental Worker
1. Performs first aid
2. Reports injury to employer
3. Reports to the designated healthcare professional for medical evaluation and follow-up care, as indicated

Employer/Infection Control Coordinator
1. Documents events in the practice setting
2. Immediately directs employee to evaluating healthcare professional
3. Sends to evaluating healthcare professional:
   - copy of standard job description of employee
   - exposure report
   - source patient's identity and bloodborne infection status (if known)
   - employee's HBV status and other relevant medical information
   - copy of the Occupational Safety and Health Administration (OSHA) Bloodborne Pathogen Standard
4. Arranges for source patient testing, if the source patient is known and has consented
5. Pays for postexposure evaluation and, if indicated, prophylaxis

Qualified Healthcare Provider
1. Evaluates exposure incident, worker, and source patient for HBV, HCV, and HIV, maintaining confidentiality
   - Arranges for collection and testing (with consent) of exposed worker and source patient as soon as feasible (if serostatus is not already known)
   - In the event that consent is not obtained for HIV testing, arranges for blood sample to arranges for blood sample to be preserved for up to 90 days (to allow time for the exposed worker to consent to HIV testing)
   - Arranges for additional collection and testing as recommended by the U.S. Public Health Service/CDC
   - Notifies worker of results of all testing and of the need for strict confidentiality with regard to source patient results
   - Provides counseling
   - Provides postexposure prophylaxis, if medically indicated
2. Assesses reported illnesses/ side effects
3. Within 15 days of evaluation, sends to the employer a Written Opinion, which contains (only):*
   - documentation that the employee was informed of evaluation results and the need for any further follow-up
   - whether HBV vaccine was indicated and if it was received

6. Receives Written Opinion from evaluating healthcare professional
   - Files copy of Written Opinion in employee's confidential medical record (if maintained by the dentist employer)
   - Provides copy of Written Opinion to exposed employee

4. Receives copy of Written Opinion

   - Provides copy of Written Opinion to exposed employee

*All other findings or diagnoses remain confidential and are not included in the written report.
Courtesy of OSAP: *From policy to practice: OSAP's guide to the guidelines,* OSAP, 2004, Annapolis, MD.

pose a threat to the health and well-being of dental personnel and potentially to patients.

Dental healthcare workers should receive the appropriate vaccines, which prevent the onset of clinical or subclinical infection, when symptoms of the disease are not apparent. The occupational risks for hepatitis B, measles, rubella, influenza, and certain other microbial infections can be minimized considerably by stimulation of artificial active immunity. Approved vaccines are available for each of these, and individuals who provide patient care should have them.

Common childhood immunizations may be given for several diseases, including diphtheria, tetanus, pertussis, polio, and rubella. Other vaccinations help prevent rubeola, mumps, and influenza. The tuberculin Mantoux test can determine whether an individual has been exposed to or has tuberculosis. This test is extremely important, because tuberculosis, once thought to be almost nonexistent in North America, is on the rise.

BARRIER PROTECTION. Although vaccines are effective at minimizing the transmission of certain infections, they are not sufficient protection against the wide variety of potential pathogens encountered during patient treatment. Physical barriers are a fundamental component of an infection control program. Disposable examination gloves, overgloves, and utility gloves should be used, and during treatment, face masks and protective clinic attire and eyewear should be worn. The administrative assistant should maintain an adequate inventory of all necessary barrier equipment. A variety of barrier covers can be used during treatment (Box 17-4).

Box 17-4
Commonly Used Barrier Covers

• Barriers coverings may be used to lessen the need for surface disinfection

Treatment Room
• Light handle covers
• On/off switch on operating light
• Plastic bag over dental chair and adjustment buttons
• Paper towel folded to cover working end of thumb forceps used to retrieve instruments from the mobile cabinetry
• Plastic tubing over hoses of unit (when accessible)
• Plastic bag attached to mobile cabinetry for debris
• Overgloves to retrieve armamentaria and charts

Radiography Treatment Room
• Plastic bag over radiographic head and PID
• Plastic covering over on/off switch
• Plastic covering over touch/control panel
• Plastic bag over dental chair
• Barrier-type film packets
• Covering over area from which each dental film is retrieved (if film is laid out on a surface before exposure, a covering placed under the film before use eliminates disinfection of the surface)

Instrument Sterilization

The processing of dental instruments and armamentarium is the primary responsibility of the clinical assistant and requires the use of utility gloves. To maintain sterility, many dental professionals bag instruments before the sterilization process. Color-coded indicators signify whether an instrument bag has reached sterilizing temperatures. Instruments are also bagged as tray setups to aid the efficiency of the clinical dental assistant.

MONITORING THE STERILIZATION PROCESS. The administrative assistant may assume a major role in monitoring the efficiency of the sterilization systems. Several factors may diminish the effectiveness of the various sterilizers used in the office. Frequent problems include improper wrapping of instruments; prevention of adequate penetration to the instrument surface; human error in timing the cycle; defective control gauges that do not reflect actual conditions inside the sterilizer; and sterilizer malfunction.

Although chemically treated tapes are available to determine color changes or biological controls as a means of checking for proper sterilizer function, the use of calibrated biological controls remains the gold standard of sterilization. A test strip with harmless active spores is placed in the sterilization chamber with a normal load of instruments. The test strip is returned to the manufacturer or a monitoring agency for verification that sterilization has occurred. The office receives written documentation that is maintained as a record.

Disposables

Disposable items are manufactured and identified for single use only. These items, which may include needles, saliva ejectors, prophylaxis cups, sealant, and composite brushes, should not be reused. Disposables are becoming even more widely available as manufacturers, distributors, and office personnel recognize their usefulness. Examples of recently marketed items include disposable prophylaxis angles, rag wheels, evacuation line traps, and HVE tips. These products pose less of a risk of cross contamination because they do not undergo recleaning and recycling; however, they must be disposed of properly.

LABORATORY ASEPSIS. Special handling is required when impressions, prosthetic devices, and the other materials are transferred from the dental office to a commercial dental laboratory. These items, which are contaminated with the patient's saliva, blood, or other substances, can be a source of disease transmission. The ADA's councils on Dental Therapeutics and Prosthetic Services and Dental Laboratory Relations updated guidelines for infection control in dental laboratories in 1988. The ADA and the CDC recommend that impressions, appliances, and other items removed from a patient's mouth be cleaned and disinfected before they are sent to the laboratory. Items received from the laboratory for delivery to a patient should be cleaned and disinfected before placement. All items must be disinfected according to product directions. Because the administrative assistant often prepares cases for and receives them from the dental laboratory, this person should have a clear understanding of the recommended guidelines.

Disinfection of dental impressions and prostheses must be done carefully to avoid distortion of impressions or damage to metal, porcelain, or acrylic surfaces of prostheses. The administrative assistant should always consult the dentist or the dental laboratory before disinfecting any material.

EDUCATING PATIENTS ABOUT INFECTION CONTROL PROGRAMS

Effective infection control must become a routine component of professional activity. The use of standard precautions in the treatment of all patients greatly minimizes occupational exposure to microbial pathogens, because it addresses the reality that most potentially infectious individuals are asymptomatic and therefore undiagnosed.

Procedures aimed at preventing the spread of infectious disease during dental treatment are constantly evaluated by the profession as well as by consumer agencies. Therefore the best course of action is to educate the staff and patients about the importance of safe practice and the use of standard precautions for all patients. You should be willing to freely discuss infection control with patients, using valid data. Remember, the two best ways to avoid potential litigation and OSHA inspections are prevention and good documentation.

> Effective infection control must become a routine component of professional activity.

The dental profession has done much in the past 35 years in the clinical application of infection control techniques and procedures. The implementation of appropriate recommendations by many dental professionals and government organizations continues to have a major impact on the way dental treatment is practiced in the 21st century. It is important for dental professionals to keep up with developments and incorporate new technology into their practices as it becomes available.

INFECTIOUS WASTE DISPOSAL IN THE DENTAL OFFICE

According to OSHA, "Infectious waste means blood and blood products, contaminated sharps, pathological wastes, and microbiological wastes." In general, all infectious waste destined for disposal should be placed in closable, leak-proof containers or bags that are color coded or labeled appropriately.

Warning labels should be affixed to containers of infectious waste, to refrigerators and freezers containing blood, to other containers used to store or transport blood or other potentially infectious materials, and to any potentially infectious materials. The labels required by OSHA should be used in the office. These labels should be fluorescent orange or orange-red or predominantly so and should have lettering or symbols in a contrasting color (see Figure 17-11, B and C).

All infectious material should be disposed of in accordance with federal, state, and local regulations. A medical waste tracking form (Figure 17-12) is completed for medical waste disposal, and a shipment log (Figure 17-13) is used to verify the mode of transport and other vital information.

MEDICAL WASTE TRACKING FORM

INSTRUCTIONS FOR COMPLETING MEDICAL WASTE TRACKING FORM

Copy 1 — GENERATOR COPY: Mailed by Destination Facility to Generator
Copy 2 — DESTINATION FACILITY COPY: Retained by Destination Facility
Copy 3 — TRANSPORTER COPY: Retained by Transporter
Copy 4 — GENERATOR COPY: Retained by Generator

As required under 40 CFR Part 259:

1. This multicopy (4-page) shipping document must accompany each shipment of regulated medical waste generated in a Covered State.
2. Items numbered 1–14 must be completed before the generator can sign the certification. Items 4, 7, 10, 11c, & 19 are optional unless required by the State. Item 22 must be completed by the destination facility.

For assistance in completing this form, contact your nearest State office or Regional EPA office, or call (800) 424-9346.

INSTRUCTIONS

TRANSPORTER

16. **Transporter 1** (Certification of Receipt of Medical Waste as described in items 11, 12, & 13)

Printed/Typed name   Signature   Date

17. **Transporter 2 or Intermediate Handler** (name and address)

18. **Telephone Number** ( )

EPA Med. Waste ID No.

19. **State Transporter Permit or ID No.**

20. **Transporter 2 or Intermediate Handler** (Certification of Receipt of Medical Waste as described in items 11, 12, & 13)

Printed/Typed name   Signature   Date

DESTINATION

21. **New Tracking Form Number** (for consolidated or remanifested waste)

22. **Destination facility** (Certification of Receipt of Medical Waste as described in items 11, 12, & 13)
☐ Received in accordance with items 11, 12, & 13

Printed/Typed name   Signature   Date
(If other than destination facility, indicate address, phone, and permit or ID no. in box 14.)

23. **Discrepancy Box** (Any discrepancies should be noted by item number and initials)

GENERATOR

1. Generator's Name and Mailing Address

2. Tracking Form Number

3. Telephone Number ( )

4. State Permit or ID No.

5. Transporter's Name and Mailing Address

6. Telephone Number ( )

7. State Transporter Permit or ID No.

EPA Med. Waste ID No.

8. Destination Facility Name and Address

9. Telephone Number ( )

10. State Permit or ID No.

11. US EPA Waste Description	12. Total No. Containers	13. Total Weight or Volume
a. Regulated Medical Waste (Untreated)		
b. Regulated Medical Waste (Treated)		
c. State Regulated Medical Waste		

14. Special Handling Instructions and Additional Information

15. **Generator's Certification:**
Under penalty of criminal and civil prosecution for the making or submission of false statements, representations, or omissions, I declare, on behalf of the generator _____ that the contents of this consignment are fully and accurately described above and are classified, packaged, marked, and labeled in accordance with all applicable State and Federal regulations, and that I have been authorized, in writing, to make such declarations by the person in charge of the generator's operation.

Printed/Typed name   Signature   Date

Figure 17-12 Medical waste tracking form.

Transporter Name and Address	Transporter State Permit or ID Number	Quantity and Category of Waste Transported		Date of Shipment	Signature of Representative Accepting Waste for Transport
		Containers	Pounds		
-------------------------		Untreated	------------	__/__/__	
-------------------------		Treated			
-------------------------		Untreated	------------	__/__/__	
-------------------------		Treated			
-------------------------		Untreated	------------	__/__/__	
-------------------------		Treated			
-------------------------		Untreated	------------	__/__/__	
-------------------------		Treated			
-------------------------		Untreated	------------	__/__/__	
-------------------------		Treated			
-------------------------		Untreated	------------	__/__/__	
-------------------------		Treated			
-------------------------		Untreated	------------	__/__/__	
-------------------------		Treated			

Figure 17-13 Generator shipment log.

LEARNING ACTIVITIES

1. Explain why it is important that each member of the dental team understand the concepts of infection control and the need for immunization.
2. Identify common barrier materials and explain their use.
3. Explain the term *standard* (formerly universal) *precautions*.
4. Describe the role the administrative assistant plays in infection control.
5. Using a sample form from the text or the office of employment, complete an accident report for the following situation.
   The clinical dental assistant, Rachel F. Thompson, experienced a needle puncture while Mr. Frank Oliver was being treated. The assistant's address is 4001 Kinect Drive, Cutlerville, MI 49545, SS# 000-00-2111, birth date 4/17/81. The accident occurred in Dr. Lake's office while the dentist was returning the syringe to the assistant at chairside, resulting in a needle poke to the middle finger of the left hand. The assistant's physician, Gerald Murphy, MD, was contacted for follow-up, but no hospitalization was necessary. The dentist is Joseph W. Lake (address and other data may be obtained from Chapter 7).
6. Review various office situations and identify incidents that might require special attention to prevent the transmission of disease-causing organisms from the treatment room or dental laboratory to the business office.

EXAMINE YOUR PROGRESS

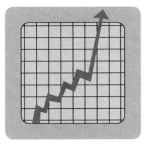

Practice by completing
Working Form 15.

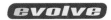

Key Terms

Acquired immunodeficiency syndrome (AIDS) A disease caused by a retrovirus known as the human immunodeficiency virus type 1 (HIV-1). A related but distinct retrovirus (HIV-2) has recently appeared in a limited number of patients in the United States.

Antiseptic An antimicrobial agent that can be applied to a body surface, usually skin or raw mucosa, to try to prevent or minimize infection in the area of application.

Autogenous infection Self-produced infection; originating within the body.

Barrier techniques Protocols used in infection control to prevent cross contamination between healthcare worker and patient or between patients.

Bioburden Any substance that interferes with the sterilization process.

Blood-borne pathogens Organisms transmitted through blood or blood products that can cause infectious diseases, such as human immunodeficiency virus (HIV) infection, AIDS, and hepatitis B virus (HBV) infection.

Centers for Disease Control and Prevention (CDC) A federal agency responsible for investigating the incidence of disease, monitoring diseases throughout the world, and conducting research directed toward controlling and preventing disease.

Communicable disease A disease that may be transmitted directly or indirectly from one individual to another.

Cross contamination The transfer of impurities, infection, or disease from one source to another.

Dental healthcare worker (DHCW) A dental professional who provides care to patients or has some contact with dental patients in the office.

Disease transmission The spread of disease-causing organisms from one person to another.

Disinfectants Chemicals used to destroy some forms of pathogenic microorganisms.

Disinfection The process of destroying some pathogenic microorganisms.

Environmental Protection Agency (EPA) A federal agency that regulates the use and disposal of hazardous materials. Workplace management of hazardous materials falls under the jurisdiction of OSHA.

Eyewash An OSHA-required device used to flush the eyes with water when exposures to unnatural contaminants has occurred.

Hazardous waste Materials identified as hazardous to human health; local, state, and federal regulations require special handling of such materials.

Hepatitis B virus (HBV) Virus that causes a form of hepatitis B that is transmitted in contaminated serum in blood transfusions, the passing of contaminated fluids, or by use of contaminated needles and instruments. *Caution:* Any DHCW who comes in contact with blood, body fluids, or body tissues has an increased risk of developing this type of hepatitis. A DHCW who does not have the protection of the HBV antigen should be immunized with a hepatitis B vaccine.

Human immunodeficiency virus (HIV) See Acquired immunodeficiency virus (AIDS).

Infection Invasion of body tissues by disease-producing microorganisms and the reaction of the tissues to these microorganisms or their toxins (or both).

Infectious waste Blood and blood products, contaminated sharps, pathological wastes, and microbiological wastes.

Occupational Safety and Health Administration (OSHA) A federal agency that establishes guidelines and regulations for worker safety. These guidelines include the storage and disposal of toxic chemicals and hazardous materials and the safe and proper use of clinical and office equipment.

Personal protective equipment (PPE) Materials used to protect the employee when occupational exposure is possible. Such equipment includes but is not limited to disposable gloves, disposable surgical masks and gowns, laboratory coats and scrubs, and face shields or eye protection with side shields.

Sanitization The act of making something sanitary, or clean and free of dirt.

Sepsis A pathological state characterized by the presence of pathogens.

Sharp containers Enclosed containers from which an article cannot be retrieved; they are used for the disposal of sharp items that may cause punctures or cuts when handled, such as broken medical glassware, needles, scalpel blades, and suture needles.

Sterilization The process of rendering an item free of germs; dental sterilization commonly is achieved by steam under pressure, dry heat, or chemical vapor.

Standard precautions Protocols used to maintain an aseptic field and to prevent cross contamination and cross infection between healthcare providers, between healthcare providers and patients, and between patients. Such measures, formerly called *universal precautions*, include but are not limited to sterilization of instruments and other equipment; isolation and disinfection of the immediate clinical environment; use of sterile disposables; scrubbing; use of personal protective equipment (e.g., mask, gown, protective eyewear, and gloves); and proper disposal of contaminated wastes.

Bibliography

American Dental Association: *ADA regulatory compliance manual,* Chicago, The Association.

Centers for Disease Control and Prevention: Guidelines for infection control in dental health-care settings, *MMWR* 52(No. RR-17), 2003.

Cottone JA, Geza TT, Molinari JA: *Practical infection control in dentistry,* Baltimore, 1996, Williams & Wilkins.

Dietz E: *Safety standards and infection control for dental assistants,* Clifton Park, NY, 2002, Delmar.

Materials for the dental team, ed 3, St. Louis, 2005, Mosby.

Miller CH, Palenik CJ: *Infection control and management of hazardous materials for the dental team,* ed 3, St. Louis, 2004, Mosby.

Molinari JA: Infection control: its evolution to the current standard (formerly universal) precautions, *JADA* 134(5):569, 2003.

Recommended Websites

www.cdc.gov/od/oc/media/pressrel/fs021025.htm (hand hygiene fact sheet)
www.ada.org (general guidelines for dentistry)
http://needlestick.mednet.ucla.edu (managing needlesticks)
www.cdc.gov/other.htm (links to CDC resources)
www.osha.gov/fso/osp/index.html (state OSHA plans)
www.hepfi.org/Hepinfo/Fact5201-99.htm

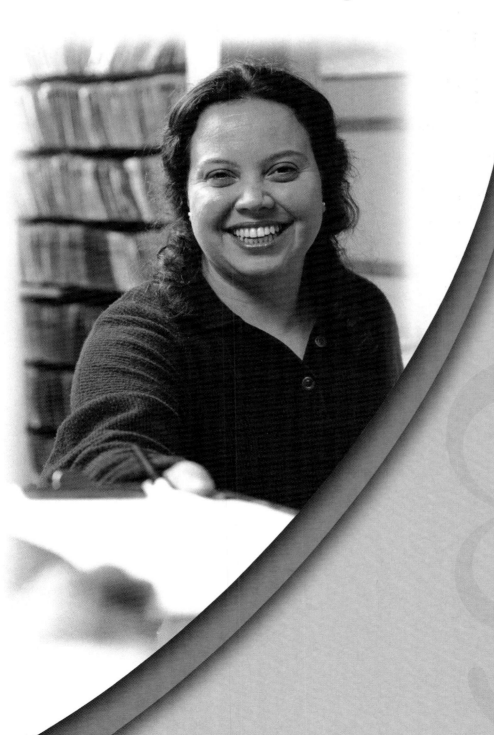

The Dental Assistant in the Workplace

Chapter Outline

Learning Outcomes

Mastery of the content in this chapter will enable the reader to:
- Determine your career goals
- Identify your personal assets and liabilities for a job
- Identify legal considerations in hiring
- Explain the use of preemployment testing
- Describe new employee orientation
- Determine desirable characteristics for a job you might seek
- Determine methods of marketing your skills
- Identify personal priorities for a potential job
- Develop a philosophy for dental assisting
- Identify factors to consider in salary negotiations
- Identify potential areas of employment

- Prepare data for job applications and interviews
- Identify potential interview questions
- List suggestions for a successful interview
- Prepare an interview follow-up letter
- Explain how to advance on the job
- List hints for success in a job on the dental team
- Describe how to terminate a job

PREPARING FOR THE JOB SEARCH

By the time you reach this chapter, you may have completed a formal educational program or course of study for clinical or administrative assistant, and you may already have passed your certification examination or other credentialing examination. Now, your thoughts are turning to finding a job.

When you apply for various jobs, your prospective employers will assume that you have completed your studies and obtained your credentials as a Certified Dental Assistant, specialty credentials as a Certified Dental Practice Management Assistant (both certifications are offered by the Dental Assisting National Board [DANB]), or even a state credential. This chapter emphasizes the tasks necessary to market your skills as a highly educated dental assistant with special training in business office management.

You sometimes may feel nervous about the prospect of taking a credentialing examination or finding a job. Even after attending formal classes or studying for a specific job, your self-confidence may falter. However, cultivating positive attitudes and taking time to reflect on career goals often help a person get on track in seeking a job. This is the time in your career when you must reflect on all the skills you have acquired. The top eight *hard skills* listed by dentist employers are

- Interpersonal skills
- Teamwork skills
- Verbal communication skills
- Critical thinking skills
- Technical skills
- Computer skills
- Written communications skills
- Leadership skills

In addition to hard skills, you have gained *soft skills,* such as value clarification, self-discipline, ethical behavior, positive attitudes, creativity, and anger and stress management. As you reflect on your skills, both hard and soft, you should analyze what they mean to your career path.

> Cultivating positive attitudes and taking time to reflect on career goals often help a person get on track in seeking a job.

Five Important Questions

Before you venture into the job market as an administrative assistant, you must identify your career goals. Obviously you are interested in the business office, because you have spent considerable time studying in this field. Therefore at this juncture, you should explore ways your career can develop in that field in the future. A career path is based on careful planning and preparation, but it can be altered by unexpected opportunities and luck. To begin preparation, you should ask yourself the series of questions shown in the job preparation ladder (Figure 18-1). Prospective employers will put your resume on the top of the job application pile if you spend some time reflecting on each of these questions: Where have I been? Where am I now? Where am I going? How am I going to get there? How will I know when I have arrived?

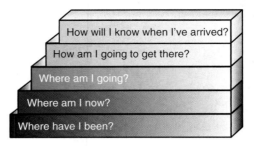

Figure 18-1 Job preparation ladder. Questions to ask yourself when preparing for a job search.

Before going to any job interviews, you should share your thoughts about these questions with peers or spend some time alone reflecting on them. This sharing and introspection can help you build confidence in your plans and goals for a career.

WHERE HAVE I BEEN? This question helps you to review your past and identify some of the reasons you arrived where you are. It is your origin and thus forms the foundation of your preparation ladder. Some individuals may find looking at the past depressing, whereas others may yearn for the comfort of the past. Regardless of the impact of your past, reflection is worthwhile. Some personal information is confidential, and certain types of questions may not be asked during a job interview; however, it is wise to be prepared for questions about your past employment. For instance, if you have worked at several jobs in the past, you may be asked about your reasons for having changed jobs frequently. You should explain your job history honestly.

WHERE AM I NOW? This question seems obvious, yet you need to reassure yourself about where you are in your career path. You have just completed a course of study, you are secure or insecure in a personal or family relationship, and you are looking forward to finding a job soon or sometime in the future. Knowing where you are at the present time enables you to continue on the career path.

WHERE AM I GOING? This is a goal-oriented question that requires you to identify what you want to do. As you progress up the preparation ladder, you must stop to think about what you want in both the near and the distant future. For some individuals, getting a job and gaining independence are their primary goals. For others, the job may be the means to a future goal. Obtaining a job now, gaining experience, and continuing with one's education may be several short-range goals that are needed to reach the ultimate goal of teaching, obtaining a business degree, or even going to dental school. Regardless of your goals, you must realize that they may change; remaining flexible in your goals enables you to accept challenges along the way.

HOW AM I GOING TO GET THERE? This question identifies the route or steps that must be taken to achieve your goals. For some, a job means independence or a sense of security and self-worth. For others, who are pursuing additional education, a short-term job supports a return to school for another degree.

HOW WILL I KNOW WHEN I HAVE ARRIVED? This is the top rung of the ladder. To answer this question, you must define what success means to you. For some people, the definition of success is always changing. Money, material goods, or a feeling of security and satisfaction can represent success. No one answer is correct for this question. It is an individual response that only you can give.

Taking time to prepare yourself for your future career can influence a job interview. When a dentist or office manager asks you to describe yourself, your background, and your career goals, you will be prepared. Simply saying, "Oh, I don't know, there isn't much to tell," indicates that you have not given your career much thought, and a potential employer might think you feel the same about employment.

SELF-ASSESSMENT

As you begin the job search, ask yourself, "What skills and characteristics can I bring to a job and to a prospective employer?" Take time to write down your skills, strengths, and weaknesses with a prospective job in mind.

As you begin this exercise, you may find that you seem to concentrate on your weaknesses; this is not uncommon. Parents, teachers, and associates share criticism willingly, thinking it improves a person, but sincere praise might not be given as freely. Criticism may be so common that when praise is offered, it might be difficult to accept. Learn to accept praise, identify your positive characteristics, and develop your assets.

> Take time to write down your skills, strengths, and weaknesses with a prospective job in mind.

Identifying Personal Assets and Liabilities

How do you begin? First, identify your positive characteristics and your skills. Then, identify your liabilities, but analyze how these weaknesses can be overcome. For instance, if you are prompt and seldom absent and you pay attention to details, you have characteristics that employers seek in a new employee (Box 18-1). You may find it difficult to use a specific type of software, or you may have a problem remembering all the American Dental Association (ADA) insurance codes; however, these skill deficiencies can be improved with experience. If a prospective employer asks about any weaknesses, you could explain that, although you have had difficulty using a specific type of software, you would like to improve this skill and are willing to spend some extra time on your own to do so. This is a positive attitude that shows an interest in improving yourself, rather than an attitude of not caring.

Box 18-1
Desirable Characteristics for an Administrative Assistant

- Promptness
- Initiative
- Dependability
- Creativity
- Flexibility
- Self-motivation
- Enthusiasm
- Honesty
- Sense of humor
- Good general health
- Willingness to accept change
- Good listener
- Willingness to work with a team
- Effective organizational skills
- Knowledge of automated equipment
- Use of proper language skills in verbal and written communications
- Attention to detail

MARKETING YOUR SKILLS

A well-educated, experienced administrative assistant with the appropriate credentials has valuable bargaining power for obtaining a job that requires these skills and provides adequate compensation. Stating that you are a graduate of a dental assistant or business program is a credible assertion; however, supporting this claim with valid data that demonstrate the positive effect you can have on the practice is likely to win you the job.

If a dentist were to state that he or she couldn't afford a well-educated administrative assistant, your response might be, "I don't believe you can afford not to have a well-educated administrative assistant." Consider the following rebuttals to the dentist's reluctance.

- Credentialed administrative assistants have proved by some form of study and perhaps by a test given by a valid national dental board that they have a basic understanding of dental knowledge and business procedures. Delegating business functions to an inexperienced person with no formal knowledge of business principles or the standards required by the Occupational Safety and Health Administration (OSHA) is opening the door to potential penalties and litigation.
- Losses caused by errors in records management, claim form management, appointment scheduling, payroll, accounts receivable, banking, accounts payable, or patient communication can be significantly reduced if a qualified, educated administrative assistant is put in charge of those elements of the practice. Although an initial orientation period is necessary in any office, an educated administrative assistant is already aware of the procedures and terminology used in business and dentistry.
- Mature students who return to school from other careers, such as homemaking, teaching, and nursing, can bring with them many life experiences that are valuable assets to an administrative assistant position.
- An educated person remains in the profession longer than an inexperienced person because the former has made a commitment to the profession through the educational process.

You must develop a caring, positive attitude about your ability to become an asset to the dental office. It is your responsibility, however, to live up to the claims you make. Your skills, knowledge of dentistry, investment in your education, and credentials are all tools that can be used to achieve compensation commensurate with that of other allied health or business professionals with similar backgrounds and responsibilities.

> You must develop a caring, positive attitude about your ability to become an asset to the dental office.

JOB PRIORITIES

Everyone dreams of the ideal job. Yet many people are so excited to be given an interview that they take the first job offer without considering their goals, needs, and priorities. Before applying for a job or preparing for a job interview, decide what you need and want in a job and what your basic philosophy is about your career.

Determining Your Career Philosophy

As mentioned earlier, before seeking employment, you should determine your needs and clarify your life goals and a philosophy that is consistent with them. Unfortunately, a dental assistant may accept the first job offer with little consideration given to how his or her philosophy coincides with the philosophy of the prospective employer. Carefully evaluate yourself and establish some realistic goals. Then ask yourself the following questions: Are my professional, moral, and social values compatible with those of my prospective employer? With what type of work environment do I want to be associated, a solo practice or a large group practice? Which of my skills in dental assisting or business do I want to use to the greatest extent? What are my strengths? What are my weaknesses? How can I compensate for my weaknesses? What do I want to be doing in 5 years, in 10 years? How important are salary, hours, and location?

Once you have written down your philosophy of life and enumerated your goals, remind yourself that these goals will be ever changing, and you undoubtedly will reevaluate your philosophy as you gain confidence from your new experiences.

After you have reviewed the various factors involved in job selection, decide your top five priorities for a job and then rate each job offer. A decision-making grid such as the one shown in Table 18-1 may be helpful for this purpose. The job offers are listed in the left vertical column, and the priorities are listed across the top. Starting on the left, the priorities are given a point value based on your personal needs. Each job is evaluated, and the points totaled. If a tie occurs, other characteristics might be added.

Remember, you may need to do more than one or two interviews to find the job that satisfies your goals, needs, and priorities, but remain steadfast in your job search.

Determining Your Worth to a Practice

Although many elements may be considered important in deciding whether to accept a job offer, for most people salary and benefits are the primary factors in job selection. The difficulty often arises when a dentist asks you during an interview what salary you expect. You need to prepare yourself for this question and not say simply, "Oh, I don't know, what have you paid your other assistants?" You need to have a firm understanding of the cost of living in your area, the comparable salaries for similar responsibilities and educational attainment, the local and national salary data available for reference, and what you are really worth in terms of your skills and knowledge. The following discussion provides ideas for formulating a benefits and salary package that could reasonably be suggested to a prospective employer. Box 18-2 lists several benefits that are commonly offered to employees.

Salary is often a difficult subject to bring up, yet it must be discussed openly before you accept a job. You need to know the beginning salary, how salary increases are obtained, and when salary increases are awarded. An employer must expect to pay a fair salary that is based on education, experience, credentials, and merit performance. The salary should be competitive with other allied health professionals who have equal responsibilities, yet it should be cost-effective.

The economics of dental assisting varies widely across the country, depending on the specific position and its responsibilities and the geographical location of the practice. According to the DANB, the average median salary of a Certified Dental Assistant in 2004 was $15.48 an hour and that

> An employer must expect to pay a fair salary that is based on education + experience + credentials + merit performance.

Table 18-1 Job Decision-Making Grid							
	Practice Environment	Salary	Benefits	Location	Challenge	Hours	Total
Point Value	6	5	4	3	2	1	
Job offer no. 1		√	√	√	√	√	15
Job offer no. 2	√		√	√			13
Job offer no. 3	√	√		√			14

Box 18-2
Potential Job Benefits

- Dress allowance
- Retirement plan
- Health insurance
- Vision insurance
- Dental care/insurance (for self and family)
- Profit sharing
- Child care
- Membership in professional organizations
- Travel and expenses for professional meetings
- Special bonuses for holidays or production achievement

---

of a noncertified assistant was $13.10 an hour.[1] (Current data are available online at www.danb.org.) Salary data also may be obtained from the ADA website (www.ada.org) for various areas of the country. Dental assistants who have a formal education, management skills, and appropriate credentials may receive significantly higher salaries. Realize that this is an average national hourly salary with no benefits included. It is sometimes stated that some dental professionals make higher hourly salaries than others. When salaries are discussed, care must be taken to determine that all factors related to the salaries compared are the same. Some dollar value must be given to each of the benefits to determine the total salary and benefits package. Determine whether the job responsibilities are equitable. Education, experience, credentials, and performance evaluations are factored into the salary. Some value is placed on job environment. No skilled administrative or clinical assistant in today's market should be making a salary that does not reflect an honest respect for the individual's productivity. It is wise to ask for a contract or an employment agreement that verifies in writing the conditions of employment. These conditions might include the salary scale, an explanation of the merit performance evaluation, and the required probationary period.

POTENTIAL AREAS OF EMPLOYMENT

An administrative assistant can choose from myriad opportunities for potential employment. These can range from a small solo practice to a large clinic; they also can include the public or the private sector, practice management consulting firms, dental manufacturers, job placement, and teaching.

Private Practice

The dental assistant may seek employment in a private practitioner's office, a group practice, or a clinic with several dentists. The practice may be a general dental practice, which means that all phases of dental treatment are rendered for a patient, or it may be limited to one of the dental specialties recognized by the ADA (i.e., endodontics, orthodontics and dentofacial orthopedics, oral and maxillofacial surgery, oral and maxillofacial pathosis, pediatric dentistry, periodontics, prosthodontics, oral and maxillofacial radiography, and dental public health). In private practice, the dental assistant may find a position that is limited specifically to clinical assisting, office management, or laboratory duties or that is a combination of all these responsibilities. Private practice affords many opportunities to work closely with the dentist and patients, as well as diversification of duties, individuality, and considerable personal responsibility. As the value of a highly skilled dental assistant continues to increase, compensation and benefits in this area will continue to rise.

Institutional Dentistry

As the federal, state, and local governments demonstrate increased interest in the delivery of dental care, more facilities are being established to provide more dental services for the public. One institution that should be considered as a source of employment is a dental school. Schools offer many areas of potential employment, such as working with undergraduate or graduate dental students at chairside, supervising clinical activities, or managing business functions. Other institutions are a part of the civil service programs and offer employment in prisons, public clinics, and Veterans Administration hospitals. Additionally, hospitals, some of which are associated closely with dental schools, offer employment in various departments. The dental assistant working in an institution has the opportunity to work with a larger staff than is possible in private dental practice. Diversification of duties, participation in newly developed techniques, potential advancement to several levels of supervision, and possibly more liberal vacations (in learning institutions, vacations are often coordinated with school calendars) may be available in this setting.

Insurance Offices

Work in insurance offices is especially appealing to the dental assistant who aspires to perform various business tasks and become involved in management. With the increase in dental insurance coverage, more companies are seeking highly qualified dental assistants to work in management positions, because a broad knowledge of dentistry is an asset to their business. A position in insurance may also involve public speaking activities and travel.

Research

Hospitals and dental schools hire many dental assistants to work in research laboratories. Individuals who enjoy working with data, mathematical computations, and details and who enjoy being independent often seek positions in research.

Dental Manufacturers

An area of potential employment that should not be overlooked is the dental manufacturers, which employ dental assistants for sales and teaching. Such employment would limit contact with dentistry to a specific type or line of products, but it also offers a great opportunity to travel throughout the country and meet people.

Management Consulting Firms

Experienced dental assistants with a broad knowledge of clinical and business concepts are turning their interest into profitable businesses. Many highly qualified administrative assistants have joined management consulting firms or created their own companies to assist dental practices in increasing their productivity through more efficient practices and marketing.

Teaching

Numerous colleges and universities have developed occupational education programs that include dental assisting. A graduate of a dental assistant program who is a Certified Dental Assistant (CDA) or Registered Dental Assistant (RDA) may transfer into a baccalaureate degree program. Anyone who has broad experience in dental assisting, is highly motivated to teach, and is patient and objective, should perhaps contact a college or university about entering their program. Another source of information is the American Dental Assistants Association (www.dentalassistant.org).

WHERE DO YOU BEGIN TO FIND EMPLOYMENT OPPORTUNITIES?

After surveying some of these potential areas of employment, where do you begin looking for the right job? Many prospects are available, and several different avenues may be used.

School Placement

The school placement office or faculty members often are notified of job opportunities in the area. Instructors frequently know employers who are interested in hiring new graduates, and they also know their students' qualifications and abilities. Most schools spend considerable time and effort obtaining information about potential job opportunities, and they take a great deal of pride in placing their graduates.

Newspaper Advertisements

Both local and out-of-area newspapers have classified sections of jobs available. Advertisements in the classified section state the qualifications required and other details about the job, including whether it is for an administrative or clinical assistant (Figure 18-2). However, in some cases the employer does not give the name of the practice or the telephone number, but instead places a **blind ad** asking the applicant to submit a resume (Figure 18-3). This type of ad should not be overlooked, because it becomes the employer's first means of screening applicants.

In composing a letter of application and a resume, always remember that although first impressions are not necessarily the most accurate, they often are the most influential. A little more initiative is required of the applicant to construct a resume than to pick up the telephone and call for an interview.

Clinical Dental Assistant needed to join a large team-oriented practice. Must have credentials for advanced functions in this state and experience in periodontics. Challenging opportunity for a skilled, ambitious professional assistant. Many benefits included. Salary commensurate to education and credentials. Send résumé to: Joseph W. Lake, 611 Main St., SE, Grand Rapids, MI 49502

Dental business manager needed for a busy orthodontic office. This position requires an energetic, ambitious person who has a broad knowledge of dentistry and business applications. For a person who enjoys a fast pace, this office provides a challenging career opportunity in practice management utilizing modern electronic business systems. Current CDPMA preferred. Write to: Ashley M. Lake, DDS, 611 Main St., SE, Grand Rapids, MI 49502

A   B

Figure 18-2 A, Job advertisement for a clinical chairside assistant. **B,** Job advertisement for a business office manager.

Dental Office Manager: Interested in an exciting position in a small, professional office? A group dental practice is expanding its clinical facilities. Position demands strong supervisory skills; ability to work effectively under pressure, use good judgment, and accept responsibility; and a working knowledge of OSHA standards. Forward your résumé to: Box #2589, Grand Rapids News, Grand Rapids, MI 49502

Figure 18-3 Blind ad.

The letter of application and the resume give the prospective employer an opportunity to evaluate the applicant's keyboarding skills, communication skills, and neatness.

Employment Agencies

Both free and private employment agencies are available. Most states provide an employment service, and applicants may register with this service without charge.

Private employment agencies, which are service enterprises, provide many good job opportunities but charge a fee. Before registering with an employment agency, always check its reputation. This can be done locally or through the National Employment Association in Washington, D.C. In fact, in many states dental professionals have begun their own employment agencies, and this type of firm is more likely to provide applicants with a dental background, determined by the agency's screening processes. After selecting a reputable agency, the applicant should find out about testing and placement procedures.

Professional Organizations and Journals

Local dental societies and dental assistant organizations frequently maintain employment placement services. By checking your local telephone directory or the Internet, you can quickly establish contact with one of these organizations. State and national professional journals generally have a classified section devoted to job offerings for dental assistants. Many of these jobs offer unique opportunities, possibly even relocation. State and local dental associations often allow new graduates to post their contact information in the association's newsletters or journals free of charge.

Internet and World Wide Web

The Internet is a group of computers connected all over the world, which allows people to communicate with each other. For instance, on the Internet you can obtain information about companies or dental offices worldwide.

If you are interested in working with a large dental manufacturing company or a dental school, you can use the Internet and the computer files of the World Wide Web (www) to find information about them. Many major companies and dental schools post company profiles and employment opportunities on the Internet. Smaller dental practices may not use this system, but several "temp" agencies and employment agencies seek prospective employees this way. Many websites are available (e.g., www. jobweb.com, www.monster.com, www.yourmissinglink.com) that can provide information for your job search or allow you to post your resume.

Personal Networks

Networking is "the process of identifying and establishing a group of acquaintances, friends, and relatives who can assist you in the job search process." This approach is one of the best strategies for finding a job. In fact, some studies have shown that as many as 80% of jobs are obtained through some form of networking. Friends, relatives, business associates, local dental assistant societies, dental associations, dental supply houses, and dental schools all offer myriad contacts, which can provide potential contacts in the profession, which may lead to a job opportunity. If a friend is leaving a job and knows you are interested in the same area of dentistry and are available for work, a good recommendation from your friend is always welcome.

How do you go about networking? If you have a part-time job or have had a clinical rotation in an office while a student, let the dentist or other staff members know that you are ready for a full-time position. If these individuals know you are interested in a full-time job, they can talk with friends in the community about your skills and often can serve as an excellent reference for you.

PREPARING EMPLOYMENT DATA

Several steps must be taken between the determination of your goals and choice of employment and the time you actually begin work. The steps include career preparation planning, searching for job information, writing the letter of application, creating a personal resume, preparing for the interview, completing a **job application,** participating in the interview, touring the facility and meeting the staff, and following up on the interview (Figure 18-4).

Preparing a Letter of Application

The **letter of application,** or *cover letter,* has three basic goals: to arouse interest, to describe your abilities, and to request an interview. The letter of application should be kept to a single page, including the date and the closing signature. Every effort must be made to customize this letter and to express your philosophy, motivations, and character in a less formal format than the resume. In fact, this letter may very well be the most important business letter you ever write.

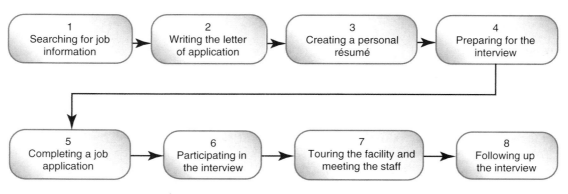

Figure 18-4 The career planning process.

AROUSE INTEREST. In the opening, introduce yourself to the prospective employer and include a brief description of your personal qualifications. This opening essentially gives you the opportunity to promote yourself. The letter should make the reader interested enough in your skills and abilities and to grant you an interview.

Example 1: "The position you have advertised in the Grand Rapids News sounds challenging. My certificate in Dental Assisting and my credential as a Certified Dental Practice Management Assistant have provided me the skills necessary to perform the job well."

Example 2: "Your employment announcement posted on my school bulletin board calls for a clinical chairside assistant who is interested in applying the latest concepts of four-handed dentistry. My education at Grand Rapids Community College has provided me with these skills."

Example 3: "Your employment announcement calls for an administrative assistant who is interested in learning the latest technology and has good computer skills. My education at Grand Rapids Community College for the past 2 years has provided me with these skills."

In each of these cases, the applicant lets the prospective employer know that she (or he) is interested in the position and believes that she (or he) has the skills needed for the job. Note that each paragraph is "you" or, reader, oriented.

DESCRIBE YOUR SKILLS AND ABILITIES. The second paragraph of the letter should describe your skills in more detail. It should also call attention to your enclosed resume, curriculum vitae, or data sheet (explained in the next section).

Example: "In August of this year I will graduate from Grand Rapids Community College. I will have completed courses in business office procedures, clinical procedures, laboratory and radiographic procedures, and dental specialties, as well as 300 hours of clinical practice in the local community. I had taken courses in accounting, management, business communications, and computers before entering the Dental Assisting Program. While in school I have worked part time as a clerical assistant in a local dental office."

This brief description includes an overview of basic skills. Further details about the skills and the dates of education and work experience are included in the attached resume.

REQUEST AN INTERVIEW. Because the purpose of a cover letter is to obtain an interview, you should ask for the interview directly.

Example: "Please give me an opportunity to discuss my qualifications with you. My telephone number is 616-999-2041."

Box 18-3 presents a list of action verbs that can be used to describe your activities. General guidelines for creating a cover letter are provided in Box 18-4.

Figures 18-5 to 18-7 show letters of application submitted by three applicants with varying backgrounds.

Contacting an Office by Telephone

If you have been informed of a job opening by an instructor or a friend, time may not allow you to write a letter of application; in such cases a telephone call is required. This situation requires a different approach. First, place a call to the office and indicate to the individual receiving your call who you are and why you are calling. Second, explain how you learned about the position. Finally, if the job is available, ask for an interview.

Whether you plan to send a letter of application or decide to contact the office by telephone, you must prepare a resume, either to enclose with the letter or to take with you to the office.

Box 18-3
Action Verbs

- Accomplished
- Achieved
- Active in
- Assisted
- Attained
- Attended
- Brought about
- Communicated
- Completed
- Conducted
- Contributed
- Cooperated
- Coordinated
- Counseled
- Created
- Demonstrated
- Designed
- Generated
- Formed
- Founded
- Graduated
- Headed
- Implemented
- Improved
- Increased
- Initiated
- Installed
- Instructed
- Interviewed
- Kept
- Lectured
- Led
- Maintained
- Managed
- Mediated
- Motivated
- Observed
- Obtained
- Operated
- Ordered
- Organized
- Originated
- Overcame
- Participated
- Perfected
- Performed
- Persuaded
- Placed
- Planned
- Prepared
- Presented
- Printed
- Processed
- Produced
- Programmed
- Proposed
- Proved
- Provided
- Publicized
- Realized
- Received
- Recognized
- Recommended
- Recruited
- Reevaluated
- Refined
- Regulated
- Represented
- Restored
- Reviewed
- Scheduled
- Secured
- Served
- Set up
- Simplified
- Sold
- Spearheaded
- Staffed
- Streamlined
- Substituted
- Trained
- Transformed
- Updated
- Validated

Box 18-4
Guidelines for Writing a Letter of Application

1. Create a professional letterhead that includes vital data; that is, your full name, address, telephone number (home, cell, and fax) and your e-mail address if you have one.
2. Use standard business letter format.
3. Use personal stationery made of quality bond paper; do not use your current employer's stationery.
4. Make sure your spelling, grammar, punctuation, and capitalization are correct. If you are composing your letter on a computer, always use the spell checker.
5. Avoid opening with "My name is…" Your name is on the letterhead and in the closing signature line.
6. Keep the letter short, three to four paragraphs. Put details in the resume.
7. Limit the letter to one page.
8. Address the letter to a specific person. Never address an application letter "To Whom It May Concern." Take time to find out the name of the employer. If it is not available, use "Dear Doctor" or, if the letter is going to a larger organization, "Dear Human Resources Manager."
9. Put the employer's needs first by making the letter "you" oriented; avoid "I."
10. Send an original letter for each application. Do not send photocopies.
11. Do not copy a letter of application from a book. Make your letter representative of your personal characteristics.
12. Consider mailing your letter and resume in a large envelope so that it will stand out from the more commonly used No. 10 envelopes on the employer's desk.

Creating a Resume

A **resume,** personal data sheet, or personal history should be prepared to accompany the letter of application or to take with you to the interview. A resume is a marketing tool, and the product is you. The objective is to capture the attention of the reader and maintain the person's interest. From the employer's point of view, the resume is a time-saver, because it gives a quick account of what you have done, what you can do, and for what you are striving. A resume needs to be a brief, well-documented account of your qualifications. A simple resume is best suited for those who are entering the job market or who have limited work experience. Remember, your objective is to be granted an interview; you therefore want to impress the reader with a resume that is a concise, positive presentation of your abilities and qualifications.

> A resume is a marketing tool, and the product is you.

When preparing your resume, it is best to create the document in word processing on the computer and then save it for future reference. Most software provides several optional templates that allow you to create a professional personal letterhead and a matching resume. Remember, you want to get the attention of the prospective employer when the person reads the letter, so take time to create an attractive professional image through your stationery. After the letter has been completed, create several original copies. If this is not possible, try to obtain the finest quality copy possible from a commercial printer. You should also keep a copy for yourself to take when going for an interview.

Jennifer M. Ellis

JE 1913 Hall Road
East Grand Rapids, MI 49506

Home: 616.111.2817
Work: 616.111.2345
FAX: 616.121.2468
E-mail: jme@juad.org

November 17, 20...

Joseph W. Lake, DDS
611 Main Street SE
Grand Rapids, MI 49502

Dear Dr. Lake:

This letter is in response to your advertisement in the Grand Rapids News, November, 12, 20...
You asked for a dental assistant who is skilled in advanced functions, is ambitious, and has
experience in Periodontics. I wish to be an applicant for this job and am forwarding my
curriculum vitae to you. I believe I possess the qualifications you desire.

You will see from the enclosed resumé that I have taken courses at Kent Community College in
Grand Rapids, Michigan, to prepare me as a Registered Dental Assistant. I have successfully
completed courses in dental assisting that will be valuable to your practice and have had
considerable clinical and business office experience. For the past three months I have been
working part-time in a periodontic practice while an assistant has been on maternity leave.

You may contact me at 616.111.2817 after 3:00 P.M. any day of the week. I am available for an
interview at your convenience.

Sincerely,

Jennifer M. Ellis, RDA

Enclosure

A

Figure 18-5 A, Letter of application for an entry-level position as a clinical assistant.

In general, your resume should be designed with the following suggestions in mind.
- Put yourself in the position of your prospective employer. Try to determine
  the qualities the person may be seeking and emphasize these qualifications.
- Be as impressive as possible but do not deviate from the truth. This is not
  the time to be shy and modest. You must tell the reader what you can do;
  no one else will do it for you.
- Review the material carefully to make sure you didn't forget anything.
  An overlooked item may be just the one the employer is seeking. Box 18-5
  presents some hints for writing a resume.

Jennifer M. Ellis

JE

1913 Hall Road
East Grand Rapids, MI 49506

Home: 616.111.2817
Work: 616.111.2345
FAX: 616.121.2468
E-mail: jme@juad.org

Objective	Obtain an entry-level dental assistant position in a periodontic practice that will utilize the skills of a highly skilled Registered Dental Assistant.
Experience	2004 to present Mark Richards, DDS, MS Rockford, MI **Clinical Dental Assistant** • Responsible for clinical assisting, infection control program, and general patient management. 2002-2004 Worthington Apparel Rockford, MI **Sales Clerk** • Responsible for sales, inventory control, and balancing daily sales receipts.
Education	Spring 2004 Kent Community College Certificate in Dental Assisting • Student representative to Dental Advisory Committee Kent Community College • Received John W. Knowles Scholarship for Dental Assistants • Graduated Summa Cum Laude.
Interests	Running, gardening, carpentry, computer graphics.
References:	Provided upon request.

B

Figure 18-5 B, Personal resume to accompany the letter applying for an entry-level position as a clinical assistant.

Every resume should have certain types of information. These include career objective, personal data, qualifications, experience, and education. Optional areas might include objectives, affiliations, and references. The arrangement of and headings for this information can vary, depending on the person's work experience, education, and general goals. It is wise to select a standard format and emphasize sections in which you have the greatest assets. Regardless of the format selected, there are do's and dont's to creating an effective resume; these are presented in Box 18-6.

1847 Sheffield
Ann Arbor, MI 48105
Home: 734.673.1235
Work: 734.768.2800
E-Mail: amy@hotmail.com

From the Desk of Amy S. March

February 5, 200—

Ashley M. Lake, DDS
611 Main St., SE
Grand Rapids, MI 49502

Dear Dr. Lake:

You will find enclosed a résumé I am sending in response to your advertisement in the Grand Rapids News for an office manager in your busy orthodontic practice. I believe, after you review this résumé, you will find that I have the qualifications needed to fill this position.

Over the past two years, I have gained a great deal of experience in a large orthodontic practice in Ann Arbor, Michigan. During the second year, I was in charge of insurance management and appointment scheduling. I have attended seminars sponsored by noted insurance companies and had an opportunity recently to attend a practice management course in Chicago on automated claim forms management.

My spouse has recently accepted a position with a law firm in the Grand Rapids area. Since our families both reside in nearby communities, we are delighted to be returning to Grand Rapids. In fact, we will be in the area looking for housing during the next thirty days, so I would welcome a call for an interview.

You may reach me at 734.673.1235 after 6 p.m. or you may leave a message on our answering machine and I will return the call as soon as possible.

Sincerely,

Amy S. March, RDA

Enclosure

A

Figure 18-6 A, Letter of application for an office manager in a specialty practice.

PERSONAL DATA Personal data include the following:
- Full name
- Address
- Telephone number
- Fax number and e-mail address (if you have one)

1847 Sheffield
Ann Arbor, MI 48105
Home: **734.673.1235**
Work: **734.768.2800**
E-Mail: amym@hotmail.com

From the Desk of Amy S. March

OBJECTIVE

I am seeking a job that will utilize me as a highly conscientious, detail-minded professional with education and clinical experience in orthodontics. Accustomed to working with a diverse patient clientele. Excellent communication and motivational skills with an interest in a challenging career in dental assisting.

EXPERIENCE

2003-Present	Orthodontic Associates Ann Arbor, MI *Business office manager*
2001-2003	Gerald Wilson, DDS, MS Ann Arbor, MI *Clinical dental assistant*
1998-2001	University of Michigan School of Dentistry Ann Arbor, MI ◆ Operative Dentistry Department ◆ Oral Diagnosis Department

EDUCATION

June 1999	Delta Midwest Insurance Lansing, MI ◆ Processing claim forms seminar
June 1998	Washtenaw Community College Ann Arbor MI ◆ Certificate, Dental Assisting ◆ WCC Dental Departmental Scholarship

CREDENTIALS

December 1998	Michigan Board of Dentistry Licensure RDA
August 1998	Dental Assisting National Board CDA

REFERENCES

Provided upon request.

B

Figure 18-6 B, Personal resume to accompany the letter applying for the position of office manager in a specialty office.

5200 Blueberry Lane
Cutlerville, MI 49509
Phone: 231.765.8899

Michelle M. Schaffer

November 7, 20—

P.O. Box 2589
Grand Rapids News
Grand Rapids, MI 49502

Dear Doctor:

Please accept my résumé directed toward the position you advertised in the *Grand Rapids News*. The position interested me since you are seeking a person with strong supervisory skills, good judgment, and ability to work under pressure, and a knowledge of OSHA standards. I have successfully managed a large clinical facility for the past six years and believe I have all of the qualifications you are seeking.

As you review my résumé you will note I am a highly motivated individual who has completed course work in numerous areas of value to your office. Since I am especially interested in infection control in a dental health care environment, I have attended a variety of seminars on this subject.

I look forward to hearing from you concerning this position and hope to meet you for an interview in the near future. You may reach me by calling in the evening at 231.675.8899. Thank you very much for your consideration of this application.

Sincerely,

Michelle M. Schaffer, CDA, CDPMA

Enclosure

E-mail: Scham6@hotmail.com
Pager: 231.789.0909

A

Figure 18-7 A, Letter of application in response to a blind advertisement for an office manager.

1913 Hall Road
East Grand Rapids, MI 49506

Michelle M. Schaffer

Objective
To obtain a management position in a team-oriented practice that will utilize my maturity, experience, communication, and motivational skills to maximum advantage and provide a setting in which safe quality care is a primary objective.

Experience

2001-Present   Hillsdale Dental Clinic   Hillsdale, MI
Office Manager

1997-2001   Kent Community College   Grand Rapids, MI
Admissions Office Clerk

1994-1997   Burlington Country Club   Rockford, MI
Dining Room Hostess

Education

July 2004   OSHA Update Seminar Presented by GRDS   Grand Rapids, MI
                Harriet Beamer, DDS, MS Lecturer

June 2003   CDC Guidelines for Dentistry   Grand Rapids, MI
                Presented by MDA John Molinari, PhD Lecturer

1998-1999   Aquinas College   Grand Rapids, MI
                B.A., Business Administration and Computer Science
                Graduated Summa Cum Laude

1996-1998   Kent Community College   Grand Rapids, MI
                Certificate in Dental Assisting

Credentials

CDPMA   Dental Assisting National Board

CDA   Dental Assisting National Board

CPR Certificate American Heart Association

References
Provided upon request.

Home: 231.789.0909   Pager: 616.757.1010   E-Mail: SchaM6@hotmail.com

Figure 18-7 B, Personal resume to accompany the letter applying for the office manager position.

Box 18-5
Hints for Preparing a Resume

- Use all the layout, formatting, and finishing techniques available to you.
- Use headings that allow the reader to find information easily.
- Be succinct.
- Use a spell checker.
- Make the resume easy to read (e.g., print size, font styles, and arrangement of information).
- Put your education and experience information in chronological order.
- Leave sufficient white space to avoid a cluttered look.

Box 18-6
Do's and Dont's for Creating an Effective Resume

Do
- Emphasize your qualities and experience.
- Substantiate your educational and experience qualifications to justify the abilities you claim.
- Be clear and concise in your descriptions.
- Choose a format that is easy to read.
- Be consistent in using the format.

Don't
- Include on the resume the date the resume was written.
- Include a physical description of yourself (e.g., height, weight, age).
- Include race or religion.
- Mention your health status.
- Include salary information (unless specifically requested; then include it in the cover letter).
- Use abbreviations or acronyms that may not be understood.

Box 18-7
Advantages and Disadvantages of a Chronological Resume

Advantages
- Highlights titles and company/dental practice names, which is advantageous when the names or tiles are relevant or impressive
- Highlights consistent progress from one position to another
- Highlights length of time in each organization

Disadvantages
- Readily shows gaps in the work history
- Shows frequent job changes
- Does not show the most impressive or relevant work experience first if it is not the most recent

CAREER OBJECTIVE. The career objective section lets the reader know about your current career goals.

Example: "Career Objective: A position as an administrative assistant with opportunities to use my technology, dental, and human relations skills."

Notice that this objective did not specify what type of dental practice, but rather emphasized the person's interest in an office management position. You might also list your long-term goals. In that case, the objective might be:

Example: "Career Objective: A position as an administrative assistant in a dental office, with a long-range goal of supervisory management."

EDUCATION. Be sure to include relevant information about your educational background. List all colleges and universities attended and the date you graduated. (List most recent schools first.) List diplomas or degrees, as well as awards and scholarships or special achievements. Courses that you took when completing the dental assistant program might be listed (e.g., dental science, dental laboratory procedures, clinical practice, dental radiography, and dental practice management).

WORK EXPERIENCE. A chronologic resume begins with your most recent job and include dates of employment, name and address of employer, position held, and a brief description of the job. Summer and part-time jobs may be lumped in a single category; however, if work experiences have been limited, you may want to list them separately. Box 18-7 presents the advantages and disadvantages of a chronologic resume.

In some instances, if your work experience is more recent than your education, the work experience should be listed before your education. At this point in your career, work experience is of greater value to a prospective employer than your education.

Optional Areas

AFFILIATIONS AND ACTIVITIES. If you have participated in school or community activities or received awards or honors, this information would be valuable to the prospective employer, and it should be included. Activities and hobbies are optional but can indicate that you are a well-rounded individual and get along well with others.

REFERENCES. Generally, references are provided upon request and not before the personal interview. Be prepared with the names, addresses, and telephone numbers of at least two people who are willing to verify your abilities and skills and one character reference. If your work experience has been limited, list instructors or clinical supervisors who can evaluate your abilities. Always obtain the individual's permission to use his or her name as a reference and be sure that person is willing to give you a good recommendation.

Remember, do not give information on the resume that might be detrimental to you. Details can be given when you are interviewed. At the interview, be prepared to discuss your weaknesses honestly, confidently, and in a way that puts your present self in the best light.

Figures 18-5, *B,* 18-6, *B,* and 18-7, *B,* show how resumes were designed to accompany each of the letters in Figures 18-5, *A,* 18-6, *A,* and 18-7, *A.*

COMPLETING THE JOB APPLICATION FORM

The type of dental assisting job for which you are applying determines the detail and complexity of the application form. The job application form is a series of questions requesting comprehensive data about you and your past education, work and professional experience. It often may require you to complete a narrative statement about yourself and give the reasons you are seeking a particular job. You may have had the opportunity to complete the application form before arriving for the interview or you may be asked to complete the form when you arrive. Figure 18-8 presents an example of an application used for private practice.

EMPLOYMENT APPLICATION

All information listed on this application will be considered and handled as personal and confidential. Please write or print legibly.

AN EQUAL OPPORTUNITY EMPLOYER

This employer provides equal opportunity to all persons without regard to handicap, race, color, religion, sex, age, or national origin.

Name:			Date of Application:
Address:	City:	State:	Zip:
Home Phone:	Cell Phone:		Social Security Number:

GENERAL INFORMATION

Position applied for: _____

Available to work: ☐ Full-Time   ☐ Part-Time   ☐ Temporary

Date available to start work: _____

Are you over 18 yrs. of age? ☐ Yes ☐ No   Will transportation be a problem for you?   ☐ Yes ☐ No

If you are not a U.S. Citizen, do you have the right to work in the United States?   ☐ Yes ☐ No

Have you ever been convicted of a felony?   ☐ Yes ☐ No

 (A conviction is not an automatic bar to employment. Each case will be considered on its own merits.)

Does the sight of blood bother you?   ☐ Yes ☐ No

EDUCATION

	Name and address of School	Major/Degree(s)	No. of Years Completed	Did you Graduate?
High School				
Community College				
4 Year Institution				
Vocational				
Other (specify)				

Describe Specialized Training, Apprenticeship, Skills, Seminars, Courses, Extra-Curricular Activities

Figure 18-8 Application for employment.

SKILLS

Task	Circle One		Task	Circle One	
Keyboarding WPM _____	Yes	No	Pour Models	Yes	No
Bookkeeping	Yes	No	Cavitron	Yes	No
Computer Operations	Yes	No	Cast Onlays	Yes	No
Handling Group Insurance	Yes	No	Plaque Control Instruction	Yes	No
Expose, Process, and Mount X-rays	Yes	No	Oral Evacuator	Yes	No
Panoramic X-Rays	Yes	No	Knowledge of Dental Instruments	Yes	No
Have you used insurance software?	Yes	No	Knowledge of Dental Terms	Yes	No

Other: (Describe if yes)

EMPLOYMENT RECORD

Beginning with your current employer, please list your work experience over the past ten years. You may include pertinent volunteer activities.

Name of Employer		Start Date	End Date
		Start Salary	End Salary
Address	Phone		
Job Title	Supervisor	Phone	
Duties			
Reason for Leaving			

Name of Employer		Start Date	End Date
		Start Salary	End Salary
Address	Phone		
Job Title	Supervisor	Phone	
Duties			
Reason for Leaving			

Name of Employer		Start Date	End Date
		Start Salary	End Salary
Address	Phone		
Job Title	Supervisor	Phone	
Duties			
Reason for Leaving			

Figure 18-8, cont'd

REFERENCES

Please provide the name, address, and phone number of at least two non employer/relatives as references.

NAME	ADDRESS	PHONE

EMERGENCY CONTACT

Name	Relationship	
Address	Phone	Alt. Phone

DUTY PERFORMANCE

Are you able to perform the essential duties of the position for which you are applying, either with or without reasonable accommodations?   ☐ Yes   ☐ No

If yes, please indicate what type(s) of reasonable accommodations are needed:

In the course of making an employment decision, this employer makes it a practice to verify with previous employers information such as dates of employment, description of job duties, attendance records, reason for leaving, etc. If there are any employers you want us to contact, please indicate their names below and reasons why:

_____

_____

_____

_____

I understand that if I am employed and any statement herein is not true, I may be released immediately, I will be paid only through the day of release and this employer may cancel any rights to accrued benefits.

_____   _____
Date   Signature

Figure 18-8, cont'd

Regardless of the job for which you are applying, you must keep several things in mind when completing the application form.

- If possible, try to obtain two forms, one to use as a working copy and the other to submit to the employer.
- Before entering data on the application form, read through the application very thoroughly and avoid asking unnecessary questions. The application form often is used as the first employment test. It tests your ability to follow directions.
- The directions may indicate that the form can be typed or written. If you are required to complete the form in your own handwriting, this may be another test of neatness and also gives the employer a sample of how well or poorly you write.
- Answer all the questions. If the question does not relate to you, write N/A (not applicable) or draw a line through the question. The employer then realizes you have read the question and have not overlooked it.
- Be truthful when answering interview questions. Dates, names, and places need to be accurate. Make a list of your former addresses, schools, family names, and references to take along when going for the interview. It is better to have the information available even if it is not needed. Be sure that no discrepancies exist between your reported date of birth and your age. If you are residing at a temporary address, be sure to give a permanent address. Be particularly careful with your spelling. A small pocket dictionary is a great item to take along as a handy reference.

> Be truthful when answering interview questions.

PREPARING FOR THE PERSONAL INTERVIEW

The day you receive a response from a prospective employer, you will be elated to know that someone is interested in your qualifications after reviewing the resume and now wishes to meet you in person. This elation is immediately followed by a feeling of fear—fear of the unknown. You may or may not know anything about this prospective position, but one thing is certain, you do know yourself. The following steps can be used to prepare for an interview. At a later time, you should go through each of these steps and apply them to your situation.

1. *Learn about the dental practice or clinic.* Once you have identified the dental practice or clinic to which you are interested in applying, spend time learning more about the office or clinic, its mission, and its vision. Find out about its reputation and how it treats its employees. This can be done in several ways:
   - Ask friends, relatives, and acquaintances what they know about this office or clinic.
   - Check the office or clinic website if one is available. For example, dental schools have a website, from which you could learn about staffing and the various types of jobs and clinics in the institution.
   - Search the dental society websites to identify professional memberships.
   - If you are a student, consult with local professional contacts or dental faculty.
   - Search the state Board of Dentistry to identify any possible disciplinary action.

2. *What do I wear?* Wear something that looks businesslike. You may have a new outfit that you would like to wear but cannot decide if it is the proper thing. If you question whether an outfit is right, don't wear it. Wash your hair and style it so that it feels comfortable and looks good on you. A moderate amount of makeup can be worn, and don't wear a perfume that is too heavy. Personal appearance is an important part of the interview, and it is prudent to follow the old adage, "First appearances are lasting ones."

You may know all the answers and have a lot of skill, but you must win the approval of the dentist before you will ever have an opportunity to display these skills.

3. *What do I take with me?* The day you receive the call for the interview, write down the time, place, and name of the interviewer. Prepare the materials to take with you to the interview. These should include a ballpoint pen, a pencil, an eraser, a small spiral notebook, a pocket dictionary, and a copy of your college transcripts and your resume. In the notebook list many of your outstanding characteristics that you may wish to bring to the attention of the dentist, a list of questions you hope to cover during the interview, and the names, addresses, and telephone numbers or e-mail addresses of your references.

Depending on the type of job for which you are applying, you may want to take a **portfolio,** which is a compilation of samples of your work. If you are applying for an administrative assistant position, a portfolio might include the following:

- Letters you have written, which show your writing style
- Spreadsheets you have prepared
- Reports, including graphics
- PowerPoint slides

Preparing a portfolio and presenting it during the job interview allows you to show what you can do rather than merely talk about it.

The Personal Interview

Plan to arrive a few minutes early at the office. Your first contact may be with the office manager. The office manager plays an important role in the office, therefore it is important to be friendly and courteous to this person. You may want to introduce yourself by saying, "Good morning, I am Jennifer Ellis (use your own name!) and I have a 10:30 appointment for an interview with Dr. Lake." The office manager will acknowledge you and may ask you to complete an application form similar to that shown in Figure 18-8. After the form is completed, the office manager may review your resume and application and will escort you to meet Dr. Lake. If you are not introduced, take the time to introduce yourself by saying, "Good morning, Dr. Lake, I am Jennifer Ellis." At this point you will be asked to be seated, and the interview will begin. Look directly at the interviewer and respond to the questions clearly and distinctly; don't be evasive. An evasive answer leaves doubt in the interviewer's mind.

In general, the applicant should be responsive and answer in complete sentences. Box 18-8 presents helpful hints on things to avoid during an interview. Box 18-9 provides a series of commonly asked interview questions.

After the series of questions, salary and job responsibilities generally are discussed. If the salary the dentist offers you is lower than you are willing to accept, you may reply that you had hoped to start at a higher salary but you are willing to accept an opportunity to demonstrate your ability and value to the practice. This undoubtedly will result in further discussion, whereupon you should be prepared to give firm answers on what you will accept. Also, you should inquire whether any benefits are included that might offset the lower salary.

After an interview that included many of the questions in Box 18-10, a prospective applicant, Jennifer Ellis, was offered an acceptable salary, although it was lower than her initial request. She replied, "I feel I have the skills you need, and it is going to save you a great deal of time in not having to teach me about all the technical skills. I would be willing to start at the lower salary if you will explain to me what the total salary scale is and how I will be evaluated for salary raises. I would like the opportunity to advance

> You may know all the answers and have a lot of skill, but you must win the approval of the dentist before you will get the opportunity to display those skills.

Box 18-8
Missteps to Avoid During a Job Interview

- Being too aggressive
- Talking about salary and hours immediately
- Chewing gum
- Lacking enthusiasm
- Lacking a neat appearance
- Using little or no eye contact
- Appearing preoccupied
- Using poor grammar
- Being vague
- Wearing too much makeup
- Lacking curiosity

---

by merit or production, since I am certain you will be pleased with my ability and production in your office." Dr. Lake explained the numerous benefits and outlined the salary system to Jennifer. Remember, as discussed earlier, salary is not the primary aspect of the job, but you must be able to earn enough to support yourself and not eliminate some of the more enjoyable things in life. Also, the benefits of a job often outweigh the basic salary, so don't overlook this aspect.

Box 18-9
Commonly Asked Interview Questions

Initial Questions
- How did you learn about this position?
- Are you familiar with our office?
- Why are you interested in this practice?
- How would you describe yourself?
- Why do you think you are qualified for this position?

Interest in the Job
- Are you currently employed? If so, does your current employer know you are seeking a new position?
- Why do you want to change jobs?
- What do you consider the ideal job for you?
- What are your long-range and short-range goals?

Education
- What formal education have you had?
- Why did you choose to study dental assisting?
- What was your academic average when you were in school?
- What do you consider your greatest strength? Your greatest weakness?

Experience
- Have you ever been fired or asked to resign from a position?
- Why did you leave your previous job?
- Which duties performed in the past have you liked the best? The least? Why?
- Why should I hire you?
- What salary do you expect?

Box 18-10
Hints for Success in a New Job

- Learn the names of staff members.
- Listen attentively.
- Establish meaningful social friendships.
- Use a notebook and calendar to record important activities and procedures.
- Use judgment in working overtime and taking breaks.
- Do not flaunt your education and abilities.
- Seek honest evaluations.
- Maintain office policies.
- Observe office hours.
- Be yourself.

Other Formats for Interviewing

Some dentists like to have team interviews, in which several members of the staff who will work with you participate in the interview. Generally a team interview in a private practice setting involves three or four people. Although this type of interview may sound intimidating, it may not be. Pay attention to the individuals' names as they are introduced so that later you can refer to them by name. Listen carefully and answer questions succinctly, giving your attention to the individual who asked the question. Make eye contact with all participants if the question or statement is meant for the group.

WORKING INTERVIEW. Often a dentist uses the working interview format to assess a clinical assistant applicant. The dentist will invite you for a day of a work at the office, for which some form of compensation is prearranged. This would serve as an opportunity to observe the office activity and give you a sense of how well the office is organized.

VIRTUAL INTERVIEW. Virtual interviews are not common in small dental practices, but some situations may warrant them. For example, if you are applying for a job in Torrance, California, and you live in Biltmore, New Jersey, it might be feasible to conduct a virtual interview. In other words, rather than having you fly to California for the interview, the dental clinic would make arrangements for you to go to a facility that has a teleconferencing center. This allows the interviewer from California to see you, and you can see the interviewer.

If you are to participate in a virtual interview, careful planning must be done in advance. Many of us get a little nervous when we know we are going to be videotaped, but a virtual interview is a two-way system that allows you to communicate with the other person as if you were in the same room. You still greet the interviewer warmly and with a smile, just as you would in person. Sit in the chair provided and avoid nervous habits. Try to forget that the camera is present and concentrate on the interviewer and the questions. Avoid wearing black, gray, or white, because they do not come across well on camera. Also avoid wearing jewelry that is distracting or that makes noise on camera.

Concluding the Interview

An interview is not a lengthy process, and it often is terminated with a tour of the office. Do not be overly flattering to the staff, but thank them for their time before you leave. You may not receive a job offer during the interview, because the dentist may have other applicants to interview. However, you may inquire as to when the dentist anticipates arriving at a decision. Remember, do not be discouraged if you do not get the job. Each interview is a learning experience, regardless of whether it produces a job offer, and it should not be treated as a disappointment.

Following Up the Interview

A good follow-up letter (Figure 18-9) should be written 1 or 2 days after the interview. This is an indication to the interviewer that you are interested in the position, and it may make you a priority applicant.

Jennifer M. Ellis

JE   1913 Hall Road
East Grand Rapids, MI 49506

Home: 616.111.2817
Work: 616.111.2345
FAX: 616.121.2468
E-mail: jme@juad.org

November 7, 2005

Joseph W. Lake, DDS
611 Main Street SE
Grand Rapids, MI 49502

Dear Dr. Lake:

Thank you for the interview you gave me yesterday. It was a privilege to see such a well-organized dental team. I was especially impressed with your facility and the infection control program you have implemented in the office.

Because of my education, I am confident that I can become an efficient dental assistant and an asset to your dental practice. After you have had a chance to review my application, you will see that I have had considerable work experience. The references I provided you yesterday will validate my reliability and quality of work.

I am available to begin work immediately. You may contact me any day of the week by calling 616.111.2817 after 3:00 p.m.

Sincerely,

Jennifer M. Ellis, RDA

Enclosure

Figure 18-9 Follow-up letter.

The follow-up letter does not have to be long. It simply restates your interest in the job and mentions some of the facts that interested you about the position.

Another type of follow-up may be necessary if you have not had a reply from the prospective employer. If the job is still available and you are interested, it is permissible to call the interviewer in a day or two after the interview. A telephone call lets the interviewer know of your continued interest; however, too many telephone calls can be annoying.

If you decide later that you are not interested in the position, you should send a letter explaining your decision. Not only is this thoughtful, but a time may come when you find yourself in a position to go back to this employer.

Regular Self-Evaluation on the Job

Regular self-evaluation is necessary to retain your position in the dental office. People often carefully evaluate themselves before they are hired but may become careless after working in the office for a time.

Don't become negligent about evaluating yourself. As a clinical or administrative assistant, you are constantly in the public eye and must maintain a good image in your employer's office. In addition, once you have obtained the position, you must maintain your skills and acquire new ones as changes occur in dentistry through expanded use of auxiliary staff. You should promptly join your professional organizations, which offer information about educational activities in relevant techniques.

HINTS FOR SUCCESS AS PART OF THE DENTAL TEAM

When you begin your new job on the dental health team, you should gear yourself for success. The following sections can help make this experience more pleasant and result in personal success. These suggestions are summarized in Box 18-10.

Learn the Names of Staff Members

Learning and remembering the names of your immediate associates should not be difficult. If the staff is large, learning the names of those not in your immediate department may be more difficult. It is wise to learn the names as quickly as possible. It may even be wise to maintain a list of names and the position of each employee until you are able to remember them.

Listen Attentively

You will be eager to learn as much as possible about your new position as quickly as possible. Listen carefully to directions and avoid talking persistently. If you relax and listen well, often the questions you are eager to ask will be answered. If not, do not hesitate to ask for clarification of a procedure.

Establish Meaningful Social Friendships

Most employers do not object if employees develop personal friendships with other employees. However, many traps can develop in your first days on a new job. One of these is developing a close relationship with one or two people too quickly, which can cost you friendship with others at a later time. Office cliques frequently create rivalry. Although you must have a friendly attitude toward other employees in the office, you need not feel you must participate in all the social activities or interests the others have. However, you should avoid a superior attitude that can be interpreted as snobbish.

Use a Notebook and Calendar to Record Important Activities and Procedures

When you begin your new job, many unfamiliar rules and regulations and other information will be given to you. To avoid misunderstandings or neglecting important information, develop the "notebook habit" and write down each bit of information. It is surprising how many successful people use this system.

Observe Office Hours

In most cases the office hours have been determined before your arrival. The efficiency of an office depends on your being prompt at all times. Your tardiness delays the work process for which you are responsible. You should ensure your means of transportation at all times. It is your responsibility to anticipate inclement weather and compensate for any potential delay. It is better to be 20 minutes early for work than 2 minutes late. The dentist will not be interested in your excuses.

> It is better to be 20 minutes early for work than 2 minutes late.

Use Judgment in Working Overtime and Taking Breaks

Employees sometimes try to impress their employer by working extra hours or skipping lunch hours or breaks. However, you should avoid continual overtime and loss of lunch hours because it may cause friction with other employees. Your actions may be misinterpreted, and other employees may make life miserable for you. This does not mean you cannot use your discretion on days when legitimate emergencies arise and your presence is necessary to maintain office efficiency.

Do Not Flaunt Your Education and Abilities

Nothing is more irritating than a new employee who constantly informs other employees of his or her exceptional abilities. It is better to prove your ability through your work than to tell everyone about your great potential. Your coworkers may have had many years of experience, and you might learn something from them if you give them a chance to help you.

Seek Honest Performance Evaluations

Most employees want to learn about their performance. Before accepting the new job, you should have asked how and when your performance would be evaluated. As time passes, periodic reviews of your performance should be obtained from the employer, and you should have an opportunity to discuss the performance evaluation and determine ways in which you are performing satisfactorily and areas that need improvement. Figure 18-10 is an example of a performance evaluation form. Such forms are reviewed periodically with you to evaluate your day to day performance. It is wise to use this evaluation form first as a self-evaluation, before your employer completes it.

Maintain Office Policies

Most offices have established policies for grooming and uniform styles. You should carefully review the office policy and adhere to it. In addition, you should take home any other handbooks the office uses for its employees and read them

Performance Evaluation Form

Employee Name _____

Job Title _____

Supervisor _____

EVALUATION

4   Excellent performance that demonstrates consistent and important contributions that meet and frequently surpass expectations of the position.

3   Performs with a very acceptable degree of skill that demonstrates the expectations of the position.

2   Performance has not met satisfactory level. Makes mistakes but usually corrects errors after further instruction. Improved performance is needed to achieve defined expectations of this position.

1   Performance indicates deficiencies that seriously interfere with attainment of the defined expectations of the position.

Attendance	**Evaluation**			
Adheres to scheduled work hours.	4	3	2	1
Uses leave appropriately.	4	3	2	1
Adjusts work schedule to office needs.	4	3	2	1
Job Knowledge				
Uses required job skills.	4	3	2	1
Updates skills periodically.	4	3	2	1
Demonstrates knowledge of procedures needed to perform the job.	4	3	2	1
Organizational Skills				
Prioritizes tasks.	4	3	2	1
Plans steps in advance to accomplish tasks.	4	3	2	1
Meets deadlines.	4	3	2	1
Work Quality				
Performs work accurately.	4	3	2	1
Demonstrates thoroughness and attention to detail.	4	3	2	1
Demonstrates neatness.	4	3	2	1
Human Relations/Communications				
Demonstrates a sense of humor.	4	3	2	1
Demonstrates good listening skills.	4	3	2	1
Maintains eye contact when speaking to another person.	4	3	2	1
Displays good manners and professional etiquette.	4	3	2	1
Conveys ideas effectively.	4	3	2	1
Responds to ideas conveyed by others.	4	3	2	1
Demonstrates sensitivity to diverse staff and patients.	4	3	2	1
Problem Solving Skills				
Remains calm in stressful situations.	4	3	2	1
Demonstrates ability to identify the problem.	4	3	2	1
Demonstrates ability to select the best solution.	4	3	2	1
Takes action to prevent future problems.	4	3	2	1
Does not require supervision to accomplish routine tasks.	4	3	2	1
Follows through on chosen solution.	4	3	2	1
Gives constructive criticism in a positive manner.	4	3	2	1
Responds to supervision in a positive manner.	4	3	2	1
Cooperation				
Respects responsibilities of others.	4	3	2	1
Provides assistance and guidance to others.	4	3	2	1
Accepts guidance from supervisor/employer.	4	3	2	1
Works as a team member.	4	3	2	1
Initiative				
Seeks work that needs to be done.	4	3	2	1
Seeks new methods and ideas to improve work.	4	3	2	1
Exhibits self-motivation to achieve team goals.	4	3	2	1
Integrity				
Respects other people and their property.	4	3	2	1
Maintains confidentiality.	4	3	2	1
Can be trusted with money that belongs to the office.	4	3	2	1
Refrains from gossip.	4	3	2	1
Is truthful regardless of potential consequences.	4	3	2	1

Supervisor/Employer Comments _____

Employee Comments _____

Employee's Signature _____   **Date** _____

Supervisor/Employer Signature _____   **Date** _____

Figure 18-10 Performance appraisal form.

carefully so that you will be well informed. If you do not understand a policy, ask for clarification to avoid making an embarrassing mistake.

Be Yourself

As you make your first impression in the office, it is wise to be yourself. Remember, you may admire characteristics in another person, but you cannot be that person. If you attempt to be someone else, you only destroy yourself and all of the finer parts of your character. Be yourself, and you will be a happier person.

ASKING FOR A RAISE

Pay increments may be discussed when you begin work, and you may find that raises are given after 6 months or 1 year of successful employment. To avoid any misunderstanding, determine how and when these raises can be obtained before accepting the job. Few dentists would consider performing extensive treatment on patients before informing them of the anticipated fees. Similarly, you should not be working unless you are aware of your potential salary and anticipated promotions. It is wise to obtain written verification of employment conditions and responsibilities and a salary scale before beginning work. This can be accomplished in an office procedures manual (see Chapter 2). However, if pay increments have not been discussed and you have completed a year of employment, you might wonder when and how the subject can be raised.

Before approaching the dentist about a raise, you should do a self-evaluation to determine that you are justified in making such a request. The questions listed in Box 18-11 might be considered in such an evaluation. A salary conference should be a two-way discussion that allows you to identify your assets for the job and explain your performance success and allows the employer to relate the performance to a monetary amount that will reward your performance and inspire increased productivity.

If you have given serious thought to the factors mentioned previously, and you feel you deserve a raise, how do you approach the dentist? Select an opportunity when the work schedule allows enough time for a discussion of the subject. Do not wait until the end of the day, when the dentist is tired and ready to leave the office. It also is not wise to start the day by asking for a raise, especially if the schedule is rather heavy.

Box 18-11
Questions to Consider Before Asking for a Raise

1. Have I performed my duties well enough to deserve a raise?
2. Have I improved or advanced my skills since beginning the job?
3. Have I been cooperative with other members of the dental team?
4. Have I continued to maintain good patient management skills?
5. Can I verify that my attendance and punctuality have been above average?
6. Have I continually maintained professional ethics, safe practice, and quality standards?
7. Can I verify that the practice's productivity has increased because of my performance?
8. Do economic factors in the practice and in the economy warrant a raise?

Let the dentist know why you believe you deserve a raise. If he or she asks why you should have one, be prepared to answer; for example, cite the rising cost of living, transportation costs, insurance, increased office production because of your efforts, or simply compensation for good performance.

Very often employees do not assert themselves enough to make the dentist aware that a raise should be given. If you become passive and content with a salary, naturally you will continue to be paid at this rate; however, if your professional skills are an asset, and because of these skills the dentist can perform the job with greater efficiency, you should be given a raise. If the employer cannot raise your salary, consider the benefits in Box 18-2 as alternatives to a salary increase.

If you are unsuccessful in getting a raise, express your appreciation for the dentist's understanding and consideration and consider your alternatives; of course, if you receive a raise, be sure to thank the responsible person.

Salary matters should be treated confidentially and are not discussed with other members of the team. Salary problems destroy positive attitudes and productivity and should be resolved as quickly as possible.

JOB TERMINATION

Terminating a job can be an obstacle for some individuals, especially when the job change is from one private practice to another in the same general locale. When you change jobs, make sure the change is to your advantage. Circumstances over which you have no control may be the reason for a change in jobs. However, an assistant who frequently changes jobs with inadequate notification or reason soon gains a poor professional reputation. Whatever the reason for terminating the job, do it ethically.

1. Give the reason for leaving the job.
2. Give sufficient notice, at least 2 weeks or longer if your job requires an extensive training period for a new assistant.
3. Write a letter of resignation as a follow-up to your verbal resignation.
4. Do not discuss the termination of your job with other members of the team until you are ready to inform the dentist that you will be leaving. The grapevine is a poor method of informing.
5. If you terminate a job where serious conflicts exist, it is best to leave these conflicts where they originated and not carry the feelings to another job. When beginning a new position, you should not make negative comments about a former employer. This is simply good ethics.

ATTITUDES FOR CONTINUED SUCCESS

A highly qualified and educated administrative assistant is the key to production, patient management, organization, accuracy, safe operation, and protection from potential litigation. The right individual can significantly reduce the stress on the dental team. As you grow past your entry-level position on the job, you will discover that your future success depends more and more on your attitude and human relations skills. Completing a course in dental practice management is only the beginning.

Your willingness to be a team player and to cooperate with patients and staff members, as well as your good communication skills, will be assets to the dental practice. Your initiative, self-motivation, creativity, and enthusiasm indicate an eagerness to accept leadership and challenges in the office. Your desire to learn, your curiosity, and your flexibility will enable you to attain new skills and to advance your career.

Continue to market your skills, maintain an interest in new technologies, and accept changes no matter where you are on your career path. Good luck!

> A highly qualified and educated administrative assistant is the key to production, patient management, organization, accuracy, safe operation, and protection from potential litigation.

LEARNING ACTIVITIES

1. Write a philosophy in which you describe who you are, where you are going, and what you hope to accomplish. This philosophy should include your goals for life, your basic values, and your strengths and weaknesses.
2. List six areas of potential employment and explain briefly the benefits of each.
3. Choose one of the advertisements in Figure 18-2 or 18-3. Respond to the advertisement by writing a letter of application for the position. Also prepare a resume to accompany the letter. Make a copy of the letter and the resume for your personal files. Assume that you have been interviewed for the position mentioned in question 3 and write an appropriate follow-up letter.
4. List five assets you have to offer that you think would attract the favorable attention of a future employer.
5. Give five ways an application form might attract unfavorable attention. List 10 questions that you might be asked during an interview.
6. Complete the application form in Figure 18-8.
7. For your personal use, review the performance evaluation form in Figure 18-10.
8. With two people assuming the roles of interviewer and applicant, answer the questions in Box 18-9. Discuss six suggestions for success on the job.
9. Discuss the procedure for the following:
   a. Asking for a raise
   b. Terminating a job

EXAMINE YOUR PROGRESS

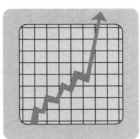

Practice by completing Working Form 16.

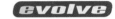

Key Terms

Blind ad   An advertisement that does not show the person or organization that placed the ad.

Job application   A form with a series of questions that request comprehensive data about the applicant, including educational background and work and professional experience.

Letter of application   The letter that accompanies a personal resume; it introduces the applicant and tries to arouse interest, prompting an interview with the prospective employer. Also called a *cover letter.*

Portfolio   A compilation of samples of the applicant's work; it may include letters, spreadsheets, reports, PowerPoint slides, or other items.

Resume   A listing of all the applicant's vital data, as well as information about the person's education and career experiences.

Reference

1. Dental Assisting National Board, Chicago, IL, 2004, Certified Press.

Bibliography

Fulton PJ: *General office procedures for colleges,* ed 12, Cincinnati, 2003, South-Western.
Locker KO: *Business and administrative communication,* ed 6, New York, 2003, McGraw Hill/Irwin.
Sabin WA: *The Gregg reference manual,* ed 10, New York, McGraw Hill/Irwin.

Appendix A

GRAMMAR

Subject and Verb Agreement

1. When the subject consists of two singular nouns or pronouns connected by *or, either ... or, neither ... nor,* or *not only ... but also,* a singular verb is required.

   > Jane or *Bob has* the letter.
   > Either *Ruth* or *Marge plans* to attend.
   > Not only a *book* but also *paper is* needed.

2. When the subject consists of two plural nouns or pronouns connected by *or, either ... or, neither ... nor,* or *not only ... but also,* a plural verb is required.

   > Neither the *secretaries* nor the *typists have* access to that information.

3. When the subject is made up of both singular and plural nouns or pronouns connected by *or, either ... or, neither ... nor,* or *not only ... but also,* the verb agrees with the last noun or pronoun mentioned before the verb.

   > Either *Ms. Rogers* or the *assistants have* access to that information.
   > Neither the *men* nor *Jo is* working.

4. Disregard intervening phrases and clauses when establishing agreement between subject and verb.

   > One of the men *wants* to go to the convention.

5. The words *each, every, either, neither, one,* and *another* are singular. When they are used as subjects or as adjectives modifying subjects, a singular verb is required.

   > Each person *is* deserving of the award.
   > Neither boy *rides* the bicycle well.

6. The following pronouns are always singular and require a singular verb: *anybody, everybody, nobody, somebody, anyone, everyone, nothing, something, anything, everything, no one, someone*

   > *Everyone plans* to attend the meeting.
   > *Anyone is* welcome at the concert.

7. *Both, few, many, others,* and *several* are always plural. When these five words are used as subjects or adjectives modifying subjects, a plural verb is required.

   Several members *were* asked to make presentations.
   Both women *are* going to apply.

8. *All, none, any, some, more,* and *most* may be singular or plural, depending on the noun to which they refer.

   Some of the *supplies are* missing.
   Some of that *paper is* needed.

9. A collective noun is a word that is singular in form but represents a group of people or things. Some examples of collective nouns are: *committee, company, department, public, class,* and *board.* The following rules determine the form of the verb to be used with a collective noun.

   a. When the members of a group are thought of as one unit, the verb should be singular.

      The *committee has voted* unanimously to begin the study.

   b. When members of the group are thought of as separate units, the verb should be plural.

      The *board are* not in agreement on the decision that should be made.

10. *The number* has a singular meaning and requires a singular verb; *a number* has a plural meaning and requires a plural verb.

    The number of requests *is* surprising.
    A number of people *are* planning to attend.

PRONOUNS

1. A pronoun agrees with its antecedent (the word for which the pronoun stands) in number, gender, and person.

   Roger wants to know if *his* book is at your house.

2. A plural pronoun is used when the antecedent consists of two nouns joined by *and.*

   Mary and *Tommie* are bringing *their* stereo.

3. A singular pronoun is used when the antecedent consists of two singular nouns joined by *or* or *nor.* A plural pronoun is used when the antecedent consists of two plural nouns joined by *or* or *nor.*

   Neither *Elizabeth* nor *Johanna* wants to do *her* part.
   Either the *men* or the *women* will do *their* share.

4. Do not confuse certain possessive pronouns and contractions that sound alike.

its (possessive)	*it's* (it is)
their (possessive)	*they're* (they are)
theirs (possessive)	*there's* (there is)
your (possessive)	*you're* (you are)
whose (possessive)	*who's* (who is)

As a test for the use of a possessive pronoun or a contraction, try to substitute *it is, they are, it has, there has, there is,* or *you are.* Use the corresponding possessive form if the substitution does not make sense.

> *Your* wording is correct.
> *You're* wording that sentence incorrectly.
> *Whose* book is it?
> *Who's* the owner of this typewriter?

5. Use *who* and *that* when referring to people.

> *He* is the boy *who* does well in keyboarding.
> *She* is the type of person *that* we like to employ.

6. Use *which* and *that* when referring to places, objects, and animals.

> The *card that* I sent you was mailed last week.
> The *fox, which* is very sly, caught the skunk.

PLURALS

In most English words, the plurals are formed by merely adding an *s* or *es,* but in Greek and Latin the plural may be designated by changing the ending.

> *-ae,* as in fasciae (singular form, fascia)
> *-ia,* as in crania (singular form, cranium)
> *-i,* as in glomeruli (singular form, glomerulus; when the singular form
>   ends in *us,* the plural form is made by adding *i* and dropping the *us.*)
> *-ata,* as in adenomata (singular form, adenoma)

SPELLING

The aforementioned rules for pronunciation and the formation of plurals are essential for spelling, but it is important that you consult a dental or medical dictionary if you are not sure. Phonetic spelling has no place in medicine or dentistry because a misspelled word may give the wrong meaning to a diagnosis. Furthermore, some terms are pronounced alike but spelled differently; for example, *ileum* is a part of the intestinal tract, but *ilium* is a pelvic bone.

From Fulton PJ: General office procedures for colleges, *ed 9, Cincinnati, 1988, South-Western.*
Adapted from Mosby: Mosby's dental dictionary, *St. Louis, 2004, Mosby.*

Appendix B

NUMBERS

1. Spell out numbers 1 through 10; use figures for numbers above 10.

   We ordered *ten* coats and *four* dresses.
   About *60* letters were keyed.

2. If there are numbers above and below 10 in correspondence, be consistent—either spell out all numbers or place all numbers in figures. If most of the numbers are below 10, spell them out. If most are above 10, express them all in figures.

   Please order *12* memo pads, *2* reams of paper, and *11* boxes of envelopes.

3. Numbers in the millions or higher may be expressed in the following manner to aid comprehension:

   3 billion (rather than 3,000,000,000)

4. Always spell out a number that begins a sentence.

   Five hundred books were ordered.

5. If the numbers are large, rearrange the wording of the sentence so that the number is not the first word of the sentence.

   We had a good year in *1976*.
   Not: Nineteen hundred and seventy-six was a good year.

6. Spell out indefinite numbers and amounts.

   A *few hundred* voters.

7. Spell out all ordinals (e.g., *first, second, third*) that can be expressed in words.

   The store's *twenty-fifth* anniversary was held this week.

8. When adjacent numbers are written in words or in figures, use a comma to separate them.

   On Car 33, 450 cartons are being shipped.

9. House or building numbers are written in figures. However, when the number *one* appears by itself, it is spelled out. Numbers one through ten in street names are spelled out; numbers above ten are written in figures.

When figures are used for both the house number and the street name, use a hyphen that is preceded and followed by a space.

101 Building
2301 Fifth Avenue
One Main Place
122 - 33rd Street

10. Ages are usually spelled out except when the age is stated exactly in years, months, and days. When ages are presented in tabular form, they are written in figures.

She is *eighteen years* old.
He is *2 years, 10 months, and 18 days* old.
Jones, Edward 19
King, Ruth 21

11. Use figures to express dates written in normal month-day-year order. Do not use *th, nd,* or *rd* after the date.

May 8, 1987
Not: May 8th, 1987

12. Fractions should be spelled out unless they are part of mixed numbers. Use a hyphen to separate the numerator and denominator of fractions written in words when the fraction is used as an adjective.

three-fourths inch
5½

13. In legal documents, numbers may be written in both words and figures.

One hundred thirty-four and 30/100 dollars
($134.30)

14. Amounts of money are usually expressed in figures. Indefinite money amounts are written in words.

$100
$3.27
several hundred dollars

15. Express percentages in figures; spell out the word *percent.*

10 percent

16. To form the plural of figures, add *s.*

Technological advances will increase in the *1980s.*

17. In times of day, use figures with A.M. and P.M.; spell out numbers with the word *o'clock.* In formal usage, all times are spelled out.

9 A.M.
10 P.M.
eight o'clock in the evening

From Fulton PJ: General office procedures for colleges, *ed 9, Cincinnati, 1988, South-Western.*

Appendix C

PREFIXES AND SUFFIXES

Prefixes

Prefixes, the most frequently used elements in the formation of medical and dental words, are one or more syllables placed before words or roots to show various kinds of relationships. They are never used independently, but when added before verbs, adjectives, or nouns, they modify the meaning. Most prefixes are a part of words in ordinary speech and do not refer specifically to medical-dental or scientific terminology, but many occur frequently in medical terminology. Studying them is an important step in learning medical terms and building a medical-dental vocabulary.

Prefix	Translation	Examples
a- (an- before a vowel)	Without, lack of	Apathy (lack of feeling), anemia (lack of blood)
ab-	Away from	Abductor (leading away from), aboral (away from mouth)
ad-	To, toward, near to	Adductor (leading toward), adhesion (sticking to)
ambi-	Both	Ambidextrous (ability to use hands equally), ambilaterally (both sides)
amphi-	About, on both sides, both	Amphibious (living on both land and water)
ampho-	Both	Amphogenic (producing offspring of both sexes)
ana-	Up, back, again, excessive	Anatomy (a cutting up)
ante-	Before, forward	Antecubital (before elbow), anteflexion (forward bending)
anti-	Against, opposed to, reversed	Antisepsis (against infection)
apo-	From, away from	Aponeurosis (away from tendon), apochromatic (abnormal color)
bi-	Twice, double	Bilateral (two sides), bifurcation (two branches)
cata-	Down, according to, complete	Catabolism (breaking down), catalepsia (complete seizure)

Continued

Prefix	Translation	Examples
circum-	Around, about	Circumference (surrounding), circumscribe (to draw around)
com-	With, together	Commissure (sending or coming together)
con-	With, together	Conductor (leading together), concentric (having a common center)
contra-	Against, opposite	Contraception (prevention of conception), contraindicated (not indicated)
de-	Away from	Dehydrate (remove water from), decompensation (failure of compensation)
di-	Twice, double	Diplopia (double vision), dichromatic (two colors)
dia-	Through, apart, across, completely	Diaphragm (wall across), diapedesis (ooze through), diagnosis (complete knowledge)
dis-	Reversal, apart from, separation	Disinfection (apart from infection), dissect (cut apart)
dys-	Bad, difficult, disordered	Dyspepsia (bad digestion), dyspnea (difficult breathing)
e-, ex-	Out, away from	Enucleate (remove from), exostosis (outgrowth of bone)
ec-	Out from	Ectopic (out of place), eccentric (away from center)
ecto-	On outside, situated on	Ectoderm (outer skin), ectoretina (outer layer of retina)
em-, en-	In	Empyema (pus in), encephalon (in the head)
endo-	Within	Endodont (within tooth)
epi-	Upon, on	Epidural (upon dura), epidermis (on skin)
exo-	Outside, on outer side, outer layer	Exogenous (produced outside)
extra-	Outside	Extracellular (outside cell)
hemi-	Half	Hemiplegia (partial paralysis), hemianesthesia (loss of feeling on one side of body)
hyper-	Over, above, excessive	Hyperemia (excessive blood), hypertrophy (overgrowth), hyperplasia (excessive formation)
hypo-	Under, below, deficient	Hypotension (low blood pressure)
im-, in-	In, into	Immersion (act of dipping in), injection (act of forcing liquid into)
im-, in-	Not	Immature (not mature), involuntary (not voluntary), inability (not able)
infra-	Below	Infraorbital (below eye), infraclavicular (below clavicle or collarbone)
inter-	Between	Intercostal (between ribs), intervene (come between)
intra-	Within	Intracerebral (within cerebrum), intraocular (within eyes)

Prefix	Translation	Examples
intro-	Into, within	Introversion (turning inward), introduce (lead into)
meta-	Beyond, after, change	Metamorphosis (change of form), metastasis (beyond original position)
opistho-	Behind, backward	Opisthotic (behind ears), opisthognathous (behind jaws)
para-	Beside, by side	Paraplegia (paralysis of both sides), paracentesis (puncture along side of)
per-	Through, excessive	Permeate (pass through), perforate (bore through)
peri-	Around	Periosteum (around bone), periatrial (around atrium)
post-	After, behind	Postoperative (after operation), postocular (behind eye)
pre-	Before, in front of	Premolar (in front of molars), preoral (in front of mouth)
pro-	Before, in front of	Prognosis (foreknowledge), prophase (appear before)
re-	Back, again, contrary	Reflex (bend back), revert (turn again to)
retro-	Backward, located behind	Retrograde (going backward), retrolingual (behind tongue)
semi-	Half	Semicartilaginous (half cartilage), semiconscious (half conscious)
sub-	Under	Subcutaneous (under skin), subungual (under nail)
super-	Above, upper, excessive	Supercilia (upper brows), supernumerary (excessive number)
supra-	Above, upon	Suprarenal (above kidney), suprascapular (on upper part of scapula)
sym-, syn-	Together, with	Symphysis (growing together), synapsis (joining together)
trans-	Across, through	Transection (cut across), transmit (send beyond)
ultra-	Beyond, in	Ultraviolet (beyond violet end of spectrum), ultrasonic (sound waves beyond the upper frequency of hearing by human ear)

Suffixes

Suffixes are one or more syllables or elements added to the *root* of a word (the part that indicates the essential meaning) to alter the meaning or indicate the intended part of speech.

To make the word pronounceable, the last letter or letters of the root to which the suffix is attached may be changed. The last vowel may be changed to an *o,* or *o* may be inserted if it is not already present before a suffix beginning with a consonant, as in *cardiology.* The final vowel in the root may be dropped before a suffix beginning with a vowel, as in *neuritis.*

Most suffixes are in common use in English, but some are peculiar to medical science. The suffixes most commonly used to indicate disease are *-itis,* meaning "inflammation," *-oma,* meaning "tumor," and *-osis,* meaning "a condition," usually morbid. The following suffixes occur often in medical-dental terminology but are also used in ordinary language:

Suffix	Use	Examples
-ise, -ize, -ate	Add to nouns or adjectives to make verbs expressing to use and to act like; to subject to; make into	Visualize (able to see), hypnotize (put into state of hypnosis)
-ist, -or, -er	Add to verbs to make nouns expressing agent or person concerned or instrument	Anesthetist (one who practices the science of anesthesia), donor (giver)
-ent	Add to verbs to make adjectives or nouns of agency	Recipient (one who receives), concurrent (happening at the same time)
-sia, -y	Add to verbs to make nouns expressing action, process, or condition	Therapy (treatment), anesthesia (process or condition of feeling)
-ia, -ity	Add to adjectives or nouns to make nouns expressing quality or condition	Septicemia (poisoning of blood), disparity (inequality), acidity (condition of excess acid), neuralgia (pain in nerves)
-ma, -mata, -men, -mina, -ment, -ure	Add to verbs to make nouns expressing result of action or object of action	Trauma (injury), foramina (openings), ligament (tough, fibrous band holding bone or viscera together), fissure (groove)
-ium, -olus, -olum, -culus, -culum, -cule, -cle	Add to nouns to make diminutive nouns	Bacterium, alveolus (air sac), follicle (little bag), cerebellum (little brain), molecule (little mass), ossicle (little bone)
-ible, -ile	Add to verbs to make adjectives expressing ability or capacity	Contractile (ability to contract), edible (capable of being eaten), flexible (capable of being bent)
-al, -c, -ious, -tic	Add to nouns to make adjectives expressing relationship, concern, or pertaining to	Neural (referring to nerve), neoplastic (referring to neoplasm), cardiac (referring to heart), delirious (suffering from delirium)
-id	Add to verbs or nouns to make adjectives expressing state or condition	Flaccid (state of being weak or lax), fluid (state of being fluid or liquid)
-tic	Add to verbs to make adjectives showing relationships	Caustic (referring to burn), acoustic (referring to sound or hearing)
-oid, -form	Add to nouns to make adjectives expressing resemblance	Polypoid (resembling polyp), plexiform (resembling a plexus), fusiform (resembling a fusion), epidermoid (resembling epidermis)
-ous	Add to nouns to make adjectives expressing material	Ferrous (composed of iron), serous (composed of serum), mucinous (composed of mucin)

The following verbs or combining forms of verbs are derived from either Greek or Latin. They may be attached to other roots to form words, or suffixes and prefixes may be added to them to form words. In the following examples, the part or root of the word to which the verb is attached is underlined, and the meaning, if not clear, is given in parentheses.

Root	Translation	Examples
-algia-	Pain	Cardialgia (heart), gastralgia (stomach), neuralgia (nerve)
-audi-, -audio-	Hear, hearing	Audiometer (measure), audiophone (voice instrument for deaf)
-bio-	Live	Biology (study of living), biogenesis (origin)
cau-, -caus-	Burn	Caustic (suffix added to make adjective), cauterization, causalgia (burning pain), electrocautery
-centesis-	Puncture, perforate	Thoracentesis (chest), pneumocentesis (lung), arthrocentesis (joint), enterocentesis (intestine)
-clas-, -claz-	Smash, break	Osteoclasis (bone), odontoclasis (tooth)
-duct-	Lead	Ductal (suffix added to make adjective), oviduct (egg uterine tube or fallopian tube), periductal (peri means "around")
-dynia-	Pain	Mastodynia (breast), esophagodynia (esophagus)
-ecta-, -ectas-	Dilate	Venectasia (dilation of vein), cardiectasis (heart), ectatic (suffix added for adjective)
-edem-	Swell	Myoedema (muscle), lymphedema (lymph), (a is a suffix added to make a noun)
-esthes-	Feel	Esthesia (suffix added to make noun), anesthesia (an is a prefix)
-flex-, -flec-	Bend	Flexion (suffix added to make noun), flexor (suffix added), anteflect (prefix added meaning "before" bending forward)
-fiss-	Split	Fissure, fission (suffixes added to make nouns)
-flu-, -flux-	Flow	Fluctuate, fluxion, affluent (abundant flowing)
-geno-, -genesis-	Produce, origin	Genotype, homogenesis (same origin), pathogenesis (disease, origin of disease), heterogenesis (prefix added meaning "other," alteration of generation)
-iatro-, -iatr-	Treat, cure	Geriatrics (old age), pediatrics (children)
-kine-, -kino-, -kineto-, -kinesio-	Move	Kinetogenic (Producing movement), kinetic (suffix added to make adjective), kinesiology (study)
-liga-	Bind	Ligament (suffix added to make noun) ligate, ligature
-logy-	Study	Parasitology (parasites), bacteriology (bacteria), histology (tissues)
-lysis-	Breaking up, dissolving	Hemolysis (blood), glycolysis (sugar), autolysis (self-destruction of cells)
-morph-, -morpho-	Form	Morphology, amorphous (not definite form), pleomorphic (more, occurring in various forms), polymorphic (many)

Continued

Root	Translation	Examples
-olfact-	Smell	Olfactophobia (fear), olfactory (suffix added to make adjective)
-op-, -opto-	See	Amblyopia (dull, dimness of vision), presbyopia (old, impairment of vision in old age), optic myopia (*myo*, to wink, half close the eyes)
-palpit-	Flutter	Palpitation
-pep-	Digest	Dyspepsia (bad, difficult), peptic (suffix added to make adjective)
-phag-, -phago-	Eat	Phagocytosis (eating of cells), phagomania (madness, mad craving for food or to eat), dysphagia (difficulty eating or swallowing)
-phan-	Appear, visible	Phanerosis (act of becoming visible), phantasia, phantasy
-pexy-	Fix	Mastopexy (fixation of breast), nephrosplenopexy (surgical fixation of kidney and spleen)
-phas-	Speak, utter	Aphasia (unable to speak), dysphasia (difficulty in speaking)
-phobia-	Fear	Hydrophobia (fear of water), claustrophobia (fear of close places)
-phil-	Like, love	Hemophilia (blood, a hereditary disease characterized by delayed clotting of blood), acidophilia (acid stain, liking or straining with acid stains), philanthropy (love of mankind)
-phrax-, -phrag-	Fence off, wall off	Diaphragm (across, partition separating thorax from abdomen), phragmoplast (formed)
-plas-	Form, grow	Neoplasm (new growth), rhinoplasty (nose operation for formation of nose), otoplasty (ear)
-plegia-	Paralyze	Paraplegia (paralysis of lower limbs), ophthalmoplegia (eye), hemiplegia (partial paralysis)
-pne-, -pneo-	Breathe	Dyspnea (difficult breathing), apnea (lack of breathing), hyperpnea (overbreathing)
-poie-	Make	Hematopoiesis (blood), erythropoiesis (red blood cells), leukopoiesis (making white cells)
-rrhagia-	Burst forth, pour	Menorrhagia (abnormal bleeding during menstruation), hemorrhage (blood)
-rrhaphy-	Suture	Herniorrhaphy (suturing or repair of hernia), hepatorrhaphy (liver), nephrorrhaphy (kidney)
-rrhea-	Flow, discharge	Leukorrhea (white discharge from vagina), rhinorrhea (nasal discharge)
-rrhexis-	Rupture	Enterorrhexis (intestines), metrorrhexis (uterus)
-schiz-	Split, divide	Schizophrenia (mind, split personality), schizonychia (nails), schizotrichia (hair)

Root	Translation	Examples
-scope-	Examine	Microscopic, cardioscope, endoscope (*endo* means "within," an instrument for examining the interior of a hollow internal organ)
-stasis-	Stop, stand still	Hematostasis (pertaining to stagnation of blood), epistasis (checking or stopping of any discharge)
-stazien-	Drop	Epistaxis (nosebleed)
-teg-, -tect-	Cover	Tegmen, tectum (rooflike structure), integument (skin covering)
-therap-	Treat, cure	Therapy, neurotherapy (nerves), chemotherapy (chemicals), physiotherapy
-tomy-	Cut, incise	Phlebotomy (incision of vein), arthrotomy (joint), appendectomy (ectomy, meaning "cutout," excision of appendix)
-topo-	Place	Topography, toponarcosis (numbing, hence numbing of a part or localized anesthesia)
-tropho-	Nourish	Hypertrophy (enlargement or overnourishment), atrophy (undernourishment), dystrophy (difficult or bad)

The following roots and combining forms are derived from Greek or Latin adjectives. Adjectives appear most often in compounds and are joined to either nouns or verbs. Suffixes may be added to make them into nouns.

In the following examples, the part or root of the word the adjective modifies is underlined, and the meaning is given in parentheses if not clear.

Root	Translation	Examples
-auto-	Self	Autoinfection, autolysis, autopathy (disease), autopsy (view, postmortem examination)
-brachy-	Short	Brachycephalia (head), brachydactylia (fingers), brachychelia (lip), brachygnathous (jaw)
-brady-	Slow	Bradypnea (breath), bradypragia (action), bradyuria (urine), bradypepsia (digestion)
-brevis-	Short	Brevity, breviflexor (short flexor muscle)
-cavus-	Hollow	Cavity, cavernous, vena cava (vein)
-coel-	Hollow	Coelarium (lining membrane of body cavity), coelom (body cavity of embryo)
-cryo-	Cold	Cryotherapy, cryotolerant, cryometer
-crypto-	Hidden, concealed	Cryptorchid (testis), cryptogenic (origin obscure of doubtful), cryptophthalmos (eye)
-dextro-	Right	Ambidextrous (using both hands with equal ease), dextrophobia (fear of objects on right side), dextrocardia (heart)
-dys-	Difficult, bad, disordered, painful	Dysarthria (speech), dyshidrosis (sweat), dyskinesia (motion), dystocia (birth), dysphasia (speech), dyspepsia (digestion)

Continued

Root	Translation	Examples
-eu-	Well, good	Euphoria (well-being), euphagia, eupnea (breath), euthyroid (normal thyroid), eutocia (normal birth)
-eury-	Broad, wide	Eurycephalic (head), euryopia (vision), eurysomatic (body, squat thickset body)
-glyco-	Sugar, sweet	Glycohemia (sugar in blood), glycopenia (poverty of sugar, low blood sugar level)
-gravis-	Heavy	Gravida (pregnant woman), gravidism (pregnancy)
-haplo-	Single, simple	Haploid (having a single set of chromosomes), haplodermatitis (simple inflammation of skin), haplopathy (simple uncomplicated disease)
-hetero-	Other, different	Heterogeneous (kind, dissimilar elements), heteroinoculation, heterology (abnormality of structure), heterointoxication
-homo-	Same	Homogeneous (same kind of quality throughout), homozygous (possessing identical pair of genes), homologous (corresponding in structure)
-hydro-	Wet, water	Hydronephrosis (kidney, collection of urine in kidney, pelvis), hydrophobia (fear of water, water causes painful reaction in this disease)
-iso-	Equal	Isocellular (similar cells), isodontic (all teeth alike), isocytosis (equality of size of cells), isochromatic (having same color throughout)
-latus-	Broad	Latitude, latissimus dorsi (muscle adducting humerus)
-leio-	Smooth	Leiomyosarcoma (smooth muscle, fleshy malignant tumor), leiomyofibroma (tumor of muscle and fiber elements), leiomyoma (tumor of unstriped muscle)
-lepto-	Slender	Leptosomatic (body), leptodactylous (fingers)
-levo-	Left	Levocardia (heart), levorotation (turning to left)
-longus-	Long	Adductor longus (muscle of thigh), longitude
-macro-	Large, abnormal size	Macrocephalic (head), macrochiria (hands), macromastia (breast), macronychia (nails)
-magna-	Large, great	Magnitude, adductor magnus (thigh muscle)
-malaco-	Soft	Malacia (softening), osteomalacia (bones)
-malus-	Bad	Malady, malaise, malignant, malformation
-medius-	Middle, median, medium	Gluteus medius (femur muscle)
-mega-	Great	Megacolon (large colon), megacephaly (head)
-megalo-	Huge	Megalomania (delusion of grandeur), hepatomegaly (enlarged liver), splenomegaly (enlarged spleen)
-meso-	Middle, mid	Mesocarpal (wrist), mesoderm (skin), mesothelium (a lining membrane of cavities)
-micro-	Small	Microglossia (tongue), microblepharia (eyelids), microorganism, microphonia (voice)
-minimus-	Smallest	Gluteus minimus (smallest muscle of hip), adductor minimus (muscle of thigh)

Root	Translation	Examples
-mio-	Less	Mio<u>plasmia</u> (plasma, abnormal decrease in plasma in blood), mio<u>pragia</u> (perform, decreased activity)
-mono-	One, single, limited to one part	Mono<u>chromatic</u> (color), mono<u>brachia</u> (arm)
-multi-	Many, much	Multi<u>para</u> (bear, woman who has borne more than one child), multi<u>lobar</u> (numerous lobes), multi<u>centric</u> (many centers)
-necro-	Dead	Necro<u>sed</u>, necro<u>sis</u>, necro<u>psy</u> (postmortem examination), necro<u>phobia</u> (fear of death)
-neo-	New	Neo<u>formation</u>, neo<u>morphism</u> (form), neo<u>natal</u> (first 4 weeks of life), neo<u>pathy</u> (disease)
-oligo-	Few, scanty, little	Oligo<u>phrenia</u> (mind), oligo<u>pnea</u> (breath), olig<u>uria</u> (urine), oligo<u>dipsia</u> (thrist)
-ortho-	Straight, normal, correct	Ortho<u>dont</u> (teeth, normal), ortho<u>genesis</u> (progressive evolution in a given direction), ortho<u>grade</u> (walk, carrying body upright), ortho<u>pnea</u> (breath, unable to breathe unless in an upright position)
-oxy-	Sharp, quick	Oxy<u>esthesia</u> (feel), oxy<u>opia</u> (vision), oxy<u>osmia</u> (smell)
-pachy-	Thick	Pachy<u>derm</u> (skin), pachy<u>sulemia</u> (blood), pachy<u>pleuritis</u> (inflammation of pleura), pachy<u>cholia</u> (bile), pachy<u>otia</u> (ears)
-paleo-	Old	Paleo<u>genetic</u> (origin in the past), paleo<u>pathology</u> (study of diseases in mummies)
-platy-	Flat	Platy<u>basia</u> (skull base), platy<u>coria</u> (pupil), platy<u>crania</u> (skull)
-pleo-	More	Pleo<u>morphism</u> (forms), pleo<u>chromocytoma</u> (tumor composed of different colored cells)
-poikilo-	Varied	Poikilo<u>derma</u> (skin mottling), poikilo<u>thermal</u> (heat, variable body temperature)
-poly-	Many, much	Poly<u>hedral</u> (many bases or faces), poly<u>mastia</u> (more than two breasts), poly<u>melia</u> (supernumerary limbs), poly<u>myalgia</u> (pain in many muscles)
-pronus-	Face down	Prone, pron<u>ation</u>
-pseudo-	False, spurious	Pseudo<u>stratified</u> (layered), pseudo<u>cirrhosis</u> (apparent cirrhosis of liver), pseudo<u>hypertrophy</u>
-sclero-	Hard	Sclero<u>sis</u> (hardening), arteriosclero<u>sis</u> (artery), sclero<u>nychia</u> (nails), sclero<u>dermatitis</u> (skin)
-scolio-	Twisted, crooked	Scolio<u>dontic</u> (teeth), scolio<u>sis</u>, scolio<u>kyphosis</u> (curvature of spine)
-sinistro-	Left	Sinistro<u>cardia</u>, sinistro<u>manual</u> (left-handed), sinistr<u>aural</u> (hearing better in left ear)
-supinus-	Face up	Supine, supin<u>ation</u>, supin<u>ator</u> longus (muscle in arm)
-steno-	Narrow	Steno<u>sis</u>, steno<u>stomia</u> (mouth), mitral steno<u>sis</u> (mitral valve in heart)
-stereo-	Solid, three dimensions	Stereo<u>scope</u>, stereo<u>meter</u>

Continued

Root	Translation	Examples
-tachy-	Fast, swift	Tachycardia (heart), tachyphrasia (speech)
-tele-	End, far away	Telepathy, telecardiogram
-telo-	Complete	Telophase
-thermo-	Heat, warm	Thermal, thermometer, thermobiosis (ability to live in high temperature)
-trachy-	Rough	Trachyphonia (voice), trachychromatic (deeply staining)
-xero-	Dry	Xerophagia (eating of dry foods) xerostomia (mouth), xerodermia (skin)

Pronunciation of Medical–Dental Terms

Medical terms are hard to pronounce, especially if you have read them but have never heard them spoken. The following are some helpful shortcuts.

ch is sometimes pronounced like *k.* Examples: *chromatin, chronic.*

ps is pronounced like *s.* Examples: *psychiatry, psychology.*

pn is pronounced with only the *n* sound. Example: *pneumonia.*

c and *g* are given the soft sound of *s* and *j,* respectively, before *e, i,* and *y* in words of both Greek and Latin origin. Examples: *cycle, cytoplasm, giant, generic.*

c and *g* have a harsh sound before other letters. Examples: *gastric, gonad, cast, cardiac.*

ae and *oe* are pronounced *ee.* Examples: *coelom, fasciae.*

e and *es,* when forming the final letter or letters of a word, are often pronounced as separate syllables. Examples: *rete (reetee), nares (nayreez).*

i at the end of a word (to form a plural) is pronounced *eye.* Examples: *alveoli, glomeruli, fasciculi.*

Appendix D

ABBREVIATIONS

A amp
@ at
āā of each (F. ana)
a.c. before meals (L., *ante cibum*)
ad Latin preposition, –to, up to
a.d. alternating days (L., *alternis diebus*)
ad lib at pleasure, as needed or desired (L., *ad libitum*)
adm admission
Ag silver (L., *argentum*)
alt. dieb. every other day (L., *alternis diebus*)
alt. hor. every other hour (L., *alternis horis*)
alt. noct. every other night (L., *alternis noctibus*)
a, am, ag amalgam
AM, a.m., A.M. before noon (L., *ante meridiem*)
amp ampule
amt amount
anat anatomy, anatomical
anes anesthesia
ant anterior
AP anteroposterior
appl applicable, application, appliance
approx approximate
aq water (L., *aqua*)
av average
bact bacterium (-ia)
BF bone fragment
bib drink (L., *bibe*)
b.i.d. twice a day (L., *bis in die*)
biol biological, biology
BP blood pressure
BS blood sugar
BW bite-wing radiograph

Bx biopsy
C centigrade
C one hundred (L., *centum*)
c̄ with (L., *cum*)
CA cardiac arrest
CA chronological age
Ca calcium
Ca carcinoma
cal calorie
caps capsules
cav cavity
CBC complete blood count
CC chief complaint
cc cubic centimeter
CDA or C.D.A. Certified Dental Assistant
cent centigrade
CHD childhood disease
CHF congestive heart failure
chr chronic
cm centimeter
c.m. tomorrow morning (L., *cras mane*)
CO₂ carbon dioxide
comp compound
conc concentrated
cond condition
CP centric position
cpd compound
Cu copper (L., *cuprum*)
cu cubic
cur curettage
CV cardiovascular
CVA cerebrovascular accident
Cx convex
CY calendar year
d dose (L., *dosis*)
D, dist distal
dbl double

Continued

dc direct current
DDS or D.D.S. Doctor of Dental Surgery/Science
deg degree
dev develop, development
Dg diagnosis
diag diagnosis
dil dilute (L., *dilue*)
DO distocclusal
dis disease
disp dispensary
dist distal
DMF decayed, missing, and filled (teeth)
DOA dead on arrival
DOB date of birth
doz dozen
Dr. doctor
d.t.d. give of such a dose (L., *datur talis dosis*)
dwt pennyweight
Dx diagnosis
EAC external auditory canal
ed effective dose
EDDA expanded duties dental assistant (auxiliary)
EENT ears, eyes, nose and throat
EFDA expanded (extended) function dental assistant (auxiliary)
e.g. for example (L., *exempli gratia*)
EKG elektrokardiogram (German)
emerg emergency
EMT emergency medical treatment
ENT ears, nose, and throat
epith epithelial
equiv equivalent
esp especially
est estimate, estimation
et and, Latin conjunction
et al. and others (L., *et alii*)
etc. and so on, and so forth, and others (L., *et cetera*)
eval evaluate, evaluation
ext extract, external
F Fahrenheit
F female
F field (of vision)
F formula
FB foreign body
FBS fasting blood sugar
FD fatal dose
ff following

FH family history
fl fluid
FLD full lower denture
fld field
fl. dr. fluid dram
fl. oz. Fluid ounce
FMX full mouth x-ray examination
frac fracture
frag fragment
freq frequent, frequency
ft foot
ft let it be made (L., *fiat/fiant*)
FUD full upper denture
func function
Fx fracture
g gram
gal gallon
ging gingiva, gingivectomy
glob globulin
gm gram
GP general practitioner
gr grain
gt drop (L., *gutta*)
gtt drops (L., *guttae*)
H, h, hr hour (L., *hora*)
H₂O water
Hb, hgb hemoglobin
Hdpc handpiece
h.d. at hour of lying down at bedtime (L., *hora decubitus*)
hosp hospital
hr hour
h.s. hour of sleep (L., *hora somni*)
ht. height
Hx history
I & D incision and drainage
IA incurred accidentally
ibid. in the same place (L., *ibidem*)
id the same (L., *idem*)
i.e. that is (L., *id est*)
IH infectious hepatitis
IM intramuscular
imp impression
in inch
inc incisal, incisive incise
in d. daily (L., *in dies*)
inf infected, inferior, infusion
inj injection, injury
inop inoperable, inoperative
int internal
IQ intelligence quotient
i.q. the same as (L., *idem quod*)
IS interspace

IV intravenous
kg, kgm kilogram
kilo kilogram
kV kilovolt
L Latin
L, l liter
lab laboratory
lac laceration
LASER (laser) light amplification by
    stimulated emission of radiation
lat lateral
lb pound (L., *libra*)
lig ligament
ling lingual
liq liquid, liquor
LN lymph node
lt left
m murmur
m meter
m. dict. as directed (L., *modo dictu*)
m male
m, mes mesial
ma milliampere
mand mandibular
MASER (maser) microwave
    amplification by stimulated
    emission of radiation
max maximum, maxillary
MDR minimum daily requirement
med medical, medicine
mg, mgm milligram
micro microscopic
min minute, minimum
ML midline
ml milliliter
MM mucous membrane
mm millimeter
MO mesiocclusal
MOD mesiocclusodistal
mo month
MS multiple sclerosis
msec millisecond
N negroid, negro
N$_2$O nitrous oxide
narc narcotic, narcotism
neg negative
non. rep. do not repeat
norm normal
NPC no previous complaint
NPH no previous history
n.p.o. nothing by mouth
    (L., *nil per os*)
NR normal record
n.r. not to be repeated (L., *non
    repetatur*)

N/S normal saline
O oxygen
O$_2$ oxygen gas
obl oblique
occ occlusal
ODC oral disease control
o.d. every day (L., *omni die*)
o.d. right eye
OH oral hygiene
o.h. every hour (L., *omni hora*)
o.m. every morning (L., *omni mane*)
o.n. every night (L., *omni nocte*)
op operation
OPC outpatient clinic
OPD outpatient department
opp opposite, opposed
OR operating room
org organism, organic
oz ounce
P pulse
P after (L., *post*)
p- para-
PA posteroanterior
Pan panoral x-ray examination
PATH pituitary adrenotropic
    hormone
path pathology
p.c. after meal (L., *post cibum*)
PCN penicillin
PDR *Physicians' Desk Reference*
perf *perforating*
PLD partial lower denture
P.M. PM, p.m. after noon
    (L., *post meridiem*)
PM after death (L., *post mortem*)
PO postoperative
p.o. by mouth (L., *per os*)
POH personal oral hygiene
pos positive
postop postoperative
prep preparation, prepare
    (for surgery)
p.r.n. as required, as the occasion
    arises (L., *pro re nata*)
prog prognosis
pt patient
PUD partial upper denture
Px prophylaxis
q every (L., *quaque*)
q.d. every day (L., *quaque die*)
q.h. every hour (L., *quaque hora*)
q.2h every second hour
    (L., *quaque secunda hora*)
q.i.d. four times a day
    (L., *quater in die*)

Continued

q.l. as much as pleased (L., *quantum libet*)

q.n. every night (L., *quaque nocte*)

q.p. at will (L., *quantum placeat*)

q.q.h. every 4 hours (L., *quaque quarta hora*)

qt quart

q.v. as much as liked (L., *quantum vis*)

r roentgen

R respiration

RX take (thou) a recipe

rad radiograph

RC retruded contact position

RC root canal

R.D.A. Registered Dental Assistant

RDH Registered Dental Hygienist

reg regular

rem(s) roentgen-equivalent-man

req requires, required

rep(s) roentgen-equivalent-physical

resp respiration

Rh Rh factor in blood (L., *Rhesus*)

RHD rheumatic heart disease

RN Registered Nurse

rt right

Rx treatment (L., *recipe*)

s without (L., *sine*)

SBE subacute bacterial endocarditis

SD sterile dressing

sec second, secondary

Sig. write on label

sol solution

spec specimen

ss one half signs and symptoms (L., *semis*)

stat immediately (L., *statim*)

std standard

stim stimulator, stimulate

strep *Streptococcus* organisms

sup superior

surg surgeon, surgery

Sx symptom

sym symmetric

symp symptom

sys system

T temperature

tab tablet

TB, TBC tuberculosis

tbsp tablespoon

temp temperature

t.i.d. three times a day (L., *ter in die*)

tinc tincture

TLC tender loving care

TM temporomandibular

TMJ temporomandibular joint

TPR temperature, pulse, respiration

tsp teaspoon

U, u unit

ung ointment (L., *unguentum*)

unk unknown

USP United States Pharmacopoeia

ut. dict. As directed

V, v volt

VD venereal disease

vert vertebra, vertical

visc viscous

VIT vitamin

viz that is, namely (L., *videlicet*)

VO verbal order

vol volume

vs versus

WF white female

wh white

WM white male

w-n well-nourished

wnd wound

wt weight

x times, 4×, four times; ×4, times four yard

xt extract, extracted

xyl, xylo Xylocaine

yd yard

YOB year of birth

yr year

Symbols

& and

* birth

† death

↓ decrease

° Degree

= equal

′ feet, minutes

♀ Female

> greater than, or indicating increase

″ inches; seconds

↑ increase

< less than, or indicating decrease

♂ male

− minus, negative

number, pound

i,ii,iii one, two, or three (as in number of grams)

ℨiss one and one-half drams

℥T one ounce

℥ss one-half ounce

/ per

% percent

+ plus, positive

Adapted from Zwemer TJ: *Boucher's clinical dental terminology*, ed 4, St Louis, 1993, Mosby.

Appendix E

DENTAL TERMINOLOGY

abrasion Mechanical wearing away of teeth by abnormal stressors. This could result from abnormal toothbrushing habits or other abnormal stress on the teeth.

accessional Permanent teeth that do not replace deciduous teeth but rather become an accession (addition) to the deciduous or succedaneous teeth, or both types.

accessory root canals Extra openings into the pulp; usually located on the sides of the roots or in the bifurcations.

acquired Pertaining to something obtained by oneself; not inherited.

ala Latin for "wing," referring to the sides of the nostrils of the nose; plural *alae*.

alignment Arrangement of teeth in a row.

allergenic Being hypersensitive to something.

allergic reaction Body's reaction to an allergen; an example of such a reaction is hives.

alveolar bone Bone that forms the sockets for the teeth.

alveolar crest Highest part of the alveolar bone closest to the cervical line of the tooth.

alveolar eminences Bulges on the facial surface of alveolar bone that outline the position of the roots.

alveolar mucosa Mucosa between the mucobuccal fold and gingiva.

alveolar process Part of the bone in the maxillae and mandible that forms the sockets for the teeth.

alveolus (alveoli) Cavity, or socket, in the alveolar process in which the root of the tooth is held.

anatomical crown That part of the tooth covered by enamel.

angle of the mandible Point at the lower border of the body of the mandible where it turns up onto the ramus.

Angle's classification System of dental classifications based primarily on the relationship of the permanent first molars to each other and to a lesser degree on the relationship of the permanent canines to each other.

ankyloglossia See *tongue-tie.*

ankylosis Fusion of the cementum of a tooth with alveolar bone.

anodontia The absence of teeth in the jaw.

anomaly Any noticeable difference or deviation from that which is ordinary or normal.

anterior Situated in front of; a term commonly used to denote the incisor and canine teeth or the area toward the front of the mouth.

anterior pillar Fold of tissue extending down in front of the tonsil.

antihistamine Drug that controls the body's histamine reaction, which causes congestion of tissues.

apex (apices) End point, or furthest tip, as of the tooth root.

apical foramen Aperture, or opening, at or near the apex of a tooth root through which the blood and nerve supply of the pulp enters the tooth.

arch, dental See *dental arch.*

atrophic Pertaining to the wasting away of a tissue, organ, or part from disease, defective nutrition, or lack of use.

atrophy Wasting away of a tissue, organ, or part from disease, defective nutrition, or lack of use.

attached gingiva Tightly adherent gingiva that extends from free gingiva to alveolar mucosa.

attrition Process of normal wear on the crown.

autonomic nervous system Automatic nervous system of the body that is not willfully controlled. It controls the functions of the glands and smooth and cardiac muscle.

bicuspid See *premolars.*

bifurcation Division into two parts or branches, as any two roots of a tooth.

body of the mandible Horizontal portion of the mandible, excluding the alveolar process.

bone Hard connective tissue that forms the framework of the body. The hardness is attributable to the hydroxyapatite crystal.

bruxism Abnormal grinding of the teeth.

bucca Latin word for cheek.

buccal Pertaining to the cheek; toward the cheek or next to the cheek. Also called *facial.*

buccal development groove Groove that separates the buccal cusps on a buccal surface.

buccal glands Small minor salivary glands in the cheek.

buccinator Muscle of facial expression that extends from the back buccal portion of the maxilla and mandible and pterygomandibular raphe forward in the cheek to the corner of the mouth.

calcification Process by which organic tissue becomes hardened by a deposit of calcium salts within its substance. The term, in a liberal sense, connotes the deposition of any mineral salts that contribute to the hardening and maturation of hard tissue.

canal Long tubular opening through a bone.

canines Third teeth from the midline, at corner of mouth; used for grasping; also called *cuspids.*

capsule Fibrous band of tissue surrounding a joint.

cell Basic functioning component of the body; capable of reproducing itself in most instances. Tissues are made up of groups of cells.

cementoenamel junction (CEJ) Junction of enamel of the crown and cementum of the root. This junction forms the cervical line around the tooth.

cementoma Cementum tumor at root tip that destroys surrounding bone.

cementum Layer of bonelike tissue covering the root of the tooth.

central developmental groove Developmental groove that crosses the occlusal surface of a tooth from the mesial to the distal side; divides the tooth into buccal and lingual parts.

centric occlusion (central occlusion) Relationship of the occlusal surfaces of one arch to those of the other when the jaws are closed and the teeth are in maximum intercuspation.

centric relation Arch-to-arch relationship of the maxilla to the mandible when the condyles are in their most upward position, the mandible is in its most posterior position, and the jaw is most braced by its musculature.

cervical Portion of a tooth near the junction of the crown and root. Pertaining to the neck region, for example, nerves of the neck.

cervical line Line formed by the junction of the enamel and cementum on a tooth.

cervical third Portion of the crown or root of a tooth at or near the cervical line.

cervicoenamel ridge Prominent ridge of enamel immediately near the cervical line on the crown of a tooth.

cervix Constricted structure; the narrow region at the junction of the crown and root of the tooth.

circumvallate papillae Large *V*-shaped row of papillae lying on the posterior dorsum of the tongue. Also called *vallate papillae*.

class I occlusal relationship Normal relationship between maxillary and mandibular molars.

class II occlusal relationship Relationship in which a mandibular molar is posterior to its normal position.

class III occlusal relationship Relationship in which a mandibular molar is anterior to its normal position.

cleft lip Gap in the upper lip that occurs during development.

cleft palate Lack of joining together of the hard or soft palates.

clinical crown Part of the tooth protruding from the gingiva.

clinical root Part of the tooth embedded in the gingiva and socket.

concavity Depression in a surface.

congenital Occurring at or before birth; may or may not be hereditary.

contact area Area of contact of one tooth with another in the same arch.

contact point Specific point at which a tooth from one arch occludes with another tooth from the opposing arch.

cross-bite Condition in which the cusps of a tooth in one arch exceed the cusps of a tooth in the opposing arch, buccally or lingually.

cross-section Cutting through a tooth perpendicular to the long axis.

crown Part of the tooth that is covered with enamel.

cusp Major pointed or rounded eminence on or near the occlusal surface of a tooth.

cusp of Carabelli Fifth lobe of a maxillary first molar.

cyst Sac of fluid lined by epithelium that may grow to varying sizes.

cytoplasm Fluid substance of cells.

debrided To have accomplished the removal (debridement) of nerve tissue and other debris from the pulp cavity to leave a surgically cleaned area.

deciduous That which will be shed; specifically, the first dentition of humans or animals.

deglutition The action of swallowing.

dental arch All teeth in either the maxillary or mandibular jaw that form an arch.

dentin (formerly dentine) Calcified tissue that forms the inside body of a tooth, underlying the cementum and enamel and surrounding the pulpal tissue.

dentinal tubule Space in the dentin occupied by the ontoblastic process.

dentinocemental junction Location in the root where the dentin joins the cementum.

dentinoenamel junction Line marking the junction of the dentin and the enamel.

dentinogenesis imperfecta Hereditary imperfect dentin formation.

dentition General character and arrangement of the teeth, taken as a whole, as in carnivorous, herbivorous, and omnivorous dentitions. *Primary dentition* refers to the deciduous teeth, and *secondary dentition* refers to the permanent teeth. *Mixed dentition* refers to a combination of permanent and deciduous teeth in the same dentition.

depression Lowering of the mandible or opening of the mouth.

developmental depression Noticeable concavity on the formed crown or root of a tooth; occurs at the junction of two lobes, as on the mesial surface of the maxillary first premolars, or at the furcation of roots.

developmental grooves Fine depressed lines in the enamel of a tooth that mark the union of the lobes of the crown.

diastema Any spacing between teeth in the same arch.

distal Distant; farthest from the median line of the face or from the origin of a structure.

distal proximal surface Proximal surface on the posterior side of a tooth.

distal third Viewed from the facial or lingual surface, the third of the surface farthest from the midline.

distobuccal developmental groove Developmental groove that extends on the buccal surface of a lower first or third molar between the distobuccal and distal cusps.

distoclusion See *class II occlusal relationship*.

dorsum of the tongue Top surface of the tongue.

edema Swelling of tissue.

edge, incisal See *incisal edge*.

embrasure Open space between the proximal surfaces of two teeth where they diverge buccally, labially, or lingually and occlusally from the contact area.

enamel Hard calcified tissue that covers the dentin of the crown portion of a tooth.

enamel dysplasia Abnormalities of enamel growth.

enamel hypocalcification Enamel that is not as dense as regular enamel.

enamel hypoplasia Enamel that is thin or pitted.

endocrine Gland or type of secretion that is carried away from the producing cells by blood vessels; the secretion is used in other parts of the body to control certain functions; has no duct system.

enzyme Agent capable of producing chemical changes in processes such as the digestion of foods.

epiglottis Cartilage that helps cover the laryngeal opening.

epinephrine Substance produced by the body or synthetically produced that causes many reactions; in dentistry, used to constrict blood flow in tissues.

epithelial Pertaining to epithelium.

epithelial attachment Substance produced by the reduced enamel epithelium that helps secure the attachment epithelium at the base of the gingival sulcus to the tooth.

epithelium Layer or layers of cells that cover the surface of the body or line the tubes or cavities inside the body; one of the four basic tissues.

equilibrium Sense of balance.

eruption Movement of the tooth as it emerges through surrounding tissue so that the clinical crown gradually appears longer.

eruptive stage Period of eruption from the completion of crown formation until the teeth come into occlusion.

exfoliation Shedding or loss of a primary tooth.

facial Term used to designate the outer surfaces of the teeth collectively (buccal or labial).

facial surface See *facial.*

facial third From a proximal view, the third of the surface closest to the facial side.

fauces Space between the left and right palatine tonsils.

FDI system The Federation Dentaire Internationale (International Dental Federation); system for tooth identification.

filiform papillae Small, pointed projections that heavily cover most of the dorsum of the anterior two thirds of the tongue.

fissure Deep cleft; developmental line fault usually found in the occlusal or buccal surface of a tooth; commonly the result of imperfect fusion of the enamel of the adjoining dental lobes.

flange Projecting edge; the edge of the denture.

fluorosis Discolored enamel resulting from excessive fluoride intake during crown development.

foliate papillae Poorly developed papillae that appear as small vertical folds in the posterior part of the sides of the tongue.

foramen Short circular opening through a bone.

fossa Round, wide, relatively shallow depression in the surface of a tooth as seen commonly in the lingual surfaces of the maxillary incisors or between the cusps of molars; also a shallow depression in bone.

free gingiva Gingiva that forms the gingival sulcus.

frenulum Little frenum or fold of tissue.

frontal sinus Air sinus in frontal bone above the eye that opens into the hiatus semilunaris in the middle meatus.

fungiform papillae Small circular papillae scattered throughout the anterior two thirds of the dorsum of the tongue.

fusion Two teeth that fuse at their dentin while developing.

gingiva Part of the gum tissue that immediately surrounds the teeth and alveolar bone.

gingival crest Most occlusal or incisal extent of the gingiva.

gingival crevice Subgingival space that, under normal conditions, lies between the gingival crest and the epithelial attachment.

gingival papillae Portion of the gingiva found between the teeth in the interproximal spaces gingival to the contact area; also called *interdental papillae.*

gingival sulcus Space between the free gingiva and the tooth surface.

gingivitis Inflammation involving the gingival tissues only.

hematoma Escape of blood from injured blood vessel into tissue spaces.

hemoglobin Component of red blood cells that carries oxygen.

hereditary Inherited through the genes of parents or grandparents.

immunity Body's resistance to certain organisms or diseases.

impacted Teeth that are not completely erupted and are fully or partly covered by bone or soft tissue.

incisal edge Edge formed at the labioincisal line angle of an anterior tooth after an incisal ridge has worn down.

incisal ridge Rounded ridge form of the incisal portion of an anterior tooth.

incisal third From a proximal, lingual, or labial view of an anterior tooth, the third of the surface closest to the incisal edge.

incisive papilla Small, rounded, oblong mound of tissue directly behind or lingual to the maxillary central incisors and lying over the incisive foramen.

incisors The four center teeth in either arch; essential for cutting.

inflammatory reaction Body's mechanism to combat harmful organisms by bringing more plasma and blood cells to the injured area.

inherited Passed on from parents or grandparents.

interdental Located between the teeth.

interdental papilla Projection of gingiva between the teeth.

interproximal Between the proximal surfaces of adjoining teeth in the same arch.

interproximal space Triangular space between adjoining teeth; the proximal surfaces of the teeth form the sides of the triangle; the alveolar bone, the base, and the contact area of the teeth form the apex.

labia Latin word for lips; singular, *labium.*

labial Of or pertaining to the lips; toward the lips.

labial frenum Fold of tissue that attaches the lip to the labial mucosa at the midline of the lips.

larynx Voice box; the trachea begins just below it.

lingual Pertaining to or affecting the tongue; next to or toward the tongue.

lingual frenum Fold of tissue that attaches the undersurface of the tongue to the floor of the mouth.

lingual glands Minor salivary glands of the tongue.

lingual groove Developmental groove on the lingual side of the tooth.

lingual surface See *lingual.*

lingual third From a proximal view, the third of the surface closest to the lingual side.

macrodontia Condition in which the teeth are too large for the jaw.

malocclusion Abnormal occlusion of the teeth.

mamelon One of the three rounded protuberances of the incisal surface of a newly erupted incisor tooth.

mandible Lower jaw.

mandibular Pertaining to the lower jaw.

mandibular arch First pharyngeal arch that forms the area of the mandible and maxilla; the lower dental arch.

mandibular condyle Rounded top of the mandible that articulates with the mandibular fossa.

mandibular foramen Opening on the medial surface of the ramus of the mandible for entrance of nerves and blood vessels to the lower teeth.

mandibular process Portion of the mandibular pharyngeal arch that forms the mandible.

mandibular tori Bony growths on the lingual cortical plate of bone opposite the mandibular canines.

marginal ridge Ridge or elevation of enamel forming the margin of the surface of a tooth; specifically, at the mesial and distal margins of the occlusal surfaces of premolars and molars, and the mesial and distal margins of the lingual surfaces of incisors and canines.

mastication Act of chewing or grinding.

maxilla Paired main bone of the upper jaw.

maxillary Pertaining to the upper arch.

maxillary arch Upper dental arch.

maxillary sinus Largest of the paired paranasal sinuses, located in the maxilla.

maxillary tuberosity Bulging posterior surface of the maxilla behind the third molar region.

median line Vertical (central) line that divides the body into right and left; the median line of the face.

mesial Toward or situated in the middle; for example, toward the midline of the dental arch.

mesial drift Phenomenon of permanent molars continuing to move mesially after eruption.

mesial third From a facial or a lingual view, the third of the surface closest to the midline.

microdontia Condition in which the teeth are too small for the jaw.

mixed dentition State of having primary and permanent teeth in the dental arches at the same time.

molars Large posterior teeth used for grinding.

mucosa Moist epithelial linings of the oral cavity and the respiratory and digestive systems.

mucous Pertaining to mucus, the thick viscous secretion of a gland.

mulberry molars Molars with multiple cusps that are caused by congenital syphilis.

multiple root Root with more than one branch.

muscle One of the four basic tissues; has the property of contraction or shortening of the fibers, which accomplishes work. The three types of muscle are skeletal, cardiac, and smooth muscle.

nasal septum Wall between the left and right sides of the nasal cavity, made up of the ethmoid and vomer bones.

nervous tissue One of the four basic tissues. Groups of cells (neurons) carry messages to and from the brain and perform many other tasks.

neuron Nerve cell.

nonsuccedaneous Permanent teeth that do not succeed or replace deciduous teeth.

occluding Contacting opposing teeth.

occlusal Articulating or biting surface.

occlusal plane Side view of the occlusal surfaces.

occlusal relationship Way in which the maxillary and mandibular teeth touch each other.

occlusal third From a proximal, lingual, or buccal view of a posterior tooth, the third of the surface closest to the occlusal surface.

occlusal trauma Injury brought about by one tooth prematurely hitting another during closure of the jaws.

occlusion Relationship of the mandibular and maxillary teeth when closed or during excursive movements of the mandible; when teeth of the mandibular arch come in contact with teeth of the maxillary arch in any functional relationship.

odontoma Tumor made up of enamel, dentin, cementum, and pulp.

opaque Not easily able to transmit light.

open bite Space left between the teeth when the jaws close.

open contact Space between adjacent teeth in the same arch; an interproximal opening instead of a contact area where the teeth touch.

overbite Relationship of teeth in which the incisal ridges of the maxillary anterior teeth extend below the incisal ridges of the mandibular anterior teeth when the teeth are in a centric occlusal relationship.

overhanging restoration Excess of filling material extending past the confines of the tooth preparation; an overextension of filling material.

overjet Relationship of teeth in which the incisal ridges or buccal cusp ridges of the maxillary teeth extend facially to the incisal ridges or buccal cusp ridges of the mandibular teeth when the teeth are in a centric occlusal relationship.

palatal Pertaining to the palate or roof of the mouth.

Palmer notation system System of coding teeth using brackets, numbers, and letters.

papillary gingiva Gingiva that forms the interdental papillae.

paramolar Small supernumerary tooth located buccally or lingually to a molar.

parasympathetic nervous system Part of the autonomic (automatic) nervous system that originates from some of the cranial nerves and some of the sacral nerves. It controls a number of functions, including stimulation of the salivary glands.

parathyroid gland Small gland embedded in the thyroid gland that helps control calcium metabolism in the body.

passive eruption Condition in which the tooth does not move but the gingival attachment moves farther apically.

peg-shaped lateral Poorly formed maxillary lateral incisor with a cone-shaped crown.

periapical Around the tip of the root of a tooth.

periodontal Surrounding a tooth.

periodontium Supporting tissues surrounding the teeth.

periosteum Fibrous and cellular layer that covers bones and contains cells that become osteoblasts.

periphery Circumferential boundary; outer border.

pharynx Throat area, from the nasal cavity to the larynx.

philtrum Small depression at the midline of the upper lip.

pillars Folds of tissue appearing in front of and behind the palatine tonsils.

pit Small pointed depression in dental enamel, usually at the junction of two or more developmental grooves; a small hole anywhere on the crown.

posterior Situated toward the back, as premolars and molars.

posterior pillars Folds of tissue behind the tonsil that contain the palatopharyngeus muscle.

posterior teeth Teeth of either jaw located to the rear of the incisors and canines.

pre-eruptive stage Period when the crown of the tooth is developing.

premature contact area Area where an upper and a lower tooth touch and hit each other before the rest of the teeth occlude.

premaxilla Bony area of the upper jaw that includes the alveolar ridge for the incisors and the area immediately behind it.

premolars Permanent teeth that replace the primary molars.

primary dentin Dentin formed from the beginning of calcification until tooth eruption.

primary dentition First set of teeth; also called *baby teeth, milk teeth,* and *deciduous teeth.*

primary palate The early developing part of the hard palate that originates from the medial nasal process and forms a *V*-shaped wedge of tissue that runs from the incisive foramen forward and laterally between the lateral incisors and canines of the maxilla.

primary teeth See *deciduous.*

prosthetic appliance Any constructed appliance that replaces a missing part.

protrusion Condition of being thrust forward, as protrusion of the anterior teeth, referring to the teeth being too far labial; the forward movement of the mandible.

proximal Nearest, next, immediately adjacent to; distal or mesial.

proximal contact areas Proximal area of a tooth that touches an adjacent tooth on the mesial or distal side.

pulp canal Canal in the root of a tooth that leads from the apex to the pulp chamber. Contains dental pulp tissue under normal conditions.

pulp cavity Entire cavity within the tooth, including the pulp canal and pulp chamber.

pulp chamber Cavity or chamber in the center of the crown of a tooth that normally contains the major portion of the dental pulp. The pulp canals lead into the pulp chambers.

pulp, dental Highly vascular and innervated connective tissue contained within the pulp cavity of the tooth. It is composed of arteries, veins, nerves, connective tissues and cells, lymph tissue, and odontoblasts.

pulp horn (horn of pulp) Extension of pulp tissue into a thin point of the pulp chamber in the tooth crown.

pulp stones Small, dentinlike calcifications in pulp.

quadrants One fourth of the dentition. The four quadrants are divided into right, left, maxillary, and mandibular.

ramus of the mandible Vertical portion of the mandible.

recession Migration of the gingival crest in an apical direction, away from the crown of the tooth.

referred pain Pain that seems to originate in one area but originates in another.

reparative dentin Localized formation of dentin in response to local trauma, such as occlusal trauma or caries.

resorption Physiological removal of tissues or body products, as of the roots of deciduous teeth, or of some alveolar process after the loss of the permanent teeth.

retromolar pad Pad of tissue behind the mandibular third molars.

retromolar triangle Triangular area of bone just behind the mandibular third molars.

retrusion Act or process of retraction or moving back, as when the mandible is placed in posterior relationship to the maxilla.

ridge Long narrow elevation or crest, as on the surface of a tooth or bone.

root Portion of a tooth that is embedded in the alveolar process and covered with cementum.

root canal See *pulp canal.*

root planing Process of smoothing the cementum of the root of a tooth.

rugae Small ridges of tissue extending laterally across the anterior of the hard palate.

sebaceous glands Small oil-producing glands that are usually connected to and lubricate hairs.

secondary dentin Dentin formed throughout the pulp chamber and pulp canal from the time of eruption.

secondary dentition Permanent dentition.

single root Root with one main branch.

slough Loss of dead cells from the surface of tissue; pronounced *sluff.*

soft tissue Noncalcified tissue, such as nerves, arteries, veins, and connective tissue.

spasm Constant contraction of muscle.

submucosa Supporting layer of loose connective tissue under a mucous membrane.

succedaneous Permanent teeth that succeed, or take the place of, deciduous teeth after the latter have been shed; that is, the incisors, canines, and premolars.

sulcus Long *V*-shaped depression or valley in the surface of a tooth between the ridges and the cusps. A sulcus has a developmental groove at the apex of its *V*-shape. Sulcus also refers to the trough around the teeth formed by the gingiva.

supplemental groove Shallow linear groove in the enamel of a tooth. It differs from a developmental groove in that it does not mark the junction of lobes; it is a secondary, or smaller, groove.

supplemental tooth Supernumerary tooth that resembles a regular tooth.

supraeruption Eruption of a tooth beyond the occlusal plane.

taste buds Small structures in vallate, fungiform, and foliate papillae that detect taste.

temporomandibular ligament Thickened part of the temporomandibular joint (TMJ) capsule on the lateral side.

tongue-tie, tongue-tied Condition in which the lingual frenum is short and attached to the tip of the tongue, making normal speech difficult. Also called *ankyloglossia.*

tonsillor pillars Vertical folds of tissue that lie in front of and behind the palatine tonsils in the lateral throat wall.

tooth germ Soft tissue that develops into a tooth.

tooth migration Movement of the tooth through the bone and gum tissue.

torus palatinus Large bony growth in the hard palate.

transverse ridge Ridge formed by the union of two triangular ridges, traversing the surface of a posterior tooth from the buccal to the lingual side.

trauma Wound; bodily injury or damage.

trifurcation Division of three tooth roots at their point of junction with the root trunk.

Universal system, Universal Code System of coding teeth using the numbers 1 to 32 for permanent teeth and the letters *A* to *T* for deciduous teeth.

uvula Small, hanging fold of tissue in back of the soft palate.

vallate papillae See *circumvallate papillae.*

vascular Relating to blood supply.

vasoconstrictor Substance that constricts blood vessels.

vermillion zone Red part of the lip where the lip mucosa meets the skin.

vestibule Space between the lips or cheeks and the teeth.

From Brand RW, Isselhard DE: Anatomy of orofacial structures, *ed 7, St Louis, 2003, Mosby.*

Index

Names of books are in italics. Page numbers followed by b indicate boxes; f, figures; and t, tables.

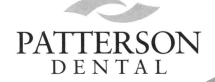
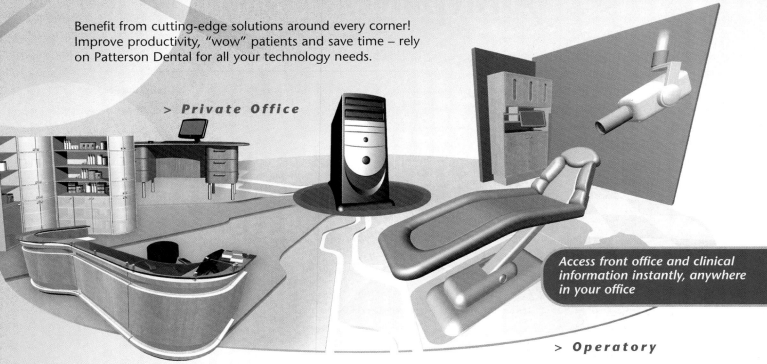
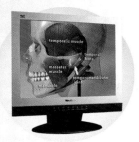
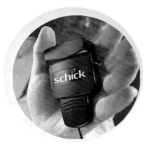
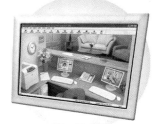

Patterson EagleSoft
Practice Management and Clinical Software

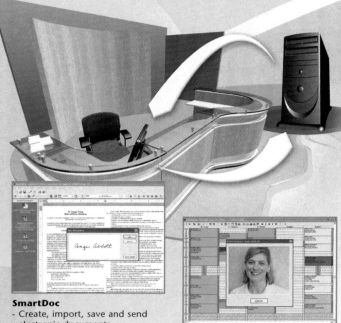

SmartDoc
- Create, import, save and send electronic documents.
- Capture digital signatures on documents.

OnSchedule
- Create an efficient, productive work schedule.

> Front Office

eBusiness
- Send insurance claims/patient statements the most reliable way.

Employee Time Clock
- Track/manage employee hours.

EagleSoft Messenger
- Send instant messages to the front office, operatory or any network computer.

End-of-Day Reporting
- Print detailed reports like "Provider Productivity," "Bank Deposit Slip" and "Audit Trail."

General Preferences
- Additional HIPAA preferences include Enable Notice of Privacy Practices Message and Enable Authorization Message.

InContact
- Make database tracking easy with an interactive contact manager.

Lab Tracking
- Simplify monitoring of lab cases and scheduling appointments.

Patient Route Sheet
- Customize patient summaries.

Payment Plan
- Set up financial arrangements.

Recalls
- Generate reports, postcards, mailing labels, envelopes, letters; e-mail recalls too.

Report Listing
- Access over 140 reports and create custom categories.

Spell Checking
- Spell check InTouch Letters, Operator Notes and Clinical Notes.

SnapShot
- Display a graphical "State-of-the-practice."

The Money Finder
- Find hidden money in your practice with this patient database query.

Treatment Plan
- Create multiple treatment plans per patient.

Trends
- Track your practice performance.

Walkout
- Process treatments and payments; generate insurance claims – all at once.

> Operatory

Advanced Imaging Tools

Sensor Images
- Acquire/edit new sensor images into templates.

EagleEye
- View tooth contrasts with spotlight diagnostics.

Update
- Update the most recent dates for full mouth series, bitewings and/or panoramic exams.

Clinical Exam
- Record/retrieve patient exam data.

Cosmetic Imaging
- Create a customized imaging report, compare before and after, whiten teeth, close a diastema, rebuild teeth; plus cosmetic imaging simulation and automatic teeth selection.

Patient Notes
- Record/manage patient notes.

Perio Chart
- Compare perio conditions of up to any three exam dates.

Digital Integration Partners
- Communicate seamlessly with digital leaders Schick®, Air Techniques®, Gendex™, Soredex®, PLANMECA®, Sirona® and GE Healthcare®.

One Patient Record
- All data in one convenient patient record. No translating programs, bridges or vendor links.

> Private Office

EveryWare™

Palm™
- Complete Palm OS® integration allows HotSync® function to import EagleSoft data.

Web
- View practice information from any Internet browser.

eReferral
- Share patient information with other offices via a Web page on the EagleSoft secure server.

eCheckup
- Compare your practice to others in your region and nationwide with this Web-based program.

Chart
- Attach images to teeth; chart conditions and services.
- Create customized draw types.

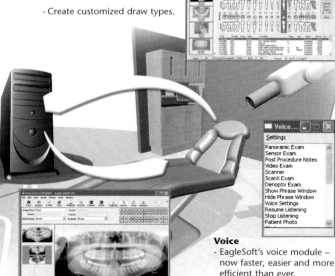

Voice
- EagleSoft's voice module – now faster, easier and more efficient than ever.

Clinical Exam
- Record and retrieve patient exam information.

Patterson EagleSoft

2202 Althoff Drive, Effingham, IL 62401
Sales 800.294.8504 | www.eaglesoft.net
Copyright ©2005 Patterson Dental Supply, Inc. All rights reserved.

E5087 (4/05)